Diagnosis and Treatment of Hepatocellular Carcinoma

Diagnosis and Treatment of Hepatocellular Carcinoma

Edited by Evangeline Hart

**hayle
medical**

New York

Hayle Medical,
750 Third Avenue, 9th Floor,
New York, NY 10017, USA

Visit us on the World Wide Web at:
www.haylemedical.com

ISBN: 978-1-63241-851-7

Cataloging-in-Publication Data

Diagnosis and treatment of hepatocellular carcinoma / edited by Evangeline Hart.
p. cm.
Includes bibliographical references and index.
ISBN 978-1-63241-851-7
1. Liver--Cancer. 2. Liver – Cancer--Diagnosis. 3. Liver – Cancer--Treatment.
I. Hart, Evangeline.
RC280.L5 D53 2020
616.994 36--dc21

Table of Contents

Preface

This book aims to highlight the current researches and provides a platform to further the scope of innovations in this area. This book is a product of the combined efforts of many researchers and scientists, after going through thorough studies and analysis from different parts of the world. The objective of this book is to provide the readers with the latest information of the field.

Hepatocellular carcinoma is a primary liver cancer. It is the most common cause of death in patients suffering from cirrhosis. Most individuals with hepatocellular carcinoma exhibit signs and symptoms consistent with chronic liver disease. Other risk factors that can contribute to an incidence of this condition include chronic hepatitis B and C, Type 2 diabetes, nonalcoholic steatohepatitis, Wilson's disease, etc. The carcinoma can be detected through blood testing and imaging evaluation, especially MRI. The treatment of hepatocellular carcinoma and its prognosis depends on factors such as tumor size, spread, histology and patient health. Surgical resection, liver transplantation, arterial catheter-based treatment and systemic therapy are certain therapies for the management of hepatocellular carcinoma. This book brings forth some of the most innovative concepts and elucidates the unexplored aspects of hepatocellular carcinoma. The objective of this book is to give a general view of the diagnosis and treatment of hepatocellular carcinoma. A number of latest researches have been included to keep the readers up-to-date with the global concepts in this area of study.

I would like to express my sincere thanks to the authors for their dedicated efforts in the completion of this book. I acknowledge the efforts of the publisher for providing constant support. Lastly, I would like to thank my family for their support in all academic endeavors.

Editor

Effectiveness and Complications of Ultrasound Guided Fine Needle Aspiration for Primary Liver Cancer in a Chinese Population with Serum α-Fetoprotein Levels ≤200 ng/ml - A Study Based on 4,312 Patients

Qi-wen Chen[1,¶,ᓂ], Chien-shan Cheng[2,¶,ᓂ], Hao Chen[1,¶,ᓂ], Zhou-yu Ning[1,¶,ᓂ], Shi-feng Tang[3,¶,ᓂ], Xun Zhang[4,¶,ᓂ], Xiao-yan Zhu[1], Sonya Vargulick[5], Ye-hua Shen[1], Yong-qiang Hua[1], Jing Xie[1], Wei-dong Shi[1], Hui-feng Gao[1], Li-tao Xu[1], Lan-yun Feng[1], Jun-hua Lin[1], Zhen Chen[1], Lu-ming Liu[1], Bo Ping[6,*], Zhi-qiang Meng[1,*]

1 Department of Integrative Oncology, Fudan University Shanghai Cancer Center, Shanghai, China, Department of Oncology, Shanghai Medical College, Fudan University, Shanghai, China, 2 School of Chinese Medicine, the University of Hong Kong, Pokfulam, Hong Kong, China, 3 First Department, Cancer Treatment Center, Weifang Hospital of Traditional Chinese Medicine, Weifang, Shandong Province, China, 4 Department of Ultrasound, Fudan University Shanghai Cancer Center, Shanghai, China, Department of Oncology, Shanghai Medical College, Fudan University, Shanghai, China, 5 Albany College of Pharmacy and Health Sciences, Albany, New York, United States of America, 6 Department of Pathology, Fudan University Shanghai Cancer Center, Shanghai, China, Department of Oncology, Shanghai Medical College, Fudan University, Shanghai, China

Abstract

Background: Hepatocellular carcinoma (HCC) can be diagnosed by noninvasive approaches with serum α-fetoprotein (AFP) levels >200 ng/ml and/or a radiological imaging study of tumor mass >2 cm in patients with chronic liver disease. Percutaneous fine needle aspiration (FNA) under ultrasound (US) guidance has a diagnostic specificity of 95% and is superior to radiological imaging studies.

Aim: The aim of this study is to elucidate the effectiveness and complications of fine needle aspiration in a Chinese population with primary liver cancer and AFP levels ≤200 ng/ml.

Materials and Methods: A retrospective study was conducted over a period of 28 years. This selection period included patients with a suspected diagnosis of primary liver cancer whose AFP levels were ≤200 ng/ml and who underwent US-FNA. This data was then analyzed with cytomorphological features correlating with medical history, radiological imaging, AFP, and follow-up information.

Results: Of the 1,929 cases with AFP ≤200 mg/ml, 1,756 underwent FNA. Of these, 1,590 cases were determined malignant and the remaining 166 were determined benign. Further, 1,478 malignant cases were diagnosed by FNA alone, and of these, 1,138 were diagnosed as PLC. The sensitivity, specificity, positive predictive value, negative predictive value, and overall accuracy of the diagnoses were 92.96%, 100%, 100%, 59.71%, and 93.62% respectively. There was no significant difference in the sensitivity, specificity, PPV and NPV between the subgroups with tumor size<2 cm and ≥2 cm. Major complications included implantation metastasis and hemorrhage.

Conclusion: Patients with PLC, especially those who present with an AFP ≤200 ng/ml, should undergo FNA. If negative results are obtained by FNA, it still could be HCC and repeated FNA procedure may be needed if highly suspicious of HCC on imaging study. The superiority of FNA in overall accuracy may outweigh its potential complications, such like hemorrhage and implantation metastasis.

Editor: Ferruccio Bonino, University of Pisa, Italy

Funding: The authors have no support or funding to report.

Competing Interests: The authors have declared that no competing interests exist.

* Email: bping2007@163.com (BP); mengzhq@gmail.com (ZM)

ᓂ These authors contributed equally to this work.

¶ QC, CC, HC, ZN, ST, and X. Zhang are co-first authors on this work.

Introduction

Primary Liver Cancer

Primary Liver Cancer (PLC) is one of the most common malignant neoplasms in the world and its incidence has risen as a result of the increased global burden of liver disease. China, which is a hepatitis B pandemic area, is also a hepatocellular carcinoma (HCC) high-incidence region, where 55% of the world's HCC occurs [1]. As a result of rather asymptomatic features, most initial diagnoses of HCC are at late stage and characterized by large tumor size and unresectable lesions, in combination with poor liver function, ultimately leading to a shortened life expectancy. Therefore, disease surveillance is not only important in high risk patients for early diagnosis, but also to have accurate diagnostic methods for further appropriate treatments.

Serum α-fetoprotein Level

Alpha-fetoprotein (AFP), a serum glycoprotein physiologically produced by the fetal liver and yolk sac, was the first recognized and is the most commonly used marker for the detection of HCC. An elevated serum AFP level may be physiologically seen in pregnancy and pathologically seen in tumors of gonadal origin, hepatoid adenocarcinoma, HCC, or nonmalignant chronic liver diseases, including acute or chronic viral hepatitis [2]. AFP is assumed to be more indicative of non-hepatitis virus infected patients in terms of HCC. According to the 2005 American Association for the Study of Liver Diseases (AASLD) practice guidelines [3], the noninvasive diagnostic approach of HCC should be based on the consideration of serum α-fetoprotein levels >200 ng/ml and/or a radiological imaging displaying tumor masses >2 cm in patients with chronic liver disease. Besides following the AASLD guidelines, the decision to use AFP > 200 ng/ml as a cut-off point in this retrospective study was based on a case-control study reported by Trevisani, et al. [4] in 2001. Trevisani, et al. reported that AFP>200 ng/ml has a substantial sensitivity and specificity for not only diagnostic and confirmatory testing for HCC, but also in a cost-effective investigation that is optimal for HCC screening. Despite the specificity of AFP, up to 40% of small HCC patients present with normal AFP levels at initial diagnosis, whereas 30% of HCC patients present with unelevated serum AFP levels [5]. As a result, other investigations such as fine needle aspiration (FNA) and radiological imaging should be used in combination with AFP levels for HCC diagnosis.

Fine Needle Aspiration

Percutaneous FNA, a minimally invasive approach used to establish the diagnosis of HCC, can obtain both cytological and histological samples via ultrasound (US) or CT guidance. Although advancements in imaging techniques have occurred in recent years, the diagnostic value of FNA should still be used for optimal sensitivity and specificity, as well as, for future guidance and determination of chemotherapy regimens and other treatment approaches. Even if the AASLD guidelines are followed closely using AFP >200 ng/ml as a diagnostic standard, there is still a possibility of a false positive diagnosis, which may result in unnecessary treatments and suffering. The possibility of a false negative diagnosis made by false interpretation of low serum AFP, should not be neglected either. Therefore, in this study, we aimed to reevaluate the significance of serum AFP ≤200 ng/ml in this patient population as a diagnostic value in the application of US-FNA to determine the overall accuracy of this procedure and to guide future clinical practice.

Materials and Methods

Patient characteristics

This study was approved by the ethics committee of Fudan University Shanghai Cancer Center. The retrospective study covered a period of 28 years, from June 1985 to December 2012. We retrospectively analyzed the medical records of 4,312 patients suspected of PLC who were admitted to Fudan University Shanghai Cancer Center, Shanghai, China. Of the patients recommended for FNA, 188 were excluded from this study due to loss of follow-up. Among the remaining patients, 1,929 presented with serum AFP levels ≤200 ng/ml. Of these, 1,756 underwent FNA, and 173 were excluded due to FNA failure. Patient characteristics of the 1,756 cases who underwent FNA are presented in Table 1.

US-FNA technique

Before the procedure, written informed consent was obtained from all patients. FNA was aborted if prothrombin time was prolonged over 5 seconds and/or if platelet counts fell below 50,000/μl. The procedures were performed under local anesthesia in the intervention room by a group of experienced oncologists, US specialized radiology technicians, and a cytotechnologist. Under ultrasonographic guidance, a safe needle pathway was determined to avoid intraparenchymal vessels and biliary structures. Tumors located near the hepatic capsule and diaphragm were avoided to prevent internal hemorrhage and diapharmatic motion. An 18-gauge guiding needle was used to aim a 22-gauge Chiba needle at the suspected lession. The Chiba needle was inserted coaxially through the guide needle into the mass with careful guidance by US imaging.

Under negative internal pressure, the needle was moved up and down within the tumor mass two to three times and cells were extracted. With the presence of a cytotechnologist, the adequacy of the sample collection was ensured to avoid failure of pathocytological findings due to lack of sample size. After FNA, the smears were fixed immediately, taken to the laboratory for H&E staining, and the final cytological diagnosis was typically made within two days. Immediately after FNA, an US examination was performed to detect any abnormalities or complications, such as intraperitoneal hemorrhage. Manual compression was made at the puncture site and a compressive bandage with a compression bag was positioned appropriately. Vital signs, including heart rate, blood pressure, respiratory frequency, blood oxygen saturation, and body temperature were monitored for 6 hours after US-FNA. Over the last five years, anhydrous ethanol has been applied to the wound as routine practice after needle removal.

Criteria for final diagnosis

In our study, final diagnosis was determined according to histopathological or initial cytological findings of malignancy, combined with imaging or clinical follow-up outcomes, including disease progression or death due to the disease. The term "primary liver cancer (PLC)" was used as a final diagnosis as most of the patients were not eligible to receive surgery or could not be further classified into a specific histopathological type. The definite diagnosis of PLC was confirmed either by post-surgical histopathological findings or positive radiological evidence, and/or increased serum AFP levels, combined with disease progression or death in clinical follow-up. Initial malignant cytological findings with positive follow-up radiological findings contributed to the final diagnosis.

Table 1. Patient characteristics of the 1,756 cases that underwent FNA.

Patient characteristics	No. of Cases
Gender	
Male	1459(83.09%)
Female	297(16.91%)
AFP Level	
<50 ng/ml	466(26.54%)
50–100 ng/ml	355(20.22%)
100–150 ng/ml	377(21.47%)
150–200 ng/ml	558(31.78%)
Tumor Size	
<20 mm	149(8.49%)
20–50 mm	209(11.90%)
50–80 mm	572(32.57%)
80–100 mm	474(26.99%)
>100 mm	352(20.05%)
Liver Cirrhosis	
Yes	932(53.08%)
No	824(46.92%)
HBsAg Status	
Positive	1038(59.11%)
Negetive	718(40.89%)

Statistical analysis

Standard methods were used and test performance was determined by calculating sensitivity, specificity, positive predictive value (PPV), negative predictive value (NPV), and overall diagnostic accuracy compared to the final diagnosis after follow-up. A chi-square test was used to compare the difference between the two groups. And P value<.05 was considered as statistically different. Cytomorphological investigation revealed atypical lesions, as well as, suspicious and unsatisfactory cases that were later diagnosed as malignancies by either clinical imaging and/or follow-up (wait-and-see). These cases were deemed as false negatives in the study.

Results

US-FNA failure cases

Of the 1,929 patients, 173 failed FNA. The most common reason for FNA failure was due to tumor location near the surface of the liver capsule or near the diaphragm, which accounted for 113 cases. Eighteen patients failed FNA and were excluded because of abnormal coagulation indexes that increased the risk of internal bleeding and could not be corrected within the short time period. Abnormal coagulation indexes included prolonged prothrombin time (>5 s), thrombocytopenia (platelet count <50,000/μl), or elevated INR >2. The procedure was not performed in six patients who failed to provide written informed consent. Infiltrative type tumors were detected in eleven patients, in which definite focal lesions could not be found. Only a small portion of failure cases (25 patients) had a contraindication for FNA. Contraindications included: low performance status (KPS<70), ascites, internal tumor liquefaction necrosis, significantly elevated total bilirubin possibly due to extrahepatic biliary obstruction and highly obstructive jaundice, severe congestive heart failure, severe infection, uncooperative patients, or coma.

Diagnostic outcome

Overall, a positive diagnosis of malignancy was confirmed in 1,478 cases, which were subclassified based on cytomorphology into tumor types. The cytological diagnoses classified as definitively malignant on aspirate material are shown in Table 2 and Table 3. Of the 1,478 cases, 1,138 were diagnosed as PLC. Twenty-three cases reported inconclusive cytology results, including fifteen cases suspicious for malignancy and eight cases containing atypical cells. Twelve cases of the suspicious group and four cases of the atypical cell group were later confirmed malignant and determined PLC. Initially, a total of 251 cases were reported negative for malignancy, however, on clinical follow-up or post-operative pathology, 92 were proven malignant. The diagnosis included 71 PLC, 19 metastatic cancer, and two sarcoma cases. There were also four additional cases in which necrotic tissue with no evidence of malignancy originally was later proven malignant by clinical and imaging follow-up. Serum AFP levels were used to analyze the sensitivity, specificity, PPV, NPV, and diagnostic accuracy of FNA (Table 4). Meanwhile, there was no significant difference in the sensitivity, specificity, PPV and NPV according to P value between the subgroups with tumor size< 2 cm and ≥2 cm (Table 5).

Hemorrhage

In this study, six cases of internal hemorrhage were diagnosed within 24 hours after FNA was performed. Most of the cases which suffered from hemorrhage after FNA occured in the early period, with two in 1980s and three in 1990s. Table 6 summarizes the characteristics of these cases. Although an intense effort was made to rescue the patients, the internal bleeding was fatal for

Table 2. Cytological diagnoses for 1,478 cases as malignant.

Final Diagnosis	No. of Cases
Primary liver neoplasm	1145
HCC	1067
CCA	63
HCC+CCA	8
Hepatoblastoma	1
Lymphoma	6
Metastatic Neoplasms	75
Adenocarcinoma	68
Squamouscell carcinoma	7
Malignancy NOS	258
Carcinoma	142
Adenocarcinoma	94
Sarcoma	21
Carcinosarcoma	1
Total	1478

NOS, not otherwise specified; HCC, hepatocellular carcinoma; CCA, cholangiocarcinoma; HCC+CCC, Mixed hepatocellular and cholangiocarcinoma.

three patients presenting with intraperitoneal hemorrhage. Sub-capsular hemorrhage was detected in three cases, but did not cause death. These patients were treated with supportive and symptomatic care.

Treatment and prognosis of implantation metastasis

The risk of needle tract metastasis implantation in this retrospective study was relatively low. Of all the patients who underwent FNA, only four cases (0.23%) of implantation metastasis were detected, and all of these cases had a history of liver cirrhosis. Two cases were detected on the thoracic wall, while the other two metastasized to the abdominal wall. The tumor size of the metastatic patients was relatively large with sizes ranging from: 8*10 cm, 11*12 cm, 16*15 cm, and 10*13 cm. The time for detection was 34, 118, 95, and 67 days respectively. Two cases received radical resection of the metastasis and two cases were performed with external radiation therapy. The survival time did not seem to be impacted by the metastasis, with 31, 11, 26 and 28 months respectively. Most likely, the patients died due to tumor progression and hepatic failure. It is worth mentioning that since 2007, after removal of the FNA needle during the procedure, manual pressure has been applied on the wound with an anhydrous alcohol cotton swab for at least 3 minutes. Since this addition, no post-procedural implantation metastases have been detected.

Discussion

Why advocate performing FNA in patients suspected of PLC with AFP ≤200 ng/ml?

The accuracy of cancer diagnosis is important since treatment regimens vary depending on cancer type and a false diagnosis can lead to unnecessary patient suffering. Over the last decade there has been a debate in the role of FNA in the detection of HCC. Advances in dynamic imaging techniques have increased the accuracy of HCC diagnosis in most nodules. Most of these dynamic imaging techniques are based on the vascular criteria. Computed tomography (CT) and magnetic resonance imaging

(MRI) have a high sensitivity (55%–91%) and specificity (77%–96%) in diagnosing HCC [6]. However, there are several limitations to the assessment of HCC using only the vascular criteria. Under various circumstances, not all HCCs radiological imaging have typical "fast-in and fast-out" patterns, nor do they always present with significant AFP elevations. This can make the differential diagnosis of HCC from metastasized liver cancer and other tumors located on the liver difficult. For example, the enhancement pattern of small HCC depends on size and cellular differentiation, and tumor size less than 2 cm may have atypical enhancement. The diagnosis of HCC based on vascular pattern may overlook the hypovascular tumors. Conversely, 52% of small early arterial-enhancing lesions decrease in time and can be considered pseudolesions [7]. Meanwhile, with liver cirrhosis at baseline, a clinical differential diagnosis of multi-nodular cirrhotic nodules from highly differentialted malignant nodules is difficult to make. This leads to differentiating HCC from benign lesions commonly seen in cirrhosis or from secondary malignancies, which remains a challenge. Serum AFP used alone can be helpful if levels are markedly elevated, which occurs in fewer than half of all cases at time of diagnosis [5]. If based on radiological images and AFP levels alone, atypical hemangiomas with diameters less than 3 cm, metastatic tumors with necrosis, cystic degeneration or rich blood supply, inflammatory pseudotumors of the liver, and focal nodular hyperplasias, may lead to a false diagnosis, causing unneccessary surgical resection, liver transplantation, or other inappropriate treatments. In this study, there was no significant difference in the sensitivity, specificity, PPV and NPV according to P value between the subgroups with tumor size<2 cm and ≥ 2 cm, which showed the advantage of FNA in the diagnostic effectiveness in small hepatic lesions.

Pathological diagnosis can provide multiple advantages to patients searching for an appropriate treatment option for their suspected malignancy. FNA can provide a pathological sample for early diagnosis and data that can be utilized in medical research. Further, for patients suspicious of small HCC, especially those with atypical lesions on radiological imaging, FNA can mitigate patients' anxiety once a liver nodule has been detected. Detecting

Table 3. Follow-up final diagnosis for cases diagnosed as metastatic neoplasm and malignancy NOS by FNA.

Cytological Diagnosis	Total	Primary Site	No. of Cases
Metastatic neoplasm	75		
adenocarcinoma	68		
		Gastrointestinal	43
		Lung	11
		Pancreatic/biliary	4
		Prostate	1
		Ovary	1
		NOS	8
Squamouscellcarcinoma	7		
		Lung	3
		Nasopharyngeal	3
		Cervix	1
Malignancy NOS	258		
Carcinoma	142		
		Liver	74
		Gastrointestinal	49
		Pancreatic/biliary	5
		Lung	10
		Breast	2
		Nasopharyngeal	2
Adenocarcinoma	94		
		Liver	64
		Gastrointestinal	23
		Pancreatic/biliary	3
		Lung	3
		Ovary	1
Sarcoma	21		
		Liver	18
		Soft tissue	3
Carcinosarcoma	1		
		Liver	1

Table 4. Diagnostic outcome of different AFP levels.

	0–200	0–50	51–100	101–150	151–200
No. of patients	1756	466	355	377	558
(malignant/benign)	(1590/166)	(422/44)	(323/32)	(341/36)	(504/54)
True positive	1478	395	299	312	472
True negative	166	44	32	36	54
False positive	0	0	0	0	0
False negative	112	27	24	29	32
Sensitivity(%)	92.96%	93.6%	92.57%	91.5%	93.65%
Specificity(%)	100%	100%	100%	100%	100%
Positive predictive value(%)	100%	100%	100%	100%	100%
Negative predictive value(%)	59.71%	61.97%	57.14%	55.38%	62.79%
Overall accuracy(%)	93.62%	94.21%	93.24%	92.31%	94.27%

Table 5. Diagnostic outcome between the subgroups with tumor size<2 cm and ≥2 cm.

	<2 cm	≥2 cm	P value
No. of patients	149	1607	-
(malignant/benign)	133/16	1457/150	-
Sensitivity	93.23%	92.93%	0.896
Specificity	100%	100%	-
PPV	100%	100%	-
NPV	64%	59.29%	0.647

PPV, positive predictive value; NPV, negative predictive value.

a liver nodule early can decrease costs that long-term imaging surveillance can accrue and provide patients with appropriate treatment options earlier.

Analysis of low NPV

The sensitivity and specificity in our study was 92.96% and 100% respectively. The sensitivities of FNA for detecting malignancy in recent large research series have ranged from 83.3% to 97.5%, with specificities approaching or achieving 100% [8]. However, the NPV of our study was approximately only 60%. The reasons are analyzed as follows. Since Shanghai Cancer Center specializes in tumor treatment, most patients who present to the hospital are highly suspicious of malignancy, and only a relatively small number of patients have benign liver diseases. Other various factors may have influenced the results of FNA. For instance, patients with tumors located too close to the diaphragmatic surface and/or who failed to keep their breathing at a low rate during aspiration may have had compromised ultrasound images. This may have led to deviations along the fine needle tract which prevented obtaining an adequate sample. Clinically, it has been recognized as relatively difficult to diagnose highly differenciated HCC from regenerative nodules. Additionally, for multiple nodular cases with background liver cirrhosis, there is a

possibility of aspirating non-malignant nodules such as liver cirrhosis nodules. Also, in the cases presenting with large tumors and cystic necrosis, the aspirated samples may have had liquefied material without malignant cells or may have failed to meet basic pathological investigation requirements.

AFP levels and diagnostic outcomes

We analyzed the FNA results of tumors with different AFP levels ranging from <50 ng/ml, 50–100 ng/ml, 100–150 ng/ml, and 150–200 ng/ml. There were no significant differences seen in regards to sensitivity and NPV of FNA results among different AFP levels. Thus, according to our study results, we interpreted that AFP levels do not influence the results of US-FNA.

It is well-known that early detection of HCC not only increases patients' chances of receiving treatment, but also improves prognosis. The most commonly used confirmatory diagnostic modality of HCC is FNA. Although FNA is only a minimally invasive diagnostic approach, it still has serious side effects and can contribute to patient suffering. Since both AFP and FNA are commonly used diagnostic approaches for the final confirmatory diagnosis for PLC, it is important to evaluate the effectiveness and relationship of these two diagnostic methods to avoid unnecessary procedures and patient suffering. Unfortunately, there are limited

Table 6. Characteristics of hemorrhage.

Case Number	1	2	3	4	5	6
Age	39	48	64	51	47	52
Gender	Male	Male	male	Male	male	Male
AFP	23.3	5.9	78.49	139	11.33	20.12
Tumor type	HCC	HCC	HCC	HCC	HCC	HCC
Tumor size (cm*cm)	12.2*13.1	13.9*11.5	9*7.7	5.7*5.5	8.9*8.2	10.4*10.8
Tumor location	Subcapsular	Subcapsular	Subcapsular	Subcapsular	Subcapsular	Subcapsular
HBsAg	+	+	—	—	+	+
Cirrhosis	+	+	+	+	+	+
Prothrombase time(s)	10.9	11.4	12.0	12.7	13.1	13.3
Platelet count (10^9/L)	78	124	185	67	96	135
Number of needle passes	1	1	2	2	2	1
Hemorrhage location	Intraperitoneal	Intraperitoneal	Intraperitoneal	Intraperitoneal	Intraperitoneal	IntraPeritoneal
Treatment outcome	dead	dead	dead	alive	alive	alive
Interval between onset and death(hour)	24	2	8	-	-	-

studies focusing on the FNA value in patients with serum AFP ≤ 200 ng/ml. Most of the studies focus on either the prognosis of different AFP levels or the recurrence and side effects of FNA in relationship to tumor size. Based on 4,312 patients, this retrospective study was the largest population of patients with AFP ≤200 mg/l and suspected PLC, in which FNA has been performed. This may prove to be valuable for future clinical practice.

Complications

As previously reported, biliary peritonitis is a serious complication of FNA [9], which fortunately, was not detected in any patients during the study. This may be related to our ability to avoid aspiration in cases where bile ducts are inevitably being punctured. The most significant complications observed in our department were hemorrhage and implantation metastasis.

Normal or only mildly reduced coagulation parameters do not prevent bleeding complications

Risk of hemorrhage is not as controversial as implantation metastasis. A mortality rate of 0.018% was reported in a multi-institutional Italian series of 10,766 US-guided FNA biopsies [10]. All of the patients in this study who presented with post-FNA hemorrhage, also presented with liver cirrhosis and platelet counts above 50,000/μl. Further, no significant abnormalities in INR, coagulation profile, and/or prothrombin time (PT) were detected. Although the doctors' skills helped avoid puncturing major liver vessels, post-FNA hemorrhage still occurred. According to our clinical experience, hemorrhage is typically associated with severe cirrhosis or large superficial tumors not covered by normal liver parenchyma, rather than coagulation profiles and platelet counts. Similar to published literature, our data suggests that normal or only mildly reduced coagulation parameters do not prevent bleeding complications [11–13]. If the tumor is covered with enough liver parenchyma, it still can be punctured and without excess risk of hemorrhage, no matter the tumor size is more than 5 cm or not. Careful monitoring for post-FNA hemorrhage should be practiced for the tumors relatively large in size or in those that have relatively small amounts of normal liver tissue coverage. Meanwhile, before the procedure of FNA, the risk of bleeding should be evaluated in every patient. If the bleeding risk is high, imaging approaches should be used to diagnose the disease to avoid hemorrhage after FNA, although we advocate every patient who is suspected with PLC should undergo FNA.

Post procedure monitoring and haemostatic agents are suggested for patients who underwent FNA

While not all reports on FNA acknowledge post-procedural hemorrhage, an acceptabley low incidence of hemorrhage does exist both theoretically and clinically. Thus, as routine practice after FNA, our department uses haemostatic agents. Until now, no prospective study has shown that using routine haemostatic agents decreases the risk of hemorrhage after FNA. It is not yet known if the use of haemostatic agents or remaining immobile for several hours following FNA increases a patient's risk of thrombosis. The incidence of hemorrhage in this retrospective study was very low with only 6 cases (3 major, 0.17% and 3 minor, 0.17%) detected in the 1,756 cases that underwent FNA. This may be due to the routine use of haemostatic agents after FNA. Meanwhile, most of the cases who suffered from hemorrhage after FNA occured in the early period, during which there were not many effective hemostatic agents. Comparatively, the newly emerged hemostatic agents may decrease the incidence of bleeding after FNA, which

make this procedure much safer than that in the early period. Additionally, an increased risk of thrombosis was not observed. Thus, based on this study, routine use of haemostatic agents is suggested after FNA.

Post-FNA monitoring should be carried out for at least 6 hours to minimize fatal complications

In all of the patients who experienced bleeding complications, including subcapsular and intraperitoneal hemorrhage, bleeding occurred within 6 hours after FNA. Thus, the experience from this study suggests that post-FNA monitoring should be carried out for at least 6 hours to minimize fatal complications. The patients that suffered from subcapsular hemorrhage were mainly treated with haemostatic agents, broad pressurizing belly bands, and blood volume expanders. The complication of subcapsular hemorrhaging resulted in no patient deaths.

For the three patients who experienced peritoneal hemorrhage, transcatheter arterial embolization was applied to two, while the other patient received a broad pressurizing belly band, blood transfusion, haemostatic agents, as well, as suppportive care. Unfortunately, peritoneal hemorrhage was fatal to all patients within 24 hours after detection. According to our study, the location of the hemorrhage site has a significant relationship with prognosis. Once peritoneal hemorrhage occurs after FNA, the condition will quickly become severe within a relatively short time period, making survival unlikely. Therefore, the patients complaining of severe abdominal pain after FNA, with signs of peritoneal irritation, significant haemoglobin decline, hemodynamic instability, and seroperitoneum detected on ultrasound investigation, should be treated for post-FNA hemorrhage immediately.

Prognosis and treatment of implantation metastasis

Implantation metastasis has always been the major argument when deciding if FNA should be performed. Risk of implantation metastasis after FNA for malignancy, in general, is considered rare. An overall incidence of 0.13% of HCC with soft tissue metastasis was reported in one large study [14] where a total of 18,227 person-times of FNA or percutaneous ethanol injections were performed on HCC patients. Sliva et al. [15] in a systemic review and meta-analysis of eight observational studies found that the incidence of needle tract seeding after FNA varied greatly from 0–5.8%. However, FNA is not the only procedure that may lead to implantation metastasis. Other procedures, including: percutaneous ethanol injection, radio frequency abalation, and percutaneous transhepaticcholangial drainage, may all potentially induce implantation metastasis. Dong-Won Ahn, et al. [16] reported that two (0.13%) of the 1,549 patients who underwent PEI, four (0.12%) of the 3,391 who underwent FNAB, and one (0.66%) of the 152 patients who underwent PTCD for HCC, experienced needle tract seeding. In animal models, Ryd et al. [17] found that FNA can implant 10^3–10^5 cells along a single needle tract. Thus, theoretically, multi-site aspiration or multi-passes may lead to an increase in the amount of malignant cells at the implantation site and needle tract, and therefore increases the possibility of implantation metastasis. Our study verifies Ryd's findings. Among the four patients who presented with implantation metastasis after FNA, three had tumors larger than 10 cm in diameter. If the initial aspiration obtained majorly liquefied necrotic material, the pathologist considered the sample inadequate, and FNA was performed on another side of the lesion, which may have negatively influenced the pathological diagnosis. These resulted in repeated aspirations with a mean of four passes and at least two sites of aspiration among the four patients. Multiple aspiration sites and several passes may increase the chance of implantation metastasis. Thus, to reduce the possibility of implantation metastasis, we suggest that needle passes during FNA be reduced to the least number possible and the puncture should ideally be performed on a single site.

Meanwhile, the decline in implantation metastasis since 2007 may be an advantage resulting from manual compression on the puncture site with an alcohol cotton swab. Interestingly, the absolute alcohol can lead to liver cancer cell lysis and degeneration, which is often used for intra-tumor injections as a treatment option for HCC. Based on our experience, we suggest routine manual compression of an anhydrous alcohol swab on the needle site for at least three minutes in every FNA case to reduce the chance of implantation metastasis.

Despite the risk of implantation metastasis in FNA, however, surgical resection of the implantation site or radiological therapy may have a satisfactory treatment outcome. In the four cases of implantation metastasis in our study, two received regional radiological therapy (2500 cGy, 100 cGy per time) and two received radical excision. All of the cases had satisfactory treatment outcomes, and implantation tumors were eradicated in three cases, with no reoccurrence detected within the survival time. One case that received radiological therapy had a significant reduction in the implanted site's size and no significant progression was seen.

Additionally, since most cases in this study were unresectable, implantation metastasis didn't influence the prognosis of these patients. The patients who suffered died because of HCC progression and hepatic failure, not implantation metastasis itself. We suspect there were additional cases of implantation metastasis, which were undetected prior to death possibly due to the progression of the disease and the short survival time of PLC patients. Implantation metastasis does not have the same

importance and influence on prognosis as metastasis has on other organs such as lung, kidney, adrenal gland, bone, etc.

However, we do not suggest patients who meet clinical diagnosis criteria and who are eligible for radical resection or liver transplantation receive FNA since the risk of needle track metastasis does exist, which may lead to unradical tumor excision.

Conclusion

Based on the large sample of patient characteristics in this retrospective study, we conclude that patients with PLC, especially those who present with AFP $\leq$200 mg/ml, should undergo FNA since a clinical diagnosis cannot be made based on serum AFP and imaging investigations alone. If negative results are obtained by FNA, it still could be HCC and repeated FNA procedure may be needed if highly suspicious of HCC on imaging study. US-FNA may be considered a relatively safe procedure with minimal side effects, however, the risk of fatal internal hemorrhage and needle track implantation metastasis should not be overlooked. Therefore, we suggest that US-FNA be performed in hospitalized patients who will receive 6 hours of routine monitoring after FNA. To our knowledge, this is the first and largest study concerning the relationship and predictive value of FNA in patients with PLC presenting with serum AFP $\leq$200 mg/l. Thus, we conclude that FNA is a necessary procedure for disease diagnosis since the benefits outweigh potential complications due to superiority in sensitivity, specificity, and overall accuracy.

Author Contributions

Conceived and designed the experiments: ZM BP. Performed the experiments: QC CC. Analyzed the data: QC CC. Contributed reagents/materials/analysis tools: HC ZN X. Zhang ST. Wrote the paper: QC CC. Involved in the FNA performance: X. Zhu YS YH JX WS HG LX LF JL ZC LL. Edited the language of this article: SV.

References

1. Parkin DM, Bray F, Ferlay J, Pisani P (2005) Global cancer statistics, 2002. CA: a cancer journal for clinicians 55: 74–108.
2. Ishiguro T, Sugitachi I, Sakaguchi H, Itani S (1985) Serum alpha-fetoprotein subfractions in patients with primary hepatoma or hepatic metastasis of gastric cancer. Cancer 55: 156–159.
3. Bruix J, Sherman M (2011) Management of hepatocellular carcinoma: an update. Hepatology 53: 1020–1022.
4. Trevisani F, D'Intino PE, Morselli-Labate AM, Mazzella G, Accogli E, et al. (2001) Serum alpha-fetoprotein for diagnosis of hepatocellular carcinoma in patients with chronic liver disease: influence of HBsAg and anti-HCV status. Journal of hepatology 34: 570–575.
5. Bialecki ES, Di Bisceglie AM (2005) Diagnosis of hepatocellular carcinoma. HPB: the official journal of the International Hepato Pancreato Biliary Association 7: 26–34.
6. Colli A, Fraquelli M, Conte D (2006) Alpha-fetoprotein and hepatocellular carcinoma. The American journal of gastroenterology 101: 1939; author reply 1940–1931.
7. Shimizu A, Ito K, Koike S, Fujita T, Shimizu K, et al. (2003) Cirrhosis or chronic hepatitis: evaluation of small (<or = 2-cm) early-enhancing hepatic lesions with serial contrast-enhanced dynamic MR imaging. Radiology 226: 550–555.
8. Bhatia KS, Lee YY, Yuen EH, Ahuja AT (2013) Ultrasound elastography in the head and neck. Part II. Accuracy for malignancy. Cancer imaging : the official publication of the International Cancer Imaging Society 13: 260–276.
9. Parajuli S, Tuladhar A, Basnet RB (2011) Ultrasound and computed tomography guided fine needle aspiration cytology in diagnosing intra-abdominal and intra-thoracic lesions. Journal of Pathology of Nepal 1:17–21.

10. Fornari F, Civardi G, Cavanna L, Di Stasi M, Rossi S, et al. (1989) Complications of ultrasonically guided fine-needle abdominal biopsy. Results of a multicenter Italian study and review of the literature. The Cooperative Italian Study Group. Scandinavian journal of gastroenterology 24: 949–955.
11. Sparchez Z (2005) Complications after percutaneous liver biopsy in diffuse hepatopathies. Romanian journal of gastroenterology 14: 379–384.
12. Piccinino F, Sagnelli E, Pasquale G, Giusti G (1986) Complications following percutaneous liver biopsy. A multicentre retrospective study on 68,276 biopsies. Journal of hepatology 2: 165–173.
13. Froehlich F, Lamy O, Fried M, Gonvers JJ (1993) Practice and complications of liver biopsy. Results of a nationwide survey in Switzerland. Digestive diseases and sciences 38: 1480–1484.
14. Tung WC, Huang YJ, Leung SW, Kuo FY, Tung HD, et al. (2007) Incidence of needle tract seeding and responses of soft tissue metastasis by hepatocellular carcinoma postradiotherapy. Liver international : official journal of the International Association for the Study of the Liver 27: 192–200.
15. Silva MA, Hegab B, Hyde C, Guo B, Buckels JA, et al. (2008) Needle track seeding following biopsy of liver lesions in the diagnosis of hepatocellular cancer: a systematic review and meta-analysis. Gut 57: 1592–1596.
16. Ahn DW, Shim JH, Yoon JH, Kim CY, Lee HS, et al. (2011) Treatment and clinical outcome of needle-track seeding from hepatocellular carcinoma. The Korean journal of hepatology 17: 106–112.
17. Ryd W, Hagmar B, Eriksson O (1983) Local tumour cell seeding by fine-needle aspiration biopsy. A semiquantitative study. Acta pathologica, microbiologica, et immunologica Scandinavica. Section A, Pathology 91: 17–21.

2

Circulating AIM as an Indicator of Liver Damage and Hepatocellular Carcinoma in Humans

Tomoko Yamazaki[1], Mayumi Mori[1], Satoko Arai[1], Ryosuke Tateishi[2], Masanori Abe[3], Mihoko Ban[4], Akemi Nishijima[1], Maki Maeda[4], Takeharu Asano[5], Toshihiro Kai[1¤], Kiyohiro Izumino[4], Jun Takahashi[4], Kayo Aoyama[1], Sei Harada[6], Toru Takebayashi[6], Toshiaki Gunji[7], Shin Ohnishi[8], Shinji Seto[4], Yukio Yoshida[5], Yoichi Hiasa[3], Kazuhiko Koike[2], Ken-ichi Yamamura[9], Ken-ichiro Inoue[4], Toru Miyazaki[1,10,11]*

1 Laboratory of Molecular Biomedicine for Pathogenesis, Center for Disease Biology and Integrative Medicine, Faculty of Medicine, The University of Tokyo, Tokyo, Japan, 2 Department of Gastroenterology, Graduate School of Medicine, The University of Tokyo, Tokyo, Japan, 3 Department of Gastroenterology and Metabology, Ehime University Graduate School of Medicine, Ehime, Japan, 4 Shunkaikai, Inoue Hospital, Nagasaki, Japan, 5 Department of Gastroenterology, Jichi Medical University, Saitama Medical Center, Omiya, Japan, 6 Department of Preventive Medicine and Public Health, School of Medicine, Keio University, Tokyo, Japan, 7 Center for Preventive Medicine, NTT Medical Center Tokyo, Tokyo, Japan, 8 National Center for Global Health and Medicine, Tokyo, Japan, 9 Center for Animal Resources and Development, Kumamoto University, Kumamoto, Japan, 10 Max Planck-The University of Tokyo Center for Integrative Inflammology, Tokyo, Japan, 11 CREST, Japan Science and Technology Agency, Tokyo, Japan

Abstract

Background: Hepatocellular carcinoma (HCC), the fifth most common cancer type and the third highest cause of cancer death worldwide, develops in different types of liver injuries, and is mostly associated with cirrhosis. However, non-alcoholic fatty liver disease often causes HCC with less fibrosis, and the number of patients with this disease is rapidly increasing. The high mortality rate and the pathological complexity of liver diseases and HCC require blood biomarkers that accurately reflect the state of liver damage and presence of HCC.

Methods and Findings: Here we demonstrate that a circulating protein, apoptosis inhibitor of macrophage (AIM) may meet this requirement. A large-scale analysis of healthy individuals across a wide age range revealed a mean blood AIM of 4.99 ± 1.8 µg/ml in men and 6.06 ± 2.1 µg/ml in women. AIM levels were significantly augmented in the younger generation (20s–40s), particularly in women. Interestingly, AIM levels were markedly higher in patients with advanced liver damage, regardless of disease type, and correlated significantly with multiple parameters representing liver function. In mice, AIM levels increased in response to carbon tetrachloride, confirming that the high AIM observed in humans is the result of liver damage. In addition, carbon tetrachloride caused comparable states of liver damage in AIM-deficient and wild-type mice, indicating no influence of AIM levels on liver injury progression. Intriguingly, certain combinations of AIM indexes normalized to liver marker score significantly distinguished HCC patients from non-HCC patients and thus could be applicable for HCC diagnosis.

Conclusion: AIM potently reveals both liver damage and HCC. Thus, our results may provide the basis for novel diagnostic strategies for this widespread and fatal disease.

Editor: Kalpana Ghoshal, The Ohio State University, United States of America

Funding: This work was supported by Grants-in-Aid for Scientific Research (A) (Japan Society for the Promotion of Science), CREST (JST), research grants by ONSENDO Co., Ltd. (to TM), Grants-in-Aid for Scientific Research (B) (Japan Society for the Promotion of Science) (to SA), research grants by The Tokyo Biochemical Research Foundation, Takeda Science Foundation and Ono Medical Research Foundation (to MM). The funders had no role in study design, data collection and analysis, decision to publish, or preparation of the manuscript.

Competing Interests: Although the authors received funding from a commercial source (ONSENDO Co., Ltd), this funding was solely for research activity, and was not used for employment, consultancy, patents, products in development, or marketed products related to either commercial source. This funding does not alter the authors' adherence to PLOS ONE policies on sharing data and materials.

* Email: tm@m.u-tokyo.ac.jp

¤ Current address: Omics Group, Genomic Science Laboratories, Dainippon Sumitomo Pharma Co., Ltd., Osaka, Japan

Introduction

Chronic liver injury is one of the most common and fatal diseases in modern society. It has multiple causes including hepatitis virus infection mostly due to hepatitis C virus (HCV) and to a lesser extent hepatitis B virus (HBV), alcohol injury, autoimmunity, and genetic disorders such as hemochromatosis [1–3]. In addition, the non-alcoholic fatty liver disease (NAFLD), which is associated with obesity, has been observed in a rapidly growing number of patients due to recent and drastic changes in lifestyle. NAFLD comprises a wide variety of disease criteria ranging from benign simple steatosis to progressive inflammation and fibrosis, called non-alcoholic steatohepatitis (NASH) [4,5]. Such chronic liver diseases exhibit continuous inflammation and fibrosis and are a prominent risk for the development of hepatocellular carcinoma (HCC) [6–8]. In contrast to patients with HCV infection, who display a high susceptibility to HCC, only a limited proportion of NAFLD patients progress to carcinoma [9–11]. Intriguingly, recent evidence has revealed that although HCC develops largely on the basis of severe liver fibrosis/cirrhosis, it often occurs without cirrhosis in NAFLD/ NASH patients exhibiting mild inflammation and fibrosis [12–18]. However, the mechanism of how each pathological background induces HCC remains to be elucidated. With such increasing risks and complicated pathogenesis, biomarkers that reflect the state of liver damage and the presence of HCC are important, particularly for the early diagnosis of HCC development. Ideally, markers that indicate an individual's susceptibility to HCC may be desirable from the prognostic and preventive views of HCC.

The circulating protein, apoptosis inhibitor of macrophage (AIM), also called CD5L, was initially identified as an apoptosis inhibitor that supports macrophage survival [19]. AIM is produced solely by tissue macrophages under transcriptional regulation by nuclear receptor liver X receptor alpha (LXRα) [20–22], and as a secreted molecule, AIM is detected in both human and mouse blood [19,23]. Interestingly, AIM associates with the immunoglobulin (Ig)M pentamer in the blood, and this association protects AIM from renal excretion, thereby maintaining circulating AIM at a relatively high concentration (approximately 2–5 μg/ml) in mice [23,24]. However, AIM's precise levels in healthy individuals and patients with various diseases remain controversial [25–28].

We recently identified that AIM is incorporated into adipocytes via CD36-mediated endocytosis where it inactivates cytoplasmic fatty acid synthase (FASN) through direct binding. This response reduces the production of lipid droplet-coating proteins such as fat-specific protein 27 (FSP27) and perilipin, thereby decreasing triacylglycerol deposition within adipocytes [29,30]. Consistent with this effect, adipocyte hypertrophy was found to be more advanced with a greater mass of visceral adipose tissue in AIM-deficient $(AIM^{-/-})$ mice than in wild-type $(AIM^{+/+})$ mice fed a high-fat diet (HFD) [29]. We also found that AIM prevents lipid storage in the liver, as in adipocytes [31]. Because a consensus has rapidly emerged that hepatocytic lipid metabolism impacts the pathogenesis of not only NAFLD but also other liver injuries, as well as HCC development, we decided to address the possible relationship in circulating AIM levels, the state of liver damage, and the presence of HCC in humans.

In this study, we first analyzed a large number of healthy individuals to determine the "normal level" of circulating AIM. We then assessed the correlation between circulating AIM levels and the state of liver damage using sera from patients with liver diseases. We also tested whether the difference in AIM levels correlated with the progression of liver damage using a mouse model. Furthermore, we investigated whether the AIM level can be applied for the diagnosis of HCC in humans.

Methods

Human subjects

Serum samples of healthy individuals were collected from volunteers who had annual medical examinations at Inoue Hospitals (Nagasaki, Japan). Serum samples of patients with liver diseases were obtained from Tokyo University Hospital, Ehime University Hospital and Jichi Medical University Hospital.

Ethic

For analysis of human subjects, informed consent in writing was obtained from each healthy volunteer and patient, and the study protocol conformed to the ethical guidelines of the 1975 Declaration of Helsinki as reflected in a priori approval by the Ethics Committee of the University of Tokyo for Medical Experiments (Permission Numbers: #3358 & #2817). In addition, all animal experiments were carried out in strict accordance with the recommendations in the Guide for the Care and Use of Laboratory Animals of the National Institutes of Health. The protocol was approved by the Committee on the Ethics of Animal Experiments of the University of Tokyo (Permit Number: P10-143). All surgery was performed under sodium pentobarbital anesthesia, and all efforts were made to minimize suffering.

Carbon tetrachloride (CCl4) administration

$AIM^{-/-}$ mice [19] had been backcrossed to C57BL/6 (B6) for 15 generations before used for experiments. Mice were intraperitoneally injected with CCl4 (Wako, Osaka, Japan) (1.6 g/kg body weight; dissolved in corn oil) twice a week for 3 or 12 wk. Mice were sacrificed 3 days after the last injection of CCl_4. All mice were maintained under a specific pathogen-free (SPF) condition.

Statistical analysis

Student's t-test was performed to compare values from two groups. Correlation coefficients and p values were calculated by Excel. Multiple linear regression analysis was performed by backward stepwise approach, with t>1.5 for entry and t<1.5 or inter-variables correlation coefficient>0.5 or probability F>0.1 for removal from the model. Multiple pairwise comparison among groups were performed by ANCOVA using JMP software (version 11).

ELISA assay

Human AIM was measured by an ELISA system using mouse anti-human AIM monoclonal antibodies (clones #6 and #7; established in our laboratory), which is now available from the Trans Genic Inc., Kumamoto, Japan. For ELISA of mouse AIM, we used two different rat anti-mouse AIM monoclonal antibodies (clones #36 and #35; established in our laboratory). Human IgM was measured by Human IgM ELISA Quantification Set (Bethyl Laboratories, Inc. Montgomery, USA).

Histology

Liver specimens were fixed overnight in 4% paraformaldehyde in phosphate buffered saline (PBS) and replaced into 30% sucrose/ PBS liquid. Samples were embedded in Tissue-Tek O.C.T. compound (Sakura Finetek Co.,Ltd., Tokyo), cut by 10 μm. For Sirius red staining, sections were washed in PBS for 5 min, counter stained with Mayer's Hematoxylin for 10 min, washed with running water for 2 min and subsequently soaked in hydrochloric acid alcohol (0.5% HCl in 70% EtOH) for 1 min. Sections were then stained with 0.03% Sirius red (Direct red 80, SIGMA-ALDRICH) in saturated picric acid solution for 15 min. HE staining was performed using Mayer's Hematoxylin (MUTO PURE CHEMICALS CO.,LTD., Tokyo) and Eosin (SIGMA-ALDRICH, St. Louis, USA).

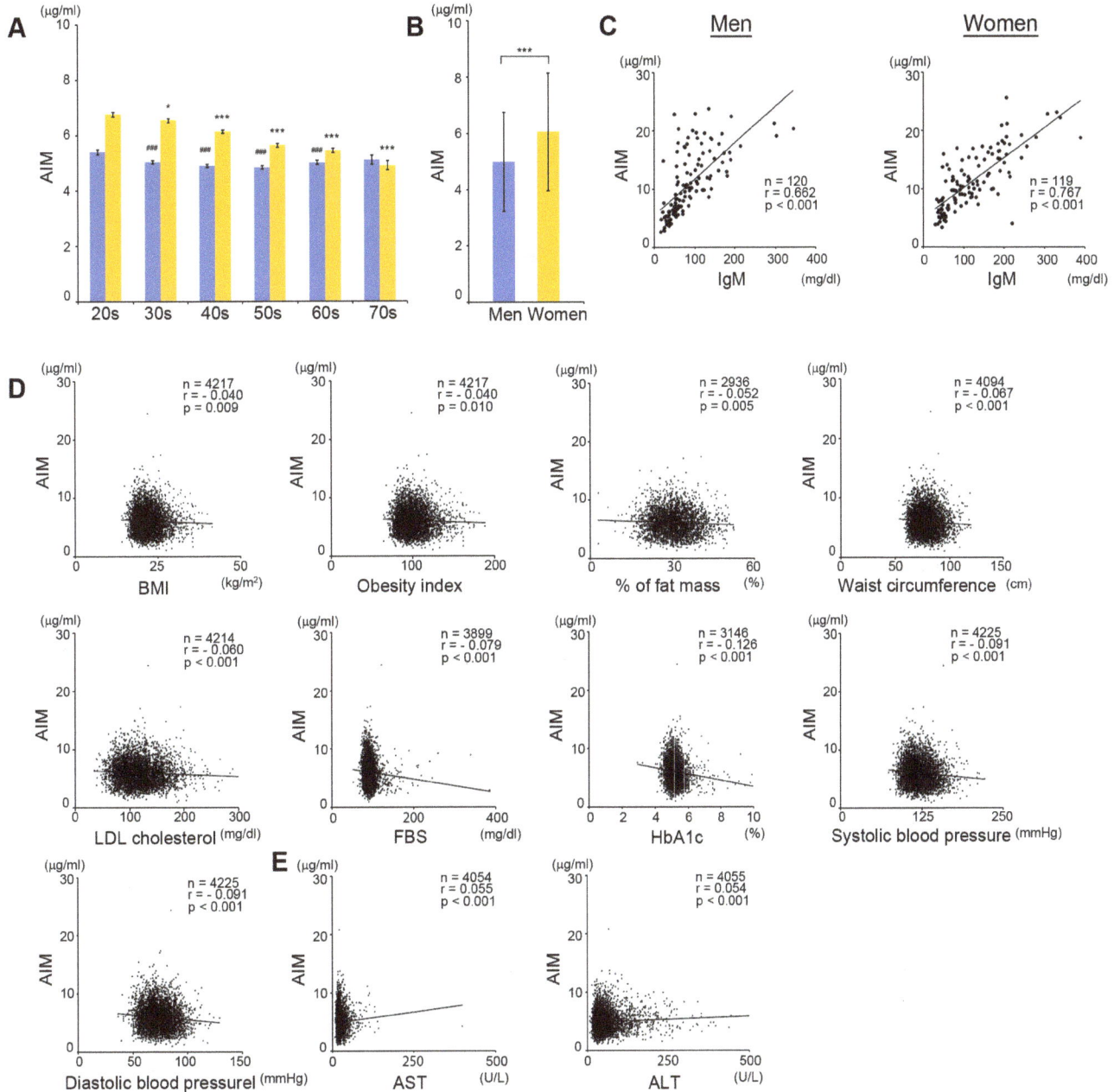

Figure 1. Circulating AIM levels in healthy indivisuals. (A) AIM levels in different generations. Error bar: SEM. ***: $p<0.001$ vs. the value of women in 20s. ###: $p<0.001$ vs. the value of men in 20s. (B) Means $\pm$ SD (μg/ml) of AIM levels in whole men and women. AIM levels were significantly higher in women than in men. (C) Correlation of AIM and IgM levels in men and women. IgM levels were analyzed by ELISA in 20 individuals exhibiting a variety of AIM levels in each generation in men and women. (D) Correlation in AIM levels and BMI, obesity index, % of fat mass or waist circumference, LDL cholesterol levels, HbA1C, FBS, systolic or diastolic blood pressure in women. (E) Correlation in AIM and AST or ALT levels in males and females. In C-E, r: correlation coefficients in single linear regression analysis, p: p value, n: number of samples. Blue dots: men, yellow dots: women.

Fibrosis analysis

Fibrosis area determined by Sirius red staining was quantified using NIH Image J software. Five areas for each sample were assessed under a microscope (FSX 100, OLYMPUS, Tokyo).

Quantitative PCR assay

The quantitative evaluation of mRNA was performed by the $\Delta\Delta C_T$ method using a 7500Fast Real-Time PCR system (Life Technologies Japan, Tokyo) and Power SYBR Green PCR Master Mix (Life Technologies). Sequences of the oligonucleotides used are below:

f-GAPDH	5'-AACTTTGGCATTGTGGAAGG-3'
r-GAPDH	5'-GGATGCAGGGGATGATGTTCT-3'
f-TNFα	5'-ACGGCATGGATCTCAAAGAC-3'
r-TNFα	5'-AGATAGCAAATCGGCTGACG-3'
f-IL1β	5'-CTGGTGTGTGACGTTCCCATTA-3'
r-IL1β	5'-CCGACAGCACGAGGCTTT-3'
f-IL 6	5'-CCAGTTGCCTTCTTGGGACT-3'

Table 1. The composition of examinees and the AIM level.

age	Male AIM (µg/ml)	n	Female AIM (µg/ml)	n
10s	5.62±1.66	28	6.39±1.65	15
20s	5.41±1.67	368	6.75±2.05	592
30s	5.04±1.69	806	6.53±2.03	791
40s	4.90±1.76	1153	6.14±2.09	1163
50s	4.84±1.78	988	5.64±1.95	977
60s	5.02±1.80	580	5.45±2.1	579
70s	5.11±1.79	120	4.91±1.57	87
80s	4.69±1.57	9	5.57±2.84	16
90s	7.55±3.60	3	4.22±2.03	5
whole	4.99±1.76	4055	6.06±2.09	4225

The AIM level is presented as mean±SD (µg/ml). n: sample number.

r-IL 6	5'-GGTCTGTTGGGAGTGGTATCC-3'
f-MCP1	5'-ACTGAAGCCAGCTCTCTCTTCCTC-3'
r-MCP1	5'-TTCCTTCTTGGGGTCAGCACAGAC-3'
f-CD11c	5'-GAGCCAGAACTTCCCAACTG-3'
r-CD11c	5'-TCAGGAACACGATGTCTTGG-3'
f-CD163	5'-CCTGGATCATCTGTGACAACA-3'
r-CD163	5'-TCCACACGTCCAGAACAGTC-3'
f-Arg-1	5'-CTCCAAGCCAAAGTCCTTAGAG-3'
r-Arg-1	5'-AGGAGCTGTCATTAGGGACATC-3'
f-MR	5'-CCACAGCATTGAGGAGTTTG-3'
r-MR	5'-ACAGCTCATCATTTGGCTCA-3'
f-TGF β	5'-TGGAGCAACATGTGGAACTC-3'
r-TGF β	5'-CAGCAGCCGGTTACCAAG-3'
f-α SMA	5'-ACTCTCTTCCAGCCATCTTCA-3'
r-α SMA	5'-ATAGGTGGTTTCGTGGATGC-3'
f-Col4a1	5'-TTAAAGGACTCCAGGGACCAC-3'
r-Col4a1	5'-CCCACTGAGCCTGTCACAC-3'
f-CTGF	5'-TGACCTGGAGGAAAACATTAAGA-3'
r-CTGF	5'-AGCCCTGTATGTCTTCACACTG-3'
f-TIMP1	5'-GCAAAGAGCTTTCTCAAAGACC-3'
r-TIMP1	5'-AGGGATAGATAAACAGGGAAACACT-3'
f-mAIM	5'-GAGGACACATGGATGGAATGT-3'
r-mAIM	5'-ACCCTTGTGTAGCACCTCCA-3'

Results

Circulating AIM levels in healthy individuals

To investigate circulating AIM levels in healthy individuals, we performed a large-scale analysis of AIM using more than 8,000 blood samples of volunteers attending annual medical examinations in 2012 and 2013. For this study, we established an ELISA system by generating monoclonal antibodies that accurately estimated human AIM levels in blood. The composition of volunteers and the mean±SD AIM level (µg/ml) are shown in Table 1. AIM levels were highest in both men and women in their 20s and decreased with age (Fig. 1A). In individuals <50 years old, AIM levels were significantly higher in women (Fig. 1A), resulting in an overall higher mean AIM level in women (Fig. 1B). Consistent with our previous report [23], a strong correlation was observed between IgM and AIM levels (Fig. 1C).

The significance of the relationships between AIM levels and various clinical parameters is presented in Table S1. In particular, we focused on obesity-related parameters because AIM has lipolytic function and thus acts as an anti-obese factor in mice [29,30]. The relationship between AIM and various parameters was more significant in women, and AIM levels correlated negatively with body mass index, obesity index, % fat mass, and

Table 2. Number of patients in each type of liver injury.

	HCC Men	Women	Non HCC Men	Women
Whole	189 (100%)	86 (100%)	90 (100%)	56 (100%)
HBV	36 (19%)	6 (7%)	28 (31%)	14 (25%)
HCV	116 (61%)	61 (71%)	30 (33%)	26 (47%)
HBV and HCV	1 (1%)	1 (1%)	0 (0%)	0 (0%)
Alcoholic hepatitis	21 (11%)	2 (2%)	4 (5%)	3 (5%)
NAFLD	0 (0%)	0 (0%)	21 (23%)	8 (14%)
NASH	3 (2%)	5 (6%)	6 (7%)	4 (7%)
Cryptogenic or other	12 (6%)	11 (13%)	1 (1%)	1 (2%)

The percentage shows the proportion in total number of each gender with or without HCC.

Table 3. Clinical features of patients analyzed for AIM.

	HCC		Non HCC	
	Men	**Women**	**Men**	**Women**
Age (year)	66±10 [32–87]	70±9 [33–87]	55±15 [23–84]	62±13 [31–80]
AIM (μg/ml)	5.7±2.8 [1.7–18.6]	5.8±2.6 [0.8–14.7]	5.1±2.7 [1.5–17.5]	5.8±2.9 [1.8–16.9]
IgM (mg/dl)	144.8±101 [24.2–708.0]	143.4±98.0 [1.6–769.2]	103.3±49.4 [18.7–216.4]	129.4±64.1 [42.8–346.0]
AST (U/L)	56.3±30.7 [14–170]	59.6±42.9 [17–312]	51.8±43.3 [13–287]	44.7±24.5 [14–139]
ALT (U/L)	53.6±37.6 [8–233]	48.0±39.5 [9–315]	60.3±66.8 [6–498]	40.4±26.6 [11–121]
TB (mg/dl)	0.98±0.54 [0.3–3.9]	1.02±0.61 [0.4–3.8]	1.13±0.85 [0.3–5.1]	1.07±1.17 [0.4–9.2]
DB (mg/dl)	0.35±0.32 [0.1–0.7]	0.38±0.32 [0.1–1.6]	0.29±0.28 [0.1–1.6]	0.25±0.13 [0.1–0.5]
ALB (g/dl)	3.69±0.46 [2.3–4.7]	3.64±0.49 [2.2–4.6]	4.06±0.49 [2.5–5.2]	3.89±0.58 [2.2–4.5]
PLT (x10⁴/mm³)	12.3±5.29 [3.0–28.3]	11.1±5.43 [4.2–31.9]	16.6±7.32 [2.1–35.6]	13.9±6.57 [2.3–26]
PT (%)	85.4±14.3 [53–100]	84.3±14.7 [42–100]	87.1±17.2 [28–100]	84.0±19.7 [32–100]
Cre (mg/dl)	0.81±0.19 [0.40–1.56]	0.61±0.14 [0.4–1.04]	0.83±0.20 [0.54–1.95]	0.66±0.26 [0.49–2.21]
ICG (%)	23.8±14.4 [2.7–72.4]	24.7±15.6 [0.9–71.2]	-	-

The mean ± SD as well as the range of diversity are presented for each parametric variable. The ICG score was only available in HCC patients.

waist circumference (Fig. 1D). In line with these results, AIM levels also correlated negatively with low-density lipoprotein (LDL) cholesterol levels (Fig. 1D) and several diabetic markers including fasting blood sugar (FBS) and glycated hemoglobin (HbA1C) (Fig. 1D), as well as with blood pressure, in women (Fig. 1D). Thus, consistent with the findings of our previous study in mice [29,30], AIM levels correlated negatively with multiple parameters related to obesity, and these correlations were more prominent in women. Intriguingly however, a weak but significant positive correlation was found between AIM levels and biomarkers of hepatocyte injury, including aspartate aminotransferase (AST) and alanine aminotransferase (ALT), particularly in men (Fig. 1E). Taken together, it is likely that AIM levels increase along with the progression of liver injury. In both men and women, a significant negative correlation was unexpectedly found between AIM levels and red blood cell numbers, but the reason underlying this correlation is unclear (Table S1).

AIM levels correlated strongly with liver function in liver injury

We next analyzed blood samples from patients with chronic hepatitis and liver cirrhosis. As depicted in Table 2, the cause of liver injury in the majority of the patients was hepatitis virus infection, whereas non-infected cases constituted a lower proportion of the patients with alcoholic liver failure and NAFLD/NASH. Patients with or without HCC were investigated. The clinical features of the patients tested are presented in Table 3 focusing on the liver function.

The positive correlation between AIM levels and AST/ALT for liver injury, which was already seen in individuals without severe liver damage (Fig. 1E) was notably more obvious in men and women with advanced liver damage. Highly significant correlations were observed between AIM and multiple biomarkers, thereby reflecting liver function, including total or direct bilirubin (TB or DB), albumin (ALB), platelet count (PLT), % prothrombin time (%PT), and the indocyanine green (ICG) test (Fig. 2). These correlations were obvious in individuals with or without hepatitis virus infection (Table S2) and in the presence or absence of HCC (Fig. 2). In HCC patients, there was no significant correlation in levels of AIM and several HCC markers including alpha

fetoprotein (AFP), des-gamma-carboxyprothrombin (DCP, also called prothrombin induced by vitamin K-absence II; PIVKA-II), and AFP fraction L3 (L3) (Fig. S1). As in healthy individuals, a significant correlation was also found between AIM and IgM levels in patients with liver injury (Fig. 3A); namely, IgM levels increased with the progression of liver damage (Fig. S2).

We then addressed which parameters correlated independently with AIM levels. To this end, we performed multiple regression analysis by the backward stepwise method including AIM. Table S3 shows the correlation coefficients between all parameters that reflect liver function and thus were candidates for determinant of AIM level. When confounding factors were eliminated, IgM, TB, ALB, and %PT in men ($R^2 = 54.0\%$) and IgM, TB, and ALB in women ($R^2 = 57.0\%$) were independent determinants of AIM in HCC patients (Table 4). In non-HCC patients, IgM, ALB, and PLT in men ($R^2 = 63.4\%$) and IgM and PLT in women ($R^2 = 53.6\%$) were the independent determinants of AIM (Table 4). In particular, in men, the t-value of TB in HCC patients was 5.39, but was not significant in non-HCC patients. In women, the t-value of ALB was −4.80 in HCC patients, but again was not significant in non-HCC patients (Table 4).

Similar results were obtained for the relationship between AIM and the grade of liver inflammation or fibrosis. Levels in inflammation (0–3) and fibrosis (F0-F4) were evaluated according to the Inuyama classification [32]. The number of patients in each category is presented in Table 5. Clinical information about inflammation and fibrosis were not available in a part of HCC patients and all of non-HCC patients. AIM levels were higher in those with liver inflammation (Fig. 3B). AIM also increased in line with the progression of liver fibrosis (Fig. 3C). Similarly, AIM levels were higher in patients with cirrhosis or ascites (Fig. 3D). Note that all cirrhotic patients tested in this study were under a compensated stage. Since some patients exhibited prominently high or low levels of AIM (>10 μg/ml or <3.0 μg/ml), we assessed relationship in levels of AIM and various parameters in these populations. However, there was no remarkable correlation in AIM and any parameter (Table S4). No significant correlation was observed between AIM levels and alcohol intake (data not shown).

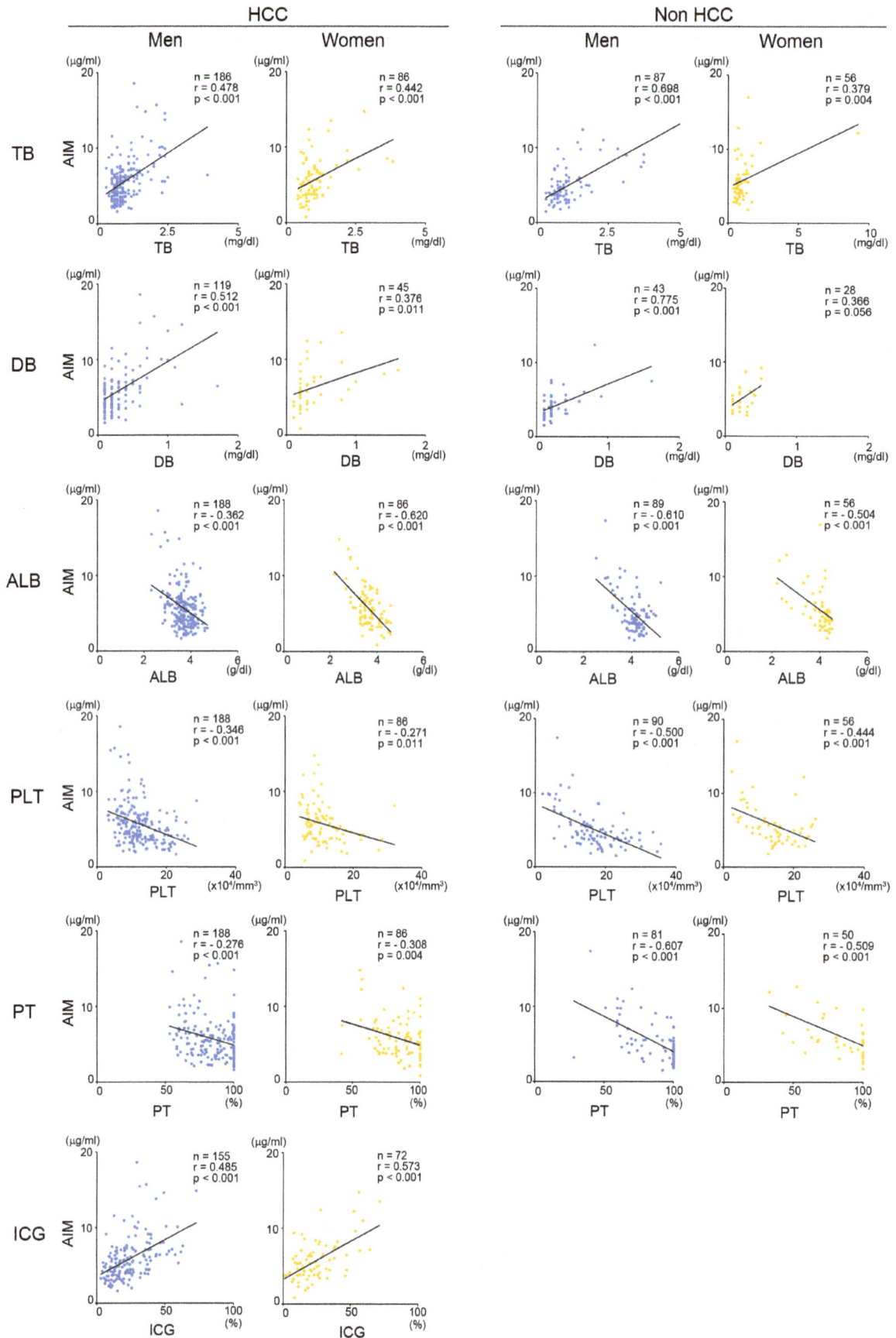

Figure 2. Correlation in the AIM level and the liver function under liver injury. Correlation in AIM levels and various biomarkers representing liver function in men (blue) and women (yellow), with or without HCC. ICG score was only available in HCC patients.

$AIM^{-/-}$ mice had comparable liver damage to wild-type mice in response to CCl4

Next, we assessed whether high AIM levels directly promote liver injury or whether AIM levels increase as a result of liver damage progression. To this end, we employed animal models of progressive liver injury induced by carbon tetrachloride. $AIM^{-/-}$ and $AIM^{+/+}$ mice were challenged with CCl4 (1.6 g/kg body weight) injected twice a week for 12 weeks, and the state of liver injury was assessed. As demonstrated in Fig. 4A, AST and ALT levels were similar at multiple time points in $AIM^{+/+}$ and $AIM^{-/-}$ mice, indicating that the liver was comparably damaged in the presence or absence of AIM. Note that the average of circulating AIM levels without CCl4 administration was 3.3 μg/ml in both males and females. Inflammatory states were investigated during the early phase (after 3 weeks of CCl4 challenge) by measuring mRNA levels for various pro-inflammatory cytokines using quantitative RT-PCR (QPCR). No significant differences were observed in the increased expression levels of *TNFα*, *IL-1β*, *IL-6*, and *MCP-1* in both types of mice (Fig. 4B). In line with this result, similar expression profiles of the M1 and M2 macrophage marker genes (*CD11c* for M1; *CD163*, *Arg-1*, and *mannose receptor (MR)* for M2) were observed in $AIM^{+/+}$ and $AIM^{-/-}$ mice (Fig. 4C), suggesting that the absence of AIM did not influence the activation state or the M1/M2 polarity of liver macrophages in response to carbon tetrachloride, resulting in comparable liver inflammation progression in both types of mice. Consistent with this finding, liver fibrosis progressed comparably in $AIM^{-/-}$ and $AIM^{+/+}$ mice, and Sirius-red staining of liver specimens showed a similar increase in fibrotic areas in both types of mice (Fig. 4D). Accordingly,

mRNA levels of various markers of fibrosis progression such as *TGFβ*, *αSMA*, *Col4a1*, and *connective tissue growth factor (CTGF)* were also comparable in $AIM^{-/-}$ and $AIM^{+/+}$ mice (Fig. 4E). Taken together, these results clearly indicate that the presence or absence of AIM did not influence the state of liver injury in response to carbon tetrachloride. Thus, it is likely that the augmented AIM levels observed in humans (Fig. 2) were the result of liver damage. Further supporting this notion is the finding that AIM levels increased markedly with progression of liver damage in $AIM^{+/+}$ mice (Fig. 4F, left). However, AIM mRNA levels in the $AIM^{+/+}$ liver did not increase in response to CCl4 (Fig. S3), suggesting that the increase in blood AIM was not brought about by enhancement of AIM production in liver Kupffer macrophages, one of the highest AIM-producing cell types [19].

Interestingly, no significant difference in increase in IgM levels was observed in both $AIM^{-/-}$ and $AIM^{+/+}$ mice, suggesting that the increase in IgM was independent of AIM (Fig. 4F, right). This result is reminiscent of our previous finding of a similar increase in IgM levels in $AIM^{-/-}$ and $AIM^{+/+}$ mice in response to a HFD [23].

Diagnostic application of AIM for HCC

As demonstrated in Fig. 2, AIM levels increased in line with the progression of liver injury in patients with or without HCC. We then wondered whether HCC and non-HCC patients who show an equivalent score of certain liver biomarkers exhibited different AIM levels. Therefore, we normalized the level of AIM (AIM index) to that of each biomarker. The AIM level was divided by a biomarker score when both correlated positively (*e.g.* AST, ALT, TB, and DB), whereas the scores were multiplied when AIM and

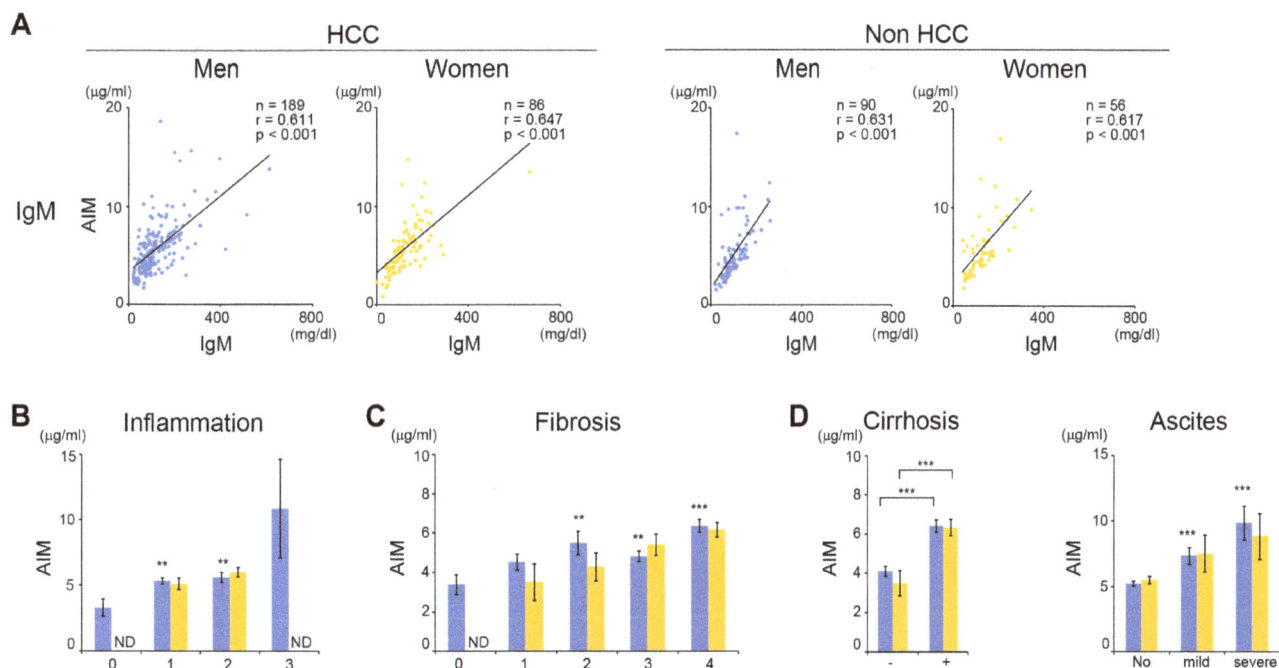

Figure 3. The AIM level increases with progression of liver inflammation and fibrosis. (A) Correlation in AIM and IgM levels in men (blue) and women (yellow), with or without HCC. (B) AIM levels in HCC patients with different inflammatory levels according to the Inuyama classification. (C) AIM levels in HCC patients with different fibrotic scores according to the Inuyama classification. (D) AIM levels in HCC patients with different grades of cirrhosis or ascites. In C-E, AIM levels are presented as means±SEM (μg/ml).

Table 4. Multiple linear regression analysis.

	HCC Men (n = 173)			Non-HCC Men (n = 89)		
	C	t	p	C	t	p
R^2	53.98%			63.44%		
Intercept	5.30	2.927	0.004	10.2	6.29	<0.001
IgM	0.0137	9.37	<0.001	0.0266	7.33	<0.001
TB	1.60	5.39	<0.001	–	–	–
ALB	−0.886	−2.53	0.012	−1.41	−3.59	<0.001
PLT	–	–	–	−0.127	−4.88	<0.001
PT	−0.0191	−1.77	0.079	–	–	–
	HCC Women (n = 86)			Non-HCC Women (n = 56)		
	C	t	p	C	t	p
R^2	57.02%			53.62%		
Intercept	9.58	4.82	<0.001	4.88	5.90	<0.001
IgM	0.0104	4.66	<0.001	0.0265	6.48	<0.001
TB	0.862	2.48	0.016	–	–	–
ALB	−2.17	−4.80	<0.001	–	–	–
PLT	–	–	–	−0.181	−4.53	<0.001

Independent determinants for AIM in men or women with or without HCC. R^2: determination coefficient, C: regression coefficient, t: t-value, p: p-value, in multiple linear regression models. _: not independent.

the biomarker correlated negatively (*e.g.* ALB, platelets, and %PT). As depicted in Fig. 5A, the ratio of the AIM-TB index to the AIM-ALB index in men was significantly higher in HCC patients than in non-HCC patients by analysis of covariance (ANCOVA), but no significant differences were observed for the ratio of the TB score to the ALB score between HCC and non-HCC patients. Similar results were obtained for the ratio of the AIM-TB index to the AIM-PLT or AIM-AST index, although TB

Table 5. Number of patients showing different levels of inflammation, fibrosis, cirrhosis, or ascites.

		Men	Women
Whole		189	86
Inflammation (in %)	0	6 (3%)	0 (0%)
	1	88 (47%)	36 (42%)
	2	50 (26%)	28 (32%)
	3	2 (1%)	0 (0%)
	unknown	43 (23%)	22 (26%)
Fibrosis (in %)	0	7 (4%)	0 (0%)
	1	14 (7%)	3 (3%)
	2	19 (10%)	13 (15%)
	3	42 (22%)	11(13%)
	4	81 (43%)	42 (49%)
	unknown	26 (14%)	17 (20%)
Cirrhosis (in %)	-	36 (19%)	6 (7%)
	+	82 (43%)	45 (52%)
	unknown	71 (38%)	35 (41%)
Ascites (in %)	No	159 (84%)	77 (90%)
	Mild (1~2L)	18 (10%)	5 (6%)
	Severe (3~5L)	10 (5%)	4 (4%)
	unknown	2 (1%)	0 (0%)

All patients here possessed HCC. The percentage shows the proportion in each level of identical phenotype. Unknown: Information was not available.

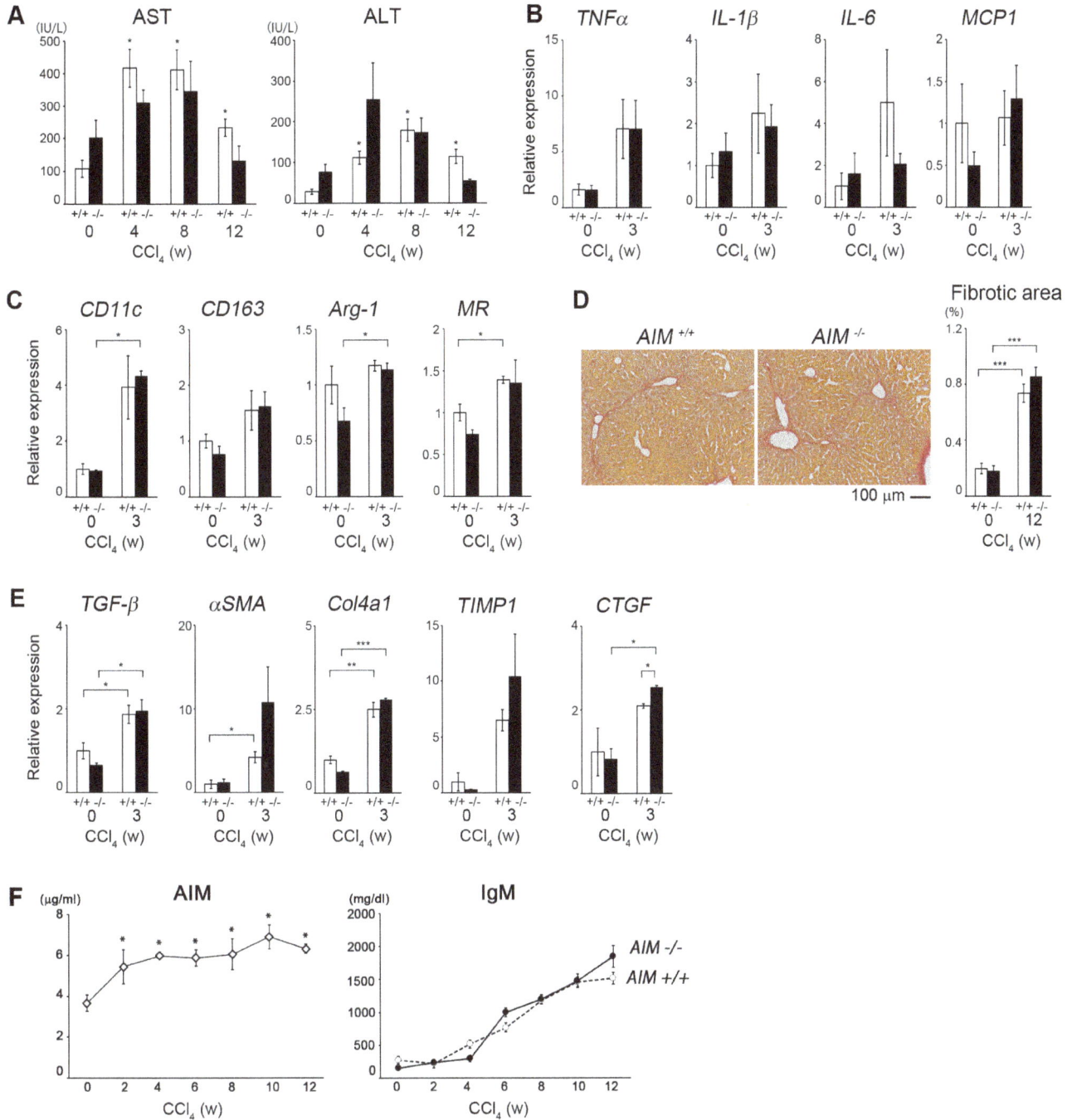

Figure 4. *AIM*[+/+] **and** *AIM*[-/-] **mice exhibit comparable liver damage in response to CCl₄.** (A) AST and ALT at 0, 4, 8, 12 wk after administration of CCl₄ (1.6 g/kg body weight, twice injection per week for 12 weeks) in *AIM*[+/+] mice (+/+) and *AIM*[-/-] mice (−/−). n = 3 for each. Error bar: SEM, *: p< 0.05 vs. before CCl4 administration (0 w). (B, C) mRNA levels of *TNFα, IL-1β, IL-6* and *MCP-1* (B); or *CD11c, CD163, Arg-1* and *MR* (C) were assessed by QPCR using RNA isolated from liver after administration of CCl₄ for 3 weeks. n = 3 for each. Error bar: SEM, *: p<0.05. (D) Sirius-red staining of the liver specimens after administration of CCl₄ for 12 weeks to *AIM*[+/+] mice (+/+) and *AIM*[-/-] mice (−/−). Bar: 100 μm. Right graph shows the quantification of fibrotic area. (E) mRNA levels of *TGFβ, αSMA, Col4a1* and *CTGF* were assessed by QPCR using RNA isolated from liver from mice after administration of CCl₄ for 3 weeks. n = 3 for each. Error bar: SEM; *: p<0.05, ***: p<0.001. (F) *Left*: Serum AIM levels were measured by ELISA from wild-type mice after administration of CCl₄. n = 6 for each. Error bar: SEM, *: p<0.05 vs. before CCl₄ administration (0 w). *Right*: Serum IgM levels were measured by semi-quantitative immunoblotting using sera from *AIM*[+/+] (+/+) mice and *AIM*[-/-] (−/−) after administration of CCl₄. Purified mouse IgM clone (3F3) was used as standard. Quantification of signals from immunoblotting was performed by using ImageQuant TL software (GE Healthcare, Little Chalfont, UK). n = 6 for each. Error bar: SEM; *: p<0.05, ***: p<0.01, vs. before CCl₄ administration (0 w) in *AIM*[+/+] (+/+) mice; ###: p<0.001 vs. before CCl₄ administration in *AIM*[-/-] mice.

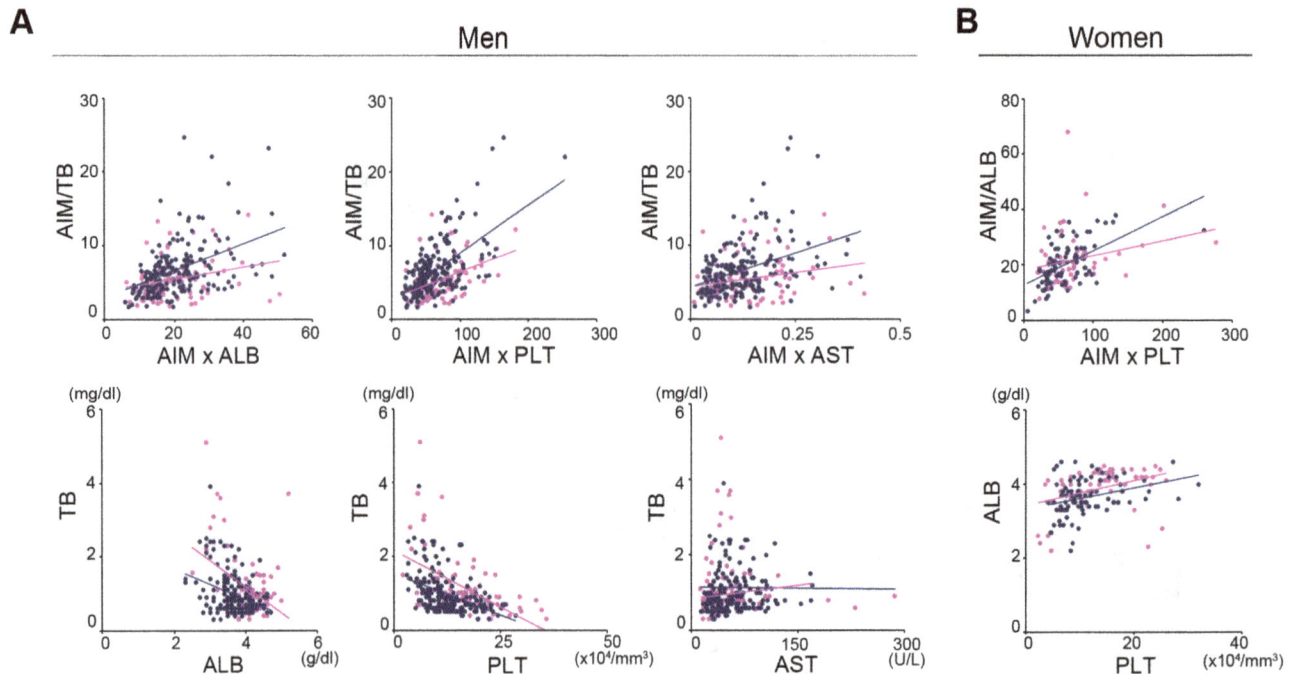

Figure 5. AIM-index distinguishes HCC and non-HCC patients. (A) AIM-TB index vs. AIM-ALB index, AIM-PLT index or AIM-AST index in men with or without HCC. TB vs. ALB, PLT or AST are also presented. (B) AIM-ALB index vs. AIM-%PT index in women with or without HCC. ALB vs. %PT is also presented. r: correlation coefficients; p: p value determined by ANCOVA. Blue dots and bars: HCC patients, red dots and bars: non-HCC patients.

correlated with neither PLT nor AST (Fig. 5A). In women, a comparison of the AIM-ALB and AIM-%PT indexes revealed similar differences between the HCC and non-HCC patients (Fig. 5B). Note that TB in male HCC patients and ALB in female HCC patients produced high t-values in multiple regression analysis when assessing the determinants of AIM (Table 3).

Discussion

This study provides the first large-scale description of the circulating AIM levels in the general population and in the context of liver function parameters in humans. A variety of new findings were obtained as follows. Firstly, relatively higher AIM levels were observed in the younger generation, especially in women, suggesting potential involvement of estrogen in the increase in circulating AIM levels. Accumulating evidence of estrogen-associated physiology including suppression of triacylglycerol (TG) storage in fat and liver tissues [33–36], reduction of expression and enzymatic activity of FASN [37], and preventive effect for foam cell formation and the development of atherosclerosis [38–41], which are all reminiscent of AIM function [20,29,30,42,43]. Although *AIM* mRNA is expressed under transcriptional regulation by LXR [20–22], the impact of estrogen on LXR activation is controversial. For instance, Wang et al. recently reported that E2 activates LXRα [41], whereas suppression of LXRα by E2 was also reported in hepatocytes [34], adipocyte [36], and pancreatic β cells [37]. Alternatively, evidence has shown that estrogen stimulates natural IgM production through B lymphocyte activation [44,45]. This effect certainly increases AIM levels based on the strong correlation between AIM and IgM. However, further studies are required to clarify the precise involvement of estrogen in the regulation of age-dependent AIM levels in humans. It is noteworthy that in individuals without advanced liver damage, AST and ALT showed a weak positive

correlation with AIM levels only in men (Fig. 1E and Table S1). It might be possible that the sex-dependent difference of AIM levels obscured the correlation in women.

Secondly, patients with advanced liver damage exhibited high AIM levels. We postulate that the mean±SD AIM level (μg/ml) in each generation in men and women presented in Table 1 can be defined as the "normal range" of AIM levels. Certainly, however, whether AIM levels that are higher or lower than this range mean pathological may depend on the type of disease. At least, patients with progressive liver damage exhibited significantly higher levels than the normal range. Based on the results of mouse experiments demonstrating that the presence or absence of AIM does not influence the state of liver injury in response to CCl4, and that AIM levels increase in response to CCl4 in wild-type mice, it is likely that AIM levels increase as a result of liver damage. Thus, AIM can be used as a novel biomarker for liver injury. The mRNA level of liver *AIM* did not increase in response to CCl4, indicating no enhanced AIM production by liver Kupffer macrophages. It remains possible, however, that inflammatory stimuli caused by carbon tetrachloride will increase *AIM* expression in macrophages in other tissues such as in the peritoneal cavity and splenic marginal zone, but additional experiments are required to assess this possibility. Alternatively, liver damage might increase AIM stability in the blood. Natural IgM is catabolized mainly in the liver [46–48]. Therefore, it is possible that the progression of liver damage prolongs the half-life of IgM, resulting in advanced accumulation of circulating AIM. This scenario can also be applied in humans, and may explain the more profound increase in AIM levels in cirrhotic patients compared with non-cirrhotic patients. A precise assessment of the half-life of IgM and AIM in the presence or absence of liver injury can evaluate this possibility.

More notably, we found that use of the AIM index, which is the blood AIM level normalized to the liver biomarker score, appeared to be useful for distinguishing HCC and non-HCC patients. The AIM-TB index of men with an equivalent AIM-ALB or AIM-PLT index was significantly higher in HCC patients than in non-HCC patients. This is not secondary effect of the correlation in TB and ALB or PLT, as there was no significance in the difference in these correlations in HCC and non-HCC groups. The same conclusion was obtained for the AIM-ALB and AIM-platelets indexes in women. Thus, the presence of HCC may increase the AIM-TB index in men and the AIM-ALB index in women. If this is the case, the AIM index can serve as a novel tumor marker and will be useful for the diagnosis of HCC. Further analysis using HCC-bearing mouse models in the presence or absence of AIM may be appropriate for evaluating this possibility. Alternatively, one could also speculate that individuals who show an enhanced increase in certain AIM indexes (*i.e.* AIM-TB index in men and AIM-ALB index in women) in response to liver injury might be more susceptible to HCC. However, further study such as prospective cohort study of HCC development in patients with similar levels of liver damage and different levels of circulating AIM is certainly needed to assess this possibility. In either case, further investigation will corroborate the applicability of the AIM index for the early detection of HCC.

Since HCC is one of the most common malignant tumors with an increasing incidence, identifying serological biomarkers are extremely needed, especially because most of HCC cases are diagnosed at a late stage. Thus, our study could be the bases of application of circulating AIM level as a diagnostic and/or prognostic marker of HCC, either solo or in combination with other biomarkers.

Supporting Information

Figure S1 Correlation between AIM levels and various HCC markers. Men: blue dots, women: yellow dots. In HCC patients, no significant correlation was observed in levels of AIM and either HCC marker.

Figure S2 Correlation between IgM levels and various biomarkers representing liver function. Men: blue dots, women: yellow dots. ICG score was only available in HCC patients.

Figure S3 *AIM* expression did not increase in the liver in response to CCl$_4$. mRNA levels of *AIM* in the liver from wild-type mice after administration of CCl$_4$ for 3 wk. n = 3 for each. Error bar: SEM.

Table S1 Correlation in AIM level and different clinical parameters. Number of samples, and the correlation coefficients and p values in the correlation with AIM levels in separate tested item. n: sample numbers.

Table S2 Correlation between AIM and liver function in patients with or without hepatitis viral infection. Number of samples, and the correlation coefficients and p values in the correlation with AIM levels in the indicated tested item, in patients with or without hepatitis viral infection. n: sample number.

Table S3 Correlation coefficients between all variables that are candidates for determinant of AIM. C: single regression coefficient, *p*: p-value. Cre: creatinine.

Table S4 AIM and various clinical markers in populations who exhibit very high or very low AIM levels. Number of samples (n), and the correlation coefficients and p values in the correlation with AIM levels in identical parameter. Low: patients who exhibited less than 3.0 μg/ml of AIM, High: patients who exhibited more than 10.0 μg/ml of AIM.

Acknowledgments

We particularly thank the staffs in the Center of Health Evaluation and Promotion, Inoue Hospital (Nagasaki) for preparation of a large number of blood samples. We also appreciate S. Jibiki, W. Murasawa and M. Shinohara for technical assistance.

Author Contributions

Conceived and designed the experiments: SA TM. Performed the experiments: TY M. Mori SA AN KA. Analyzed the data: TY TK M. Mori. Contributed reagents/materials/analysis tools: RT MA MB M. Maeda TA K. Izumino JT SH TT TG SO SS YY YH KK KIY K. Inoue. Wrote the paper: TM.

References

1. Jemal A, Bray F, Center MM, Ferlay J, Ward E, et al. (2011) Global cancer statistics. CA Cancer J Clin 61: 69–90.
2. Bosch FX, Ribes J, Cleries R, Diaz M (2005) Epidemiology of hepatocellular carcinoma. Clin Liver Dis 9: 191–211.
3. El-Serag HB, Rudolph KL (2007) Hepatocellular carcinoma: epidemiology and molecular carcinogenesis. Gastroenterology 132: 2557–2576.
4. Baffy G, Brunt EM, Caldwell SH (2012) Hepatocellular carcinoma in non-alcoholic fatty liver disease: an emerging menace. J Hepatol 56: 1384–91.
5. Angulo P (2002) Nonalcoholic fatty liver disease. N Engl J Med 346: 1221–1231.
6. Hytiroglou P, Park YN, Krinsky G, Theise ND (2007) Hepatic precancerous lesions and small hepatocellular carcinoma. Gastroenterol Clin North Am 36: 867–887, vii.
7. He G, Karin M (2011) NF-κB and STAT3 - key players in liver inflammation and cancer. Cell Res 21: 159–168.
8. Park EJ, Lee JH, Yu GY, He G, Ali SR, et al. (2010) Dietary and genetic obesity promote liver inflammation and tumorigenesis by enhancing IL-6 and TNF expression. Cell 140: 197–208.
9. Powell EE, Cooksley WG, Hanson R, Searle J, Halliday JW, et al. (1990) The natural history of nonalcoholic steatohepatitis: a follow-up study of forty-two patients for up to 21 years. Hepatology 11: 74–80.
10. Day CP, Saksena S (2002) Non-alcoholic steatohepatitis: definitions and pathogenesis. J Gastroenterol Hepatol 17: S377–S384.
11. Harrison SA, Torgerson S, Hayashi PH (2003) The natural history of nonalcoholic fatty liver disease: a clinical histopathological study. Am J Gastroenterol 98: 2042–2047.
12. Torres DM, Harrison SA (2012) Nonalcoholic steatohepatitis and noncirrhotic hepatocellular carcinoma: fertile soil. Semin Liver Dis 32: 30–38.
13. Starley BQ, Calcagno CJ, Harrison SA (2010) Nonalcoholic fatty liver disease and hepatocellular carcinoma: a weighty connection. Hepatology 51: 1820–1832.
14. Kawada N, Imanaka K, Kawaguchi T, Tamai C, Ishihara R, et al. (2009) Hepatocellular carcinoma arising from non-cirrhotic nonalcoholic steatohepatitis. J Gastroenterol 44: 1190–1194.
15. Chagas AL, Kikuchi LO, Oliveira CP, Vezozzo DC, Mello ES, et al. (2009) Does hepatocellular carcinoma in non-alcoholic steatohepatitis exist in cirrhotic and non-cirrhotic patients? Braz J Med Biol Res 42: 958–962.
16. Ertle J, Dechêne A, Sowa JP, Penndorf V, Herzer K, et al. (2011) Non-alcoholic fatty liver disease progresses to hepatocellular carcinoma in the absence of apparent cirrhosis. Int J Cancer 128: 2436–2443.
17. Paradis V, Zalinski S, Chelbi E, Guedj N, Degos F, et al. (2009) Hepatocellular carcinomas in patients with metabolic syndrome often develop without significant liver fibrosis: a pathological analysis. Hepatology 49: 851–859.
18. Takuma Y, Nouso K (2010) Nonalcoholic steatohepatitis-associated hepatocellular carcinoma: our case series and literature review. World J Gastroenterol 16: 1436–1441.
19. Miyazaki T, Hirokami Y, Matsuhashi N, Takatsuka H, Naito M (1999) Increased susceptibility of thymocytes to apoptosis in mice lacking AIM, a novel

murine macrophage-derived soluble factor belonging to the scavenger receptor cysteine-rich domain superfamily. J Exp Med 189: 413–422.

20. Arai S, Shelton JM, Chen M, Bradley MN, Castrillo A, et al. (2005) A role of the apoptosis inhibitory factor AIM/Spα/Api6 in atherosclerosis development. Cell Metab 1: 201–213.

21. Joseph SB, Bradley MN, Castrillo A, Bruhn KW, Mak PA, et al. (2004) LXR-dependent gene expression is important for macrophage survival and the innate immune response. Cell 119: 299–309.

22. Valledor AF, Hsu LC, Ogawa S, Sawka-Verhelle D, Karin M, et al. (2004) Activation of liver X receptors and retinoid X receptors prevents bacterial-induced macrophage apoptosis. Proc Natl Acad Sci USA 101: 17813–17818.

23. Arai S, Maehara N, Iwamura Y, Honda S, Nakashima K, et al. (2013) Obesity-associated autoantibody production requires AIM to retain IgM immune complex on follicular dendritic cells. Cell Rep 3: 1187–1198.

24. Tissot JD, Sanchez JC, Vuadens F, Scherl A, Schifferli JA, et al. (2002) IgM are associated to Sp alpha (CD5 antigen-like). Electrophoresis 23: 1203–1206.

25. Gangadharan B, Antrobus R, Dwek RA, Zitzmann N (2007) Novel serum biomarker candidates for liver fibrosis in hepatitis C patients. Clin Chem 53: 1792–1799.

26. Gray J, Chattopadhyay D, Beale GS, Patman GL, Miele L, et al. (2009) A proteomic strategy to identify novel serum biomarkers for liver cirrhosis and hepatocellular cancer in individuals with fatty liver disease. BMC Cancer 9: 271.

27. Kim WK, Hwang HR, Kim do H, Lee PY, In YJ, et al. (2008) Glycoproteomic analysis of plasma from patients with atopic dermatitis: CD5L and ApoE as potential biomarkers. Exp Mol Med 40: 677–685.

28. Mera K, Uto H, Mawatari S, Ido A, Yoshimine Y, et al. (2014) Serum levels of apoptosis inhibitor of macrophage are associated with hepatic fibrosis in patients with chronic hepatitis C. BMC Gastroenterol 13: 14–27.

29. Kurokawa J, Arai S, Nakashima K, Nishijima A, Miyake K, et al. (2010) AIM is endocytosed into adipocytes and decreases lipid droplets via inhibition of fatty acid synthase activity. Cell Metab 11: 479–492.

30. Iwamura Y, Mori M, Nakashima K, Mikami T, Murayama K, et al. (2012) Apoptosis inhibitor of macrophage (AIM) diminishes lipid droplet-coating proteins leading to lipolysis in adipocytes. Biochem Biophys Res Commun 422: 476–481.

31. Arai S, Miyazaki T (2014) Impacts of the apoptosis inhibitor of macrophage (AIM) on obesity-associated inflammatory diseases. Semin Immunopathol 36: 3–12.

32. Ichida F, Tsuji T, Omata M, Ichida T, Inoue K, et al. (1996) New Inuyama classification; new criteria for histological assessment of chronic hepatitis. Int hepatol commun 6: 112–119.

33. Bryzgalova G, Lundholm L, Portwood N, Gustafsson J-Å, Khan A, et al. (2008) Mechanisms of antidiabetogenic and body weight-lowering effects of estrogen in high-fat diet-fed mice. Am J Physiol Endocrinol Metab 295: E904–E912.

34. Gao H, Bryzgalova G, Hedman E, Khan A, Efendic S, et al. (2006) Long-term administration of estradiol decreases expression of hepatic lipogenic genes and improves insulin sensitivity in ob/ob mice: a possible mechanism is through direct regulation of signal transducer and activator of transcription 3. Mol Endocrinol 20: 1287–1299.

35. Han SI, Komatsu Y, Murayama A, Steffensen KR, Nakagawa Y, et al. (2014) Estrogen receptor ligands ameliorate fatty liver through a nonclassical estrogen receptor/Liver X receptor pathway in mice. Hepatology 59: 1791–1802.

36. Lundholm L, Movérare S, Steffensen KR, Nilsson M, Otsuki M, et al. (2004) Gene expression profiling identifies liver X receptor alpha as an estrogen-regulated gene in mouse adipose tissue. J Mol Endocrinol 32: 879–892.

37. Tiano JP, Mauvais-Jarvis F (2012) Molecular mechanisms of estrogen receptors' suppression of lipogenesis in pancreatic β-cells. Endocrinology 153: 2997–3005.

38. Hage FG, Oparil S (2013) Ovarian hormones and vascular disease. Curr Opin Cardiol 28: 411–416.

39. Grodstein F, Manson JE, Colditz GA, Willett WC, Speizer FE, et al. (2000) A prospective, observational study of postmenopausal hormone therapy and primary prevention of cardiovascular disease. Ann Intern Med 133: 933–941.

40. Grady D, Herrington D, Bittner V, Blumenthal R, Davidson M, et al. (2002) Cardiovascular disease outcomes during 6.8 years of hormone therapy: Heart and Estrogen/progestin Replacement Study follow-up (HERS II). JAMA 288: 49–57.

41. Wang H, Liu Y, Zhu L, Wang W, Wan Z, et al. (2014) 17β-estradiol promotes cholesterol efflux from vascular smooth muscle cells through a liver X receptor α-dependent pathway. Int J Mol Med 33: 550–558.

42. Hamada M, Nakamura M, Tran MT, Moriguchi T, Hong C, et al. (2014) MafB promotes atherosclerosis by inhibiting foam-cell apoptosis. Nat Commun 5: 3147.

43. Miyazaki T, Kurokawa J, Arai S (2011) AIMing at Metabolic Syndrome: Towards the development of novel therapies for metabolic diseases via apoptosis inhibitor of macrophage (AIM). Cir J 75: 2522–2531.

44. Xu Y, Fan H, Li X, Sun L, Hou Y (2012) 17β-Estradiol enhances response of mice spleen B cells elicited by TLR9 agonist. Cell Immunol 278: 125–135.

45. Li X, Xu Y, Ma L, Sun L, Fu G, et al. (2009) 17beta-estradiol enhances the response of plasmacytoid dendritic cell to CpG. PLoS One 4: e8412.

46. Bazin H, Malet F (1969) The metabolism of different immunoglobulin classes in irradiated mice. Immunology 17: 345–365.

47. Vieira P, Rajewsky K (1988) The half-lives of serum immunoglobulins in adult mice. Eur J Immunol 18: 313–316.

48. Kai T, Yamazaki T, Arai S, Miyazaki T (2014) Stabilization and augmentation of circulating AIM in mice by synthesized IgM-Fc. PLoS One 9: e97037.

3

Functional Short Tandem Repeat Polymorphism of PTPN11 and Susceptibility to Hepatocellular Carcinoma in Chinese Populations

Xiankun Zhao[1], Shuxiang Hu[1], Lu Wang[1], Qing Zhang[1], Xiaodan Zhu[1], Hua Zhao[2], Chaoqun Wang[1], Ruiyang Tao[1], Siping Guo[1], Jing Wang[1], Jiejie Xu[3], Yan He[4]*, Yuzhen Gao[1]*

1 Department of Forensic Medicine, Medical College of Soochow University, Suzhou, Jiangsu, P.R. China, 2 Department of General Surgery, the First Affiliated Hospital of Soochow University, Suzhou, Jiangsu, P.R. China, 3 Key Laboratory of Medical Molecular Virology, MOE & MOH, School of Basic Medical Sciences, Shanghai Medical College, Fudan University, Shanghai, China, 4 Department of Epidemiology, Medical College of Soochow University, Suzhou, Jiangsu, P. R. China

Abstract

Background: *PTPN11*, which encodes tyrosine phosphatase Shp2, is a critical gene mediating cellular responses to hormones and cytokines. Loss of Shp2 promotes hepatocellular carcinoma (HCC), suggesting that PTPN11 functions as a tumor suppressor in HCC tumorgenesis. The aim of this study was to evaluate the effects of the short tandem repeat (STR) polymorphism (rs199618935) within 3'UTR of *PTPN11* on HCC susceptibility in Chinese populations.

Methodology/Principal Findings: We analyzed the associations in 400 patients from Jiangsu province of China, validating the findings in an additional 305 patients from Shanghai of China. Unconditional logistic regression was used to analyze the association between rs199618935 and HCC risk. Additional biochemical investigations and *in-silico* studies were used to evaluate the possible functional significance of this polymorphism. Logistic regression analysis showed that compared with individuals carrying shorter alleles (11 and 12 repeats), those subjects who carry longer alleles (13 and 14 repeats) had a significantly decreased risk of HCC [adjusted odds ratio (OR) $= 0.63$, 95% confidence interval (CI) $= 0.53$–0.76, $P = 2.00 \times 10^{-7}$], with the risk decreased even further in those carrying allele 15 and 16 (adjusted OR $= 0.46$, 95% CI $= 0.34$–0.62, $P = 1.00 \times 10^{-7}$). Biochemical investigations showed that longer alleles of rs199618935 conferred higher PTPN11 expression *in vivo* and *in vitro*. The altered luciferase activities in reporter gene system suggested that STR regulation of PTPN11 expression could be a transcriptional event. Finally, *in-silico* prediction revealed that different alleles of rs199618935 could alter the local structure of PTPN11 mRNA.

Conclusions/Significance: Taken together, our findings suggested that the STR polymorphism within *PTPN11* contributes to hepatocarcinogenesis, possibly by affecting PTPN11 expression through a structure-dependent mechanism. The replication of our studies and further functional studies are needed to validate our findings.

Editor: Xin-Yuan Guan, The University of Hong Kong, China

Funding: This study is supported by grants from National Natural Science Foundation of China (No. 81171893 and No. 81201574), Priority Academic Program Development of Jiangsu Higher Education Institutions as well as Hui-Chun Chin and Tsung-Dao Lee Chinese Undergraduate Research Endowment (CURE). The funders had no role in study design, data collection and analysis, decision to publish, or preparation of the manuscript.

Competing Interests: The authors have declared that no competing interests exist.

* Email: yuzhengao@suda.edu.cn (YG); yhe@suda.edu.cn (YH)

❾ These authors contributed equally to this work.

Introduction

Hepatocellular carcinoma (HCC) is one of the most common malignancies and the third leading cause of cancer death [1]. Approximately 80% of HCCs occur in developing countries where hepatitis B virus (HBV) infection is endemic, with the highest incidences being in the Asia-Pacific region, and sub-Saharan Africa [2]. In addition, chronic alcoholism, and long-term exposure to aflatoxin B1 are well-established risk factors for HCC [3]. Molecular biology of carcinogenesis and tumor progression of HCC have been increasingly elucidated with intense research in recent years. However, the molecular and cellular mechanisms of HCC pathogenesis are still poorly understood. Compelling evidence suggests the involvement of host genetic factors in HCC carcinogenesis and genome-wide association studies (GWAS) have greatly contributed to the identification of common genetic variants related to HCC [4,5]. Thus, it is of particular interest in identifying HCC-related genetic variations, which will definitely benefit the prediction of HCC risks, and the exploration of approaches to prevent HCC development.

Protein tyrosine phosphatase, non-receptor type 11 (*PTPN11*) encodes the non-receptor protein tyrosine phosphatase SHP2, which is critical for RAS/ERK pathway activation in most receptor tyrosine kinase, cytokine receptor, and integrin signaling pathways [6]. SHP2 is widely expressed in most tissues and plays a regulatory role in various cell signaling events that are important for a diversity of cell functions, such as mitogenic activation, metabolic control, transcriptional regulation, and cell migration. Activating mutations in *PTPN11* have been shown to be directly associated with the pathogenesis of Noonan syndrome and childhood leukemias [7,8]. Several lines of evidence have indicated that PTPN11 is involved in development of multiple cancers [9–12], including HCC. PTPN11 is first identified as a proto-oncogene in leukemia [13]. However, most recent findings suggest an unexpected tumor suppressor role of PTPN11 in HCC [14,15], implying its dual faces in tumorigenesis.

Previous studies have reported genetic variation within *PTPN11*, either dependent or independent of interaction with *helicobacter pylori*, is associated with the risks of gastric cancer and/or atrophic gastritis that precede carcinoma [16]. While the contributions of *PTPN11* polymorphisms to HCC susceptibilities has not been investigated. Considering the important roles of PTPN11 in HCC, we hypothesize that genetic variations in *PTPN11* may modulate its expression thus involve in HCC carcinogenesis. In the current study, we selected one trinucleotide short tandem repeat (STR) polymorphism (rs199618935) and conducted a two-stage case-control study to analyze the genetic effect of the polymorphism on the susceptibilities to HCC in Chinese populations. Additional experimental and *in-silico* studies were used to evaluate the possible functional significance of this polymorphism.

Materials and Methods

Ethics Statement

This study was approved by the Ethical Committee of Soochow University. Written informed consent was obtained from each participant before investigation.

Study Populations

The case-control study was performed on genomic DNA extracted from peripheral blood of 705 newly diagnosed incident HCC cases together with 723 controls after obtaining informed consent. All subjects recruited were unrelated ethnic Han Chinese. For the Jiangsu's case-control study (Panel I), the case series were comprised of 400 HCC patients diagnosed, hospitalized and treated in the affiliated hospitals of Soochow University from 2007 to 2011. For the Shanghai's case-control study (Panel II), 305 HCC patients were recruited at Nantong Tumor Hospital from 2003 to 2005. Controls were cancer-free individuals selected from a community nutritional survey that was conducted in the same regions during the same period as the recruitment of cancer patients. Controls without clinical evidence of liver disease were frequency matched for age (±5 years) and sex to each set of HCC individuals. The diagnosis of the cases, the inclusion and exclusion criteria for the cases and controls, and the definition of smokers and drinkers were described previously in details [17,18]. Briefly, the diagnosis of these patients was confirmed by a pathological examination combined with positive imaging (Magnetic resonance imaging and/or computerized tomography). Tumor stages were assigned according to a modified American Joint Committee on Cancer (AJCC) and international union against cancer (UICC) standard. The "current smokers" were individuals who had kept smoking almost every day for more than one year till the time of interview; and the "former smokers" were those who experienced the same degree of smoking as the "current smokers", but stopped

smoking at least one year prior to the interview; the non-smokers were those either never smoked or seldom did. Subjects were considered as "light drinkers", if they consumed 1–2 alcohol drinks per week for more than one year. Those who consumed more than 2 alcohol drinks per week for more than one year were categorized as "heavy drinkers". "Non-drinkers" were those either never drank or seldom did.

Additional 48 tumor tissues and adjacent non-HCC tissues from patients with a diagnosis of HCC were collected from Department of General Surgery, the First Affiliated Hospital of Soochow University from 2011 to 2012. All cases had histological confirmation of their tumor diagnosis and none of these patients had received preoperative chemotherapy or radiotherapy. After surgical resection, the fresh tissues were immediately stored at −80°C until the DNA/RNA extraction was processed.

DNA Extraction and Genotyping

Genomic DNA of peripheral blood samples, tissue samples and HCC cell lines were isolated using genomic DNA purification kit (Qiagen). DNA fragments containing rs199618935 were amplified with a pair of genotyping primers (Forward primer: 5′-GTGTCCCTTCTACTTCCCTCT-3′, Reverse primer: 5′-GCTGGGCTTGTGACTTGTTT-3′). The PCR products were analyzed by 7% non-denaturing polyacrylamide gel electrophoresis (PAGE) and visualized by silver staining [19]. For the six different alleles we observed, a direct sequencing method was used to determine the number of repeat motif. The nomenclature of allele was determined according to the recommendations of the DNA commission of the International Society for Forensic Haemogenetics [20]. The genotypes of all samples were analyzed using a homemade allelic ladder, a mixture of all six different alleles. Approximately 10% of the samples were randomly selected and examined in blind duplicates by independent researchers, and the reproducibility was 100%.

Real-Time RT-PCR Analysis

The Hep-G2, Hep3B and Huh7 hepatoma cell lines were obtained directly from Shanghai Cell Bank of Chinese Academy of Sciences. Cells were cultured in Dulbecco's Modified Eagle's Medium (DMEM) supplemented with 10% fetal bovine serum (FBS) and 1% penicillin-streptomycin at 37°C in a humidified 5% CO2 incubator before RNA extraction. Total RNA was isolated from hepatoma cell lines and tissue samples using RNA isolation kit (Qiagen). cDNA was generated using random primers and Superscript II reverse transcriptase (Invitrogen). A SYBR Green real-time PCR was performed using Roche LightCycler 480 to quantify relative PTPN11 expression in these samples. GAPDH was chosen as the internal control. Primer sequences used for PTPN11 and GAPDH were as follows: PTPN11-F: 5′-TCAG-CACAGAAATAGATGTG-3′, PTPN11-R: 5′- TGCTTATCA-AAAGGTAGTCA-3′, GAPDH-F: 5′-CTCTCTGCTCCTCC-TGTTCGAC-3′, GAPDH-R: 5′-TGAGCGATGTGGCTCGG-CT-3′. The 25 μl total volume final reaction mixture consisted of 1 μM of each primer, 12.5 μl of Master Mix (Applied Biosystems), and 50–100 ng of cDNA. The negative control experiments were performed with distilled H_2O as template. The expression levels of target genes were normalized with GAPDH using a $2 - \Delta\Delta CT$ method [21]. In addition, the melting curve analysis was performed for the PCR products to verify the specificity of primer.

Construction of Reporter Plasmids and Luciferase Assays

The partial structures (~570 bp) of human PTPN11-3′UTR containing allele 12, 14 and 15 of rs199618935 were amplified with forward primer 5′-GATCTCTAGACCCCAACTGT-

Table 1. Demographic characteristics among HCC cases and controls.

Characteristics	Overall			Jiangsu (Panel I)			Shanghai (Panel II)		
	Case	Control	P	Case	Control	P	Case	Control	P
	(n = 705)	(n = 723)		(n = 400)	(n = 408)		(n = 305)	(n = 315)	
Age(mean±SD)	49.8±11.7	51.1±11.6	0.45[a]	52.8±12.1	52.5±11.9	0.48[a]	49.2±10.7	50.5±11.5	0.42[a]
Gender, N (%)									
Male	462(0.66)	488(0.68)	0.43[b]	261(0.65)	274(0.67)	0.57[b]	201(0.66)	214(0.68)	0.5[b]
Female	243(0.34)	235(0.32)		139(0.35)	134(0.33)		104(0.34)	101(0.32)	
Smoking Status									
Nonsmokers	485(0.69)	510(0.71)	0.47[b]	276(0.69)	286(0.70)	0.68[b]	209(0.69)	224(0.71)	0.53[b]
Former Smokers	106(0.15)	104(0.14)		59(0.15)	60(0.15)		47(0.15)	44(0.14)	
Current smoker	114(0.16)	109(0.15)		65(0.16)	62(0.15)		49(0.16)	47(0.15)	
Drinking status									
Nondrinker	392(0.56)	410(0.57)	0.27[b]	217(0.54)	224(0.55)	0.45[b]	175(0.57)	186(0.59)	0.43[b]
Light Drinker	186(0.26)	206(0.28)		113(0.28)	126(0.31)		73(0.24)	80(0.25)	
Heavy Drinker	127(0.18)	107(0.15)		70(0.18)	58(0.14)		57(0.19)	49(0.16)	
Tumor stages									
Ia+Ib	487(0.69)			275(0.69)			212(0.70)		
IIa+IIb	156(0.22)			85(0.21)			71(0.23)		
IIIa+IIIb	62(0.09)			40(0.10)			22(0.07)		
HBsAg, N (%)									
Positive	517(0.73)	71(0.10)	<0.0001[b]	296(0.74)	42(0.10)	<0.0001[b]	221(0.72)	29(0.09)	<0.0001[b]
Negative	188(0.27)	652(0.90)		104(0.26)	366(0.90)		84(0.28)	286(0.91)	

Cases indicate patients with HCC and controls are non-cancerous patients.
[a]Two-sided two-sample t-test between cases and controls.
[b]χ^2 test for differences between cases and controls.

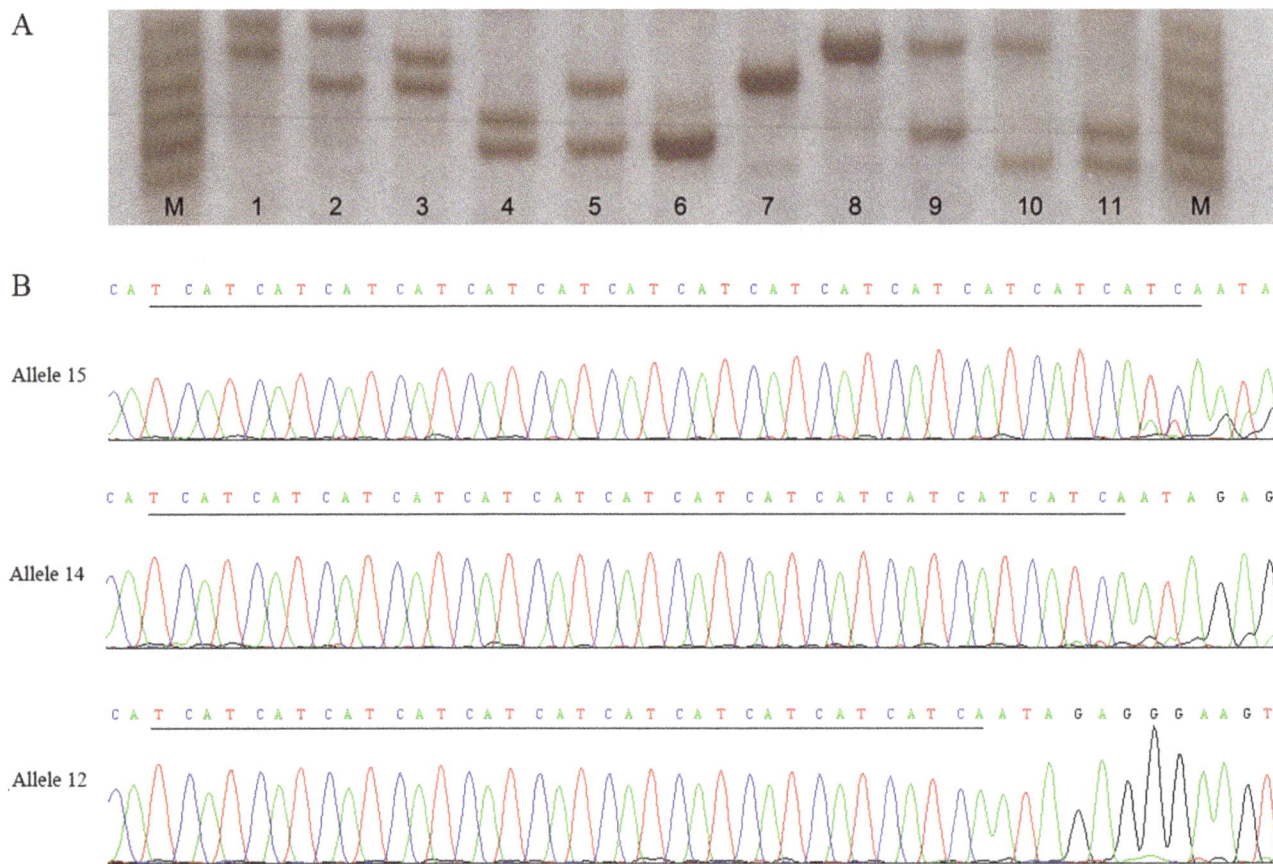

Figure 1. Example sequencing and genotyping output for rs199618935. The upper panel showed an example of the genotyping assay results. DNA was run in 7% non-denaturing polyacrylamide gel electrophoresis (PAGE) and visualized by silver staining (the genotypes from lane 1 to 11 was 15/16, 14/16, 14/15, 12/13, 12/14, 12/12, 14/14, 15/15, 12/15, 11/15 and 11/12, respectively). The lower panel displayed the sequences of the most three common alleles (allele 12, 14 and 15). The underlined base-pairs indicated the "TCA" repeat polymorphism.

TAGTCAATCTGAGC-3′ and reverse primer 5′- CATG-GATCCTTGTCCCAGCTACTGTAAGCAGC-3′ from three homozygous human genomic DNA samples. The PCR products were separated in agarose gel and extracted, purified, and cloned with TA cloning Kit (Promega). The repeat numbers of different alleles were confirmed by sequencing. Finally, the 3′UTR of Renilla luciferase in the vector pRL-SV40 (Promega) was replaced with the cloned 3′UTR of *PTPN11* by restriction enzymes XbaI and BamHI. The resulting constructs were verified by sequencing.

The Hep-G2, Hep3B, sk-Hep-1 and Huh7 hepatoma cell lines were seeded at 1×10^5 cells per well in 24-well plates (BD Biosciences). Twenty-four hours after the plating, cells were transfected by Lipofectamine 2000 according to manufacturer's manual. In each well, 500 ng constructed pRL-SV40 vector and 50 ng pGL3 control vector were cotransfected. Six replicates were performed for each group and each experiment was repeated at least three times. After transfection for 24 hr, cells were harvested by the addition of 100 μl passive lysis buffer. Renilla luciferase activities in cell lysate were measured with the Dual Luciferase assay system (Promega) in TD-20/20 luminometer (Turner Biosystems) and were normalized with the firefly luciferase activities.

In-silico Predicting Effects of STR Polymorphism on PTPN11 Folding Structures

As certain conserved structures more likely serve important biological functions, a 60-bp region covering the polymorphism

was analyzed using RNAfold to predict the putative influence of different alleles on local folding structures of PTPN11 using default parameters [22].

Statistical Analysis

The genotype distribution was analyzed by Hardy-Weinberg equilibrium using χ^2 test. Since rs199618935 is a multi-allele polymorphism, the genotypic frequencies were calculated by a specific counting method based on different alleles. The samples would be classified into specific genotypic groups provided it has one or two specific alleles. Genotypic and allelic frequencies for each allele between HCC patients and controls were compared by χ^2 test. To facilitate analysis, alleles with frequencies lower than 3% were combined with the adjacent alleles (e.g. allele 11 and 12, allele 13 and 14, allele 15 and 16). Unconditional logistic regression was used to analyze the association between rs199618935 and HCC risk, adjusted by gender, age, smoking, drinking and HBV infection status. As HBV infection was one of the major risk factors, a stratified analysis by HBV infection status for overall population was performed using binary logistic regression model. Student's t test was used to examine the differences in luciferase reporter gene expression. The normalized expression values of PTPN11 in tissue samples and hepatoma cell lines were compared with student's t test and one-way ANOVA, respectively. These statistical analyses were implemented in Statistic Analysis System software (version 8.0, SAS Institute).

Table 2. Genotypic and allelic frequencies of the trinucleotide STR in HCC patients and controls.

Panel	Repeat number	Genotypic frequency				OR (95% C.I.)[a]	P	Allelic frequency				OR (95% C.I.)	P
		Cases	%	Controls	%			Cases	%	Controls	%		
Panel I	11/12	375	93.8	341	83.6	1.00 (Reference)		580	72.5	506	62.0	1.00 (Reference)	
	13/14	160	40.0	192	47.1	0.76(0.58–0.99)	0.034	175	21.9	228	27.9	0.67(0.53–0.85)	6.19×10^{-4}
	15/16	45	11.3	78	19.1	0.52(0.35–0.79)	1.22×10^{-3}	45	5.6	82	10.0	0.48(0.32–0.71)	1.26×10^{-4}
Panel II	11/12	287	94.1	260	82.5	1.00 (Reference)		450	73.8	382	60.6	1.00 (Reference)	
	13/14	115	37.7	153	48.6	0.68(0.50–0.92)	0.010	127	20.8	183	29.0	0.59(0.45–0.77)	8.04×10^{-5}
	15/16	33	10.8	62	19.7	0.48(0.30–0.78)	1.42×10^{-3}	33	5.4	65	10.3	0.43(0.27–0.68)	1.31×10^{-4}
Overall	11/12	662	93.9	601	83.1	1.00 (Reference)		1030	73.0	888	61.4	1.00 (Reference)	
	13/14	275	39.0	345	47.8	0.72(0.59–088)	1.01×10^{-3}	302	21.4	411	28.4	0.63(0.53–0.76)	2.00×10^{-7}
	15/16	78	11.1	140	19.3	0.51(0.37–0.69)	5.70×10^{-6}	78	5.5	147	10.2	0.46(0.34–0.62)	1.00×10^{-7}

[a]Adjusted for sex, age, smoking status, drinking status and HBV infection.

Table 3. Logistic regression analyses for the association between rs199618935 and risk of HCC in HBV positive and negative groups.

Genotype	HBV positive				OR[a] (95% c.i.)	P	HBV negative				OR [a] (95% c.i.)	P
	Case	%	Control	%			Case	%	Control	%		
11/12	480	92.8	59	83.1	1.00(Reference)		173	92.0	538	82.5	1.00(Reference)	
13/14	198	38.3	33	46.5	0.79(0.49–1.28)		73	38.8	313	48.0	0.74(0.54–1.02)	
15/16	66	12.8	15	21.1	0.60(0.31–1.19)		24	12.8	128	19.6	0.61(0.38–1.00)	
P_{trend}						$P = 0.086$						$P = 0.011$

[a]Adjusted for sex, age, smoking status, drinking status and HBV infection.

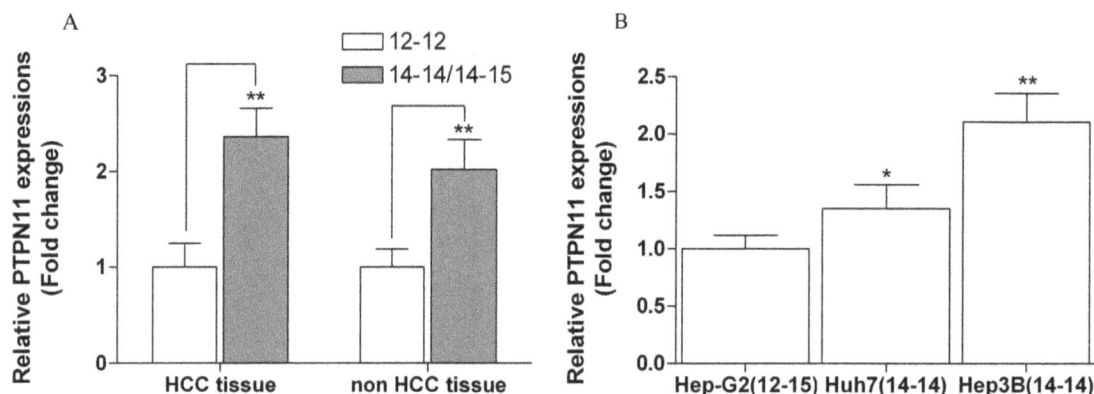

Figure 2. Expression of PTPN11 in HCC tissues and cell lines with different genotypes. (A) PTPN11 mRNA expression (mean ±SEM.) in HCC tissue and adjacent non-HCC tissues samples, by rs199618935 genotype. N=39 for genotype 12–12, N=5 for genotype 14–14, N=4 for genotype 14–15. ** indicates $P<0.01$ compared with 12–12 genotype within the same group. (B) PTPN11 mRNA expression (mean ±SD) in cell lines with different rs199618935 genotypes. * indicates $P<0.05$, ** indicates $P<0.01$ compared with Hep-G2 carrying one 12 allele.

$P<0.05$ was used as the criterion of statistical significance. All statistical tests were two sided.

Results

The Associations of STR Polymorphism with HCC Susceptibility

The demographic characteristics of the 705 HCC patients and 723 controls from two independent case-control sets were summarized in Table 1. There were no statistically significant differences in terms of the frequency distribution of sex, age, smoking and drinking status, suggesting that the frequency matching was adequate. Approximately 73.0% of the cases and 10.0% of the controls were HBsAg-positive, in accordance with the fact that HBV infection was a major risk factor for HCC. Example output from sequencing and genotyping assay of the STR polymorphism were shown in Figure 1. The observed genotypic frequencies for rs199618935 were consistent with those expected from the Hardy-Weinberg equilibrium in both cases and controls (all P values >0.05).

Six different alleles (11, 12, 13, 14, 15 and 16) were detected corresponding to 11–16 repeats (allele nomenclature rule is described in methods) and there were totally 11 and 12 different genotypes observed in overall cases and controls, respectively. Genotypic and allelic frequencies of rs199618935 as well as its

associations with HCC susceptibility were presented in Table 2. The carriage of allele 11 and 12 was significantly more common (72.5%) in HCC patients, whereas allele 13, 14, 15 and 16 was more common (37.9%) in controls. For the Jiangsu's case-control study, compared with the 11/12 genotype, subjects of 13/14 or 15/16 genotypes of rs199618935 had a significantly decreased risk of HCC in a dose dependent manner (adjusted OR=0.76, 95%C.I.=0.58–0.99; adjusted OR=0.52, 95%C.I.=0.35–0.79, respectively). Similar trends were observed in the Shanghai's case-control study. Furthermore, based on HBV stratification analysis, no obvious difference was observed between HBV positive and negative population (Table 3).

The Genotype-Phenotype Correlations Between the STR Polymorphism and *PTPN11* Expression

To further explore the effect of rs199618935 on the expression of PTPN11, we used different genotypic HCC tissue samples as well as their adjacent non-tumor tissues to examine PTPN11 expression. As shown in Figure 2A, results of q-PCR demonstrated that the PTPN11 expression level was significantly correlated with the genotypes of the STR polymorphism. Compared with 12–12 genotype, the PTPN11 expression of 14–14 or 14–15 genotypes

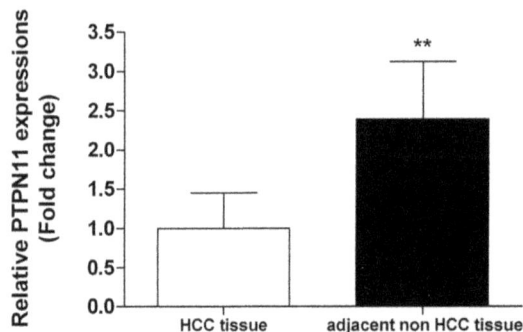

Figure 3. Relative PTPN11 expression in HCC tumor tissues *vs.* adjacent non-tumor tissues. ** indicates $P<0.01$ compared with paired HCC tumor tissue. N=48.

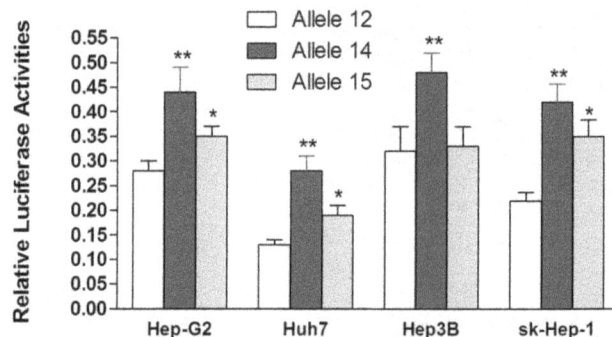

Figure 4. The effects of rs199618935 on PTPN11 transcriptional activity as determined by luciferase reporter assay. In three tested cell lines, significant difference was observed for the relative luciferase activity among allele 12, 14 and 15 constructs. * indicates $P<0.05$, ** indicates $P<0.01$ compared with construct containing allele 12 within the same group.

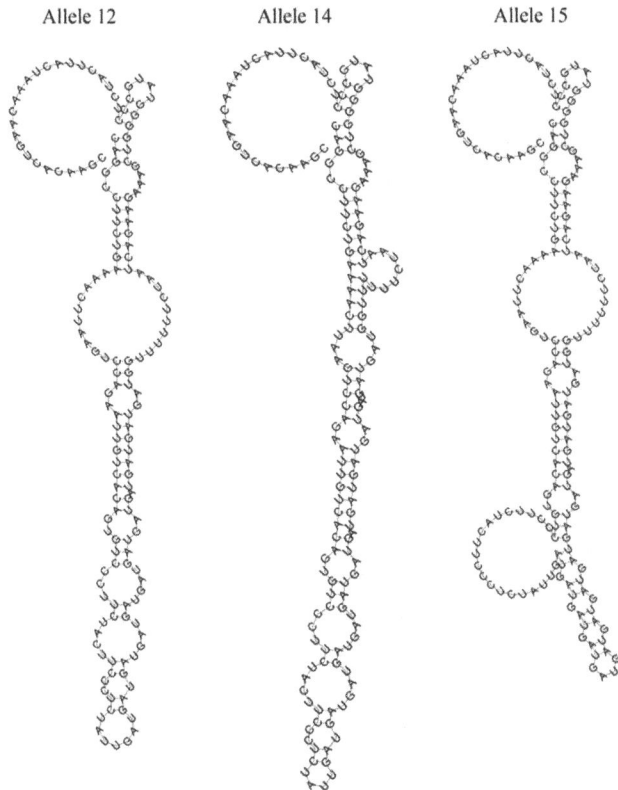

Figure 5. Influence of rs199618935 on PTPN11 mRNA local folding structures. The local structure changes were illustrated by RNAfold using default parameters.

was dramatically increased in both HCC tissues and adjacent non-tumor tissues (fold change $= 2.36$ and 2.02, respectively, $P<0.01$). To validate our findings in tissue samples, we further examined the genotype-phenotype correlations in three common hepatoma cell lines (Huh7, Hep3B and Hep-G2). Compared with Hep-G2 cell lines carrying 12–15 genotype, the PTPN11 mRNA expression levels of Huh-7 (14–14 genotype) and Hep3B (14–14 genotype) were significantly increased (Figure 2B). Thus, we observed a differential PTPN11 expression pattern in a STR genotype-dependent manner *in vivo* and *in vitro*. Finally, the expression level of PTPN11 in adjacent non-tumor tissues was 2.39-fold higher than that of HCC tumor tissues (Figure 3).

Effects of the STR Polymorphism on Transcriptional Activity

We further investigated the molecular mechanism underlying correlations between the STR polymorphism and PTPN11 expression. Since rs199618935 was located within 3′UTR of *PTPN11*, two luciferase reporter gene constructs were framed by PCR, and they were used to transiently transfect HCC cell lines. As shown in Figure 4, we found that the constructs containing allele 14 and allele 15 drove an increased reporter expression compared with the constructs containing allele 12 in all four hepatoma cell lines. Of note, allele 14 displayed the highest luciferase expression, which was significantly higher than that of allele 12 and allele 15.

In-silico Analysis of the STR Polymorphism on PTPN11 Folding

Considering the fact that the STR polymorphism is located within 3′UTR of *PTPN11*, it is plausible that different allele may

affect the folding structures of PTPN11, which in turn influence its expression through a structure-dependent mechanism. Using RNAfold algorithms, we predicted the local structure changes of PTPN11 caused by different alleles. As shown in Figure 5, the different "TCA" repeat motif displayed different local structures. Specifically, the allele 12 and 15 appeared to disrupt a highly base paired region which could be formed by the allele 14.

Discussion

We presented here the first case control study evaluating the association between the novel STR polymorphism within 3′UTR of *PTPN11* and HCC susceptibility. On the basis of our current findings, we propose a schematic model to illustrate the molecular mechanism and functional basis for polymorphism-associated hepatocarcinogenesis conferred by PTPN11 expression. Therefore, the novel STR polymorphism may serve as a potential marker for genetic susceptibility to HCC in Chinese populations.

Most recent experimental data suggest that in contrast to the proto-oncogene effect of dominant-active mutants, PTPN11 may act as a tumor suppressor in hepatocarcinogenesis [14]. Further studies confirmed the tumor suppressor roles of PTPN11 in HCC tumorgenesis and decreased PTPN11 expression has been shown to be a prognostic marker in HCC [15]. Our results also demonstrated that PTPN11 expression was significantly higher in self-matched adjacent non-tumor tissues compared with that of HCC tissues ($P<0.01$), which validated the tumor-inhibiting effect of PTPN11 in HCC. Similarly, Ptpn11 has also been proved to be a tumor suppressor in cartilage and involved in metachondromatosis by inducing hedgehog signaling [23]. Given the critical link between protein-tyrosine kinases (PTKs) activation and oncogenesis, the opposing functions of PTPN11 within different cellular context remain to be fully elucidated.

To test whether the different allele in human *PTPN11* 3′UTR regulates mRNA level, we transfected three different constructs containing different alleles (e.g. 12, 14 and 15) into Huh7, Hep3B, sk-Hep-1 and Hep-G2 cells and then assayed luciferase levels. Our data provided first evidence that the construct containing allele 14 displayed the highest luciferase activity, which was significantly higher than that of constructs containing allele 12 and 15. The altered luciferase activities we observed in the reporter gene system suggested that STR regulation of PTPN11 expression can be a transcriptional event, such as changed RNA stability in a post-transcriptional level. Early studies have shown that STR polymorphism in the 3′UTR formed structural elements (stem-loops) and contributed to mRNA regulation [24]. Indeed, our *in-silico* studies have shown different structures formed by sequences containing different alleles (Figure 5). Based on the results of our current study, we hypothesized that different alleles of the STR may act as an enhancer or repressor to regulate PTPN11 gene expression. Coordinately controlled by PTKs and protein tyrosine phosphatases (PTPs), PTPN11 is a feature of many important signaling pathways that are involved in cell proliferation, adhesion, and migration [25,26]. Our results showed that longer alleles (14 and 15) conferred higher PTPN11 expression, which was consistent with the fact that longer alleles were associated with decreased HCC risks.

Deregulation of PTPN11 causes hyperactivation of ERK, leading to growth abnormality. Gain-of-function *PTPN11* mutations have been found in various types of human cancer [27–29]. It has been shown that the activating SHP2 mutant promotes lung tumorigenesis [30]. Additional data suggest that targeting SHP2 may represent an effective strategy for treatment of epidermal growth factor receptor (EGFR) inhibitor resistant non-small cell lung cancer [31]. Therefore, the STR polymorphism identified in our study may serve as a potential marker for individualized diagnosis or treatment of cancers.

Although this is the first report for the possible association between *PTPN11* STR polymorphism and HCC risk, the significance of this finding is limited by the relative small sample size used in this study. However, result from our genetic association analysis provides a preliminary data and evokes the need for future study with different or expanded case-control populations to confirm our observations. Furthermore, the underlined molecular mechanisms between the STR polymorphism and PTPN11 expression still need to be fully investigated both at genetic and functional levels.

In summary, we have provided initial evidence that the length variation of the "TCA" repeats within human PTPN11 3′UTR may play a functional role in regulating the expression of PTPN11

and subsequently affect development of HCC. Therefore, PTPN11 may be a promising marker for personalized diagnosis and therapy of HCC.

Acknowledgments

We gratefully acknowledge the participation of patients with HCC and cancer-free individuals.

Author Contributions

Conceived and designed the experiments: YG. Performed the experiments: XZ SH LW QZ XZ HZ. Analyzed the data: CW RT SG JW. Contributed reagents/materials/analysis tools: YG HZ JX YH. Contributed to the writing of the manuscript: YG. Contributed to manuscript editing: XZ SH CW RT.

References

1. Yang JD, Roberts LR (2010) Hepatocellular carcinoma: A global view. Nat Rev Gastroenterol Hepatol 7: 448–458.
2. El-Serag HB (2012) Epidemiology of viral hepatitis and hepatocellular carcinoma. Gastroenterology 142: 1264–1273.
3. Monto A, Wright TL (2001) The epidemiology and prevention of hepatocellular carcinoma. Semin Oncol 28: 441–449.
4. Kumar V, Kato N, Urabe Y, Takahashi A, Muroyama R, et al. (2011) Genome-wide association study identifies a susceptibility locus for HCV-induced hepatocellular carcinoma. Nat Genet 43: 455–458.
5. Clifford RJ, Zhang J, Meerzaman DM, Lyu MS, Hu Y, et al. (2010) Genetic variations at loci involved in the immune response are risk factors for hepatocellular carcinoma. Hepatology 52: 2034–2043.
6. Grossmann KS, Rosário M, Birchmeier C, Birchmeier W (2010) The tyrosine phosphatase Shp2 in development and cancer. Adv Cancer Res 106: 53–89.
7. Tartaglia M, Gelb BD (2005) Germ-line and somatic PTPN11 mutations in human cancer. Eur J Med Genet 48: 81–96.
8. Loh ML, Vattikuti S, Schubbert S, Reynolds MG, Carlson E, et al. (2004) Mutations in PTPN11 implicate the SHP-2 phosphatase in leukemogenesis. Blood 103: 2325–2331.
9. Mohi MG, Neel BG (2007) The role of Shp2 (PTPN11) in cancer. Curr Opin Genet Dev 17: 23–30.
10. Leibowitz MS, Srivastava RM, Andrade Filho PA, Egloff AM, Wang L, et al. (2013) SHP2 is overexpressed and inhibits pSTAT1-mediated APM component expression, T-cell attracting chemokine secretion, and CTL recognition in head and neck cancer cells. Clin Cancer Res 19: 798–808.
11. Liu X, Zheng H, Qu CK (2012) Protein tyrosine phosphatase Shp2 (Ptpn11) plays an important role in maintenance of chromosome stability. Cancer Res 72: 5296–5306.
12. Chang W, Gao X, Han Y, Du Y, Liu Q, et al. (2013) Gene expression profiling-derived immunohistochemistry signature with high prognostic value in colorectal carcinoma. Gut (doi: 10.1136/gutjnl-2013-305475).
13. Chan RJ, Feng GS (2007) PTPN11 is the first identified proto-oncogene that encodes a tyrosine phosphatase. Blood 109: 862–867.
14. Bard-Chapeau EA, Li S, Ding J, Zhang SS, Zhu HH, et al. (2011) Ptpn11/Shp2 acts as a tumor suppressor in hepatocellular carcinogenesis. Cancer Cell 19: 629–639.
15. Jiang C, Hu F, Tai Y, Du J, Mao B, et al. (2012) The tumor suppressor role of Src homology phosphotyrosine phosphatase 2 in hepatocellular carcinoma. J Cancer Res Clin Oncol 138: 637–646.
16. He C, Tu H, Sun L, Xu Q, Li P, et al. (2013) Helicobacter pylori-related host gene polymorphisms associated with susceptibility of gastric carcinogenesis: a two-stage case-control study in Chinese. Carcinogenesis 34: 1450–1457.
17. Zhu Z, Gao X, He Y, Zhao H, Yu Q, et al. (2012) An insertion/deletion polymorphism within RERT-lncRNA modulates hepatocellular carcinoma risk. Cancer Res 72: 6163–6172.
18. Wan J, Huang M, Zhao H, Wang C, Zhao X, et al. (2013) A novel tetranucleotide repeat polymorphism within KCNQ1OT1 confers risk for hepatocellular carcinoma. DNA Cell Biol 32: 628–634.
19. Allen RC, Graves G, Budowle B (1989) Polymerase chain reaction amplification products separated on rehydratable polyacrylamide gels and stained with silver. Biotechniques 7: 736–744.
20. Lincoln PJ (1997) DNA recommendations–further report of the DNA Commission of the ISFH regarding the use of short tandem repeat systems. Forensic Sci Int 87: 181–184.
21. Livak KJ, Schmittgen TD (2001) Analysis of relative gene expression data using real-time quantitative PCR and the 2(-Delta Delta C(T)) Method. Methods 25: 402–408.
22. Gruber AR, Lorenz R, Bernhart SH, Neuböck R, Hofacker IL (2008) The Vienna RNA Nucleic Acids Res 36(Web Server issue): W70–74.
23. Yang W, Wang J, Moore DC, Liang H, Dooner M, et al. (2013) Ptpn11 deletion in a novel progenitor causes metachondromatosis by inducing hedgehog signalling. Nature 499: 491–495.
24. Mooers BH, Logue JS, Berglund JA (2005) The structural basis of myotonic dystrophy from the crystal structure of CUG repeats. Proc Natl Acad Sci USA 102: 16626–16631.
25. Chan G, Kalaitzidis D, Neel BG (2008) The tyrosine phosphatase Shp2 (PTPN11) in cancer. Cancer Metastasis Rev 27: 179–192.
26. Feng GS (2012) Conflicting roles of molecules in hepatocarcinogenesis: paradigm or paradox. Cancer Cell 21: 150–154.
27. Bentires-Alj M, Paez JG, David FS, Keilhack H, Halmos B, et al. (2004) Activating mutations of the noonan syndrome-associated SHP2/PTPN11 gene in human solid tumors and adult acute myelogenous leukemia. Cancer Res 64: 8816–8820.
28. Taylor BS, Schultz N, Hieronymus H, Gopalan A, Xiao Y, et al. (2010) Integrative genomic profiling of human prostate cancer. Cancer Cell 18: 11–22.
29. Ding L, Getz G, Wheeler DA, Mardis ER, McLellan MD, et al. (2008) Somatic mutations affect key pathways in lung adenocarcinoma. Nature 455: 1069–1075.
30. Schneeberger VE, Luetteke N, Ren Y, Berns H, Chen L, et al. (2014). SHP2E76K mutant promotes lung tumorigenesis in transgenic mice. Carcinogenesis 2014 (in press).
31. Xu J, Zeng LF, Shen W, Turchi JJ, Zhang ZY. (2013) Targeting SHP2 for EGFR inhibitor resistant non-small cell lung carcinoma. Biochem Biophys Res Commun 439: 586–590.

4

Aberrant Upregulation of 14-3-3σ and EZH2 Expression Serves as an Inferior Prognostic Biomarker for Hepatocellular Carcinoma

Yi Zhang[1], Yang Li[4], Changwei Lin[2], Jie Ding[3], Guoqing Liao[1]*, Bo Tang[4]*

1 Department of Gastrointestinal Surgery, Xiangya Hospital, Central South University, Changsha, P.R. China, **2** Department of Gastrointestinal Surgery, Third Xiangya Hospital, Central South University, Changsha, P.R. China, **3** Department of Gastrointestinal Surgery, Guizhou Provincial People's Hospital, Guiyang, P.R. China, **4** Department of Hepatobiliary Surgery, Affiliated Hospital of Guilin Medical University, Guilin, P.R. China

Abstract

Hepatocellular carcinoma (HCC) is the fifth most common malignancy in the world. It is of important significance to find biomarkers for the prognostic monitoring of HCC. The 14-3-3σ and EZH2 proteins are involved in cell cycle regulation and epigenetic silencing. We herein examined the significance of 14-3-3 σ and EZH2 in HCC (n = 167) by immunohistochemistry, RT-PCR and qRT-PCR. The correlation between 14-3-3σ and EZH2 expression and patients' clinicopathologic features were examined, as was the correlation between 14-3-3σ and EZH2 expression and the prognosis of HCC patients. We found that 14-3-3σ and EZH2 were highly expressed in HCC (71% and 90%), the expression of EZH2, but not 14-3-3σ, is associated with vascular invasion and tumor differentiation ($p < 0.01$). The coexistence of 14-3-3σ and EZH2 overexpression is associated with a relatively unfavorable prognosis ($p < 0.01$), suggesting that aberrant upregulation of 14-3-3σ and EZH2 expression serves as an inferior prognostic biomarker for HCC.

Editor: Erica Villa, University of Modena & Reggio Emilia, Italy

Funding: This research was supported by the National Natural Science Foundation of China (81360367), Science and technology research projects focused on universities in Guangxi (2013ZD046), Guangxi Health Department self-funded project, and the National Natural Science Foundation of Hunan province (08JJ5009) (Z2013464). The funders participated in study design, data collection and analysis.

Competing Interests: The authors have declared that no competing interests exist.

* Email: liaoguoqing@medmail.com.cn (GL); dytangbo@163.com (BT)

Introduction

Hepatocellular carcinoma (HCC) is the fifth most common malignancy in the world, and the estimated number of HCC-related deaths exceeds 500,000 per year [1]. The genetic mechanism behind HCC formation is unclear, but it can be concluded that genetic alterations may include cyclins, p27, and p21. However, the functions of some of the associated genes have not been proven, so it is of significant importance for the diagnosis and treatment of liver cancer to explore and study the relationship between associated genes and the generation and development of liver cancer.

The 14-3-3σ protein, which belongs to the 14-3-3 protein family, was originally characterized as an epithelial-specific marker, HME1, which was shown to be responsible for G2 cell cycle checkpoint control by p53 in response to DNA damage in human cells [2]. Moreover 14-3-3σ has been defined as a new class of Cdk inhibitor, as it can bind Cdk2, Cdc2 and Cdk4 and sequester them in the cytoplasm through altered nuclear exporting activities [3]. The 14-3-3σ protein plays important roles in a wide range of regulatory processes, such as mitogenic signal transduction, cell cycle control, and apoptotic cell death [4]. Up- or down-regulation of 14-3-3σ has been found in human cancers. For example, 14-3-3σ expression is lost in breast cancer cells due to

promoter hypermethylation [5]. The loss of 14-3-3σ expression was also found in partial HCC tissue, and a significant correlation was found between methylation and loss of expression [6].

Enhancer of zeste homolog 2 (EZH2) is a member of the Polycomb Group (PcG) of proteins. The gene maps to chromosome 7q35 and contains 20 exons and 19 introns [7]. EZH2, the catalytic subunit of PRC2, has a SET domain, which is a typical structural signature of histone methyltransferase activity [8], and gives rise to the methylated version of lysine residue 27 within histone H3 [9]. Moreover, EZH2 is capable of exhibiting DNA methyltransferase activity and can repress the activities of certain genes by gene methylation [10]. Studies have found that the expression of the EZH2 gene in cancer was significantly higher than in paraneoplastic or normal tissue [11]. Silencing EZH2 expression in liver cancer cells attenuated liver cancer proliferation and metastasis [12].

The expression of 14-3-3σ is determined by the methylation status of the gene, and EZH2 is also a methylation-regulated gene. Is there a correlation between 14-3-3σ and EZH2 expression? What type of relationship exists between the gene expression and the clinicopathological features and prognosis of HCC? Our study further investigates the above issues. We determined that there is no correlation between 14-3-3σ and EZH2 expression and that EZH2 is associated with tumor differentiation and vascular infiltration. In addition, the combination of 14-3-3σ and EZH2 can predict the prognosis of HCC, which suggests that no regulatory relationship exists between 14-3-3σ and EZH2 expression, but the combination of the two genes could become candidate indicators for monitoring the prognosis of HCC.

Materials and Methods

Patient samples

The study was reviewed and approved by ethics committee of affiliated hospital of Guilin medical university and written informed consent was obtained from all patients. The study included 167 patients with HCC aged from 25 to 74 years; all patients underwent curative surgery from 2006 to 2008 at the Department of Hepatobiliary Surgery, The Affiliated Hospital of Guilin Medical University. No patients underwent palliative resection, preoperative chemotherapy, or radiotherapy. Clinico-pathological features examined included age, gender, etiology, presence of liver cirrhosis, AFP, tumor size, tumor differentiation, vascular invasion, and tumor stage. Tumors were classified and graded based on the pTNM classification advocated by the International Union Against Cancer. All 167 patients were followed for 5 years with computed tomography and ultrasonography every six months after discharge.

Immunohistochemistry

Specimens were fixed with 10% formaldehyde, embedded in paraffin, and sectioned into 4-μm-thick slices. Sections were deparaffinized by prolonged incubation in xylene (3–4 min), followed by prolonged washing and rehydration in ethanol (96% ethanol for 2–3 min, 80% ethanol for 3 min, and 70% ethanol for 3 min). After deparaffinization, endogenous peroxidase was blocked by a 0.3% hydrogen peroxidase-methanol solution for 30 minutes. For antigen retrieval, sections were pretreated with citrate buffer for 15 minutes at 100°C in a microwave oven. After blocking with phosphate-buffered saline (PBS) plus 3% skim milk at room temperature for 2 h, the blocked sections were incubated overnight at 4°C with primary antibody for 14-3-3σ (sc-7681, Santa Cruz, USA) or EZH2 (ab189201, abcam, USA) at a dilution of 1 : 100. After washing, the sections were reacted with biotinylated rabbit anti-goat IgG (Santa Cruz, USA) or goat anti-rabbit IgG (Santa Cruz, USA) at a dilution of 1 : 500, followed by incubation with an avidin–biotin peroxidase complex. The immune complex was visualized with diaminobenzidine as the substrate. The sections were rinsed briefly in water, counterstained with hematoxylin, and mounted. In addition, sections incubated without the primary antibody were used as the negative controls.

If the HCC accompany with liver fibrosis. The METAVIR scoring system was used to stage liver fibrosis as follows: F1, portal fibrosis without septa; F2, portal fibrosis and few septa; F3, numerous septa without cirrhosis; F4, cirrhosis [13]. Scores of F3 or F4 were considered to indicate advanced fibrosis.

Two investigators independently evaluated the immunohisto-chemical staining. Ten high power fields (×200) were randomly selected for quantification. The percentage of 14-3-3σ or EZH2 positive tumor cells were estimated as follows: 0 point, <1%; 1 point, 1–25%; 2 points, 26–50%; 3 points, 51–75%; 4 points, > 75%. The score of the staining intensity was presented as follows: 0 point, no staining; 1 point, weak staining; 2 point, moderate staining; 3 point, strong staining. Then, the two scores were multiplied to obtain a combination score ranging from 0 to 12, with 0 representing no staining (-), 1–3 points representing weak intensity (+); 4–6 points representing moderate intensity (++); 8–12 points representing strong intensity (+++). Protein expression was defined as high when the combination scores were >3 and low when combination scores were≤3.

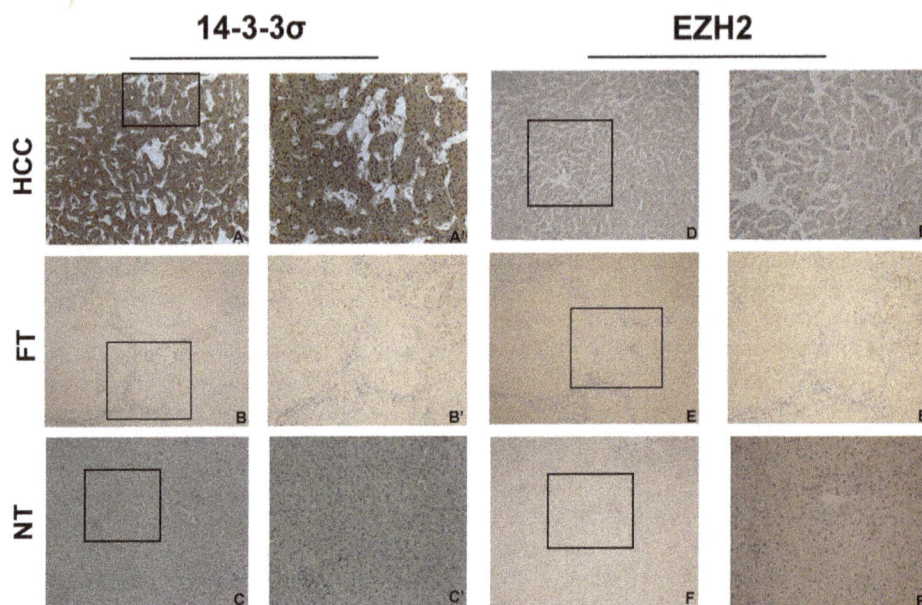

Figure 1. Immunohistochemical staining for 14-3-3σ and EZH2 in hepatocellular carcinoma, fibrotic tissues and normal adjacent tissues. (A) 14-3-3σ was strong stained in hepatocellular carcinoma tissue, (B) nearly negative expression of 14-3-3σ in fibrotic tissue, (C) with an almost negative expression level in paired normal adjacent tissue (100×); (D) EZH2 was overexpressed in the cytoplasm in hepatocellular carcinoma tissue, (E) almost negative expression of EZH2 in fibrotic tissue, (F) nearly absent in paired normal tissues from the same case (100×). (A', B' and C') and (D', E' and F') demonstrated the higher magnification (200×) from the area of the box in (A, B and C) and (D, E and F), respectively.

A

B

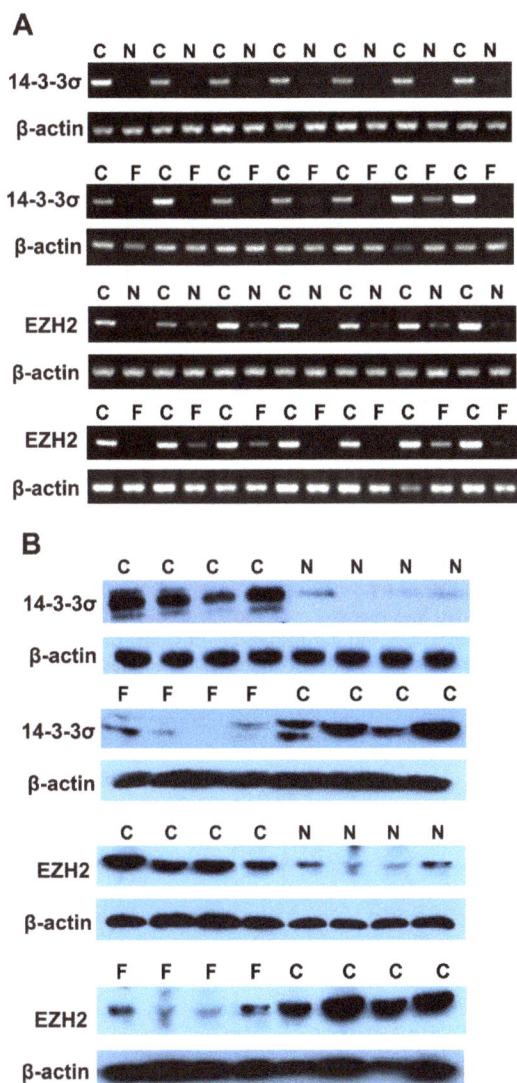

Figure 2. The expression of 14-3-3σ and EZH2 in hepatocellular carcinoma, fibrotic tissues and normal adjacent tissues as determined by RT-PCR and Western blot. (A) The expression of 14-3-3σ and EZH2 was detected by RT-PCR, C: Cancer tissue, N: Noncancerous tissue, F: fibrotic tissues. (B) The immunoblot analysis of 14-3-3σ and EZH2. β-actin was used as endogenous reference.

Western blot

Frozen tissues were homogenized and lysed with lysis buffer (50 mM Tris–HCl, 137 mM NaCl, 10% glycerol, 100 mM sodium orthovanadate, 1 mM phenylmethylsulphonyl fluoride (PMSF), 10 mg/ml aprotinin, 10 mg/ml leupeptin, 1% Nonidet P-40, 5 mM protease inhibitor cocktail; pH 7.4). After the determination of the protein concentration using BCA kit assay, β-mercaptoethanol and bromophenol blue were added to the sample buffer for electrophoresis. Proteins was separated by 10% PAGE and transferred to polyvinylidene difluoride membranes (Bio-Rad, USA). The membranes were incubated with primary antibody overnight at 4 °C. After incubation with secondary antibody for another 2 h, reactive bands were visualized using the enhanced chemiluminescence system. The band intensity was quantified using an image analysis system (Quantity One v4.62).

RNA extraction and reverse transcriptase PCR (RT-PCR)

Total RNA from tissue was prepared using RNAisoTM Plus (Takara, Japan) according to the manufacturer's instructions. The concentration of the total RNA samples was determined with a spectrophotometer (Beckman Coulter, USA). The primers specific for 14-3-3σ and EZH2 were synthesized by Invitrogen Biotechnology Co. Ltd., China. The primers for amplification were as follows: Human 14-3-3σ forward (5'-AGAAGCGCATCATT-GACTCA-3'), reverse (5'-CTGTTGGCGATCTCGTAGTG-3'); EZH2 forward (5'-GCCAGACTGGGAAGAAATCTG-3'), reverse (5'-TGTGCTGGAAAATCCAAGTCA-3'). The RT-PCR was performed using an RT-PCR kit (TaKaRa, Japan) according to the manufacturer's instructions. PCR was performed with the following conditions: initial denaturation at 94 °C for 2 min, then 35 cycles at 95°C for 30 s, 55 °C for 45 s and 72 °C for 70 s, and a final extension at 72 °C for 5 min. The PCR products were separated on 1.5% agarose gels by electrophoresis and visualized with UV light.

Quantitative real time RT-PCR (qRT-PCR)

Gene expression was evaluated again by the quantitative real-time RT-PCR method. Total RNA was prepared from HCC specimens using an RNeasy Mini Plus Kit (Qiagen, Holland) and the quality was evaluated using an Agilent 2100 Bioanalyzer (Agilent Technologies, USA) as described above. One microgram of total RNA per 20 μl of reaction mixture was converted to cDNA using a High Capacity cDNA Reverse Transcription Kit (Life Technologies, USA). Quantitative real-time PCR was performed with SYBR Premix Ex Taq (Takara, Japan) on a GeneAmpV R 7300 Sequence Detection System (Life Technologies, USA) in accordance with the manufacturer's protocol. The primers for amplification were as follows: Human 14-3-3σ forward (5'-AGAAGCGCATCATTGACTCA-3'), reverse (5'-CTGTTG-GCGATCTCGTAGTG-3'); EZH2 forward (5'-GCCAGACTG-GGAAGAAATCTG-3'), reverse (5'-TGTGCTGGAAAATCCA-AGTCA-3').

Statistical analysis

Statistical analysis was performed using SPSS 17.0 software (SPSS Inc., USA). χ^2 tests were used to evaluate the relationship between the expression and clinicopathological variables. Spearman's correlation coefficient was used to calculate correlations between 14-3-3σ and EZH2. The Kaplan-Meier analysis was employed for survival analysis, and differences in survival probabilities were estimated using the log-rank test. The Cox proportional hazards model was used to determine the independent factors of survival. $p < 0.05$ was considered statistically significant.

Results

14-3-3σ and EZH2 expression in normal tissue, fibrotic tissue and liver cancer

Many HCC often arise within the background of liver fibrosis, so we detected the expression of 14-3-3σ and EZH2 in liver cancer with normal tissue and liver fibrotic tissue as control by RT-PCR, qRT-PCR, Western blot and immunohistochemistry. 14-3-3σ was detected in the cytoplasm of cells in 71% (119/167) of HCC patients, whereas adjacent normal tissue and liver fibrosis tissues showed negative expression. On the contrary, EZH2 immunostaining was detected in a nuclear staining pattern. Out of all HCC tissues, 90% (150/167) were immunopositive for EZH2, whereas the adjacent normal tissues and liver cirrhosis tissues were immunonegative or weak for EZH2 (Figure 1). The results of

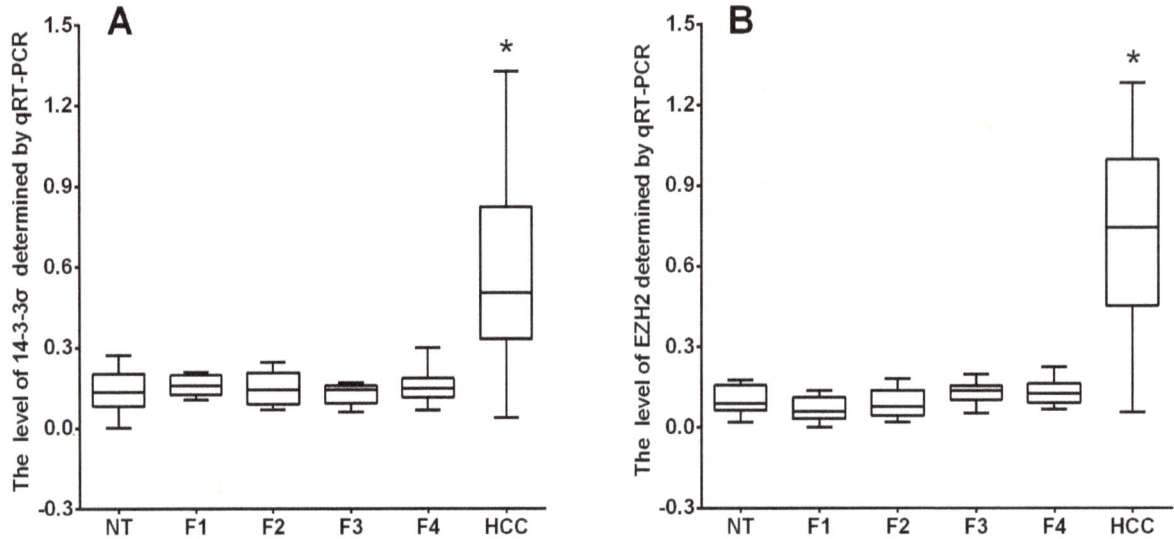

Figure 3. Expression levels of 14-3-3σ and EZH2 quantitatively determined by real-time RT–PCR. (A) Expression levels of 14-3-3σ in hepatocellular carcinoma, fibrotic tissues and normal adjacent tissues, liver fibrosis was classified into four stages, F1 to F4, according to METAVIR scoring system. (B) Expression levels of EZH2 quantitatively in hepatocellular carcinoma, fibrotic tissues and normal adjacent tissues. The correction values were calculated by dividing the 14-3-3σ and EZH2 amounts by the amount of β-actin concurrently examined on the same samples (*, $p<0.05$).

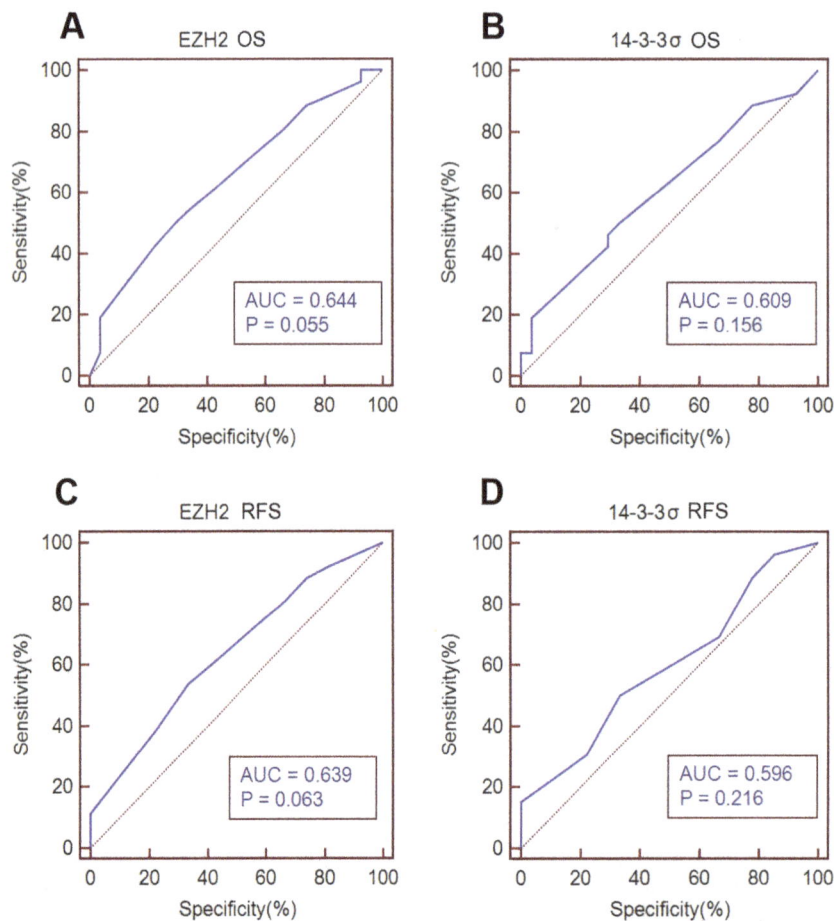

Figure 4. ROC curve analysis to determine cutoff score for 14-3-3σ and EZH2 expression. (A, C) EZH2 cutoff point of OS and DFS, the EZH2 cutoff score for OS and DFS was 4 ($p=0.055$) and 4 ($p=0.063$). (B, D) 14-3-3σ cutoff point for OS and DFS. The 14-3-3σ cutoff scores for OS and DFS were 3 ($p=0.156$) and 3 ($p=0.216$), respectively. At each immunohistochemical score, the sensitivity and specificity for the outcome being studied was plotted, thus generating a ROC curve.

Table 1. Relationship between 14-3-3σ and EZH2 and clinicopathological parameters in 167 HCC patients.

Variables	All cases	14-3-3σ expression		χ²	P*	EZH2 expression		χ²	P*
		High	Low			high	low		
Age(years)									
≥50	93	59	34			70	23		
<50	74	39	35	0.041	0.161	57	17	1.581	0.791
Gender									
Male	120	70	50			92	28		
Female	47	28	19	2.464	0.883	35	12	1.408	0.765
Liver cirrhosis									
Positive	110	68	42			86	24		
negative	57	30	27	0.104	0.252	41	16	0.231	0.369
Etiology									
viral	109	66	43			79	30		
Non-viral	58	32	26	0.458	0.502	48	10	0.030	0.138
Serum AFP(ng/ml)									
≤200	93	57	36			66	27		
>200	74	41	33	0.345	0.443	61	13	0.011	0.085
Tumor stage									
I	30	19	4			23	7		
II	49	28	21			31	18		
III	67	38	29			55	12		
IV	21	13	8	0.694	0.125	18	3	0.484	0.079
Tumor size(cm)									
≤5	29	13	16			20	9		
>5	138	85	53	0.014	0.096	107	31	0.176	0.326
Tumor differentiation									
Well	34	17	17			25	9		
Moderate	101	57	44			84	17		
Poor	32	24	8	0.192	0.092	18	14	0.015	0.007
Vascular invasion									
Yes	72	45	27			61	11		
No	95	53	42	0.250	0.383	66	29	0.000	0.022
14-3-3σ	EZH2					rs			p

* Probability, P, from χ² test.

Table 2. Correlation analysis between expression of 14-3-3σ and EZH2 in HCC.

14-3-3σ	EZH2					rs	p
	+++	++	+	-	Total		
+++	8	15	10	4	37	-0.054	0.492
++	17	35	8	1	61		
+	7	9	2	3	21		
-	21	15	4	8	48		
total	53	74	24	16	167		

Overall survival　　　Relapse-free survival

RT-PCR and Western blot also revealed similar findings (Figure 2). Furthermore, we divided liver fibrosis into four stages according to METAVIR scoring system, and detect the expression of 14-3-3σ and EZH2 in different stage of liver fibrosis (n = 110), normal tissue (n = 57) and liver cancer by qRT-PCR(Figure 3). The results indicated that there was no significant difference in 14-3-3σ expression between different stages F1 to F4, 14-3-3σ expression in HCC was significantly higher than other group. Interestingly, in EZH2 expression group, we found an increase trend from F1 to F4 stage, but no significant difference existed between each stage and normal tissue.

To further assess the survival analysis and to avoid the problems of multiple cutpoint selection, ROC curve analysis was employed to determine the cutoff score for 14-3-3σ and EZH2 expression. As shown in Figure 4, the 14-3-3σ cutoff scores for OS and DFS were 3 ($p = 0.156$) and 3 ($p = 0.216$), respectively; the EZH2 cutoff scores for OS and DFS were 4 ($p = 0.055$) and 4 ($p = 0.063$). We thus selected a 14-3-3σ expression score of 3 (> 3 VS ≤3) and EZH2 expression score of 4 (>4 VS≤4) as the uniform cutoff point for survival analysis (Figure 3).

14-3-3σ and EZH2 expression and clinicopathologic features

The association of 14-3-3σ and EZH2 expression with pathological variables was examined. 14-3-3σ expression in HCC was not statistically associated with clinicopathologic features. On the other hand, the incidence of vascular invasion and poor tumor differentiation was higher in the high EZH2 group than in the EZH2 low group. No significant differences in host factors, such as the patient's age, gender, tumor stage, tumor size, etc. were observed between the high and low EZH2 groups (Table 1).

Relationship between 14-3-3σ and EZH2 expression

We wondered whether EZH2 could regulate the expression of 14-3-3σ by methylation, so we examined the relationship between 14-3-3σ and EZH2. The results showed that the Spearman's correlation coefficient between 14-3-3σ and EZH2 was -0.054 ($p = 0.492$), suggesting no association between the two parameters (Table 2).

14-3-3σ and EZH2 expression and survival analysis

We carried out follow-up for patients out to five years. Kaplan-Meier analysis shows that the five-year OS rates were 32.65% and 40% in the 14-3-3σ positive and negative groups, respectively, and the five-year RFS were 24.49% and 21.74% in both groups. Although the OS rate of the 14-3-3σ negative group was better than the positive group (40% vs. 32.65%). No significant differences were detected between the two groups (Figure 5, $p = 0.348$). Kaplan-Meier analysis also shows that the OS of the EZH2 high and low groups were 32.28% and 45%, respectively, and the RFS of EZH2 was 22.05% and 27.5%. There is no significant difference between the EZH2 high and low groups (Figure 5, $p = 0.172$).

Then, the presence of 14-3-3σ and EZH2 overexpression was investigated to verify their correlation with patients' survival. We found that the five-year OS and RFS of coexistent high 14-3-3σ and EZH2 groups were 23.75% and 13.75%, significantly worse than three other groups (Figure 5, p for OS and RFS were 0.001 and 0.001). This difference is statistically significant.

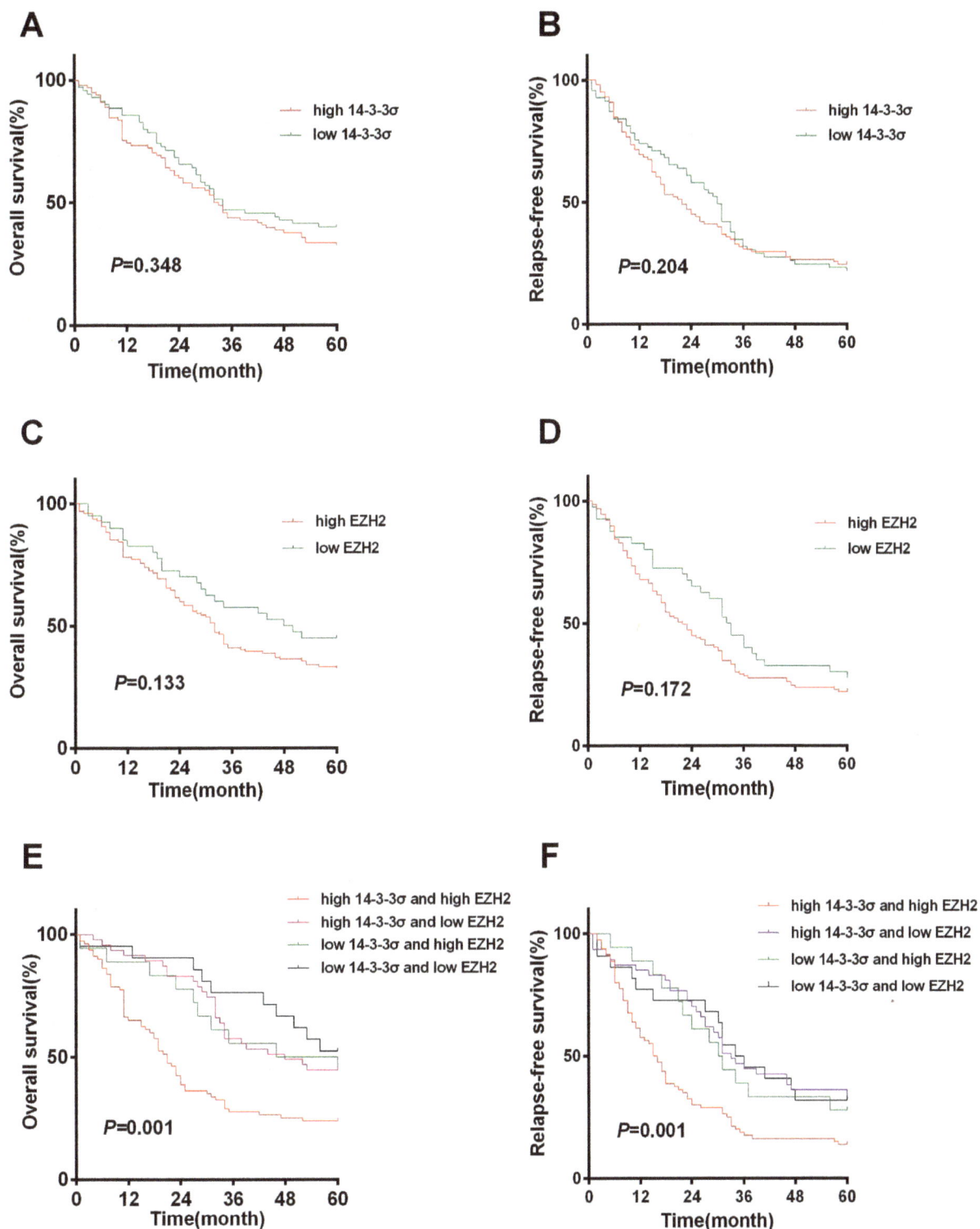

Figure 5. Kaplan-Meier survival curves with regard to disease-free-survival and overall survival according to 14-3-3σ and EZH2 expression. (A) There are no significant differences in OS between patients with positive (32.65%) and negative (40%) staining for 14-3-3σ. (B) There are no significant differences in RFS between patients with positive (24.49%) and negative (21.74%) expressions of 14-3-3σ. (C) There are no significant differences in OS between patients with positive (32.28%) and negative (45%) expressions of EZH2. (D) There are no significant differences in RFS between patients with positive (24.49%) and negative (21.74%) expressions of EZH2. (E) The five-year OS of the coexpressed high 14-3-3σ and EZH2 group were 23.75%, significantly worse than the three other groups ($p<0.05$). (F) The five-year OS of coexpressed high 14-3-3σ and EZH2 group were 23.75%, significantly worse than three other groups ($p<0.05$).

Table 3. Multivariate survival analysis of five-year overall and relapse-free survival in 167 patients with hepatocellular carcinoma.

variable	Overall survival			Relapse-free survival		
	Hazard Ratio	95% confidence interval	P	Hazard Ratio	95% confidence interval	P
Age	0.801	0.437–1.529	0.501	0.865	0.345–2.155	0.748
Gendar	0.937	0.617–1.434	0.752	1.175	0.539–2.601	0.696
Liver cirrhosis	1.558	1.020–2.357	0.035	2.056	1.113–3.766	0.025
etiology	1.554	0.542–4.510	0.424	1.755	0.693–4.434	0.245
AFP	1.241	0.451–2.031	0.490	1.438	0.743–2.743	0.281
Stage	3.358	2.090–5.398	0.001	2.913	1.878–4.698	0.001
size	2.608	1.093–6.211	0.035	2.040	1.062–2.889	0.036
differentiation	1.443	0.969–2.184	0.089	1.454	0.977–2.171	0.074
Vascular invasion	3.505	2.157–5.724	0.000	2.973	1.835–4.825	0.000
14-3-3σ	1.410	0.590–3.353	0.442	1.213	0.604–2.449	0.594
EZH2	1.843	0.645–5.310	0.262	1.993	0.925–4.351	0.082

Multivariate Cox regression analysis

Multivariate analysis showed the following factors to be significantly related to survival: liver cirrhosis, stage, size, and vascular invasion. Multivariate regression analysis indicated that expression of EZH2 and expression of 14-3-3σ were not independent prognostic factors (Table 3).

Discussion

Several reports have noted that EZH2 was over-expressed in most HCC resection tissues by immunohistochemistry, whereas it was negatively expressed in nearly all of the corresponding non-tumor tissues [14,15], which was consistent with our findings. We found that the expression rate of EZH2 was 90% in 167 HCC specimens and that the staining intensity was significantly higher than in liver fibrotic tissues and normal tissues. However, the expression level of 14-3-3σ in our study was inconsistent with an investigation by Norikazu Iwata, whose finding showed 5/19 HCC tissues have 14-3-3σ expression [6]. We found that the expression rate of 14-3-3σ was 71%, significantly higher than 5/19. The reason may be the differences in the number of samples; a sample size of 19 is too small compared to 167 samples in our study. Our findings also suggested that EZH2 and 14-3-3σ may become hopeful biomarkers to distinguish liver cancer from non-tumor tissues.

Although the association between clinicopathological variables and 14-3-3σ has been well documented for gastric cancer [16,17] and breast cancer [18], little is known about the association in liver cancer. We examined the clinicopathological features of 14-3-3σ expression in HCC. We observed no statistically significant association between 14-3-3σ expression and clinicopathological features. Increased expression of EZH2 in HCC has been documented in many studies [19]; our study found that EZH2 expression was closely associated with tumor differentiation and vascular infiltration. These findings are compatible with a previous study in which upregulated EZH2 was shown to be associated with tumor progression, especially facilitating portal vein invasion in human HCC [20]. The association of EZH2 with tumor differentiation may be related to the major biological function of EZH2 which is to maintain the undifferentiated stage of cells [21]. Molecular mechanisms linking high EZH2 expression with increased vascular infiltration in HCC has not been well defined, but Au SL et al. reported that EZH2 overexpression can activate Rho/ROCK signaling by inactivating DLC1 to promote liver metastasis [22].

One important role of EZH2 in cancer is the epigenetic repression of tumor suppressor genes by histone modification and promoter methylation. Emmanuelle et al. demonstrated that EZH2 is required for DNA methylation of EZH2-target promoters via interactions with DNA methyltransferases [23]. Additionally, 14-3-3σ is regarded as tumor suppressor gene that is a negative regulator of the cell cycle G2-M phase checkpoint [24]. Norikazu et al. provide evidence that hypermethylation results in the loss of the 14-3-3σ in HCC [11]. Therefore, we examined whether 14-3-3σ expression is regulated by EZH2. We examined the association between 14-3-3σ and EZH2, and no correlation was found between their expression levels, which indicated the methylation of 14-3-3σ might be controlled by factors other than EZH2.

We also investigated the correlation of EZH2 and 14-3-3σ expression with the prognosis of HCC. Although the OS rate in the 14-3-3σ -negative group was better than the positive group, this difference was not statistically significant. This finding appears to be consistent with previous studies [9]. As a possible explanation, EZH2 expression is strongly associated with prognosis only in patients with malignancies from hormonally regulated tissues, such as breast and prostate [25]. The correlation between 14-3-3σ and prognosis has not been reported to date, and we found no significant differences in the OS and RFS rates between the low and high group. Then, the combination of 14-3-3σ and EZH2 was applied to investigate their correlation with prognosis. Interestingly, the coexistence of 14-3-3σ and EZH2 high groups have the worst survival relative to the other three groups. The presence of 14-3-3σ and p53 overexpression may be considered as a significant predictor of OS and RFS in HCC.

In conclusion, we demonstrated in a large study population with HCC that 14-3-3σ and EZH2 are immunopositive in 71% and 90% of the patients correspondingly. Additionally, we found that 14-3-3σ has no correlation with clinicopathological features and that EZH2 was associated with tumor differentiation and vascular infiltration. Moreover, the presence of 14-3-3σ and EZH2 overexpression identifies a population of patients with an unfavorable prognosis, which can be considered a significant predictor of OS and RFS in HCC. However, the precise function of EZH2 and 14-3-3σ in HCC remains unclear, and further investigation is needed to clarify the relationship between EZH2, 14-3-3σ and HCC progression.

References

1. Okuda K (2000) Hepatocellular carcinoma. J Hepatol 32:225–237.
2. Kino T, Gragerov A, Valentin A, Tsopanomihalou M, Ilyina-Gragerova G, et al. (2005) Vpr protein of human immunodeficiency virus type 1 binds to 14-3-3 proteins and facilitates complex formation with Cdc25C: implications for cell cycle arrest. J Virol 79:2780–2787.
3. Laronga C, Yang HY, Neal C, Lee MH (2000) Association of the cyclin-dependent kinases and 14-3-3 sigma negatively regulates cell cycle progression. J Biol Chem 275:23106–23112.
4. Chan TA, Hermeking H, Lengauer C, Kinzler KW, Vogelstein B (1999) 14-3-3Sigma is required to prevent mitotic catastrophe after DNA damage. Nature 401:616–620.
5. Luo J, Feng J, Lu J, Wang Y, Tang X, et al. (2010)Aberrant methylation profile of 14-3-3 sigma and its reduced transcription/expression levels in Chinese sporadic female breast carcinogenesis. Med Oncol 27:791–797.
6. Iwata N, Yamamoto H, Sasaki S, Itoh F, Suzuki H, et al. (2000) Frequent hypermethylation of CpG islands and loss of expression of the 14-3-3 sigma gene in human hepatocellular carcinoma. Oncogene 19:5298–5302.
7. Cardoso C, Mignon C, Hetet G, Grandchamps B, Fontes M, et al. (2000) The human EZH2 gene: genomic organisation and revised mapping in 7q35 within the critical region for malignant myeloid disorders. Eur J Hum Genet 8:174–180.
8. Sewalt RG, van der Vlag J, Gunster MJ, Hamer KM, den Blaauwen JL, et al. (1998) Characterization of interactions between the mammalian polycomb-group proteins Enx1/EZH2 and EED suggests the existence of different mammalian polycomb-group protein complexes. Mol Cell Biol 18:3586–3595.
9. Cao R, Wang L, Wang H, Xia L, Erdjument-Bromage H, et al. (2002) Role of histone H3 lysine 27 methylation in Polycomb-group silencing. Science 298:1039–1043.
10. Viré E, Brenner C, Deplus R, Blanchon L, Fraga M, et al. (2006) The Polycomb group protein EZH2 directly controls DNA methylation. Nature 439:871–874.
11. Sudo T, Utsunomiya T, Mimori K, Nagahara H, Ogawa K, et al. (2005) Clinicopathological significance of EZH2 mRNA expression in patients with hepatocellular carcinoma. Br J Cancer 92: 1754–1758.
12. Sasaki M, Ikeda H, Itatsu K, Yamaguchi J, Sawada S, et al. (2008) The overexpression of polycomb group proteins Bmi1 and EZH2 is associated with the progression and aggressive biological behavior of hepatocellular carcinoma. Lab Invest 88: 873–882.
13. Bedossa P, Poynard T (1996) An algorithm for the grading of activity in chronic hepatitis C. The METAVIR Cooperative Study Group. Hepatology 24:289–93.
14. Sudo T, Utsunomiya T, Mimori K, Nagahara H, Ogawa K, et al. (2005) Clinicopathological significance of EZH2 mRNA expression in patients with hepatocellular carcinoma. Br J Cancer 92:1754–1758.
15. Sasaki M, Ikeda H, Itatsu K, Yamaguchi J, Sawada S, et al. (2008) The overexpression of polycomb group proteins Bmi1 and EZH2 is associated with the progression and aggressive biological behavior of hepatocellular carcinoma. Lab Invest 88:873–882.
16. Zhou WH, Tang F, Xu J, Wu X, Feng ZY, et al. (2011) Aberrant upregulation of 14-3-3σ expression serves as an inferior prognostic biomarker for gastric cancer. BMC Cancer 11:397.
17. Gheibi A, Kazemi M, Baradaran A, Akbari M, Salehi M (2012) Study of promoter methylation pattern of 14-3-3 sigma gene in normal and cancerous tissue of breast: A potential biomarker for detection of breast cancer in patients. Adv Biomed Res 1:80.
18. Zurita M, Lara PC, del Moral R, Torres B, Linares-Fernández JL, et al. (2010) Hypermethylated 14-3-3-sigma and ESR1 gene promoters in serum as candidate biomarkers for the diagnosis and treatment efficacy of breast cancer metastasis. BMC Cancer 10:217.
19. Hajósi-Kalcakosz S, Dezső K, Bugyik E, Bödör C, Paku S, et al. (2012) Enhancer of zeste homologue 2 (EZH2) is a reliable immunohistochemical marker to differentiate malignant and benign hepatic tumors. Diagn Pathol 7:86.
20. Sudo T, Utsunomiya T, Mimori K, Nagahara H, Ogawa K (2005) Clinicopathological significance of EZH2 mRNA expression in patients with hepatocellular carcinoma. Br J Cancer 92:1754–1758.
21. Pirrotta V (1998) Polycombing the genome: PcG, trxG, and chromatin silencing. Cell 93:333–336.
22. Au SL, Wong CC, Lee JM, Wong CM, Ng IO (2013) EZH2-Mediated H3K27me3 Is Involved in Epigenetic Repression of Deleted in Liver Cancer 1 in Human Cancers. PLoS One 8:e68226.
23. Viré E, Brenner C, Deplus R, Blanchon L, Fraga M (2006) The Polycomb group protein EZH2 directly controls DNA methylation. Nature 439:871–874.
24. Laronga C, Yang HY, Neal C, Lee MH (2000) Association of the cyclin-dependent kinases and 14-3-3 sigma negatively regulates cell cycle progression. J Biol Chem 275:23106–23112.
25. Kleer CG, Cao Q, Varambally S, Shen R, Ota I, et al. (2003) EZH2 is a marker of aggressive breast cancer and promotes neoplastic transformation of breast epithelial cells. Proc Natl Acad Sci U S A 100:11606–11611.

Author Contributions

Conceived and designed the experiments: BT GL. Performed the experiments: YZ YL. Analyzed the data: CL. Contributed reagents/materials/analysis tools: JD. Contributed to the writing of the manuscript: YZ.

5

HBx Inhibits CYP2E1 Gene Expression via Downregulating HNF4α in Human Hepatoma Cells

Hongming Liu[1ⓢ], Guiyu Lou[2ⓢ], Chongyi Li[2], Xiaodong Wang[3,4], Arthur I. Cederbaum[3], Lixia Gan[2]*, Bin Xie[1]*

1 Department of Hepatobiliary Surgery, Daping Hospital & Institute of Surgery Research, The Third Military Medical University, Chongqing, China, 2 Department of Biochemistry and Molecular Biology, The Third Military Medical University, Chongqing, China, 3 Department of Pharmacology and Systems Therapeutics, Icahn School of Medicine at Mount Sinai, New York, New York, United States of America, 4 Chongqing Biomean Technology Co., Ltd, Chongqing, China

Abstract

CYP2E1, one of the cytochrome P450 mixed-function oxidases located predominantly in liver, plays a key role in metabolism of xenobiotics including ethanol and procarcinogens. Recently, down-expression of CYP2E1 was found in hepatocellular carcinoma (HCC) with the majority to be chronic hepatitis B virus (HBV) carriers. In this study, we tested a hypothesis that HBx may inhibit CYP2E1 gene expression via hepatocyte nuclear factor 4α (HNF4α). By enforced HBx gene expression in cultured HepG2 cells, we determined the effect of HBx on CYP2E1 mRNA and protein expression. With a bioinformatics analysis, we found a consensus HNF-4α binding sequence located on -318 to -294 bp upstream of human CYP2E1 promoter. Using reporter gene assay and site-directed mutagenesis, we have shown that mutation of this site dramatically decreased CYP2E1 promoter activity. By silencing endogenous HNF-4α, we have further validated knockdown of HNF-4α significantly decreased CYP2E1expression. Ectopic overexpression of HBx in HepG2 cells inhibits HNF-4α expression, and HNF-4α levels were inversely correlated with viral proteins both in HBV-infected HepG2215 cells and as well as HBV positive HCC liver tissues. Moreover, the HBx-induced CYP2E1 reduction could be rescued by ectopic supplement of HNF4α protein expression. Furthermore, human hepatoma cells C34, which do not express CYP2E1, shows enhanced cell growth rate compared to E47, which constitutively expresses CYP2E1. In addition, the significantly altered liver proteins in CYP2E1 knockout mice were detected with proteomics analysis. Together, HBx inhibits human CYP2E1 gene expression via downregulating HNF4α which contributes to promotion of human hepatoma cell growth. The elucidation of a HBx-HNF4α-CYP2E1 pathway provides novel insight into the molecular mechanism underlining chronic HBV infection associated hepatocarcinogenesis.

Editor: Wang-Shick Ryu, Yonsei University, Republic of Korea

Funding: This work was supported by grants from the National Natural Science Foundation of China (NSFC) No. 30772464, 81372270 (to Bin Xie), and NSFC No. 81270482 (to Lixia Gan). The funders had no role in study design, data collection and analysis, decision to publish, or preparation of the manuscript.

Competing Interests: The authors have declared that no competing interests exist.

* Email: ganlixia@yahoo.com (LG); xiebin313@126.com (BX)

ⓢ These authors contributed equally to this work.

Introduction

Hepatocellular carcinoma (HCC) is the fifth most common cancer globally and the second leading cause of cancer death in China, a country with the largest HCC population in the world [1–3]. The risk factors for HCC have been well defined and included hepatitis virus infection, cirrhosis, and alcohol consumption. More than 50% of HCC patients are Hepatitis B Virus (HBV) carriers, and chronic HBV infection has been regarded as the major etiological factor of HCC [4]. However, the mechanism by which HBV contributes to the development of HCC remains incompletely understood. Increasing evidence suggests that the X protein encoded by HBV genome plays a critical pathogenic role in HCC development [5,6].

Cytochrome P450 2E1 (CYP2E1), a member of the cytochrome P450 mixed-function oxidase system, plays an important role in the metabolism of xenobiotics including ethanol, acetone, drugs and procarcinogens [7,8]. So far, at least 18 families of CYP genes

and 43 subfamilies have been identified [8], which account for almost 75% of the total drug metabolism in humans. CYP2E1 is one of the most abundant isoforms among all P450s [9]. In human liver, CYP2E1 is constitutively expressed and is induced under a wide variety of physiological or pathophysiologic conditions such as alcohol consumption, fasting, obesity and diabetes [10,11]. Regulation of CYP2E1 expression is complex and could occur at transcriptional, translational and post-translational levels [12]. Genetic polymorphism in the 5'- regulatory region of CYP2E1 has also been shown to alter its gene expression [13,14]. Although CYP2E1 has been extensively studied for many years, lots of this research effort has been focused on its role in drug metabolism and alcoholic liver diseases. Therefore, our knowledge of CYP2E1 in HCC is limited. Recently, gene array studies revealed that CYP2E1 was significantly down-expressed in HCC liver tissue [15]. Using a chemical-induced rat HCC model, Man et al showed that CYP2E1 expression declined along with the initiation, promotion and progression of HCC [16]. In clinical specimens from 85 HCC patients, Ho et al. found that 70% of the tumor tissues showed lower expression of CYP2E1, and decreased CYP2E1 is associated with poor prognosis of HCC [17]. These studies suggest that down-regulation of CYP2E1 may play an important role in HCC tumorigenesis. However, the mechanism of CYP2E1downregulation in HCC has so far not been elucidated.

Hepatocyte nuclear factors (HNFs) are liver-enriched transcription factors controlling multiple liver-specific gene expression and maintaining hepatocyte differentiation. These proteins belong to the nuclear hormone receptor superfamily which currently consist HNF1, HNF3, C/EBP, HNF4, and HNF6 [18]. As a key member of the HNF4 family, HNF-4α is indispensable for the hepatic epithelium formation during embryonic development and for epithelial phenotype maintenance of hepatocytes in mature liver [19,20]. Expression of HNF-4α has been found to be at lower levels in HCC tissues compared to para- or non-cancerous liver tissue [21,22]. Loss of HNF-4α accelerates HCC progression [21], whereas introduction of HNF-4α dramatically blocked the development of HCC in rats subjected to diethylinitrosamine administration [23,24]. Thus, HNF-4α has been implicated as a key tumor suppressor in HCC development. Recent studies showed that it also plays important roles in regulating the expression and replication of HBV by stimulating the transcription of HBV pregenomic RNA [25,26]. Overexpression of HNF4α enables replication of the HBV genome even in nonhepatic cell lines [25]. A reduction in the expression of HNF4α in liver cells reduces HBV replication in primary human hepatocytes [27] and in transgenic mice [28]. Currently, it is not clear whether expression of CYP2E1 is regulated by HNF-4α. It is also not known whether HNF-4α expression can be regulated by HBV viral protein in hepatocytes.

In this study, a hypothesis was proposed that HBx may inhibit CYP2E1 gene expression via HNF-4α. We found that ectopic overexpression of HBx inhibits CYP2E1 gene expression via downregulating HNF4α in cultured HepG2 cells and promotes hepatoma cell growth. Furthermore, using proteomics analysis,the changed proteins in the liver tissue from CYP2E1 knockout mice were evaluated. As overexpression of CYP2E1 dramatically inhibits hepatoma cell growth, our observation implies that down-regulation of CYP2E1 during chronic HBV infection may promote hepatocarcinogenesis.

Materials and Methods

Patients and mice tissue samples

Ethical Statement. Informed written consent was obtained from the patients for the collection of liver specimens, and the study protocol was approved by the Medical Ethics Committee in Daping Hospital, the Third Military Medical University.

5 pairs of primary HCC tissues and their adjacent tissues, and 5 cases of non-hepatitis B virus infection liver tissues from liver hemangioma (used as normal liver controls) were obtained from surgical resection in the Department of Hepatobiliary Surgery of the Daping Hospital, the Third Military Medical University. Each tissue was frozen immediately after surgery and stored in liquid nitrogen for later extraction of RNA/DNA and protein. All tumors were independently confirmed as HCC on haematoxylin and eosin (HE) stained sections by two pathologists. 5 cases of HCC tissues and their adjacent tissues, and 5 cases of normal liver tissues were processed into paraffin slides and stained for immunohischemistry.

The mice received humane care, and experiments were carried out according to the criteria outlined in the Guide for the Care and Use of Laboratory Animals and with approval of the Mount Sinai Animal Care and Use Committee.

Materials

Human hepatocarcinoma cell lines HepG2 were maintained by our laboratory. HepG2.2.15, a cell line with HBV DNA sequences chromosomally integrated into HepG2 cells and capable of consistently expressing all the HBV encoded proteins, was kindly provided by the Infection Diseases Center of Southwest Hospital in our university. E47 and C34 cells, two stably transfected HepG2 cell lines harboring CYP2E1 recombinant gene or its empty vector as a control, respectively, were kindly gifts from Dr. Arthur Cederbaum in Mount Sinai Medical Center. The recombinant adenoviruses of AdHNF4α and AdGFP (control) were gifts from Dr. Wei-Fen Xie in the Second Military Medical University. The pGL3- Basic plasmid and the transfection reagent Lipofectamine 2000TM were bought from Invitrogen (USA). pMD18-T vector was purchased from TaKaRa Biotechnology (Dalian Co.). The pCMV-2B–FLAG-X (HBx gene expression vector) was a gift from the Institute of Viral Hepatitis affiliated to Chongqing Medical University. Anti-HBx, -CYP2E1 and –HNF4α antibodies were purchased from Abcam (USA) for both western blotting and immunochemistry.

Cells and cell culture

HepG2 cell lines were maintained in 10% fetal bovine serum (Life Technologies, Inc.) in DMEM (Life Technologies, Inc.) and grown at 37°C in a 5% CO_2 incubator. Before the experiment, cells were trypsinized and inoculated at a density of 1×10^5 cells in a 24-well plate or 4×10^5 cells in a 6-well plate.

Construction for pGL3-CYP2E1 promoter reporter plamids

Human CYP2E1 (Gene ID: 219567) promoter DNA was amplified by PCR using primers listed in Table 1. The 1.4 kilobase pairs of the CYP2E1 promoter DNA was ligated into the pMD18-T vector using T4 DNA ligase and then transformed into E. coli. The pGL3-Basic vector was used to construct the expression vectors by subcloning PCR-amplified DNA of the CYP2E1 promoter into the XhoI/HindIII site of the pGL3-Basic vector (pGL3-CYP2E1-P). Similarly, deletion constructs were synthesized, annealed, and cloned into the EcoRV site in the pMD18-T vector, and then subcloned into pGL3-Basic vector. The PCR products were validated by their size with electrophoresis, and confirmed by DNA sequencing. Ten of the human CYP2E1 promoter constructs harboring sequential deletion of about 100-bp fragments from the 5'-ends were made with the corresponsive primers shown in Table 1.

Western blot analysis

Liver samples from HCC patients and control individuals were processed to protein extraction and analyzed by Western blot. Antibodies against HBx, CYP2E1 or HNF4α were incubated at 4°C overnight, followed by washing 5 min for 3 times with TBST (0.05% Tween-20 in Tris-buffered saline, TBS) and incubation with horseradish peroxidase conjugated secondary antibody (Zhongshan company Co., Beijing, China) for 2 h at room temperature. The membranes were washed again as described above, and the bands were detected by chemiluminescence for visualization. β-actin was used as an internal control. The expression level of CYP2E1 or HBx was represented by the optical density (OD) ratio to β-actin.

Table 1. Primers used for making CYP2E1 promoter luciferase reporter gene constructs.

Construct Name	Sense (5'→3')	Antisense (5'→3')
CYP2E1-P-Luc	CATTGTCAGTTCTCACCTC	GGACACCAGCAGGAGGAAG
CYP2E1-P1-Luc	CAATGACTTGCTTATGTGG	GGACACCAGCAGGAGGAAG
CYP2E1-P2-Luc	CCACAAGTGATTTGGCTGG	GGACACCAGCAGGAGGAAG
CYP2E1-P3-Luc	TGCCAGTTAGAAGACAGAATG	GGACACCAGCAGGAGGAAG
CYP2E1-P4-Luc	CATAGAAGGTGGAAGAGGG	GGACACCAGCAGGAGGAAG
CYP2E1-P5-Luc	CCGGGATCAACAAAGACAAG	GGACACCAGCAGGAGGAAG
CYP2E1-P6-Luc	CTACAGCCAGAATATATACC	GGACACCAGCAGGAGGAAG
CYP2E1-P7-Luc	CTGGGGGCTGCTCAGACAAACC	GGACACCAGCAGGAGGAAG
CYP2E1-P8-Luc	TATGGGTTGGCAACATGTTCCT	GGACACCAGCAGGAGGAAG
CYP2E1-P9-Luc	GTGCTAGCAACCAGGGTGTTGA	GGACACCAGCAGGAGGAAG
CYP2E1-P10-Luc	CTGGGGGCCACCATTGCGGGAA	GGACACCAGCAGGAGGAAG

RNA extraction, reverse transcription (RT) and PCR

Total RNA was isolated from cultured cells by TRIzol (Invitrogen, USA) according to the manufacturer's instructions. Cells were lysed directly in the flasks, and RNA samples were stored at −70°C for later extraction. RNA concentrations were determined by absorbance at 260 nm, and the 260/280 nm absorption ratio of the samples was >1.9. The synthesis of cDNA and amplification of target gene was performed using a one-step RT-PCR kit (Takara, Dalian) using the specific primers listed in Table 2. The cDNA of GAPDH was adopted as an internal standard during RT-PCR analysis.

Real time quantitative PCR

To quantitate the expression of CYP2E1 in human tissues or cultured cells, real time quantitative PCR was also performed. Preparation of RNA and synthesis of cDNA were carried out as described above. PCR amplication was performed with an Applied Biosystems PRISM 7500 Sequence Detector (Applied Biosystems, Foster City, CA, USA), using the Platinum SYBR Green qPCR SuperMix-UDG kit (Invitrogen, Carlsbad, CA, USA). The PCR procedure was heat at 94°C for 5 min followed by 40 cycles of 94°C for 30 s, 57°C 30 s and 72°C 45 s. The level of CYP2E1 expression was expressed as the ratio of CYP2E1 relative to GAPDH levels using the formula of $2^{-\Delta\Delta Ct}$.

CYP2E1 promoter activity assay

HepG2 cells were plated into six-well plates at a density of 10^5 cells/well and grown overnight. The next day, cells were cotransfected with 1 μg of pCMV-2B–FLAG-X plasmid, 1 μg of CYP2E1 promoter luciferase reporter construct, and 1 μg of β-galactosidase reporter plasmid by the lipofectamine method (Invitrogen, USA) in the presence or absence of HBx expression

vector. At 24 h post-transfection, cells were harvested for reporter gene assay. Activities of luciferase or β-galactosidase in the cell lysates were detected using the luciferase/β-galactosidase enzyme assay system (Promega). Luciferase activity was normalized to the β-galactosidase activity and calculated as an average of three independent experiments. To study the effect of HNF4α consensus site on CYP2E1 expression, mutations of this binding site on the CYP2E1 promoter were generated using the Quick Change Site-Directed Mutagenesis Kit (Stratagene, La Jolla, CA), and were named pGL3-mut-HNF4α. Transfection of mutant construct into HepG2 cells were performed as above and controlled to wild-type construct.

HNF4α knockdown by RNA interference

Human HNF4α-specific siRNA (si- HNF4α): 5'-GGCAGUGC-GUGGUGGACAAdTdT-3' and 5'-UUGUCCACCACGCA-CUGCCdGdG-3' and the scrambled control RNA (siNC): 5'-UUCUCCGAACGUGUCACGUdTdT-3' and 5'-ACGUGA-CACGUUCGGAGAAdTdT-3' was provided by GenePharma (Shanghai, China). HepG2 cells were transfected using Lipofectamine RNAiMAX (Invitrogen, USA) following the manufacturer's instructions. After 24 h of transfection with siRNA, the samples were prepared for assays of RT-PCR and western blotting as indicated.

E47 and C34 cell growth test

E47 cells, a human hepatoma cell line that constitutively expresses CYP2E1 (HepG2 cells transfected with plasmid pCI-neo containing CYP2E1 cDNA in the sense orientation), and C34 cells (HepG2 cells transfected with pCI-neo), which do not express CYP2E1 were used as an vitro model to test the effect of CYP2E1 expression level on hepatoma cell growth. E47 and C34 cells with

Table 2. RT-PCR and real-time PCR primers for CYP2E1, HBV RNA and GAPDH.

Genes	Sense (5'→3')	Antisense (5'→3')
CYP2E1	AATGGACCTACCTGGAAGGAC	CCTCTGGATCCGGCTCTCATT
HBV RNA	AGCAATGTCAACGACCGACC	GTGCGCAGACCAATTTATGCC
GAPDH	TCTGCTGATGCCCCCATGTTC	GGATGATGTTCTGGAGAGCCC

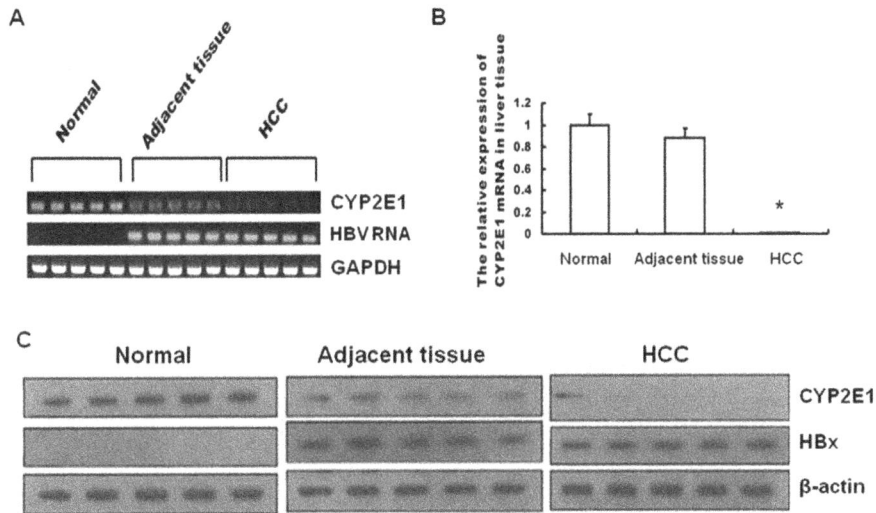

Figure 1. Enhanced HBx expression correlates with lowered CYP2E1 level in livers of HCC patients. (A) CYP2E1 and HBV RNA were determined by RT-PCR using GAPDH as an internal control in surgically resected human normal hepatic tissue, HCC tissue and its adjacent tissues. (B) CYP2E1 mRNA level was detected by real time quantitative PCR. (C) CYP2E1 and HBx protein were measured by Western blotting using β-actin as an internal control. The values were represented as the mean±standard deviation; *, P<0.001 vs. normal tissue or the adjacent tissue.

the same density of 2×10^4 cells/well were seeded in triplicate on 96-well plates and cultured for up to 6 days. Each day, the triplicate of cultured cells was harvested and subjected to CCK-8 assay at 450 nm. The amount of the formazan dye, generated by the activities of dehydrogenases in the HepG2 cells, is directly proportional to the number of living cells.

Caspase-3 activity assay in C34 and E47 cells

Caspase-3 activities were determined in cell lysate by measuring proteolytic cleavage of the proluminescent substrates AC-DEVD-AMC (Calbiochem, La Jolla, CA). The fluorescence was detected to reflect the amount of released AMC (caspase-3, $\lambda ex = 380$, $\lambda em = 460$). The results were expressed as arbitrary units of fluorescence (AUF) per milligram of lysate protein.

In vivo mouse models and liver proteomics analysis

SV129 background CYP2E1 knockout mice were kindly provided by Dr. Frank J Gonzalez (Laboratory of Metabolism, National Cancer Institute, Bethesda, MD), and breeding colonies establoshed at Mount Sinai. SV129 wild type mice were purchased from Charles River Laboratory. Animal experiments were performed in Mount Sinai. Mice used in this study were all males at the age of 8 weeks, with body weight of 20–25 g, and fed with liquid dextrose diet (Bio-Serv, Frenchtown, NJ). When sacrificed, liver tissues were collected and rapidly excised into small fragments and washed with cold saline. With the use of the iTRAQ technique, a multifactorial comparative proteomic study between wild type and CYP2E1 knockout mice can be performed. MALDI plates were analyzed with a TOF/TOF 5800 mass spectrometer (AB Sciex). Functional annotation of protein was conducted using DAVID Bioinformatics Resources 6.7 (NIAID/NIH). For molecular pathway and network analysis of significantly changed proteins, the quantitative data were analyzed using Ingenuity Pathways Analysis (IPA).

Statistical analysis

Data are presented as mean values ± SD. Differences between groups were analyzed by one-way ANOVA (SPSS 10.0 statistical software package, SPSS Inc., Chicago, IL) in all assays. P<0.05 was considered statistically significant.

Results

Enhanced HBx expression correlates with lowered CYP2E1 level in livers of HCC patients

Since previous studies show that viral proteins play a critical role in HCC development, we analyzed the expression levels of HBV RNA and CYP2E1 in liver tissues from HCC patients. 5 pairs of HBV-positive primary HCC tissues, adjacent tissue of HCC and 5 cases of HBV-negative normal liver tissues were freshly resected from surgery. RT-PCR, real-time quantitative PCR, and western blot were performed to measure HBV RNA and CYP2E1 mRNA with a focus on correlation of HBx proteins levels and CYP2E1 amount. Results showed that expression of HBV RNA (Fig. 1A) and HBx protein (Fig. 1C) were higher in HBV-positive HCC livers. Conversely, CYP2E1 mRNA and protein levels were markedly lower compared to those of the normal livers (Fig. 1B and Fig. 1C). The inverse correlations between two proteins suggest that HBx may down-regulate CYP2E1 expression.

Enforced expression of HBx decreases CYP2E1 gene expression in HepG2 cells

To test whether HBx functions to inhibit CYP2E1 expression, a HBx-coding plasmid, pCMV-2B–FLAG-X, was introduced into HepG2 cells via transient transfection. Results showed that ectopic gene transfer increased mRNA of HBx in HepG2 cells (Fig. 2A). Overexpression of HBx significantly lowered CYP2E1 mRNA compared to the non-transfected cells or pGL3 empty vector transfected cells as shown by RT-PCR (P<0.001) (Fig. 2A) and real-time quantitative PCR (Fig. 2B). These results demonstrate that CYP2E1 gene expression can be negatively regulated by HBx at the transcription level.

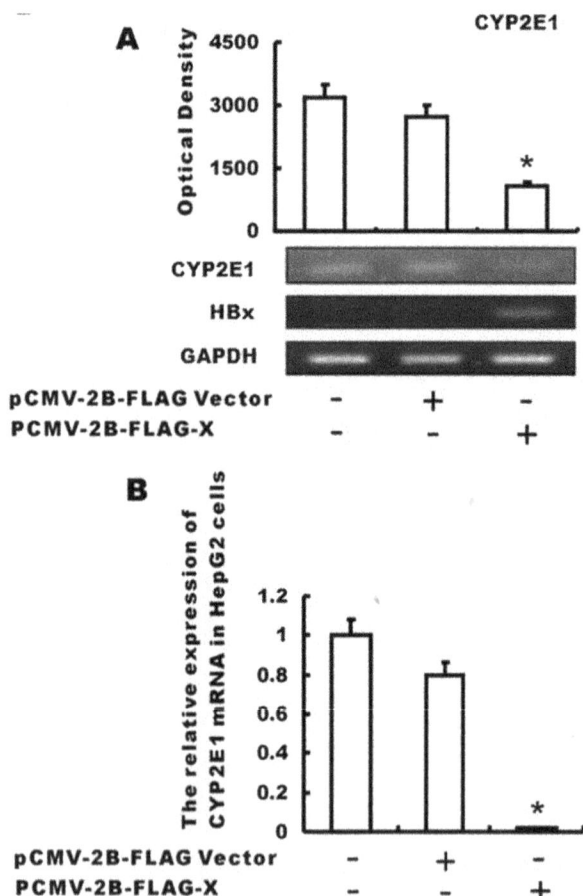

Figure 2. Enforced expression of HBx inhibits CYP2E1 gene expression in HepG2 cells. Plasmid expressing HBx (pCMV-2B–FLAG–X) or a control plasmid (pGL3 empty vector) was transfected into HepG2 cells. (A) Overexpression of HBx significantly inhibited CYP2E1 mRNA compared to the non-transfected cells or pGL3 empty vector transfected cells by RT-PCR with GAPDH as an internal control. (B) Effect of ectopic overexpression of HBx on CYP2E1 mRNA level was determined by real time quantitative PCR in HepG2 cells. The values were represented as the mean standard deviation; *, $P<0.001$ vs. the control group or the empty vector group.

HNF4α plays a crucial role in controlling CYP2E1 expression

To molecularly define how HBx inhibits CYP2E1 expression, the human CYP2E1 promoter ($-1360 \sim +100$) was amplified and cloned onto the luciferase reporter plasmid pGL3 and named as pGL3-CYP2E1-P. Based on this plasmid, a series of pGL3 reporter plasmids harboring various lengths of the 5′-flanking region, spaced at 64–210 base pairs of the human CYP2E1 promoter were constructed and designated as pGL3-CYP2E1-P1 to –P10 (Fig. 3A). HepG2 cells were cotransfected with HBx expression vector and each of the reporter plasmids. As shown in Fig. 3B, HBx significantly inhibits CYP2E1 promoter activity in constructs pGL3-CYP2E1-P1 to –P7, but not pGL3-CYP2E1-P8 to –P10. These results indicate that the 5′-flanking region located at $-483 \sim -274$ base pairs upstream of the human CYP2E1 gene transcriptional start site is required for HBx to repress the human CYP2E1 promoter activity.

To precisely define the transcription factor mediating this inhibition effect, CYP2E1 promoter sequence was subjected to transcription factor binding sites search using an online software of MatInspector professional analysis (http://www.genomatix.de/en/index.html), and a consensus element for HNF4α was found at -318 to -294. As previous studies demonstrated that HNF4α regulates CYP2C9 and CYP2C19 gene expression [29], we tested if this HNF4α consensus site plays a role in CYP2E1 expression. Site-directed mutagenesis was subsequently performed on the construct pGL3-CYP2E1-p7 and the corresponding mutant was designated as pGL3-mut- HNF4α (Fig. 3C). Results showed that mutation of this site disrupted the basal CYP2E1 promoter activity by 77% (Fig. 3D), indicating that this DNA element is critical in controlling CYP2E1 transcription in HepG2 cells. To validate the role of HNF4α in the regulation of CYP2E1 expression, endogenous HNF4α expression was silenced with small interfering RNA (siRNA) in HepG2 cells, and the HNF4α knockdown effects was confirmed both on the mRNA and protein level (Fig. 3E and 3G). CYP2E1 mRNA and protein level markedly decreased when HNF4α was silenced (Fig. 3F and 3G). Together, these results showed that HNF4α plays a crucial role in controlling CYP2E1 expression in hepatocytes.

Down-regulatory effect of HBx on CYP2E1 expression is mediated through HNF4α

As previous studies from animal and clinical tissues showed that HNF4α levels were markedly decreased in HCC liver tissues [21,22], we tested whether infection of HBV affects HNF4α levels in hepatocytes. For this purpose, we turned to HepG2.2.1.5, a cell line with HBV DNA sequences chromosomally integrated into HepG2 cells and capable of consistently expressing all the HBV encoded proteins. Western Blotting showed the stable overexpression of viral protein (HBx) in HepG2.2.15 was inversely correlated with significantly lower levels of HNF4α and CYP2E1 proteins compared to HepG2 cells (Fig. 4A). To confirm the role of viral protein HBx in regulating HNF4α expression, HBx-expression plasmid was transiently expressed into HepG2 cells. Western Blotting showed over-expression of HBx significantly inhibited HNF4α as well as CYP2E1 expression (Fig. 4B). To further validate that the down-regulatory effect of HBx on CYP2E1 gene expression was mediated through HNF-4α, we applied the adenovirus mediated overexpression of HNF-4α(AdHNF4α) with AdGFP as control in the presence or absence of HBx expression plasmid, respectively, in HepG2 cells. Western Blotting showed that CYP2E1 protein levels could be recovered, at least partially, by ectopic supplement of HNF-4α (Fig. 4C). Taken together, these results confirmed that HBx-induced CYP2E1 reduction could be rescued by ectopic supplement of HNF-4α protein expression.

Expression of HNF4α and CYP2E1 inversely correlates with HBV infection in HCC liver tissues

To determine whether HNF4α and CYP2E1 are coordinately regulated in vivo, immunohistochemical (IHC) staining was performed in normal and HCC tissue. Morphological and IHC changes of liver tissues are shown in Fig. 5. HE showed the normal structure of liver tissue (panel 1), adjacent paracarcinoma tissue (panel 2) and typical carcinoma tissue (panel 3). HBx staining showed that normal liver tissue is absent of HBV infection (panel 4), whereas intensive HBx expression was observed in HBV positive HCC liver tissue (panel 6), and expression of HBx was much higher compared to the paracarcinoma area (panel 5). Conversely, HNF-4α levels were inversely correlated with HBx expression (panel 7 to panel 9) and positively correlated with CYP2E1 expression (panel 10 to panel 12). These results provide in vivo evidence for a synergistic change of HNF-4α and CYP2E1 expression under chronic HBV infection in human livers.

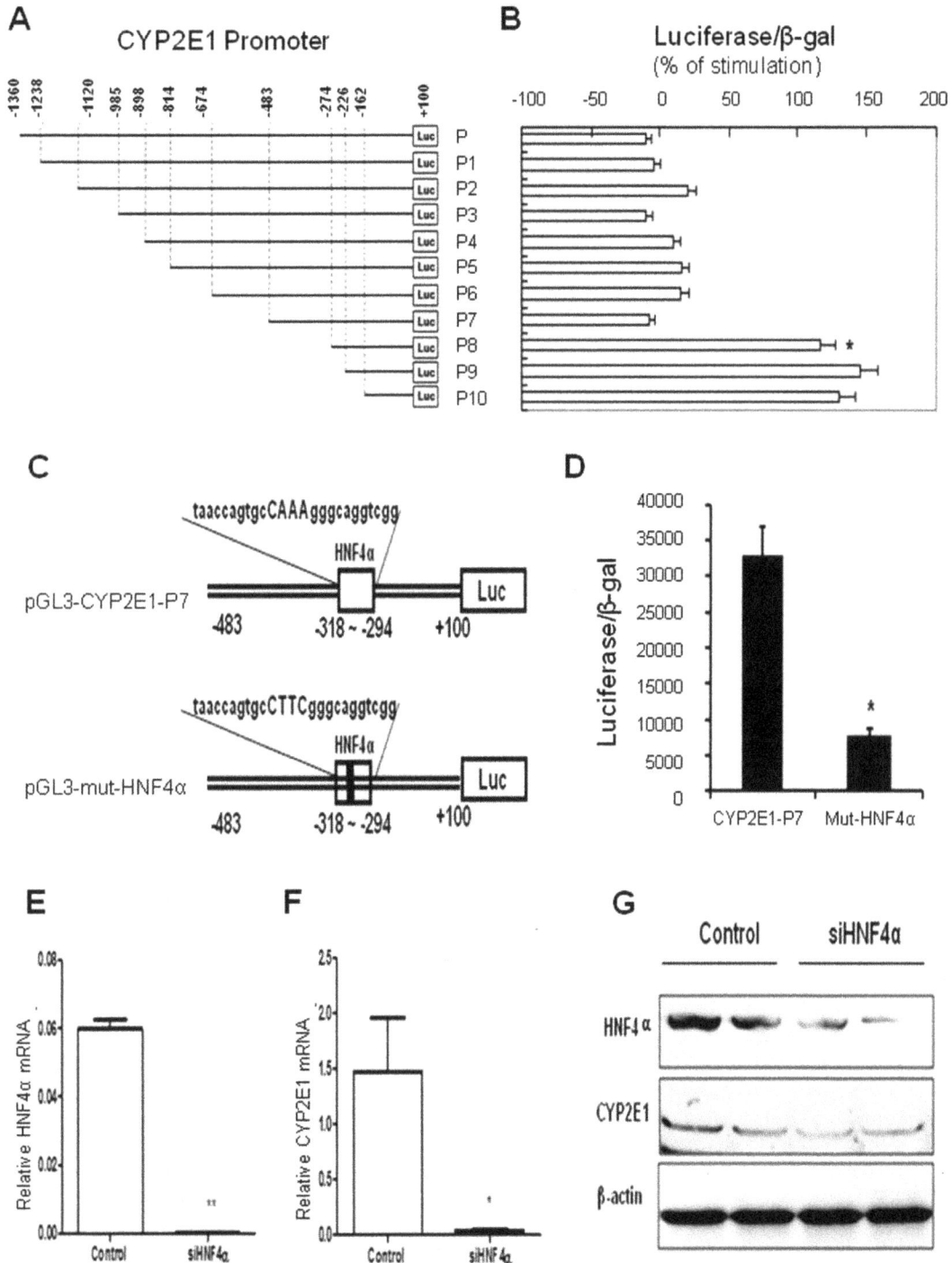

Figure 3. HNF-4α plays a critical role in CYP2E1 gene expression. (A) A schematic depiction of different human CYP2E1 promoter regions cloned into the pGL3-basic plasmid. The constructs were designated as CPY2E1-P-luc and its various deletion constructs CPY2E1-P1-luc to -P10. (B) Effects of HBx overexpression on promoter activities of different CYP2E1 promoter constructs and identification of a specific promoter region localized at −483~−274 bp on the CYP2E1 gene 5′-flanking region upstream of the transcription start site which mediates the inhibition effect of HBx to repress CYP2E1 expression. HepG2 cells were cotransfected with one of the CYP2E1 promoter constructs and HBx expression plasmid or control plasmid. At 24 h post-transfection, cells were harvested for determination of relative luciferase activities. Results are expressed as percent of the corresponding control in the absence of HBx expression and represent mean±standard deviation. Results are expressed as percent of the corresponding untreated control cells and represent as mean±standard deviation; *, P<0.001 vs. construct CPY2E1-P7-luc. (C) Schematic representation of the consensus HNF4α binding element and its mutant forms on the human CYP2E1 gene promoter. Site-directed mutagenesis on HNF4α consensus binding was performed, and the mutant constructs were named pGL3-mut-HNF4α; (D) Effects of HNF4α binding site mutation on CYP2E1 promoter activity. (E–F) Effects of silencing HNF4α on endogenous HNF4α and CYP2E1 mRNA expression by real-time PCR, and (G) on their protein expressions by Western Blotting with β-action as internal control.

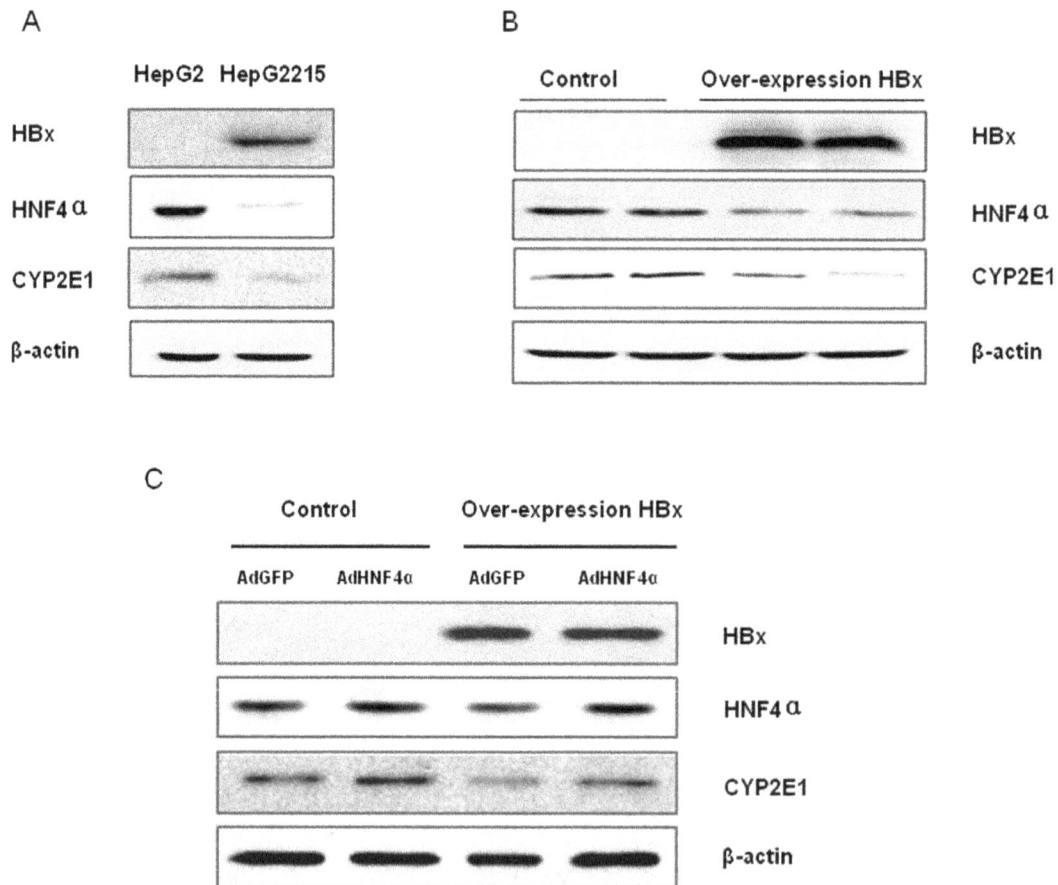

Figure 4. HBx inhibits CYP2E1 expression via downregulation of HNF4α. (A) HBV virus downregulated HNF4α and CYP2E1. HepG2215 cells, a cell line with the HBV genome integrated into the chromosome of HepG2 cells and capable of producing all HBV proteins, was used. Expression of HBx, CYP2E1 and HNF4α levels were measured with Western blotting. (B) Enforced expression of HBx protein downregulates CYP2E1 and HNF4α. HepG2 cells were transiently transfected with HBx-expression plasmid, and 24 hours post transfection, cells were harvested and cell lysate were used to determine HNF4α expression with Western Blotting. (C) HBx-induced CYP2E1 reduction could be rescued by HNF4α. HepG2 cells were transiently transfected with HBx-expression plasmid for 24 hours, then were infected with 1×10^9 plaque-forming units of AdHNF4α, or the same amount of AdGFP as control for one more day, respectively, in HepG2 cells. Cells were harvested and protein expression of HBx, CYP2E1 and HNF4α levels were measured with Western blotting.

Increased CYP2E1 inhibits HepG2 cell growth

In order to understand the consequences of decreased CYP2E1 in hepatocarcinogenesis, we tested the effect of CYP2E1 levels on hepatoma cell growth. E47 cells, a stably transfected HepG2 cell line with CYP2E1 overexpression was compared with C34 cells harboring only empty vector in the same host cell as the control. Cells were loaded with the same amount in 96 wells and were cultured up to 6 days. Cell growth rate was determined each day with a CCK8 kit. Result showed that E47 cells demonstrated significantly lower growth rate compared to C34 cells (Fig. 6A), indicating that the decreased expression of CYP2E1 promotes hepatoma cell growth. As a strong generator of reactive oxygen species (ROS), elevated CYP2E1 expression participates in promoting cell apoptosis [34,35], we tested whether this CYP2E1-induced reduction in cell growth was due to enhanced cell apoptosis. Activities of caspase-3 were determined in C34 and E47 cells post-seeding onto 96-well plates on day 1, 3 and 6. Results showed that activities of caspase-3 were increased in E47 cells compared to C34 cells and the difference was statistically significant on day 6 (Fig. 6B), indicating that decreased cell growth in E47 cells may be attributed, at least in part, to enhanced cell apoptosis.

Impacts of CYP2E1 absence on multiple cellular pathways

To better understand the effects of decreased CYP2E1 on hepatocyte functions at the molecular level, liver tissues from adult CYP2E1-knockout mice were collected and subjected to proteomics analysis to be compared with wild type mice as the control. Principal component analysis (PCA) was conducted with Matlab statistical software. All identified proteins with quantitative data were tested with $p < 0.05$. The quantitative mass spectrometry data from CYP2E1 knockout mice which was compared to control showed that, 23 proteins were significantly increased with the fold > 1.5. Among the up-regulated proteins, 5 are involved in protein synthesis which includes small and large ribosomal proteins as well as initiation factor with 2 of those demonstrating the highest fold change (Table 3). Proteins which are involved in amino acid or carbohydrate catabolism, electron transfer and ATP synthase were also increased, all of which may act to supply increased energy production for protein synthesis. In addition, some of the increased proteins were also those participating in other aspects of liver functions, such as biotransformation or xenobiotics metabolism, serum protein for transportation, and histone as a chromosome constituent. In particular, some of the increased proteins such as

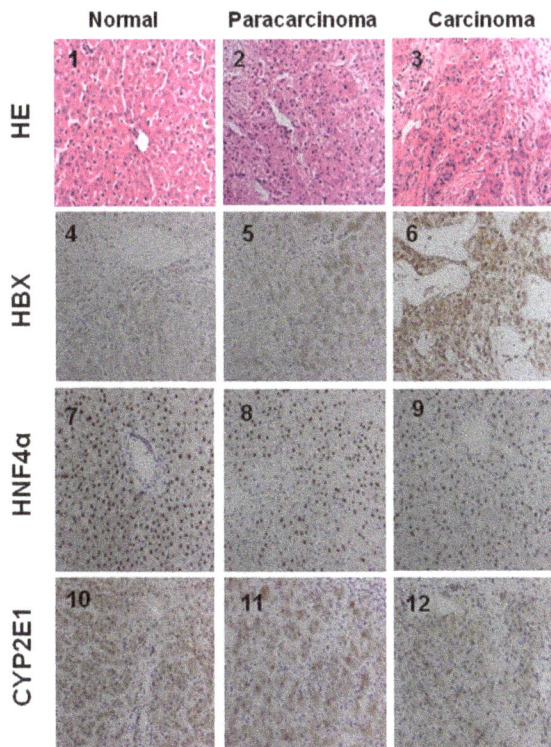

Figure 5. Immunohistochemical staining of HNF4α, CYP2E1 and HBx in human liver tissues. Row 1, morphology observation with HE staining. Row 2, HBx immunochemical staining. Row 3, HNF4α immunochemical staining. Row 4, CYP2E1 immunochemical staining. All HE staining or immunochemical staining were shown as typical fields from five cases of human normal, and five cases of paracarcinoma or HCC liver tissues.

keratins and cdc42 functions to maintain epithelial hepatocyte structure or cell cycle control. Enhanced levels of these proteins were previously shown in HCC [30,31].

On the other hand, 18 proteins were shown to be significantly decreased with the fold<0.5 (Table 4). Among the down-regulated proteins, 2 of the most significantly decreased proteins are CYP2E1 and aldehyde dehydrogenase, both of which were known to be critical players in ethanol metabolism [10]. Notably, among the significantly decreased are 4 proteins encoded by Ogdh, Hadha, Acadm, Hmgcs2, which participating in metabolism of long-chain or medium-chain fatty acids, krebs cycle or ketogenesis. In particular, all of these are mitochondria proteins involved in lipid metabolism. There are also decreases in proteins with functions such as glucose or amino acid metabolism, serum protein and DNA binding proteins.

Discussion

It is well known that CYP2E1 is a highly inducible enzyme whose expression changes under various circumstances. For example, CYP2E1 is induced by acute and chronic alcohol consumption resulting in the enhancement of their metabolism and also induced by ketone bodies such as acetone in diabetic patients [11]. During the biotransformation of exogenous and endogenous compounds by this enzyme, various reactive oxygen species (ROS) are produced which could lead to tissue damages [32,33]. As CYP2E1 is a potent generator of ROS, the finding that CYP2E1 actually decreased in HCC is rather intriguing and may raise a number of questions. First, what is the function of decreased CYP2E1 in HCC development? Over expression of CYP2E1 in HepG2 cells and CYP2E1 knockin mice showed increased oxidative stress and cytotoxicity to the cell and liver injury [33], and stable transfection of CYP2E1 in E47 cells showed increased apoptosis compared to C34 cells upon ethanol treatment [34,35]. In addition, other pathological changes, such increased

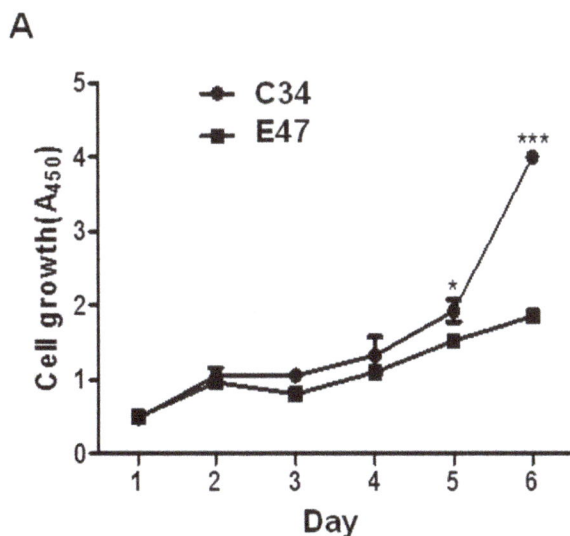

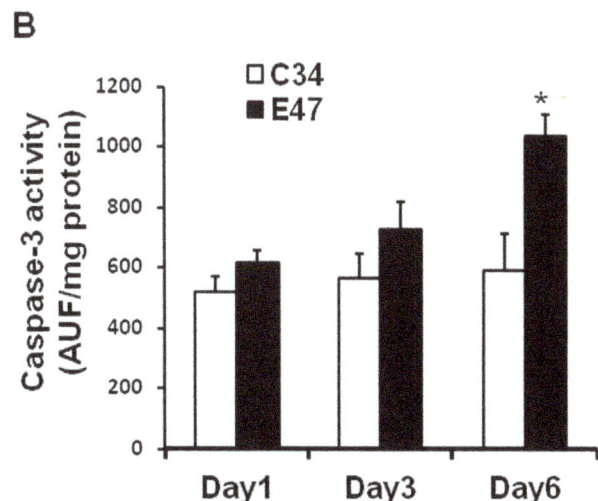

Figure 6. Cell proliferation and caspase-3 activity assay. (A) Stable overexpression of CYP2E1 inhibits the cell growth of HepG2 cells. E47 and C34 cells, two stably transfected HepG2 cell lines harboring CYP2E1 recombinant gene or its empty vector respectively, were seeded with the same number in triplicate on 96-well plates and cultured for up to 6 days. Each day, the triplicate of cultured cells was harvested and subjected to CCK-8 assay at 450 nm. The amount of the formazan dye, generated by the activities of dehydrogenases in cells, is directly proportional to the number of living cells. (B) Activities of caspase-3 increased in HepG2 cells which stably expresses ectopic CYP2E1. E47 and C34 cells were seeded in triplicate on 96-well plates. Cells were harvested on day 1, 3 and 6, and cell lysates were used to test the activities of caspase-3 by measuring proteolytic cleavage of the proluminescent substrates AC-DEVD-AMC. The fluorescence was detected to reflect the amount of released AMC (caspase-3, $\lambda ex = 380$, $\lambda em = 460$). The results were expressed as arbitrary units of fluorescence (AUF) per milligram of lysate protein.

Table 3. Proteomic results: increased.

Accession	Gene Symbol	Protein description	KO/WT
Protein synthesis			
P60843	Eif4a1	Eukaryotic initiation factor 4A–I	99.083
P62849	Rps24	40 S ribosomal protein S24	36.644
P62908	Rps3	40 S ribosomal protein S3	9.036
P14148	Rpl7	60 S ribosomal protein L7	5.495
P47963	Rpl13	60 S ribosomal protein L13	1.770
Protein/amino acid catabolism			
P46471	Psmc2	26 S protease regulatory subunit 7	83.176
Q9QXF8	Gnmt	Glycine N-methyltransferase	4.285
Q8QZR5	Gpt	Alanine amino transferase 1	1.820
Carbohydrate catabolism			
A2AJL3	Fggy	FGGY carbohydrate kinase domain containing protein	84.723
Q91×44	Gckr	Glucokinase regulatory protein	1.977
Electron transfer/energy production			
P03930	Mtatp8	ATP synthase protein 8	9.462
Q9D0M3	Cyc1	Cytochrome c1	6.668
Biotransformation/xenobiotics metabolism			
P24456	Cyp2d10	Cytochrome P450 2D10	11.803
P37040	Por	NADPH–cytochrome P450 reductase	7.447
Q9DBG1	Cyp27a1	Sterol 26-hydroxylase	4.656
Q9DCM2	Gstk1	Glutathione S-transferase kappa 1	3.467
Hepatocyte structure maintenance			
P11679	Krt8	Keratin, type II cytoskeletal 8	12.474
P05784	Krt18	Keratin	5.649
Transport/signaling/chromosome			
Q00724	Rbp4	Retinol-binding protein 4	84.723
P29391	Ftl1	Ferritin light chain 1	9.727
P60766	Cdc42	Cell division control protein 42 homolog	2.938
Q64374	Rgn	Regucalcin	1.542
P62806	Hist1h4a	Histone H4	4.699

The proteins whose levels are increased in CYP2E1 knockout versus wild type (WT) mice and directly related to carbohydrate, protein or amino acid catabolism, or biotransformation are listed. The relative protein expression level in knockout versus wild-type mice (KO/WT) is shown.

ethanol-toxicity and accumulation of fat, were also documented in CYP2E1 knockin mice but not in CYP2E1 knockout mice [36]. Therefore it is reasonable to speculate that decreased level of CYP2E1 may cause lower cytotoxicity and apoptotic rate, thus favoring tumor growth. Indeed, decreased CYP2E1 has been previously shown in rat and human HCC tissues, and associated with poor prognosis of HCC [15–17]. In this study, we have shown that CYP2E1 was decreased in HCC tissues, thus adding further proof for downregulation of CYP2E1 in HCC. We have shown E47 cells with CYP2E1 expression have a significantly lower growth rate compared to C34 cells without ectopic CYP2E1 gene (Figure 6), suggesting that decreased CYP2E1 promotes hepatoma cells growth. With proteomics analysis, we have identified significantly differently expressed liver proteins that have not been previously reported in CYP2E1 knockout mice which may play a role in promoting hepatocarcinogenesis. For example, lack of CYP2E1 in HCC may decrease hepatic metabolism for xenobiotics including ethanol and procarcinogens, and a prolonged effect of this change may predispose liver to

enhanced cytotoxicity. Also, decreased lipid metabolism (as shown in Table 4) may exacerbate liver steatosis and oxidative stress. Meanwhile, enhanced protein synthesis as evident by significant increases of multiple ribosomal proteins and initiation factors (see Table 3) may promote cell growth. Our study thus broadens the current understanding for the role of CYP2E1 in HCC development. The impacts of all these changes associated with lack of CYP2E1 on HCC development are currently unclear and merits further investigation.

How is CYP2E1 downregulated in HCC? It is known that CYP2E1 has been a focus in alcoholic liver diseases which has been intensively investigated in the past two decades. Regulation of this enzyme occurs at transcriptional, post-transcriptional and post-translational levels [12]. Multiple transcriptional factors have been identified to activate the CYP2E1 promoter, such as HNF-1α in rat [37], Sp1 and NF-κB in rabbit [38], and STAT5, STAT6, NFATc1 [39,40] and GATA4 and NR5A2 (fetoprotein transcription factor) in human [41]. In adult animals, CYP2E1 is post-transcriptionally regulated through mRNA and protein stabiliza-

Table 4. Proteomic results: decreased.

Accession	Gene Symbol	Protein description	KO/WT
Biotransformation/xenobiotics metabolism			
Q05421	Cyp2e1	Cytochrome P450 2E1	0.047
Q9CPU0	Glo1	Lactoylglutathione lyase	0.061
P47738	Aldh2	Aldehyde dehydrogenase	0.394
Fatty acid catabolism/ketogenesis			
Q60597	Ogdh	2-oxoglutarate dehydrogenase	0.437
Q8BMS1	Hadha	Trifunctional enzyme subunit alpha	0.258
P45952	Acadm	Medium-chain specific acyl-CoA dehydrogenase	0.251
P54869	Hmgcs2	Hydroxymethylglutaryl-CoA synthase	0.101
Glucose/amino acid metabolism			
Q05920	Pc	Pyruvate carboxylase	0.331
O35490	Bhmt	Betaine–homocysteine S-methyltransferase 1	0.078
O08749	Dld	Dihydrolipoyl dehydrogenase	0.011
P97328	Khk	Ketohexokinase	0.492
Transport/cell motility/chromosome			
Q92I11	Tf	Serotransferrin	0.340
Q60597	Ogdh	2-oxoglutarate dehydrogenase	0.437
P07724	Alb	Serum albumin	0.449
Q8VDD5	Myh9	Myosin-9	0.125
RRsp|A	Ttn	REVERSED Titin	0.011

The proteins whose levels are decreased in CYP2E1 knockout versus wild type (WT) mice and directly related to carbohydrate, lipids, protein or amino acid catabolism, or biotransformation are listed. The relative protein expression level in knockout versus wild-type mice (KO/WT) is shown.

tion [39]. In this study, we have identified HNF-4α as a critical activator controlling CYP2E1 expression. Supported for this concept are: (1) a consensus HNF-4α binding site was found at −318 to −294 bp on the CYP2E1 promoter region; (2) mutation of this site dramatically disrupted CYP2E1 promoter activity; (3) silencing of endogenous HNF-4α in HepG2 cells significantly decreased CYP2E1 expression both at mRNA and protein levels. To the best of our knowledge, this is the first evidence showing that HNF-4α plays a critical role in regulation of CYP2E1 expression. HNF-4 α is one of the critical hepatocyte enriched nuclear factors in the maintenance of liver architecture and function, and down-regulation of which has been repeatedly shown in rodent and human HCC [21,22]. Importantly, forced expression of HNF-4α dramatically inhibits the epithelial mesenchymal transition (EMT) of hepatocyte, generation of the cancer stem/progenitor cells [23] and proliferation of HCC cells, thus preventing hepatocarcinogenesis in rats [23,24]. Therefore, identification of CYP2E1 as a new target of HNF-4α expands our understanding for its function in HCC.

What provokes HNF-4α downregulation in HCC? As the majority of chronic hepatitis and cirrhosis patients are at high risk of liver cancer, substantial evidence has revealed that HBV proteins, in particular HBx, play an important role in the development of HCC. Several studies showed that HNF4α promotes HBV replication by binding to the core promoter of virus genes [25]. On the other hand, expression of HNF4α differs with different outcome of HBV infection, being significantly higher in patients with severe hepatitis B(SHB) than those with chronic hepatitis B(CHB) and liver cirrhosis(LC) [26], two well-established risks factors for CHB-associated hepatocarcinogenesis. In the current study, we demonstrated that HNF-4α was decreased by enforced expression of HBx in cultured HepG2 cells, and that the level of HNF-4α was significantly lower in HepG2.2.15 cell line and in HBV positive human HCC liver tissues. Our results thus identify HNF-4α as a mediator for chronic HBV infection-associated CYP2E1 down-regulation in promoting HCC development.

As chronic HBV infection is also associated with hepatic inflammation, and there is decreased expression of CYP2E1 by pro-inflammatory cytokines, such as IL-1β, IL-6 and TNF-α [42,43], the possibility of its downregulation by HBV-induced immune responses cannot be excluded. In addition, HBV is known to encode four major proteins, HBs, HBc, HBp and HBx. HBs has also been suggested to play a pathogenic role in HCC [44]. Whether HNF-4α and CYP2E1 can be downregulated by HBs is yet to be determined. The increased CYP2E1 levels in para-cancerous HCC tissue have been suggested to promote tissue damage and cancerous transformation possibly due to increased production of ROS [17]. Therefore, functions of CYP2E1 at different stage in the development of HCC merits more detailed investigation.

In addition, previous study in liver-specific HNF4α knockout mouse model proved that HNF4α plays a critical role in controlling a subset of sexually dimorphic P450 gene expression via the altered expression of liver transcription factors both positively for HNF1α, C/EBPα, and C/EBPβ and negatively for HNF3α, HNF3β, HNF6 and the HNF4α coactivator PGC-1α [45]. Besides, androgen pathway was demonstrated in vitro and in vivo to increase HBV transcription, including HBx mRNA synthesis and subsequent protein expression [46–48]. Therefore, the findings of HBx/HNF4α/CYP2E1 pathway proposed in this study may be differently modulated by sex hormones. Future studies of the molecular mechanism(s) for HNF4α and other liver factors in regulation of CYP2E1 expression in condition of HBV infection should include both genders, which may help to better understand the gender disparity in HBV-related HCC.

In conclusion, our results demonstrate that CYP2E1 is controlled by HNF-4α, and both of these proteins are down-regulated by HBx. Elucidation of the novel pathway of HBx/ HNF-4α/CYP2E1 might provide insight into molecular mecha-

nisms for hepatocarcinogenesis, particularly, under chronic HBV infection.

Author Contributions

Conceived and designed the experiments: BX LG. Performed the experiments: HL GL CL XW. Analyzed the data: BX LG HL GL. Contributed reagents/materials/analysis tools: AC. Contributed to the writing of the manuscript: BX LG AC.

References

1. Schutte K, Bornschein J, Malfertheiner P (2009) Hepatocellular carcinoma epidemiological trends and risk factors. Dig Dis 27: 80–92.
2. El-Serag HB, Rudolph KL (2007) Hepatocellular carcinoma: epidemiology and molecular carcinogenesis. Gastroenterology 132: 2557–2576.
3. Chen M, Therneau T, Orsini LS, Qiao YL (2011) Design and rationale of the HCC BRIDGE study in China: a longitudinal, multicenter cohort trial in hepatocellular carcinoma. *BMC* Gastroenterol 11: 53–60.
4. Kew MC (2010) Epidemiology of chronic hepatitis B virus infection, hepatocellular carcinoma, and hepatitis B virus-induced hepatocellular carcinoma. Pathol Biol (Paris) 58: 273–277.
5. Brechot C, Kremsdorf D, Soussan P, Pineau P, Dejean A, et al. (2010) Hepatitis B virus (HBV)-related hepatocellular carcinoma (HCC): molecular mechanisms and novel paradigms. Pathol Biol (Paris) 58: 278–287.
6. Ng SA, Lee C (2011) Hepatitis B virus X gene and hepatocarcinogenesis. J Gastroenterol 46: 974–990.
7. Cederbaum AI (2010) Role of CYP2E1 in ethanol-induced oxidant stress, fatty liver and hepatotoxicity. Dig Dis 28: 802–811.
8. Wang JF, Chou KC (2010) Molecular modeling of cytochrome P450 and drug metabolism. Curr Drug Metab 11: 342–346.
9. Bie'che I, Narjoz C, Asselah T, Vacher S, Marcellin P, et al. (2007) Reverse transcriptase-PCR quantification of mRNA levels from cytochrome (CYP)1, CYP2 and CYP3 families in 22 different human tissues. Pharmacogenet Genomics 17: 731–742.
10. Cederbaum AI (2012) Alcohol metabolism. Clin Liver Dis 16: 667–685.
11. Wang Z, Hall SD, Maya JF, Li L, Asghar A, et al. (2003) Diabetes mellitus increases the in vivo activity of cytochrome P450 2E1 in humans. Br J Clin Pharmacol 55: 77–85.
12. Novak RF, Woodcroft KJ (2000) The alcohol-inducible form of cytochrome P450 (CYP2E1): role in toxicology and regulation of expression. Arch Pharm Res 23: 267–282.
13. Hayashi S, Watanabe J, Kawajiri K (1991) Genetic polymorphisms in the 5′-flanking region change transcriptional regulation of the human cytochrome P450IIE1 gene. J Biochem 110: 559–565.
14. Zeng T, Guo FF, Zhang CL, Song FY, Zhao XL, et al. (2013) Roles of cytochrome P4502E1 gene polymorphisms and the risks of alcoholic liver disease: a meta-analysis. PLoS One 8: e54188.
15. Kinoshita M, Miyata M (2002) Underexpression of mRNA in human hepatocellular carcinoma focusing on eight loci. Hepatology 36: 433–438.
16. Man XB, Tang L, Qiu XH, Yang LQ, Cao HF, et al. (2004) Expression of cytochrome P4502E1 gene in hepatocellular carcinoma. World J Gastroenterol 10: 1565–1568.
17. Ho JC, Cheung ST, Leung KL, Ng IO, Fan ST (2004) Decreased expression of cytochrome P450 2E1 is associated with poor prognosis of hepatocellular carcinoma. Int J Cancer 111: 494–500.
18. Schrem H, Klempnauer J, Borlak J (2002) Liver-enriched transcription factors in liver function and development. Part I: the hepatocyte nuclear factor network and liver-specific gene expression. Pharmacol Rev 54: 129–158.
19. Parviz F, Matullo C, Garrison WD, Savatski L, Adamson JW, et al. (2003) Hepatocyte nuclear factor 4α controls the development of a hepatic epithelium and liver morphogenesis. Nat Genet 34: 292–296.
20. Battle MA, Konopka G, Parviz F, Gaggl AL, Yang C, et al. (2006) Hepatocyte nuclear factor 4α orchestrates expression of cell adhesion proteins during the epithelial transformation of the developing liver. Proc Natl Acad Sci U S A 103: 8419–8424.
21. Lazarevich NL, Cheremnova OA, Varga EV, Ovchinnikov DA, Kudrjavtseva EI, et al. (2004) Progression of HCC in mice is associated with a downregulation in the expression of hepatocyte nuclear factors. Hepatology 39: 1038–1047.
22. Lazarevich NL, Shavochkina DA, Fleishman DI, Kustova IF, Morozova OV, et al. (2010) Deregulation of hepatocyte nuclear factor 4 (HNF4) as a marker of epithelial tumors progression. Exp Oncol 32: 167–171.
23. Ning BF, Ding J, Yin C, Zhong W, Wu K, et al. (2010) Hepatocyte nuclear factor 4 alpha suppresses the development of hepatocellular carcinoma. Cancer Res 70: 7640–7651.
24. Yin C, Lin Y, Zhang X, Chen YX, Zeng X, et al. (2008) Differentiation therapy of hepatocellular carcinoma in mice with recombinant adenovirus carrying hepatocyte nuclear factor-4alpha gene. Hepatology 48: 1528–1539.
25. Long Y, Chen E, Liu C, Huang F, Zhou T, et al. (2009) The correlation of hepatocyte nuclear factor 4 alpha and 3 beta with hepatitis B virus replication in the liver of chronic hepatitis B patients. J Viral Hepat 16: 537–546.
26. Chen EQ, Sun H, Feng P, Gong DY, Liu C, et al. (2012) Study of the expression levels of Hepatocyte nuclear factor 4 alpha and 3 beta in patients with different outcome of HBV infection. Virol J 9: 23–28.
27. Hösel M, Quasdorff M, Wiegmann K, Webb D, Zedler U, et al. (2009) Not interferon, but interleukin-6 controls early gene expression in hepatitis B virus infection. Hepatology 50: 1773–1782.
28. Li L, Oropeza CE, Sainz B Jr, Uprichard SL, Gonzalez FJ, et al. (2009) Developmental regulation of hepatitis B virus biosynthesis by hepatocyte nuclear factor 4alpha. PLoS One 4: e5489.
29. Chen Y, Goldstein JA (2009) The transcriptional regulation of the human CYP2C genes. Curr Drug Metab 10: 567–578.
30. Lee CW, Kuo WL, Yu MC, Chen TC, Tsai CN, et al. (2013) The expression of cytokeratin 19 in lymph nodes was a poor prognostic factor for hepatocellular carcinoma after hepatic resection. World J Surg Oncol 11: 136–147.
31. Chen YW, Chu HC, Lin ZS, Shiah WJ, Chou CP, et al. (2013) P16 Stimulates CDC42-dependent migration of hepatocellular carcinoma cells. PLoS One 8: e69389.
32. Cederbaum AI, Lu Y, Wu D (2009) Role of oxidative stress in alcohol-induced liver injury. Arch Toxicol 83: 519–548.
33. Lu Y, Wu D, Wang X, Ward SC, Cederbaum AI (2010) Chronic alcohol-induced liver injury and oxidant stress are decreased in cytochrome P4502E1 knockout mice and restored in humanized hepatic cytochrome P4502E1 knock-in mice. Free Radic Biol Med 49: 1406–1416.
34. Chen Q, Galleano M, Cederbaum AI (1997) Cytotoxicity and apoptosis produced by arachidonic acid in Hep G2 cells overexpressing human cytochrome P4502E1. J Biol Chem 272: 14532–14541
35. Wu D, Cederbaum AI (1999) Ethanol-induced apoptosis to stable HepG2 cell lines expressing human cytochrome P-4502E1. Alcohol Clin Exp Res 23: 67–76
36. Wu D, Cederbaum AI (2013) Inhibition of autophagy promotes CYP2E1-dependent toxicity in HepG2 cells via elevated oxidative stress, mitochondria dysfunction and activation of p38 and JNK MAPK. Redox Biol 1: 552–565
37. Liu SY, Gonzalez FJ (1995) Role of the liver-enriched transcription factor HNF-1 alpha in expression of the CYP2E1 gene. DNA Cell Biol 14: 285–293.
38. Peng HM, Coon MJ (2000) Promoter function and the role of cytokines in the transcriptional regulation of rabbit CYP2E1 and CYP2E2. Arch Biochem Biophys 382: 129–137.
39. Gonzalez FJ, Gelboin HV (1990) Transcriptional and posttranscriptional regulation of CYP2E1, an N-nitrosodimethylamine demethylase. Princess Takamatsu Symp 21: 157–164.
40. Wang J, Hu Y, Nekvindova J, Ingelman-Sundberg M, Neve EP (2010) IL-4-mediated transcriptional regulation of human CYP2E1 by two independent signaling pathways. Biochem Pharmacol 80: 1592–1600.
41. Akiyama TE, Gonzalez FJ (2003) Regulation of P450 genes by liver-enriched transcription factors and nuclear receptors. Biochim Biophys Acta 1619: 223–234.
42. Abdel-Razzak Z, Loyer P, Fautrel A, Gautier JC, Corcos L, et al. (1993) Cytokines down-regulate expression of major cytochrome P-450 enzymes in adult human hepatocytes in primary culture. Mol Pharmacol 44: 707–715.
43. Hakkola J, Hu Y, Ingelman-Sundberg M (2003) Mechanisms of down-regulation of CYP2E1 expression by inflammatory cytokines in rat hepatoma cells. J Pharmacol Exp Ther 304: 1048–1054.
44. Hsu JL, Chuang WJ, Su IJ, Gui WJ, Chang YY, et al. (2013) Zinc-dependent interaction between JAB1 and pre-S2 mutant large surface antigen of hepatitis B virus and its implications for viral hepatocarcinogenesis. J Virol 87: 12675–12684.
45. Wiwi CA, Gupte M, Waxman DJ (2004) Sexually dimorphic P450 gene expression in liver-specific hepatocyte nuclear factor 4alpha-deficient mice. Mol Endocrinol 18: 1975–1987.
46. Wang SH, Yeh SH, Lin WH, Wang HY, Chen DS, et al. (2009) Identification of androgen response elements in the enhancer I of hepatitis B virus: a mechanism for sex disparity in chronic hepatitis B. Hepatology 50: 1392–1402.
47. Wu MH, Ma WL, Hsu CL, Chen YL, Ou JH, et al. (2010) Androgen receptor promotes hepatitis B virus-induced hepatocarcinogenesis through modulation of hepatitis B virus RNA transcription. Sci Transl Med 2: 32ra35.
48. Tian Y, Kuo CF, Chen WL, Ou JH (2012) Enhancement of hepatitis B virus replication by androgen and its receptor in mice. J Virol 86: 1904–1910.

6

TIMP-3 Expression Associates with Malignant Behaviors and Predicts Favorable Survival in HCC

Xuefeng Gu[1,9], Maoying Fu[1,9], Yuqin Ding[1], Huihui Ni[1], Wei Zhang[1], Yanfang Zhu[1], Xiaojun Tang[2], Lin Xiong[3], Jiang Li[4], Liang Qiu[4], Jiaren Xu[5]*, Jin Zhu[2,6]*

1 Department of Infectious Diseases, The First People's Hospital of Kunshan Affiliated with Jiangsu University, Suzhou, China, 2 The Key Laboratory of Cancer Biomarkers, Prevention & Treatment Cancer Center and The Key Laboratory of Antibody Technique of Ministry of Health, Nanjing Medical University, Nanjing, China, 3 Department of Pathology, The Second Affiliated Hospital of Nanjing Medical University, Nanjing, China, 4 Department of Pathology, Jiangsu Province Geriatric Institute, Nanjing, China, 5 Department of Hematology and Oncology, Jiangsu Provincial Hospital, Nanjing, China, 6 Huadong Medical Institute of Biotechniques, Nanjing, China

Abstract

The tissue inhibitors of metalloproteinases (TIMPs) are proteins that specifically inhibit the proteolytic activity of the matrix metalloproteinases (MMPs). TIMP-3, the only member of the TIMPs that can tightly bind to the extracellular matrix, has been identified as a unique tumor suppressor that demonstrates the ability to inhibit tumor angiogenesis, invasion, and metastasis. This study aimed to detect the expression of TIMP-3 in hepatocellular carcinoma (HCC) and investigate the association between TIMP-3 expression and its clinicopathological significance in HCC patients. In the current study, reverse transcription-polymerase chain reaction (RT-PCR) and Western blotting of HCC cell lines and one-step quantitative reverse transcription PCR (qPCR) and immunohistochemistry (IHC) analyses in HCC tissues were performed, to characterize the TIMP-3 expression. Kaplan-Meier survival and Cox regression analyses were utilized to evaluate the prognosis of 101 HCC patients. The results showed that the expression of TIMP-3 in HCC was significantly decreased relative to that of non-cancerous cells and tissues. Furthermore, the TIMP-3 expression was statistically associated with malignant behaviors of HCC, including portal vein invasion (p = 0.036) and lymph node metastasis (p = 0.030). Cox regression analysis revealed that TIMP-3 expression was an independent prognostic factor for disease-free survival (p = 0.039) and overall survival (p = 0.049). These data indicate that TIMP-3 expression is a valuable prognostic biomarker for HCC and that TIMP-3 expression suggests a favorable prognosis for HCC patients.

Editor: William B. Coleman, University of North Carolina School of Medicine, United States of America

Funding: The authors received no specific funding for this work.

Competing Interests: The authors have declared that no competing interests exist.

* Email: xujiaren@tom.com (JRX); zhujin1968@njmu.edu.cn (JZ)

⑨ These authors contributed equally to this work.

Introduction

Hepatocellular carcinoma (HCC), the most common primary malignancy of the liver, represents one of the leading causes of cancer mortality worldwide, with over 20,000 deaths in the United States in 2013 [1]. Most HCC cases develop in East and Southeast Asia, however, as China alone accounts for more than 50% of newly diagnosed cases globally (approximately 400,000 cases) [2,3] and the township of Qidong in the Jiangsu Province in China is one of the highest endemic regions for HCC in the entire world [4]. HCC tumorigenesis is a multistep process, and various factors are associated with HCC development, including hepatitis B (HBV) and hepatitis C (HCV) viral infections, chronic alcohol consumption and nonalcoholic fatty liver disease [5,6]. Despite various therapeutic strategies for HCC treatment that have improved in the last two decades, such as surgical resection, radiofrequency, microwave ablation, chemotherapy, and transplantation, HCC remains a highly fatal disease because of the high recurrence and metastasis rates [7]; the overall 5-year survival rate of HCC patients has recently been reported to be only 16% [8].

Given the poor prognosis for patients with HCC and the complexity of outcome prediction, it is vital to identify useful prognostic factors for HCC in order to optimize the therapeutic approach for each case.

The tissue inhibitors of metalloproteinases (TIMPs) are proteins that specifically inhibit the proteolytic activity of matrix metalloproteinases (MMPs), and they have been generally recognized as potential suppressors of angiogenesis and tumorigenesis [9,10]. Among the TIMPs, TIMP-3 has been identified as a unique tumor suppressor and is the only member of the TIMPs that could tightly bind to the extracellular matrix. TIMP-3 has been demonstrated to inhibit tumor angiogenesis, invasion, and metastasis [11–13]. TIMP-3 promotes apoptosis in tumor cells through the stabilization of cell surface death receptors and the activation of caspase-8 [14]. Additionally, a large number of clinical studies have evaluated TIMP-3 expression and its clinical significance in a variety of malignant tumors [15–17]. Reduced TIMP-3 expression was associated with poor outcomes in esophageal adenocarcinoma and lung cancer patients [18–20]. The above data suggest that TIMP-3 operates as a tumor suppressor and that the inhibition of

TIMP-3 expression indicates poor survival in human cancer. However, an early report suggested a positive relationship between TIMP-3 promoter methylation and better survival in lung cancer patients [21], and high TIMP-3 expression has been linked to an unfavorable prognosis in head and neck cancer [22]. Hence, the prognostic value of TIMP-3 in human cancers, including HCC, needs to be further elucidated.

In this study, we detected TIMP-3 expression in HCC cell lines via reverse transcription-polymerase chain reaction (RT-PCR) and Western blotting analyses. Furthermore, we examined the TIMP-3 expression in HCC tissues with one-step quantitative-polymerase chain reaction (qPCR) and immunohistochemistry (IHC) analysis of a tissue microarray (TMA). Finally, we evaluated the correlation of TIMP-3 expression with the clinicopathologic features and prognostic significance in HCC.

Materials and Methods

Ethics statement

The Ethics Committee of Nanjing Medical University and each local hospital approved the study protocol. Written informed consent was acquired from all of the patients who were enrolled in this study.

Cell lines

Four HCC cell lines (BEL-7402, SMMC-7721, HepG2 and SK-HEP-1), and one human liver cell line (LO-2) were purchased from the cell bank of the Chinese Academy of Science (Shanghai, China). All cells were cultured in DMEM medium (Gibco, Invitrogen, Carlsbad, CA, USA) supplemented with 10% fetal bovine serum (FBS; Gibco), penicillin (100 U/mL) and strepto-mycin (100 µg/mL).

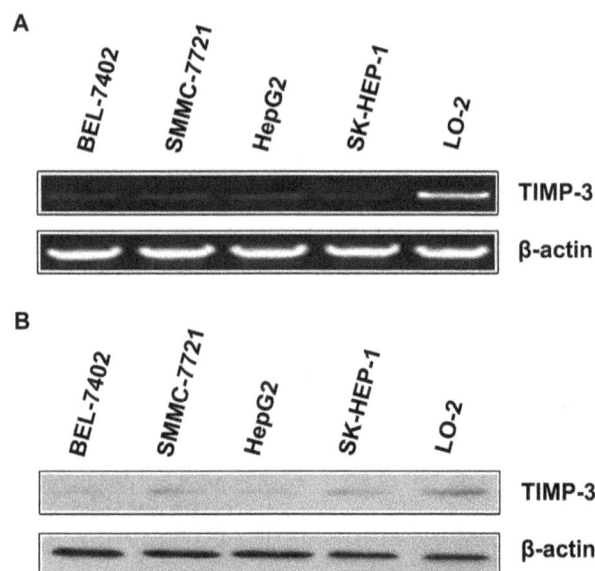

Figure 1. TIMP-3 expression in four hepatocellular carcinoma (HCC) cell lines and one non-cancerous cell line. A. Reverse transcription-polymerase chain reaction (RT-PCR) revealed that TIMP-3 mRNA expression in HCC cell lines was detected at a low intensity when compared to TIMP-3 expression in the human liver cell line, LO-2. B. Western blotting illustrated that TIMP-3 protein expression in the HCC cell lines BEL-7402, SMMC-7721, HepG2 and SK-HEP-1 are decreased relative to the non-cancerous human liver cell line LO-2.

Patient tissue samples

A total of 20 fresh HCC tissues and corresponding adjacent non-cancerous tissues were obtained for this study from the Affiliated Hospital of Nantong University and the First People's Hospital of Kunshan, affiliated with Jiangsu University. Archival tissue samples (101 formalin-fixed, paraffin-embedded HCC tissues and 100 matched tumor-adjacent normal tissues) were obtained from the Affiliated Hospital of Nantong University and the First People's Hospital of Kunshan, affiliated with Jiangsu University, dating from 2003 to 2010. Before surgical therapy, none of the patients had received neoadjuvant chemotherapy, radiation therapy or immunotherapy. Representative and impor-tant clinical data, such as gender, age, tumor size, hepatitis B virus (HBV) infection, liver cirrhosis, pathological grade, portal vein invasion, lymph node metastasis, distant metastasis and TNM stage, were collected for further analyses. The TNM stage of all HCC samples was confirmed according to the 2002 American Joint Committee on Cancer/International Union Against Cancer TNM staging system [23].

RT-PCR and Western blotting analysis in HCC cell lines

For RT-PCR testing, total RNA was extracted from four HCC cell lines (BEL-7402, SMMC-7721, HepG2 and SK-HEP-1) and one human liver cell line (LO-2) using the Trizol reagent (Life Technologies, Inc., Grand Island, NY, USA) according to the manufacturer's guidelines. The prepared RNA (5 µg) was mixed with oligo-dT primers and reverse-transcribed with MMLV reverse transcriptase (Promega, USA). The primers for TIMP-3 were as follows: forward primer 5'- TCT GCA ACT CCG ACA TCG T-3'; reverse primer 5'- TTG GTG AAG CCT CGG TAC AT-3'. β-actin was used as a loading control, and the primers for β-actin were as follows: forward 5'- CTC CAT CCT GGC CTC GCT GT-3', reverse 5'- GCT GCT ACC TTC ACC GTT CC-3'. PCR amplification was executed in 20 µL using a thermocycler (Biometra, Germany). Total RNA extraction, amplification conditions and RT-PCR procedures were described in our previous publication [24,25].

For Western blotting analysis, the cells were washed and lysed with cell lysis buffer. Equal amounts of proteins were separated by 10% SDS-PAGE and transferred onto nitrocellulose membranes. The membranes were first incubated with primary anti-TIMP-3 antibody (Abcam, Cambridge, MA, USA), then a secondary antibody, and finally detected with an ECL kit and autoradiog-raphy using X-ray film. β-actin blotting was used as an internal control.

One-step qPCR test and IHC analysis in HCC tissues

For qPCR analysis, 20 fresh HCC tissues and corresponding adjacent non-cancerous tissues were collected. Total RNA was extracted from HCC tissues and non-cancerous tissues following the protocols mentioned above. The glyceraldehyde 3-phosphate dehydrogenase (GAPDH) mRNA level was used to standardize the measurements of the target gene and, with the primers for GAPDH as follows: forward primer 5'-TGC ACC ACC AAC TGC TTA GC-3'; reverse primer 3'-GGC ATG GAC TGT GGT CAT GAG-5'. A SensiMixTM One-Step Kit (Quantace, Berlin, Germany) was used to execute qPCR analysis with a real time PCR system (Bio-Rad Laboratories, Hercules, CA, USA). The one-step qPCR procedure was described in our previous publication [26].

For IHC analysis, 101 HCC tissues and matched non-cancerous tissues were prepared and arranged in a TMA by Alenabio Biotech Co., Ltd (Xi'an, China). The TMA was cut into 4 µm-thick sections and placed on Superfrost charged glass microscope

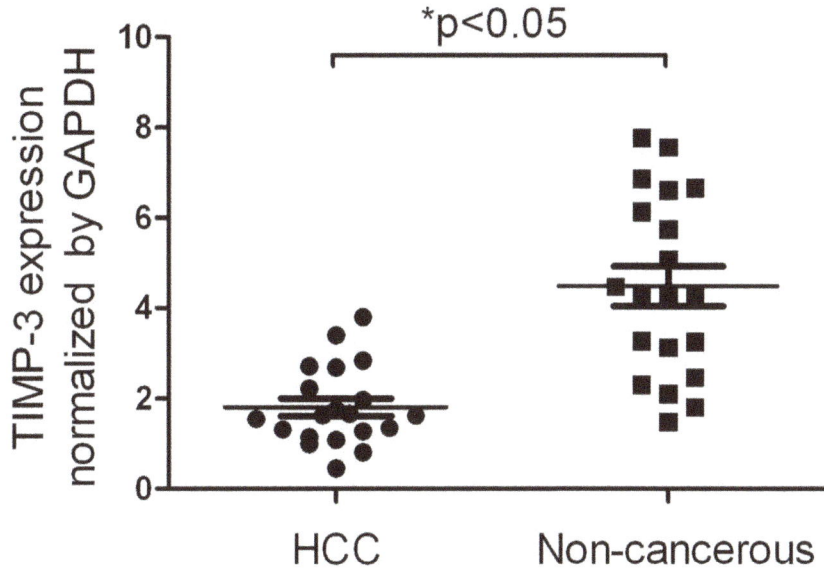

Figure 2. TIMP-3 expression in hepatocellular carcinoma (HCC) tissues and tumor-adjacent, non-cancerous tissues. One-step quantitative real-time polymerase chain reaction (qPCR) demonstrated that the mRNA expression of TIMP-3 in HCC tissues (1.81 ± 0.197) was significantly lower than in matched non-cancerous tissues (4.49 ± 0.446) after normalization with the GAPDH internal control. *$p<0.05$.

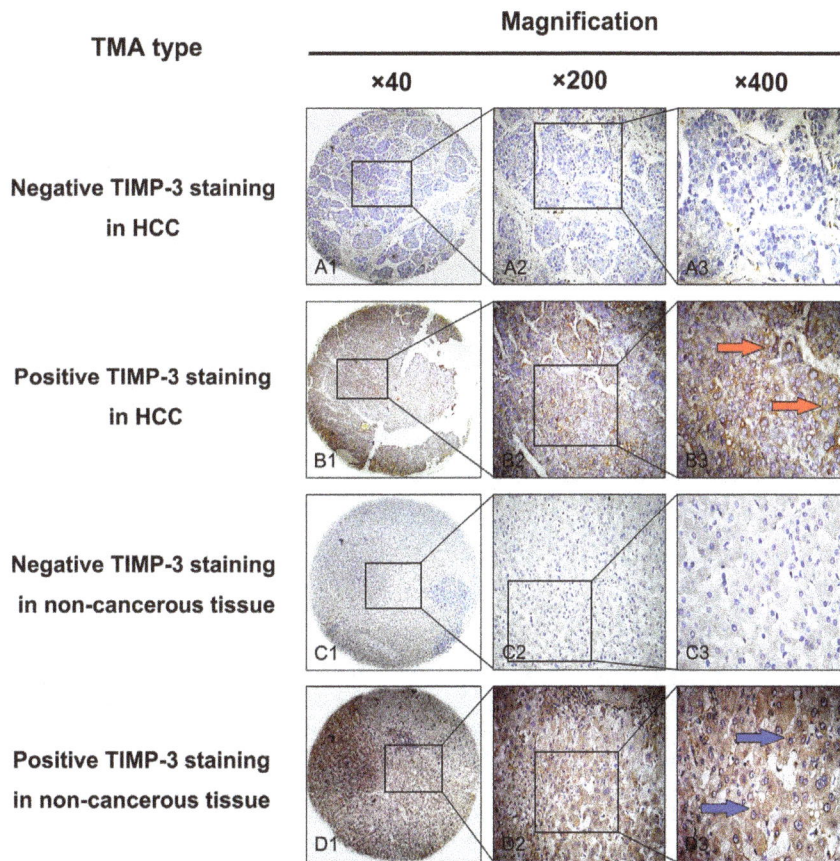

Figure 3. Representative staining pattern of TIMP-3 protein expression in HCC and corresponding non-cancerous tissues in a tissue microarray (TMA). A1, A2 and A3. Negative immunohistochemical (IHC) staining of TIMP-3 in HCC samples. B1, B2 and B3. Positive IHC staining of TIMP-3 in HCC samples. The red arrow highlights positive staining in the cytoplasm of cancer cells. C1, C2 and C3. Negative IHC staining of TIMP-3 in non-cancerous tissue samples. D1, D2 and D3. Positive IHC staining of TIMP-3 in non-cancerous tissue samples. The blue arrow highlights positive staining in the cytoplasm of non-cancerous cells. Original magnification ×40 in A1, B1, C1 and D1; ×200 in A2, B2, C2 and D2; ×400 in A3, B3, C3 and D3.

Table 1. Relationship of high TIMP-3 expression with clinicopathological characteristics in HCC.

Groups	No.	TIMP-3		χ^2	p value
		+	%		
Total	101	36	35.6		
Gender					
Male	84	28	33.3	1.16	0.281
Female	17	8	47.1		
Age (years)					
<60	77	26	33.8	0.50	0.480
≥60	24	10	41.7		
Tumor size (cm)					
>5	59	20	33.9	0.19	0.664
≤5	42	16	38.1		
Hepatitis B virus infection					
Positive	67	22	32.8	0.68	0.408
Negative	34	14	41.2		
Liver cirrhosis					
Positive	43	16	37.2	0.08	0.777
Negative	58	20	34.5		
Pathological grade					
Grade 1	11	3	27.3	2.42	0.298
Grade 2	72	29	40.3		
Grade 3	18	4	22.2		
Portal vein invasion					
Positive	39	9	23.1	4.37	0.036*
Negative	62	27	43.5		
Lymph node metastasis					
Positive	27	5	18.5	4.71	0.030*
Negative	74	31	41.9		
Distant metastasis					
Positive	7	1	14.3	1.50	0.221
Negative	94	35	37.2		
TNM stage					
Stage I	13	4	30.8	5.27	0.153
Stage II	37	17	45.9		
Stage III	45	15	33.3		
Stage IV	6	0	0.0		

*$p<0.05$.

slides. IHC analysis was performed as described previously [24–26]. TMA sections were incubated with a primary anti-TIMP-3 antibody (Abcam) in phosphate-buffered saline (PBS), washed and then incubated with a horseradish peroxidase-conjugated antibody (Santa Cruz Biotechnology, Santa Cruz, CA, USA). Negative controls were included by replacement of the primary antibody with PBS. TIMP-3 immunostaining was defined according to the intensity and percentage of TIMP-3-positive tumor cells. The staining intensity was scored as follows: 0 (negative), 1 (weakly positive), 2 (moderately positive), and 3 (strongly positive). The percentage of TIMP-3-positive cells was also classified into 4 categories, in which a score of 1 was given for 0–10%, 2 for 11–50%, 3 for 51–80%, and 4 for 81–100%. The product of the intensity and percentage scores led to the ultimate staining score.

The degree of TIMP-3 staining was quantified using a two-level grading system as follows: <3 indicates negative expression while 3–9 indicates positive expression.

Statistical analysis

The TIMP-3 mRNA expression in fresh HCC tissues relative to the matched non-cancerous tissues was analyzed with the Wilcoxon signed rank nonparametric test. The significance of TIMP-3 protein expression in clinical data from HCC patients was calculated by the chi-square test. Both univariate and multivariate analyses were performed with Cox proportional hazards regression models to identify important factors that were associated with disease-free and overall survival status. The Kaplan-Meier method was utilized to analyze the relationship

Table 2. Univariate and multivariate analysis of prognostic factors in HCC for disease-free survival.

	Univariate analysis			Multivariate analysis		
	HR	p>|z|	95% CI	HR	p>|z|	95% CI
TIMP-3 expression						
High versus Low	0.40	0.004*	0.217–0.749	0.50	0.039*	0.257–0.967
Gender						
Male versus Female	1.18	0.640	0.582–2.409			
Age (years)						
<60 versus ≥60	1.68	0.137	0.848–3.317			
Tumour size (cm)						
>5 versus ≤5	1.79	0.035*	1.042–3.075	1.18	0.581	0.655–2.128
Hepatitis B virus infection						
Positive versus Negative	1.23	0.465	0.706–2.142			
Liver cirrhosis						
Positive versus Negative	0.90	0.701	0.536–1.523			
Pathological grade						
Grade 1 and 2 versus Grade 3	2.15	0.001*	1.344–3.342	1.67	0.044*	1.015–2.761
Portal vein invasion						
Positive versus Negative	3.21	0.001*	1.909–5.396	1.93	0.030*	1.066–3.510
Lymph node metastasis						
Positive versus Negative	2.64	0.001*	1.543–4.516	1.71	0.086	0.927–3.159
Distant metastasis						
Positive versus Negative	2.34	0.038*	1.049–5.207	0.63	0.334	0.247–1.609
TNM stage						
Stage I–II versus Stage III–IV	0.32	0.001*	0.184–0.564	0.56	0.093	0.282–1.103

*p<0.05.

between TIMP-3 expression and the outcome of HCC patients. The significance level for statistical analysis was set at p<0.05. All statistical analyses were conducted by using SPSS 16.0 (SPSS Inc, Chicago, IL, USA).

Results

Summarization of the clinical information from 101 HCC patients

A patient sample of 84 males and 17 females, with a median age of 54.23 years (range 27–73 years), was enrolled in this study. The tumor diameter of 59 patients was >5 cm, while that of the remaining of 42 patients was ≤5 cm. Sixty-seven patients experienced HBV infection and 43 patients encountered liver cirrhosis in their medical history. In terms of the pathological grade of disease, 11 patients were at grade 1, 72 were at grade 2, and 18 were at grade 3. Portal vein invasion was witnessed in 39 patients, lymph node metastasis was detected in 27 patients, and distant metastasis was observed in 7 patients. With regard to the TNM stage among all 101 HCC cases, 13 patients were in stage I, 37 patients were in stage II, 45 patients were in stage III, and the last 6 patients were in stage IV.

Detection of TIMP-3 expression in HCC cell lines by RT-PCR and Western blotting analysis

TIMP-3 expression was detected in four HCC cell lines (BEL-7402, SMMC-7721, HepG2 and SK-HEP-1) and one non-cancerous cell line (LO-2) by performing RT-PCR and Western

blotting analyses. As shown in Figure 1, RT-PCR and Western blotting analysis revealed that TIMP-3 expression was decreased in four HCC cell lines relative to that of the non-cancerous cell line.

Detection of TIMP-3 expression in HCC tissues by qPCR

TIMP-3 expression was examined in 20 fresh HCC tissues and their corresponding non-cancerous tissues by qPCR. As shown in Figure 2, the TIMP-3 expression in HCC tissues (1.81 ± 0.197) was significantly lower than that of the corresponding non-cancerous tissues (4.49 ± 0.446) when normalized to GAPDH (p<0.05).

IHC Detection of TIMP-3 expression in an HCC TMA

TIMP-3 expression in HCC tissues was evaluated by IHC analysis. High TIMP-3 expression was exhibited in only 36 of 101 (35.6%) HCC tissue samples, whereas 64 of 101 cases of non-cancerous normal tissues (63.4%) showed positive TIMP-3 expression. The TIMP-3 protein expression level was significantly decreased in HCC tissues when compared to that of non-cancerous tissues (p<0.05). Positive staining was mainly localized in the cytoplasm of HCC cells; representative IHC staining for TIMP-3 expression in HCC is shown in Figure 3. The relationship between TIMP-3 protein expression and clinicopathological characteristics are illustrated in Table 1. It is of note that positive TIMP-3 expression was more prevalent in patients with a lack of portal vein invasion and no lymph node metastasis. Additionally, the statistical results revealed that positive TIMP-3 expression was

Table 3. Univariate and multivariate analysis of prognostic factors in HCC for overall survival.

	Univariate analysis			Multivariate analysis		
	HR	p>|z|	95% CI	HR	p>|z|	95% CI
TIMP-3 expression						
High versus Low	0.41	0.005*	0.220–0.759	0.52	0.049*	0.267–0.997
Gender						
Male versus Female	1.20	0.512	0.691–2.097			
Age (years)						
<60 versus ≥60	1.73	0.113	0.877–3.428			
Tumour size (cm)						
>5 versus ≤5	1.78	0.036*	1.037–3.062	1.27	0.422	0.709–2.272
Hepatitis B virus infection						
Positive versus Negative	1.20	0.512	0.691–2.097			
Liver cirrhosis						
Positive versus Negative	0.86	0.563	0.508–1.446			
Pathological grade						
Grade 1 and 2 versus Grade 3	2.19	0.001*	1.369–3.511	1.60	0.052	0.996–2.556
Portal vein invasion						
Positive versus Negative	3.27	0.001*	1.939–5.501	2.04	0.019*	1.124–3.712
Lymph node metastasis						
Positive versus Negative	2.42	0.001*	1.420–4.132	1.40	0.285	0.789–2.557
Distant metastasis						
Positive versus Negative	2.07	0.072	0.936–4.594			
TNM stage						
Stage I–II versus Stage III–IV	0.35	0.001*	0.199–0.606	0.66	0.237	0.338–1.307

*p<0.05.

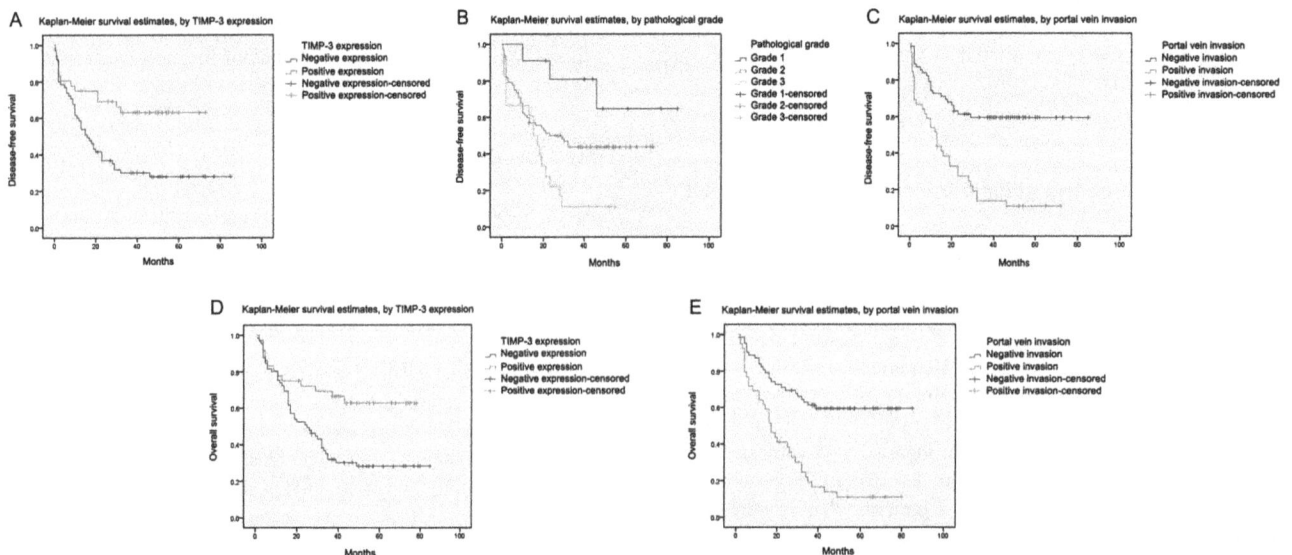

Figure 4. Survival analysis of HCC patients by the Kaplan-Meier method. A. The disease-free survival rate in patients with negative TIMP-3 expression (blue line) was significantly lower than that of patients with positive TIMP-3 expression (green line). B. The disease-free survival rate in patients with pathological grade 1 (blue line) and 2 (green line) was significantly higher than that of patients with pathological grade 3 (yellow line). C. The disease-free survival rate in patients with positive portal vein invasion (green line) was significantly lower than that of patients without portal vein invasion (blue line). D. The overall survival rate in patients with negative TIMP-3 expression (blue line) was significantly lower than that in patients with positive TIMP-3 expression (green line). D The overall survival rate in patients with positive portal vein invasion (green line) was significantly lower than that of patients without portal vein invasion (blue line).

negatively correlated with portal vein invasion (p = 0.036) and lymph node metastasis (p = 0.030).

Survival analysis

According to univariate analysis, several items were correlated with both disease-free survival and overall survival of HCC, including TIMP-3 expression, tumor size, portal vein invasion, lymph node metastasis and the TNM stage. In addition, distant metastasis also affected disease-free survival, but not overall survival (Tables 2 and 3). Moreover, by using multivariate analysis with Cox regression model, we found that TIMP-3 expression (p = 0.039, p = 0.049) and portal vein invasion (p = 0.030, p = 0.019) were associated with disease-free survival and overall survival, respectively. Additionally, portal vein invasion (p = 0.044) was also correlated with disease-free survival of HCC (Tables 2 and 3). Kaplan-Meier survival curves subsequently indicated that HCC patients with positive TIMP-3 expression and negative portal vein invasion displayed a statistically better duration of disease-free survival and overall survival (Figure 4). Meanwhile, HCC patients with an advanced pathological grade encountered unfavorable disease-free survival time (Figure 4).

Discussion

The MMPs, a family of extracellular proteolytic enzymes, and their cognate inhibitors (TIMPs) are both known to play significant roles during tumor development. A proper balance between MMPs and TIMPs seems to be of great importance for influencing cancer metastasis and invasion [9,27–29]. Tumor cells can synthesize MMPs and influence cellular properties, including cell growth, death and migration, as well as contribute to the invasion, angiogenesis, and establishment of metastatic lesions in the tumor environment [28,30]. TIMPs, which are natural inhibitors of MMPs and contain four members (denoted TIMP-1 to -4), is reported to ameliorate the invasion and metastasis of tumor cells induced by MMPs [20,31]. As for TIMP-3, a large number of studies have shown that the expression of TIMP-3 was reduced in various cancer tissues when compared to non-cancerous tissues or in the advanced stages of cancer relative to the early stages of cancer. The decreased expression of TIMP-3 was significantly associated with pathologic stage, nodal involvement, and poor survival [16–20]. The possible mechanisms of TIMP-3 function are a subject of much investigation. TIMP-3 suppresses tumorigenesis and angiogenesis by interacting with Integrin α7 and angiotensin II type 2 receptor [32,33]. TIMP-3 induces endothelial apoptosis in lung cancer by inhibiting p-AKT and inducing p-ERK1/2 pathways [13]. The expression of TIMP-3 could be repressed by zeste homolog 2 and result in cancer cell migration [34]. TIMP-3 expression in tumors can also be modulated through the regulation of microRNAs, as TIMP3 is a positive target of several microRNAs including miR21, miR181b, miR221 and 222 [35–37]. All data suggest that the inhibitory effect of TIMP-3 in cancer development could identify TIMP-3 as a novel and useful biomarker in human cancer. However, the clinicopathological significance, particularly the prognostic role of TIMP-3 in HCC, has not been investigated. The potential of TIMP-3 as a candidate for targeted therapy in HCC requires further exploration.

The RT-PCR and Western blotting analyses illustrated that TIMP-3 mRNA and protein expression was significantly reduced in four HCC cell lines when compared to that of non-cancerous cell lines. Subsequently, qPCR further illustrated that the TIMP-3 mRNA expression levels in HCC tissues were lower than those in normal non-cancerous tissues. Furthermore, IHC analysis of an HCC TMA similarly showed a reduced cytoplasmic expression of TIMP-3 protein in cancer cells relative to normal non-cancerous cells. These results are similar to the studies that indicated that the expression of TIMP-3 was inhibited in malignant cancers [16,18,20,38]. Moreover, positive TIMP-3 expression in HCC was negatively correlated with certain clinical pathologic items, including portal vein invasion and lymph node metastasis. Likewise, Zhang et al. reported that high TIMP-3 expression inhibited tumorigenic and metastatic potential in HCC xenografts [39]. Wang et al. concluded that the upregulation of hepatic miR-181b promoted hepatocarcinogenesis by inhibiting TIMP-3 [36]. Our results are in line with previous studies and further confirm that the positive expression of TIMP-3 may play a critical role in inhibiting malignant behaviors in HCC, including portal vein invasion and lymph node metastasis.

Univariate analysis and multivariate analysis demonstrated that TIMP-3 expression and portal vein invasion were both correlated with life span in the disease-free survival and the overall survival of HCC patients. Moreover, Kaplan-Meier analysis analogously demonstrated that the life span of patients with positive TIMP-3 expression was longer than that of patients with negative expression. These data are also consistent with previous reports that low TIMP-3 expression facilitated tumor development and predicted poor survival in several human cancers [18–20]. Conclusively, we believe that TIMP-3 significantly exerts anti-oncogenic roles and that positive TIMP-3 expression critically suspends malignant activities associated with cancer invasion. It is rational to presume that TIMP-3 could be used as a novel candidate for cancer therapy. To date, several therapeutic strategies targeting TIMP-3 have already shown promising effectiveness in cancer treatment [40,41].

However, some contradictory results imply that TIMP-3 expression is increased in certain types of cancers and that high TIMP-3 expression is linked poor prognosis in head and neck cancer [21,42,43]. A possible explanation for the conflicting data may be attributed to differences in tumor origins and antibody quality [42]. Further studies that enroll a larger number of clinical HCC patients are necessary to validate our results that characterize TIMP-3.

In summary, this is the first study to illustrate that positive TIMP-3 expression is correlated with the malignant phenotype of HCC. The data from the current study imply that TIMP-3 could be defined as a novel biomarker for HCC prognosis and that targeting TIMP-3 may provide a promising strategy for HCC treatment.

Author Contributions

Conceived and designed the experiments: JRX JZ. Performed the experiments: XFG MYF HHN XJT LX JL LQ. Analyzed the data: XFG MYF XJT YQD WZ. Contributed reagents/materials/analysis tools: YQD HHN WZ YFZ. Contributed to the writing of the manuscript: XFG. Supervised the study: JRX JZ.

References

1. Siegel R, Naishadham D, Jemal A (2013) Cancer statistics, 2013. CA Cancer J Clin 63: 11–30.
2. Jemal A, Bray F, Center MM, Ferlay J, Ward E, et al. (2011) Global cancer statistics. CA Cancer J Clin 61: 69–90.
3. Nguyen VT, Law MG, Dore GJ (2009) Hepatitis B-related hepatocellular carcinoma: epidemiological characteristics and disease burden. J Viral Hepat 16: 453–463.
4. Qu LS, Liu JX, Liu TT, Shen XZ, Chen TY, et al. (2014) Association of hepatitis B virus pre-s deletions with the development of hepatocellular carcinoma in qidong, china. PLoS One 9: e98257.
5. Ding J, Wang H (2014) Multiple interactive factors in hepatocarcinogenesis. Cancer Lett 346: 17–23.
6. Li W, Chen G, Yu X, Shi Y, Peng M, et al. (2013) Accumulation of the mutations in basal core promoter of hepatitis B virus subgenotype C1 increase

the risk of hepatocellular carcinoma in Southern China. Int J Clin Exp Pathol 6: 1076–1085.

7. Fong ZV, Tanabe KK (2014) The clinical management of hepatocellular carcinoma in the United States, Europe, and Asia: A comprehensive and evidence-based comparison and review. Cancer. [Epub ahead of print].

8. Wong RJ, Devaki P, Nguyen L, Cheung R, Nguyen MH (2014) Ethnic disparities and liver transplantation rates in hepatocellular carcinoma patients in the recent era: results from the surveillance, epidemiology, and end results registry. Liver Transpl 20: 528–535.

9. Brew K, Nagase H (2010) The tissue inhibitors of metalloproteinases (TIMPs): an ancient family with structural and functional diversity. Biochim Biophys Acta 1803: 55–71.

10. Bourboulia D, Stetler-Stevenson WG (2010) Matrix metalloproteinases (MMPs) and tissue inhibitors of metalloproteinases (TIMPs): Positive and negative regulators in tumor cell adhesion. Semin Cancer Biol 20: 161–168.

11. Mahller YY, Vaikunth SS, Ripberger MC, Baird WH, Saeki Y, et al. (2008) Tissue inhibitor of metalloproteinase-3 via oncolytic herpesvirus inhibits tumor growth and vascular progenitors. Cancer Res 68: 1170–1179.

12. Zhang Y, Qian H, Lin C, Lang J, Xiang Y, et al. (2008) Adenovirus carrying TIMP-3: a potential tool for cervical cancer treatment. Gynecol Oncol 108: 234–240.

13. Chetty C, Lakka SS, Bhoopathi P, Kunigal S, Geiss R, et al. (2008) Tissue inhibitor of metalloproteinase 3 suppresses tumor angiogenesis in matrix metalloproteinase 2-down-regulated lung cancer. Cancer Res 68: 4736–4745.

14. Kallio JP, Hopkins-Donaldson S, Baker AH, Kahari VM (2011) TIMP-3 promotes apoptosis in nonadherent small cell lung carcinoma cells lacking functional death receptor pathway. Int J Cancer 128: 991–996.

15. Lin H, Zhang Y, Wang H, Xu D, Meng X, et al. (2012) Tissue inhibitor of metalloproteinases-3 transfer suppresses malignant behaviors of colorectal cancer cells. Cancer Gene Ther 19: 845–851.

16. Guan Z, Zhang J, Song S, Dai D (2013) Promoter methylation and expression of TIMP3 gene in gastric cancer. Diagn Pathol 8: 110.

17. Liu HQ, Song S, Wang JH, Zhang SL (2011) Expression of MMP-3 and TIMP-3 in gastric cancer tissue and its clinical significance. Oncol Lett 2: 1319–1322.

18. Ninomiya I, Kawakami K, Fushida S, Fujimura T, Funaki H, et al. (2008) Quantitative detection of TIMP-3 promoter hypermethylation and its prognostic significance in esophageal squamous cell carcinoma. Oncol Rep 20: 1489–1495.

19. Wu DW, Tsai LH, Chen PM, Lee MC, Wang L, et al. (2012) Loss of TIMP-3 promotes tumor invasion via elevated IL-6 production and predicts poor survival and relapse in HPV-infected non-small cell lung cancer. Am J Pathol 181: 1796–1806.

20. Mino N, Takenaka K, Sonobe M, Miyahara R, Yanagihara K, et al. (2007) Expression of tissue inhibitor of metalloproteinase-3 (TIMP-3) and its prognostic significance in resected non-small cell lung cancer. J Surg Oncol 95: 250–257.

21. Gu J, Berman D, Lu C, Wistuba, II, Roth JA, et al. (2006) Aberrant promoter methylation profile and association with survival in patients with non-small cell lung cancer. Clin Cancer Res 12: 7329–7338.

22. De Schutter H, Geeraerts H, Verbeken E, Nuyts S (2009) Promoter methylation of TIMP3 and CDH1 predicts better outcome in head and neck squamous cell carcinoma treated by radiotherapy only. Oncol Rep 21: 507–513.

23. Varotti G, Ramacciato G, Ercolani G, Grazi GL, Vetrone G, et al. (2005) Comparison between the fifth and sixth editions of the AJCC/UICC TNM staging systems for hepatocellular carcinoma: multicentric study on 393 cirrhotic resected patients. Eur J Surg Oncol 31: 760–767.

24. Fu M, Fan W, Pu X, Ni H, Zhang W, et al. (2013) Elevated expression of SHIP2 correlates with poor prognosis in non-small cell lung cancer. Int J Clin Exp Pathol 6: 2185–2191.

25. Mao Y, Zhang DW, Lin H, Xiong L, Liu Y, et al. (2012) Alpha B-crystallin is a new prognostic marker for laryngeal squamous cell carcinoma. J Exp Clin Cancer Res 31: 101.

26. Fu M, Gu X, Ni H, Zhang W, Chang F, et al. (2013) High expression of inositol polyphosphate phosphatase-like 1 associates with unfavorable survival in hepatocellular carcinoma. Int J Clin Exp Pathol 6: 2515–2522.

27. Wu ZS, Wu Q, Yang JH, Wang HQ, Ding XD, et al. (2008) Prognostic significance of MMP-9 and TIMP-1 serum and tissue expression in breast cancer. Int J Cancer 122: 2050–2056.

28. Coussens LM, Fingleton B, Matrisian LM (2002) Matrix metalloproteinase inhibitors and cancer: trials and tribulations. Science 295: 2387–2392.

29. Cruz-Munoz W, Sanchez OH, Di Grappa M, English JL, Hill RP, et al. (2006) Enhanced metastatic dissemination to multiple organs by melanoma and lymphoma cells in timp-3-/- mice. Oncogene 25: 6489–6496.

30. Bashash M, Shah A, Hislop G, Treml M, Bretherick K, et al. (2013) Genetic polymorphisms at TIMP3 are associated with survival of adenocarcinoma of the gastroesophageal junction. PLoS One 8: e59157.

31. Destouches D, Huet E, Sader M, Frechault S, Carpentier G, et al. (2012) Multivalent pseudopeptides targeting cell surface nucleoproteins inhibit cancer cell invasion through tissue inhibitor of metalloproteinases 3 (TIMP-3) release. J Biol Chem 287: 43685–43693.

32. Tan LZ, Song Y, Nelson J, Yu YP, Luo JH (2013) Integrin alpha7 binds tissue inhibitor of metalloproteinase 3 to suppress growth of prostate cancer cells. Am J Pathol 183: 831–840.

33. Kang KH, Park SY, Rho SB, Lee JH (2008) Tissue inhibitor of metalloproteinases-3 interacts with angiotensin II type 2 receptor and additively inhibits angiogenesis. Cardiovasc Res 79: 150–160.

34. Xu C, Hou Z, Zhan P, Zhao W, Chang C, et al. (2013) EZH2 regulates cancer cell migration through repressing TIMP-3 in non-small cell lung cancer. Med Oncol 30: 713.

35. Song B, Wang C, Liu J, Wang X, Lv L, et al. (2010) MicroRNA-21 regulates breast cancer invasion partly by targeting tissue inhibitor of metalloproteinase 3 expression. J Exp Clin Cancer Res 29: 29.

36. Wang B, Hsu SH, Majumder S, Kutay H, Huang W, et al. (2010) TGFbeta-mediated upregulation of hepatic miR-181b promotes hepatocarcinogenesis by targeting TIMP3. Oncogene 29: 1787–1797.

37. Garofalo M, Di Leva G, Romano G, Nuovo G, Suh SS, et al. (2009) miR-221&222 regulate TRAIL resistance and enhance tumorigenicity through PTEN and TIMP3 downregulation. Cancer Cell 16: 498–509.

38. Turner SL, Mangnall D, Bird NC, Bunning RA, Blair-Zajdel ME (2012) Expression of ADAMTS-1, ADAMTS-4, ADAMTS-5 and TIMP3 by hepatocellular carcinoma cell lines. Int J Oncol 41: 1043–1049.

39. Zhang H, Wang YS, Han G, Shi Y (2007) TIMP-3 gene transfection suppresses invasive and metastatic capacity of human hepatocarcinoma cell line HCC-7721. Hepatobiliary Pancreat Dis Int 6: 487–491.

40. Zhang L, Zhao L, Zhao D, Lin G, Guo B, et al. (2010) Inhibition of tumor growth and induction of apoptosis in prostate cancer cell lines by overexpression of tissue inhibitor of matrix metalloproteinase-3. Cancer Gene Ther 17: 171–179.

41. Chen YY, Brown NJ, Jones R, Lewis CE, Mujamammi AH, et al. (2014) A peptide derived from TIMP-3 inhibits multiple angiogenic growth factor receptors and tumour growth and inflammatory arthritis in mice. Angiogenesis 17: 207–219.

42. Kornfeld JW, Meder S, Wohlberg M, Friedrich RE, Rau T, et al. (2011) Overexpression of TACE and TIMP3 mRNA in head and neck cancer: association with tumour development and progression. Br J Cancer 104: 138–145.

43. Rohrs S, Dirks WG, Meyer C, Marschalek R, Scherr M, et al. (2009) Hypomethylation and expression of BEX2, IGSF4 and TIMP3 indicative of MLL translocations in acute myeloid leukemia. Mol Cancer 8: 86.

7

Association of Serum MicroRNA Expression in Hepatocellular Carcinomas Treated with Transarterial Chemoembolization and Patient Survival

Mei Liu[1♉], Jibing Liu[2♉], Liming Wang[3], Huiyong Wu[2], Changchun Zhou[4], Hongxia Zhu[1], Ningzhi Xu[1]*, Yinfa Xie[2]*

1 Laboratory of Cell and Molecular Biology & State Key Laboratory of Molecular Oncology, Cancer Institute & Cancer Hospital, Chinese Academy of Medical Sciences & Peking Union Medical College, Beijing, PR China, 2 Department of Interventional Surgical Oncology, Cancer Hospital of Shandong Province, Shandong Academy of Medical Sciences, Jinan, Shandong, China, 3 Department of Abdominal Surgery, Cancer Institute & Cancer Hospital, Chinese Academy of Medical Sciences & Peking Union Medical College, Beijing, PR China, 4 Clinical Laboratory, Cancer Hospital of Shandong Province, Shandong Academy of Medical Sciences, Jinan, Shandong, China

Abstract

Background and Aim: Hepatocellular carcinoma (HCC) is one of the most deadly tumors. Transarterial chemoembolization (TACE) is effective for unresectable HCC. In recent years, miRNAs have been proposed as novel diagnostic and prognostic tools for HCC. This study aimed to identify whether microRNAs (miRNAs) can serve as biomarkers to reliably predict outcome before HCC patients are treated with TACE.

Methods: Eleven miRNAs (miR-, miR-19a, miR-101-3p, miR-199a-5p, miR-200a, miR-21, miR-214, miR-221, miR-222, miR-223 and miR-, -5p) were quantified by quantitative real-time PCR (qRT-PCR) in 136 HCC patients' serum before they received TACE therapy. Univariate and multivariate analysis were used to identify the prognostic value of clinical parameters and miRNAs. Area under the receiver operating characteristic curve (AUC) was used to evaluate the prediction potency.

Results: The levels of some miRNAs were dramatically associated with clinicopathologic features regarding Child-Puge class, AFP, tumor size and satellite nodules. Univariate analysis revealed that miR-200a, miR-21, miR-122 and miR-224-5p were significantly associated with patients' survival. Multivariate analysis demonstrated that AFP, satellite nodules and miR-200a were the independent prognostic factors associated with survival in this cohort ($p = 0.000$, 0.001, 0.000, respectively). The probability of the prognostic accuracy of miR-200a was 81.64% (74.47% specificity and 88.76% sensitivity), which was higher than the classifier established by combination of AFP and satellite nodules (76.87% probability, 70.21% specificity and 69.66% sensitivity). Furthermore, the combination of AFP, satellite nodules and miR-200a demonstrated as a classifier for HCC prognosis, yielding a ROC curve area of 88.19% (93.62% specificity and 68.54% sensitivity).

Conclusions: Our study indicated that serum miR-200a may prognosticate disease outcome in HCC patients with TACE therapy. Therefore, miR-200a can potentially guide individualized treatment for HCC patients with a high risk of TACE treatment failures.

Editor: Lian-Yue Yang, Xiangya Hospital of Central South University, China

Funding: This work was supported by State Key Laboratory of Molecular Oncology program (SKL-2013-14), Development projects of Shandong province science and technology (2012GSF11837) and Beijing Hope Run Special Fund (LC2012B19), PR China. The funders had no role in study design, data collection and analysis, decision to publish, or preparation of the manuscript.

Competing Interests: The authors have declared that no competing interests exist.

* Email: xningzhi@public.bta.net.cn (NX); Laoxie6996@163.com (YX)

♉ These authors contributed equally to this work.

Introduction

Hepatocellular carcinoma (HCC) is the most common type of malignancy of liver cancer. An estimated 748,300 new liver cancer cases and 695,900 cancer deaths occurred worldwide. Half of these cases and deaths were estimated to occur in China [1]. A great many HCC patients diagnosed at advanced tumor stages when standard surgery is not operable. Transarterial chemoembolization (TACE) treatment represents a first-line noncurative therapy for HCC and has been thought to be effective in improving survival of HCC patients with good liver function [2]. Most HCC patients receive TACE treatment. However, clinical outcomes vary significantly and are difficult to predict. The lack of effective outcome prediction models makes it difficult to apply individualized treatment protocols to HCC patients. A biomarker to accurately predict disease outcome before TACE therapy would be important for the early identification of patients with a high risk of treatment failures. For the high-risk patients, modified therapy or adjuvant therapy may potentially be applied to improve their survival.

MicroRNA (miRNA) is a type of endogenous non-coding RNA (ncRNA). They are responsible for post-transcriptional regulation and participate in nearly all biological processes [3]. The use of miRNA as cancer biomarker is of particular interest because it could be detected in blood plasma or serum with high stability [4]. In recent years, the therapeutic potential of miRNAs in HCC has been reported in various studies [5–7]. miRNAs have been proposed as novel diagnostic tools for classification and prognostic stratification of HCC. In light of reports from independent studies, consistent deregulation of miR-122, miR-199a-5p, miR-221 and miR-21 appears to be particularly important in HCC [8–10].

In this study, we selected 11 miRNAs to further validate in 136 HCC patients' serum. All serum samples were collected before the HCC patients had been treated with TACE. The 11 miRNAs were selected based on the mining of public literatures that have been reported by different study cohorts of liver disease [11–19]. They were miR-122, miR-199a-5p, miR-221, miR-21, miR-101-3p, miR-200a, miR-214, miR-222, miR-223, miR-19a and miR-224-5p. Our study suggested that serum miRNAs can be considered as useful biomarkers that could help to stratify the prognosis and monitor follow-up in TACE-treated HCC patients. And the classifier of serum miR-200a outperforms the classifier established by the combination of AFP and satellite nodules in predicting the prognosis of TACE-treated HCC.

Materials and Methods

Patients with HCC

From January 2010 to July 2012, a total of 136 unresectable HCC patients who underwent TACE for the first time at Cancer Hospital of Shandong Province were included in this study. HCC was diagnosed according to the NCCN (National Comprehensive Cancer Network) guidelines. Status with respect to hepatitis B virus (HBV) infection was determined on the basis of HBsAg, HBsAb, HBcAb, HBeAg and HBeAg using commercially available immunoassay kits (Roche Diagnostics, Germany). AFP levels were determined by immunoenzymatic chemiluminescence (Roche Diagnostics, Germany). Clinicopathologic informations of the patient were summarized in Table 1. All serum samples were collected before the patients had received TACE. All of the patients were followed-up until November 2013.

This study was approved by the medical ethics committee of Cancer Hospital of Shandong Province, and all the participants signed written informed consent forms.

Treatment of Transarterial chemoembolization

Selective angiography was performed to identify the major arterial supply to HCC. TACE was conducted using a mixture of adriamycin, lipiodol and contrast agent. The dose of adriamycin and lipiodol were dependent on the tumor size and vascularity with 20–50 mg of adriamycin and 5–20 ml lipiodol per session. Subsequently, embolization was performed using gelatin sponge particles after TACE, and occlusion of target vessels and absence of additional tumor blood supply was confirmed.

RNA isolation and qRT-PCR assay

Eleven candidate miRNAs were characterized in the serum samples by using SYBR-based real-time PCR (Quantobio Technology, Beijing, China). The QuantoBio Total RNA Isolation Kit was used to isolate RNA from the serum samples. The miR-Quanto System is composed with three reaction steps to convert and quantify levels of miRNA expression. Firstly, a

polyadenine tail was attached to miRNA at their 3′ end. This is followed by a retro-transcription step that converts miRNA into cDNA and attaches a universal DNA tag at the 5′ end of synthesized cDNA. After the first strands of cDNA synthesized, qPCR was performed by using the miRNA specific forward primer and a reverse universal primer mix. The data were normalized using the external controls Quanto EC1 and Quanto EC2 which were added when the samples were extracted. All of the reactions were performed according to the manufacturer's instructions.

Survival analysis

Univariate Cox proportional hazards regression analysis were done to evaluate the association of each miRNA or clinical parameters to overall patient survival. The p values were calculated using the Wald test. Multivariate Cox proportional hazards regression analysis were done to evaluate the independent prognostic value of the miRNA signature or clinical parameters. The Kaplan-Meier estimator was used to evaluate the median survival time of the OS that was based on miRNA expression signature or clinical parameters. The p value of the Kaplan-Meier analysis was calculated with the log-rank test. Overall survival was defined as the time interval from the date of the first treatment of TACE to death or censored on the last follow-up.

Statistical analysis

SPSS16.0 software was used for the statistical analysis. Statistical descriptions were used to describe the clinical pathological features, and the t test (Student's t test) or ANOVA (analysis of variance) was used to analyze the measurement data. The p value was bilaterally tested, and values less than 0.05 were regarded as statistically significant. Logistic regression analysis was performed to analyze various combinations of clinical parameters and miRNA. The receiver operating characteristic (ROC) curve and the area under the curve (AUC) were used to determine the feasibility. The Youden's Index was used to identify the optimal cut-off point. As defined, the corresponding sensitivity and specificity was showed.

Results

Association of clinical parameters with overall survival of HCC treated with TACE

The characteristics of this patient cohort were summarized in Table 1. The prognostic values of multiple commonly used clinicopathologic features were analyzed with univariate analysis. AFP, BCLC stage, Child-Puge class and satellite nodules were significantly associated with survival (Figure 1 & Table 2), whereas other features, including gender, age at diagnosis, tumor size, HBV, relapse and tumor multiplicity, were not.

According to the "diagnosis and treatment norms of primary hepatic carcinoma" that was issued by ministry of health of the PRC in 2011, AFP level of more than 400 ng/mL is a cut-off value to diagnose primary hepatic carcinoma. Here, HCC patients were divided into three AFP groups: normal ($\leq$20 ng/mL), elevated (21–400 ng/mL), and diagnostic (>400 ng/mL). As shown in Figure 1A, for the AFP-normal HCC patients (n = 45), the median OS was 37.20 month, AFP-elevated HCC patients (n = 37), the median OS was 28.57 month, and AFP-diagnostic HCC patients (n = 54), the median OS was 12.00 month. The OS of the AFP-normal patients was statically longer than AFP-elevated and AFP-diagnostic HCC patients (p = 0.000). The group of patients with BCLC stage A and B had a longer OS than the group with BCLC stage C, the median OS was 28.56 month and

Table 1. Clinicopathologic features in 136 HCC patients treated with TACE.

Parameters	Patients with HCC (n = 136)
Gender	
Male	118(86.8%)
Female	18(13.2%)
Age (years)	
≤60	86(63.2%)
>60	50(36.8%)
BCLC Stage	
A	9(6.6%)
B	82(60.3%)
C	45(33.1%)
Child-Puge Class	
A	85(62.5%)
B	51(37.5%)
HBV	
Yes	129(94.9%)
No	7(5.1%)
Tumor size	
≦5 cm	52(38.2%)
>5 cm	84(61.8%)
AFP(ng/ml)	
<20	45(33.1%)
20–400	37(27.2%)
>400	54(39.7%)
Statellite nodules	
Present	54(39.7%)
Absent	82(60.3%)
Relapse	
Yes	15(11.0%)
No	121(89.0%)
Tumor multiplicity	
Present	36(26.5%)
Absent	100(73.5%)

12.00 month, respectively (p = 0.008) (Figure 1B). The median OS of patients with Child-Puge A as 33.77 month and the median OS of patients with Child-Puge B was 15.77 month (p = 0.002) (Figure 1C). The group of patients with satellite nodules had a lower median OS (12.00 month) than the group without satellite nodules (33.77 month) (p = 0.000) (Figure 1D).

Multivariate Cox proportional hazard regression analysis revealed that AFP and satellite nodules were the independent prognostic factors associated with survival (Table 2).

The expression of serum miRNAs was associated with HCC survival treated with TACE

Eleven miRNAs were analyzed in 136 HCC patients' serum to identify prognostic factors for outcome. By summarizing available data from independent studies, the selected miRNAs may have potential prognostic significance. The expression of individual miRNAs was correlated to overall patient survival with univariate analysis. We divided the 136 patients into two groups based on the median value of the expression level of each miRNA. Among the 11 miRNAs, four miRNAs (miR-200a, miR-21, miR-122 and miR-224-5p) were significantly associated with cancer survival, while the OSs of other groups were not significantly different (p> 0.05). The Kaplan-Meier curves of OS according miR-200a, miR-21, miR-122 and miR-224-5p were plotted in Figure 2A–D. Comparing each miRNA expression in HCC serum with patient's survival time revealed two group: those with predominantly higher expression of miR-200a, miR-21, miR-122, miR-224-5p and poor survival and those with predominantly lower expression of miR-200a, miR-21, miR-122, miR-224-5p and good survival (p = 0.000, 0.026, 0.025, 0.041, respectively). The relative expression level of each miRNA between the high and low group was showed in Figure 2E. The Multivariate Cox proportional hazard regression analysis revealed that miR-200a was the independent prognostic factor associated with survival (Table 3).

To further understand the significance of miRNAs in the prognosis of TACE-treated HCC patients, whether the 11 miRNAs expression were significantly associated with the clinico-

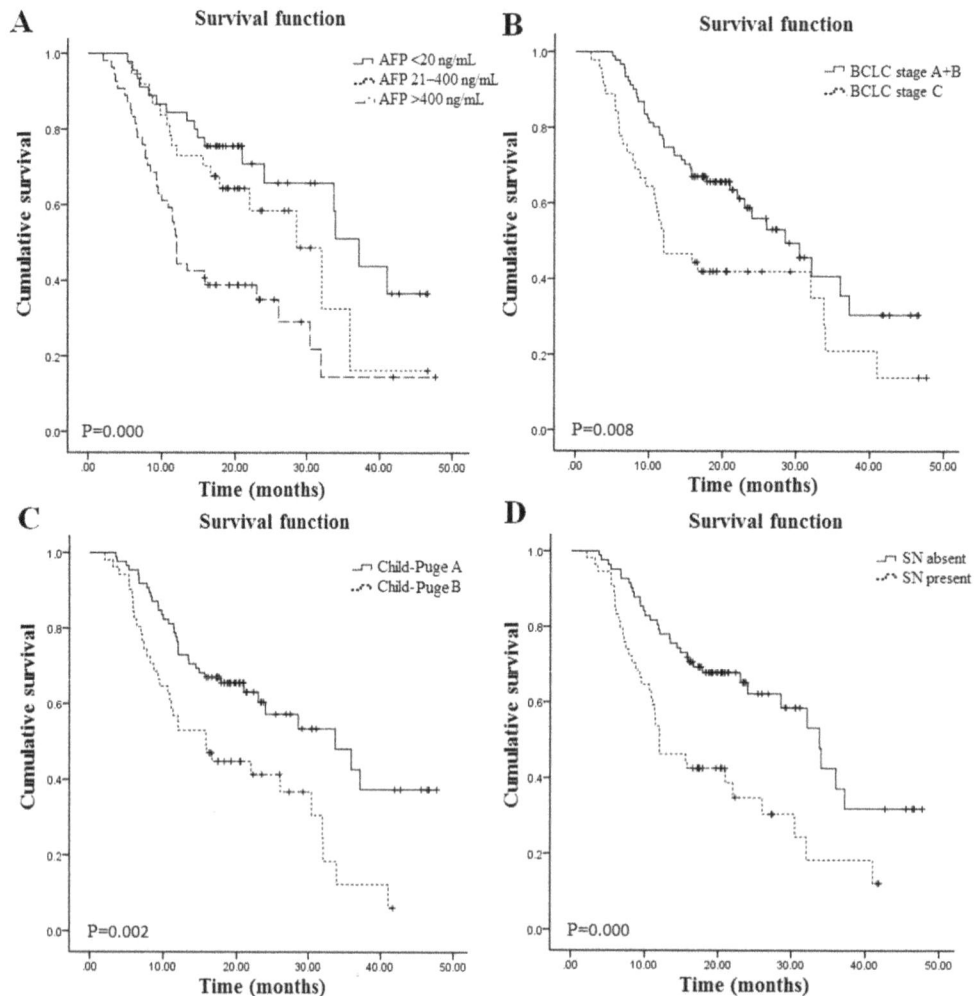

Figure 1. Association of clinical parameters with overall survival by Kaplan-Meier curves and the log-rank test. A. AFP-normal, AFP-elevated or AFP-diagnostic patients. **B.** Patients with BCLC stages A+B or C. **C.** Patients with Child-Puge class A or B. **D.** Patients with or without satellite nodules. SN: satellite nodules.

pathologic features were analyzed. As shown in table 4, univariate analysis showed that the expression of miR-101-3p, miR-199a-5p and miR-221 were considerably associated with Child-Puge stage, miR-21, miR-222 and miR-224-5p were associated with tumor size, miR-122, miR-200a, miR-214, miR-21 and miR-224-5p

were associated with AFP, and miR-101-3p, miR-19a and miR-222 were associated with satellite nodules (p<0.05).

Table 2. Univariate and Multivariate Cox proportional hazards regression analysis of clinical parameters in relation to disease outcome.

Clinical variable	Overall survival			
	Univariate analysis		Multivariate analysis	
	HR(95%CI)	p value	HR(95%CI)	p value
BCLC Stage	1.871(1.167–3.000)	0.009		
Child-Puge Class	2.079(1.303–3.316)	0.002		
AFP	1.001(1.000–1.001)	0.000	1.001(1.000–1.001)	0.000
Satellite nodules	2.298(1.439–3.670)	0.000	2.240(1.403–3.578)	0.001

HR, hazard ratio; CI, confidence interval; BCLC, Barcelona Clinic Liver Cancer; AFP, alpha-fetoprotein.

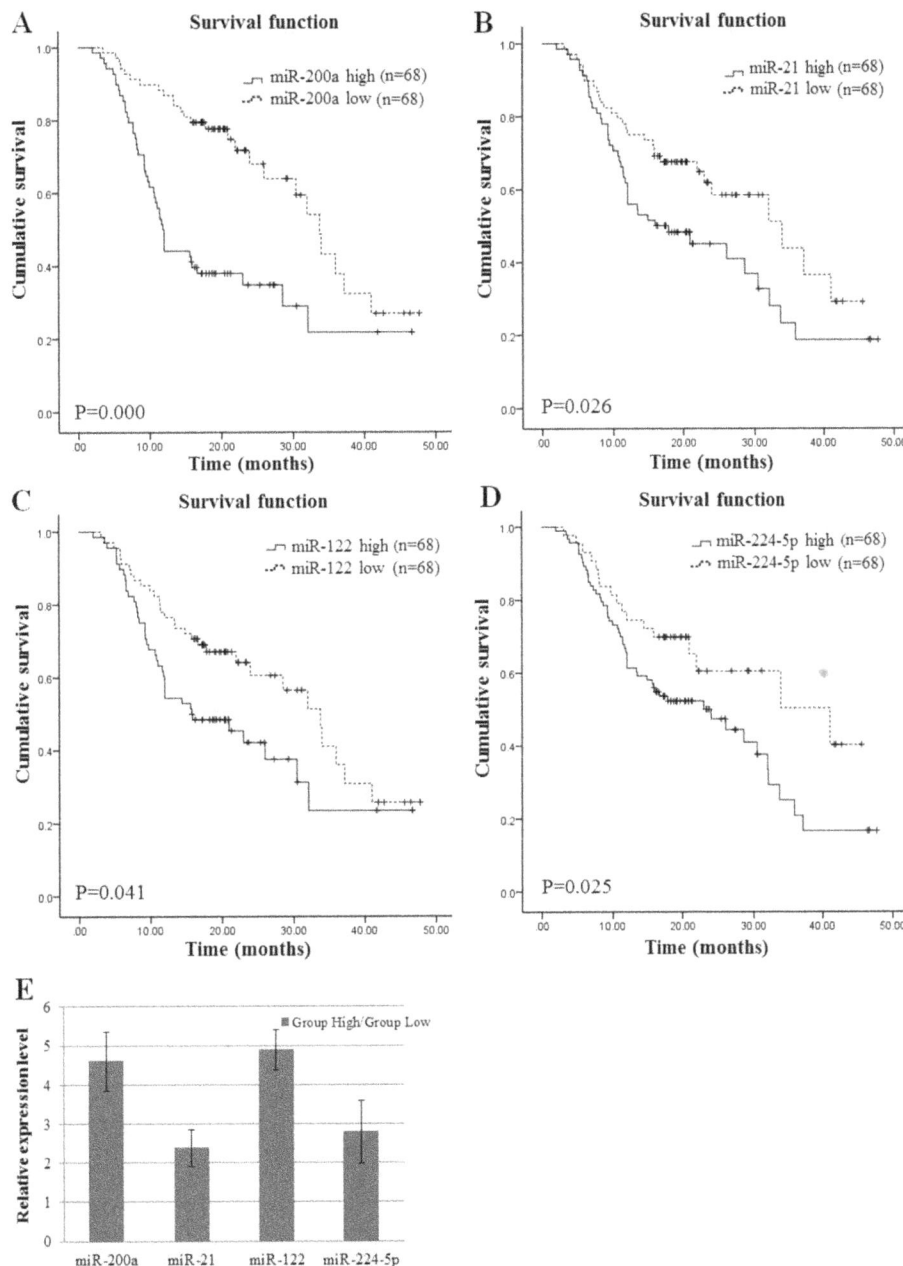

Figure 2. The levels of serum miRNAs were associated with overall survival. A. Patients with low or high expression of miR-200a (Cutoff value: Delta CT = 16.02). **B.** Patients with low or high expression of miR-21 (Cutoff value: Delta CT = 6.08). **C.** Patients with low or high expression of miR-122 (Cutoff value: Delta CT = 6.88). **D.** Patients with low or high expression of miR-224-5p (Cutoff value: Delta CT = 14.22). **E.** The relative expression level of serum miR-200a, miR-21, miR-122 and miR-224-5p in the group of HCC patients with high expression level was normalized by the group of patients with low expression level (set as 1), respectively. Mean ± s.d.

The classifiers for predicting prognosis of hepatocellular carcinoma with TACE treatment

Multivariate analysis revealed that AFP, satellite nodules and miR-200a were the independent predict factor associated with patient survival. Then, the discriminative power of these factors in predicting the outcome before TACE-treatment to HCC patients was verified. According to the OS, the patients were stratified into two subgroups, including a sensitive group (>12 months) and a resistant group (≤12 months). To evaluate the diagnostic value, the ROC curve was used to analyze the sensitivity and specificity. As shown in Figure 3, the ROC curve of the combination of AFP and satellite nodules showed an AUC of 76.87% (69.66% sensitivity and 70.21% specificity) (Figure 3A). The ROC curve of miR-200a had an AUC of 81.64% (88.76% sensitivity and 74.47% specificity). Meanwhile, the combination of AFP, satellite nodules and miR-200a, yielding an AUC of 88.19% (68.54% sensitivity and 93.62% specificity), was proved to be a powerful discrimination tool.

These classifiers were tested in the subgroups of patients with normal-, elevated- and diagnostic-AFP, respectively. As shown in Figure 3, the AUC of miR-200a was 81.20% (sensitivity = 84.21%, specificity = 85.71%) in the normal AFP (≤20 ng/

Table 3. Univariate and Multivariate Cox proportional hazards regression analysis of miRNAs in relation to HCC outcome.

Variable	Overall survival				
	Univariate analysis			Multivariate analysis	
	HR(95%CI)	p value		HR(95%CI)	p value
miR-200a	0.572(0.474–0.690)	0.000		0.572(0.474–0.690)	0.000
miR-21	0.700(0.528–0.926)	0.013			
miR-224-5p	0.700(0.553–0.886)	0.003			
miR-122	0.804(0.686–0.942)	0.007			

HR, hazard ratio; CI, confidence interval; miR, microRNA.

ml) group. In the elevated AFP (21–400 ng/mL) group, the AUC of miR-200a was 78.89% (sensitivity = 74.07%, specificity = 80.00%). In diagnostic (>400 ng/mL) group, the AUC of miR-200a was 81.39% (sensitivity = 91.67%, specificity = 80.00%). The analysis demonstrated that the miR-200a classifier was more powerful than the combination of AFP and satellite nodules in all three subgroups, especially in the normal AFP one.

Discussion

In recent years, the clinical value of miRNAs has been assessed because of its tumor-specific expression and stability in tissues and in the circulation. Although miRNA expression signatures have been applied to the outcome prediction of HCC, no study to date has been reported for the application of miRNAs to patients with HCC that received TACE treatment. TACE is recommended as a single treatment modality in unresectable HCC. There are a few

predictors of OS, including AFP and BCLC stage [20,21], which are consistent with our study. Previous studies have reported the prognostic effect of AFP status after TACE and the dynamic change after locoregional therapy, including TACE [21,22]. However, the prognostic significance of baseline AFP levels before treatment in HCC patients has not been well clarified. Our study demonstrated the prognostic value of AFP in HCC patients before TACE treatment. Patients with high AFP expression display significantly lower overall survival. Meanwhile, univariate analysis showed that the expression of miR-122, miR-214 and miR-200a were associated with AFP. It has been demonstrated that miR-122, a liver-specific miRNA, could regulate AFP via miR-122/CUX1/miR-214/ZBTB20 pathway [23]. A recent study showed that ASB4 is regulated by miR-200a directly in HCC and the level of ASB4 is associated with serum AFP [24]. These studies provide clues to support our results, although the exact molecular

Table 4. Correlation between the expression of 11 miRNAs and clinical parameters of 136 HCC patients with TACE treatment.

Parameters	miRNAs	P value
Gender	None	
Age	None	
BCLC stage	None	
	miR-101-3p	0.026
Child-Puge class	miR-199a-5p	0.004
	miR-221	0.036
HBV	None	
	miR-21	0.018
Tumor size	miR-222	0.044
	miR-224-5p	0.046
	miR-122	0.017
	miR-200a	0.005
AFP	miR-214	0.022
	miR-21	0.023
	miR-224-5p	0.000
	miR-101-3p	0.005
Satellite nodules	miR-19a	0.010
	miR-222	0.039
Relapse	None	
Tumor multiplicity	None	

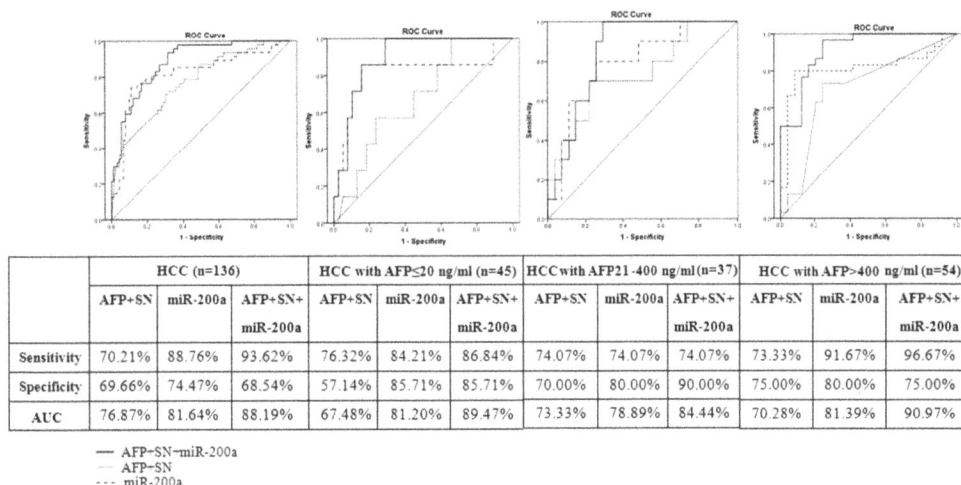

	HCC (n=136)			HCC with AFP≤20 ng/ml (n=45)			HCC with AFP21-400 ng/ml (n=37)			HCC with AFP>400 ng/ml (n=54)		
	AFP+SN	miR-200a	AFP+SN+ miR-200a	AFP+SN	miR-200a	AFP+SN+ miR-200a	AFP+SN	miR-200a	AFP+SN+ miR-200a	AFP+SN	miR-200a	AFP+SN+ miR-200a
Sensitivity	70.21%	88.76%	93.62%	76.32%	84.21%	86.84%	74.07%	74.07%	74.07%	73.33%	91.67%	96.67%
Specificity	69.66%	74.47%	68.54%	57.14%	85.71%	85.71%	70.00%	80.00%	90.00%	75.00%	80.00%	75.00%
AUC	76.87%	81.64%	88.19%	67.48%	81.20%	89.47%	73.33%	78.89%	84.44%	70.28%	81.39%	90.97%

— AFP-SN-miR-200a
--- AFP-SN
--- miR-200a

Figure 3. Receiver operating characteristic curve analysis for predicting prognostic accuracy of hepatocellular carcinoma with TACE treatment. ROC curves for the combination of AFP and satellite nodules, miR-200a and the combination of AFP, satellite nodules and miR-200a in total 136 patients and subgroup of HCC patients with normal (≤20 ng/ml), elevated (20–400 ng/ml) and diagnostic (>400 ng/ml) AFP level, respectively. The sensitivity, specificity and AUC were indicated below each ROC graph. SN: satellite nodules.

mechanisms that mediate AFP expression are needed to be elucidated.

When correlated the above 11 miRNAs with patient's survival, we found that the higher presence of miR-200a, miR-21, miR-122 and miR-224-5p in HCC following TACE was associated with a decreased overall survival. The association at the tissue level between HCC and these four miRNAs has been previously reported. Huang et al demonstrated that miR-200a and miR-200b plays important roles in HCC migration by regulating E-cadherin expression [25]. Petrelli A et al showed that activation of the nuclear factor erythroid related factor 2 (NRF2) pathway and up-regulation of the miR-200 family were among the most prominent changes of early molecular changes in HCC. Further, miR-200a is known to negatively regulate the NRF2 pathway [26]. The findings of the above studies emphasized the important role of miR-200a in HCC. A recent study showed that miR-200a was significantly down-regulated in HCC tissue [27]. Our present study showed that HCC patients with higher serum miR-200a expression experienced worse survival. Thus, serum miR-200a maybe served as a marker to present disease severity-dependent change of HCC patients. Moreover, miR-21 has been reported as a potent oncogene that overexpressed in HCC and plays a key role in resisting programmed cell death in cancer cells [28,29]. Consistent with the present findings, a newly published report suggested that circulating miR-21 has a prognostic value in patients with cancer [30]. miR-122 has been shown to be liver-specific and highly expressed in the normal liver. Previous reports showed that serum miR-122 may serve as a potential biomarker for liver injury [31–33]. Elevated miR-122 in the serum of patients may be released from the damage of hepatocytes caused by virus infection or cancer. This might explain why miR-122 is down-regulated in HCC tissue but elevated in serum of HCC patients. And, the change in miR-122 concentration appeared earlier than the increase in aminotransferase activity in the blood [31]. Li et al validated that miR-224 was overexpressed in HCC tissues and regulated cell migration and invasion by miR-224/HOXD10/p-PAK4/MMP-9 signaling pathway in HCC [34,35]. These studies strongly support the importance of these four miRNAs in HCC development, although the roles of them need to be further studied.

In the present study, we have found that miR-200a was a robust classifier in predicting prognosis of HCC treated with TACE and outperformed the classifier of the combination of AFP and satellite nodules as biomarker with positive predictive value. When we combined AFP, satellite nodules and miR-200a together to predict the prognosis, the probability could be further improved (from 81.6% to 88.2%). Furthermore, the accuracy of the combination of AFP and satellite nodules in normal-AFP subgroup was 67.48%, lower than the 70% value that is considered highly useful. However, the classifier of miR-200a in normal-AFP subgroup presented an AUC of 81.20% with a sensitivity of 84.21% and a specificity of 85.71%, confirming the potential role of miR-200a in predicting the prognosis of HCC.

This study was a retrospective study with a relatively small sample size and the application of the classifier in TACE-treated HCC patients is yet to be further validated, but the aim is clearly different from previous. There has no study to date reporting the association of miRNA expression with HCC prognosis following TACE therapy. Our evidences highlight that serum miR-200a may be a promising prognostic biomarker in HCC patients. Patients with a high risk of TACE treatment failure may benefit from measurement of miR-200a in serum.

In summary, the AFP status, satellite nodules and miR-200a in serum before TACE may help us to predict patients' survival, and it may also enables pretherapeutic stratification of HCC patients in designing a treatment strategy.

Author Contributions

Conceived and designed the experiments: ML JL YX NX. Performed the experiments: ML HZ JL CZ LW. Analyzed the data: LW. Contributed reagents/materials/analysis tools: ML JL HW CZ YX NX. Contributed to the writing of the manuscript: ML LW JL YX NX. Serum samples and followed-up the patients: JL CZ HW.

References

1. Jemal A, Bray F, Center MM, Ferlay J, Ward E, et al. (2011) Global cancer statistics. CA Cancer J Clin 61: 69–90.
2. Llovet JM, Real MI, Montana X, Planas R, Coll S, et al. (2002) Arterial embolisation or chemoembolisation versus symptomatic treatment in patients with unresectable hepatocellular carcinoma: a randomised controlled trial. Lancet 359: 1734–1739.
3. Bartel DP (2004) MicroRNAs: genomics, biogenesis, mechanism, and function. Cell 116: 281–297.
4. Mitchell PS, Parkin RK, Kroh EM, Fritz BR, Wyman SK, et al. (2008) Circulating microRNAs as stable blood-based markers for cancer detection. Proc Natl Acad Sci U S A 105: 10513–10518.
5. Krutzfeldt J, Rajewsky N, Braich R, Rajeev KG, Tuschl T, et al. (2005) Silencing of microRNAs in vivo with 'antagomirs'. Nature 438: 685–689.
6. Elmen J, Lindow M, Schutz S, Lawrence M, Petri A, et al. (2008) LNA-mediated microRNA silencing in non-human primates. Nature 452: 896–899.
7. Park JK, Kogure T, Nuovo GJ, Jiang J, He L, et al. (2011) miR-221 silencing blocks hepatocellular carcinoma and promotes survival. Cancer Res 71: 7608–7616.
8. Negrini M, Gramantieri L, Sabbioni S and Croce CM (2011) microRNA involvement in hepatocellular carcinoma. Anticancer Agents Med Chem 11: 500–521.
9. Ferracin M, Veronese A and Negrini M (2010) Micromarkers: miRNAs in cancer diagnosis and prognosis. Expert Rev Mol Diagn 10: 297–308.
10. Minguez B and Lachenmayer A (2011) Diagnostic and prognostic molecular markers in hepatocellular carcinoma. Dis Markers 31: 181–190.
11. Tsai WC, Hsu PW, Lai TC, Chau GY, Lin CW, et al. (2009) MicroRNA-122, a tumor suppressor microRNA that regulates intrahepatic metastasis of hepatocellular carcinoma. Hepatology 49: 1571–1582.
12. Coulouarn C, Factor VM, Andersen JB, Durkin ME and Thorgeirsson SS (2009) Loss of miR-122 expression in liver cancer correlates with suppression of the hepatic phenotype and gain of metastatic properties. Oncogene 28: 3526–3536.
13. Fornari F, Gramantieri L, Ferracin M, Veronese A, Sabbioni S, et al. (2008) MiR-221 controls CDKN1C/p57 and CDKN1B/p27 expression in human hepatocellular carcinoma. Oncogene 27: 5651–5661.
14. Gramantieri L, Fornari F, Ferracin M, Veronese A, Sabbioni S, et al. (2009) MicroRNA-221 targets Bmf in hepatocellular carcinoma and correlates with tumor multifocality. Clin Cancer Res 15: 5073–5081.
15. Meng F, Henson R, Wehbe-Janek H, Ghoshal K, Jacob ST, et al. (2007) MicroRNA-21 regulates expression of the PTEN tumor suppressor gene in human hepatocellular cancer. Gastroenterology 133: 647–658.
16. Murakami Y, Yasuda T, Saigo K, Urashima T, Toyoda H, et al. (2006) Comprehensive analysis of microRNA expression patterns in hepatocellular carcinoma and non-tumorous tissues. Oncogene 25: 2537–2545.
17. Gramantieri L, Ferracin M, Fornari F, Veronese A, Sabbioni S, et al. (2007) Cyclin G1 is a target of miR-122a, a microRNA frequently down-regulated in human hepatocellular carcinoma. Cancer Res 67: 6092–6099.
18. Jiang J, Gusev Y, Aderca I, Mettler TA, Nagorney DM, et al. (2008) Association of MicroRNA expression in hepatocellular carcinomas with hepatitis infection, cirrhosis, and patient survival. Clin Cancer Res 14: 419–427.
19. Han ZB, Zhong L, Teng MJ, Fan JW, Tang HM, et al. (2012) Identification of recurrence-related microRNAs in hepatocellular carcinoma following liver transplantation. Mol Oncol 6: 445–457.
20. Farinati F, Marino D, De Giorgio M, Baldan A, Cantarini M, et al. (2006) Diagnostic and prognostic role of alpha-fetoprotein in hepatocellular carcinoma: both or neither? Am J Gastroenterol 101: 524–532.
21. Wang Y, Chen Y, Ge N, Zhang L, Xie X, et al. (2012) Prognostic significance of alpha-fetoprotein status in the outcome of hepatocellular carcinoma after treatment of transarterial chemoembolization. Ann Surg Oncol 19: 3540–3546.
22. Riaz A, Ryu RK, Kulik LM, Mulcahy MF, Lewandowski RJ, et al. (2009) Alpha-fetoprotein response after locoregional therapy for hepatocellular carcinoma: oncologic marker of radiologic response, progression, and survival. J Clin Oncol 27: 5734–5742.
23. Kojima K, Takata A, Vadnais C, Otsuka M, Yoshikawa T, et al. (2011) MicroRNA122 is a key regulator of alpha-fetoprotein expression and influences the aggressiveness of hepatocellular carcinoma. Nat Commun 2: 338.
24. Au V, Tsang FH, Man K, Fan ST, Poon RT, et al. (2014) Expression of ankyrin repeat and SOCS box containing 4 (ASB4) confers migration and invasion properties of hepatocellular carcinoma cells. Biosci Trends 8: 101–110.
25. Hung CS, Liu HH, Liu JJ, Yeh CT, Chang TC, et al. (2013) MicroRNA-200a and -200b mediated hepatocellular carcinoma cell migration through the epithelial to mesenchymal transition markers. Ann Surg Oncol 20 Suppl 3: S360–368.
26. Petrelli A, Perra A, Cora D, Sulas P, Menegon S, et al. (2014) MicroRNA/gene profiling unveils early molecular changes and nuclear factor erythroid related factor 2 (NRF2) activation in a rat model recapitulating human hepatocellular carcinoma (HCC). Hepatology 59: 228–241.
27. Dhayat SA, Mardin WA, Kohler G, Bahde R, Vowinkel T, et al. (2014) The microRNA-200 family-A potential diagnostic marker in hepatocellular carcinoma? J Surg Oncol 110: 430–438.
28. Callegari E, Elamin BK, Sabbioni S, Gramantieri L and Negrini M (2013) Role of microRNAs in hepatocellular carcinoma: a clinical perspective. Onco Targets Ther 6: 1167–1178.
29. Buscaglia LE and Li Y (2011) Apoptosis and the target genes of microRNA-21. Chin J Cancer 30: 371–380.
30. Wang Y, Gao X, Wei F, Zhang X, Yu J, et al. (2014) Diagnostic and prognostic value of circulating miR-21 for cancer: a systematic review and meta-analysis. Gene 533: 389–397.
31. Zhang Y, Jia Y, Zheng R, Guo Y, Wang Y, et al. (2010) Plasma microRNA-122 as a biomarker for viral-, alcohol-, and chemical-related hepatic diseases. Clin Chem 56: 1830–1838.
32. Xu J, Wu C, Che X, Wang L, Yu D, et al. (2011) Circulating microRNAs, miR-21, miR-122, and miR-223, in patients with hepatocellular carcinoma or chronic hepatitis. Mol Carcinog 50: 136–142.
33. Wang K, Zhang S, Marzolf B, Troisch P, Brightman A, et al. (2009) Circulating microRNAs, potential biomarkers for drug-induced liver injury. Proc Natl Acad Sci U S A 106: 4402–4407.
34. Li Q, Wang G, Shan JL, Yang ZX, Wang HZ, et al. (2010) MicroRNA-224 is upregulated in HepG2 cells and involved in cellular migration and invasion. J Gastroenterol Hepatol 25: 164–171.
35. Li Q, Ding C, Chen C, Zhang Z, Xiao H, et al. (2013) miR-224 promotes cell migration and invasion by modulating p-PAK4 and MMP-9 via targeting HOXD10 in human hepatocellular carcinoma. J Gastroenterol Hepatol.

8

Autophagy and Apoptosis in Hepatocellular Carcinoma Induced by EF25-(GSH)$_2$: A Novel Curcumin Analog

Tao Zhou[1], Lili Ye[1], Yu Bai[1], Aiming Sun[2,3], Bryan Cox[2], Dahai Liu[1,5], Yong Li[1,5], Dennis Liotta[2,3], James P. Snyder[2,3], Haian Fu[4], Bei Huang[1,5]*

1 School of life Sciences, Anhui University, Hefei, China, **2** Department of Chemistry, Emory University, Atlanta, Georgia, United States of America, **3** Emory Institute for Drug Development (EIDD), Emory University, Atlanta, Georgia, United States of America, **4** Department of Pharmacology and Emory Chemical Biology Discovery Center, Emory University, Atlanta, Georgia, United States of America, **5** Center for Stem Cell and Translational Medicine, Anhui University, Hefei, China

Abstract

Curcumin, a spice component as well as a traditional Asian medicine, has been reported to inhibit proliferation of a variety of cancer cells but is limited in application due to its low potency and bioavailability. Here, we have assessed the therapeutic effects of a novel and water soluble curcumin analog, 3,5-bis(2-hydroxybenzylidene)tetrahydro-4H-pyran-4-one glutathione conjugate [EF25-(GSH)$_2$], on hepatoma cells. Using the MTT and colony formation assays, we determined that EF25-(GSH)$_2$ drastically inhibits the proliferation of hepatoma cell line HepG2 with minimal cytotoxicity for the immortalized human hepatic cell line HL-7702. Significantly, EF25-(GSH)$_2$ suppressed growth of HepG2 xenografts in mice with no observed toxicity to the animals. Mechanistic investigation revealed that EF25-(GSH)$_2$ induces autophagy by means of a biphasic mechanism. Low concentrations (<5 µmol/L) induced autophagy with reversible and moderate cytoplasmic vacuolization, while high concentrations (>10 µmol/L) triggered an arrested autophagy process with irreversible and extensive cytoplasmic vacuolization. Prolonged treatment with EF25-(GSH)$_2$ induced cell death through both an apoptosis-dependent and a non-apoptotic mechanism. Chloroquine, a late stage inhibitor of autophagy which promoted cytoplasmic vacuolization, led to significantly enhanced apoptosis and cytotoxicity when combined with EF25-(GSH)$_2$. Taken together, these data imply a fail-safe mechanism regulated by autophagy in the action of EF25-(GSH)$_2$, suggesting the therapeutic potential of the novel curcumin analog against hepatocellular carcinoma (HCC), while offering a novel and effective combination strategy with chloroquine for the treatment of patients with HCC.

Editor: Yu-Jia Chang, Taipei Medicine University, Taiwan

Funding: Support was provided by the Natural Science Foundation of the Education Department in Anhui Province, China (KJ2012A030, to Bei Huang) and NCI 5 P50 CA128613 SPORE in Head and Neck Cancer (to Haian Fu and J. P. Snyder). The funders had no role in study design, data collection and analysis, decision to publish, or preparation of the manuscript.

Competing Interests: The authors have declared that no competing interests exist.

* Email: beihuang@163.com

Introduction

Hepatocellular carcinoma (HCC) is the fifth most common cancer and the third leading cause of cancer death worldwide [1]. Certain regions in Asia and Africa are disproportionally affected, while China alone accounted for half of the new liver cancer cases occurring worldwide during 2008 [2]. Chemotherapy plays a crucial role in the treatment of HCC especially at advanced stages when curative therapies like resection and liver transplantation are inapplicable [3,4]. However, since most widely used chemotherapeutic drugs show severe side effects, development of novel and safe agents is mandatory.

Curcumin, a natural compound isolated from the commonly used spice turmeric, has been shown to inhibit cell proliferation in various types of cancer cells *in vitro* and *in vivo* [5]. Numerous curcumin derivatives and analogues have been developed in recent years in order to enhance anti-tumor efficacy and overcome limitations such as poor aqueous solubility, relative low bioavailability and intense yellow staining [6,7]. The compounds 3,5-bis(2-flurobenzylidene)piperidin-4-one (EF24) and 3,5-bis(pyridin-2-ylmethylene)piperidin-4-one (EF31), synthetic structural analogues of curcumin [8], exhibit improved anticancer activity and a safety

profile similar to curcumin [8–11]. Synthetic manipulation of these agents generates EF24-(GSH)$_2$ and EF31-(GSH)$_2$, double glutathione conjugates with no less anticancer capability compared to EF24 and EF31. However the conjugates exhibit superior stability in solution, water solubility and lack of color [8]. The structurally related compound 3,5-bis(2-hydroxybenzylidene)tetrahydro-4H-pyran-4-one (EF25) and its double glutathione conjugate EF25-(GSH)$_2$, are under investigation and reported here for the first time.

Although much of the research into the anti-cancer mechanisms of curcumin has focused on its ability to induce apoptosis, curcumin has also been found to induce other types of cell death including autophagic cell death, mitosis catastrophe and paraptosis [5,12–14]. By testing different cell lines, it has been found that the mode of cell death induced by curcumin varies among different cell lines, and the mechanisms of different cellular responses remains a mystery [14].

Here we show that *in vitro* EF25-(GSH)$_2$ exhibits preferential toxicity to malignant liver cancer cells compared with immortalized human hepatic cells. In parallel, *in vivo* EF25-(GSH)$_2$ significantly suppresses the growth of hepatocellular carcinoma

(HepG2) xenografts and is relatively nontoxic to mice. Further investigation into the mechanism of action reveals that EF25-$(GSH)_2$ induces a mixed mode of cell death in hepatoma cells in which autophagy, cell cycle arrest, cytoplasmic vacuolization, caspase-dependent and caspase-independent apoptosis all take place.

Materials and Methods

1. Ethics Statement

All procedures involving mice were approved by Anhui Medical University Animal Care Committee, which follows the protocol outlined in The Guide for the Care and Use of Laboratory Animals published by the USA National Institute of Health (NIH publication No. 85-23, revised 1996). The details of animal welfare and steps taken to ameliorate suffering were in accordance with the recommendations in The Guide for the Care and Use of Laboratory Animals, and all efforts were made to minimize suffering.

2. Reagents

Cisplatin was purchased from the National Institutes for Food and Drug Control (China). Curcumin and other reagents were purchased from Sigma-Aldrich. Antibodies against microtubule-associated protein 1 light chain 3B (LC3B), caspase-3, caspase-8 and actin were obtained from Cell Signaling Technology. mCherry-GFP-LC3B plasmid was kindly provided by Dr. Mian Wu (University of Science and Technology of China). Lentivirus-based shRNA constructs targeting the human Atg5 gene (pLKO.1-shAtg5-D8 and pLKO.1-shAtg5-D9, targeting different sequences), human Beclin-1 gene (pLKO.1-shBeclin-1-C2 and pLKO.1-shBeclin-1-C3, targeting different sequences) were kindly provided by Dr. Qinghua Shi (University of Science and Technology of China), and negative control targeting LacZ (pLKO.1-shLacZ) was obtained from the National RNAi Core Facility (Taiwan). Three helper plasmids (pLP1, pLP2 and pLP/VSVG) of lentiviral systems were kindly provided by Dr. Yong Li (Anhui University).

3. Synthesis of EF25 and EF25-$(GSH)_2$

EF25 was prepared as previously reported where it was originally named "compound 11" [15], while EF25-$(GSH)_2$ was obtained by a procedure identical to that for EF24-$(GSH)_2$ [8]. It should be noted that EF25 combined with glutathione much more slowly by comparison with EF24. EF25 (64.0 mg, 0.2 mmol, 1.0 eq.) in CH_3CN (0.2 ml) was added dropwise to a solution of GSH (123.0 mg, 0.4 mmol, 2.0 eq.) in water at room temperature. The reaction mixture was refluxed for 2 hr until the disappearance of both the yellow color and EF25 by LC/MS. Evaporation of the solvent delivered the product as a white powder in quantitative yield. HR-ESI-MS (m/z): $[M+H]^+$ calcd for $C_{39}H_{51}O_{16}N_6S_2$ 923.28053, found, 923.28121 (= 00068 amu) (Fig. S1).

The ^1H NMR spectrum of EF25-$(GSH)_2$ in DMSO-d6 and D_2O (buffer pH7) are complex due to the presence of diastereo-isomers resulting from GSH conjugation at the two C = C bonds of EF25. The ^1H NMR spectrum of the unconjugated EF25 in DMSO-d6 exhibits a sharp singlet at 7.89 ppm assigned to the olefinic(C =)C–H proton and sharp aromatic signals at 6.8–7.3 ppm. The intensity of the olefinic signal decreases for the conjugated EF25-$(GSH)_x$, and the sharp aromatic signals observed for unconjugated EF25 are broadened for EF25-$(GSH)_x$. These observations indicate a mixture of the mono- and bis-conjugates EF25-(GSH) and EF25-$(GSH)_2$, respectively, and possibly rapid exchange between them (Fig. S2). The comparison of the ^1H

NMR spectra of EF25 in DMSO-d6 and EF25-$(GSH)_2$ in D_2O (pH7) illustrates the absence of observable quantities of unconjugated EF25 (Fig. S3). Thus, in these solvents, the equilibrium lies primarily on the side of the conjugates, although in biological tissues it is shifted to the unconjugated form as the hydrophobic EF25 interacts with its target proteins.

4. Cell culture

The three human hepatocellular carcinoma cell lines (HepG2, SMMC-7721 and BEL-7402) and one immortalized human hepatic cell line (HL-7702) were kindly supplied by Dr. Hui Zhong (Academy of Military Medical Sciences) [16–19]. The other three human tumor cell lines (HCT116 human colon cancer cell line, A549 human lung carcinoma cell line and Hela human cervical carcinoma cell line) and HEK293FT cell line were kindly supplied by Dr. Qinghua Shi (University of Science and Technology of China) [20,21]. The HepG2, HCT116, A549, Hela, BEL-7402 and HEK293FT cells were grown in DMEM (Gibco). The SMMC-7721 cells and HL-7702 cells were grown in RPMI 1640 (Gibco). Both media were supplemented with 10% fetal bovine serum (FBS; Gibco), 100 units/mL penicillin and 100 μg/mL streptomycin at 37°C in a humidified incubator containing 5% CO_2.

5. Cell viability assay

Cells (8×10^3 per well) were seeded onto 96-well plates in supplemented DMEM and incubated overnight. Then the cells were treated in triplicate for the indicated time with increasing doses of EF25-$(GSH)_2$ in 10% FBS containing DMEM or RPMI 1640 without antibiotic. Treated cells were then incubated in the presence of 0.5 mg/mL 3-(4,5-Dimethylthiazol-2-yl)-2,5-diphenyl-tetrazoliumbromide (MTT) for 4 h. The formazan crystals were dissolved in DMSO and monitored at an absorbance of 490 nm. Absorbance values were normalized to those obtained for the untreated cells to determine percentage survival. All experiments were repeated at least three times. IC_{50} values (50% inhibition concentration) were then calculated using the Statistical Package for the Social Sciences (SPSS, Inc.).

6. Colony formation assay

Twenty-four-well plates were seeded with 500 viable cells in complete medium and incubated overnight. The cells were then treated in triplicate with EF25-$(GSH)_2$ in 10% FBS containing DMEM without antibiotic for 24 h. The compound-containing medium was then removed, and the cells were washed with PBS twice and incubated in complete medium for another two weeks. Medium was replaced once at the end of the first week. The cell colonies formed were fixed in 10% formalin for 10 min and visualized by staining with Giemsa [22].

7. DNA content analysis

5×10^6 HepG2 cells were seeded into six-well plates and incubated overnight. The cells were treated with EF25-$(GSH)_2$ and then collected by trypsinization and fixed in precooled 70% ethanol overnight. Cells were then stained with 50 μg/mL propidium iodide (PI) in the presence of 100 μg/mL RNase A. DNA content was analyzed by FACSCalibur (Becton Dickinson), and data were analyzed by the Flowjo software. The percentage of cells in sub-G_1-G_0 was used to represent the apoptosis rate.

8. HepG2 cell tumor xenograft in mice

Five-week-old male athymic mice were obtained from Beijing Vital River Laboratory Animal Co., Ltd. Animals were given ad

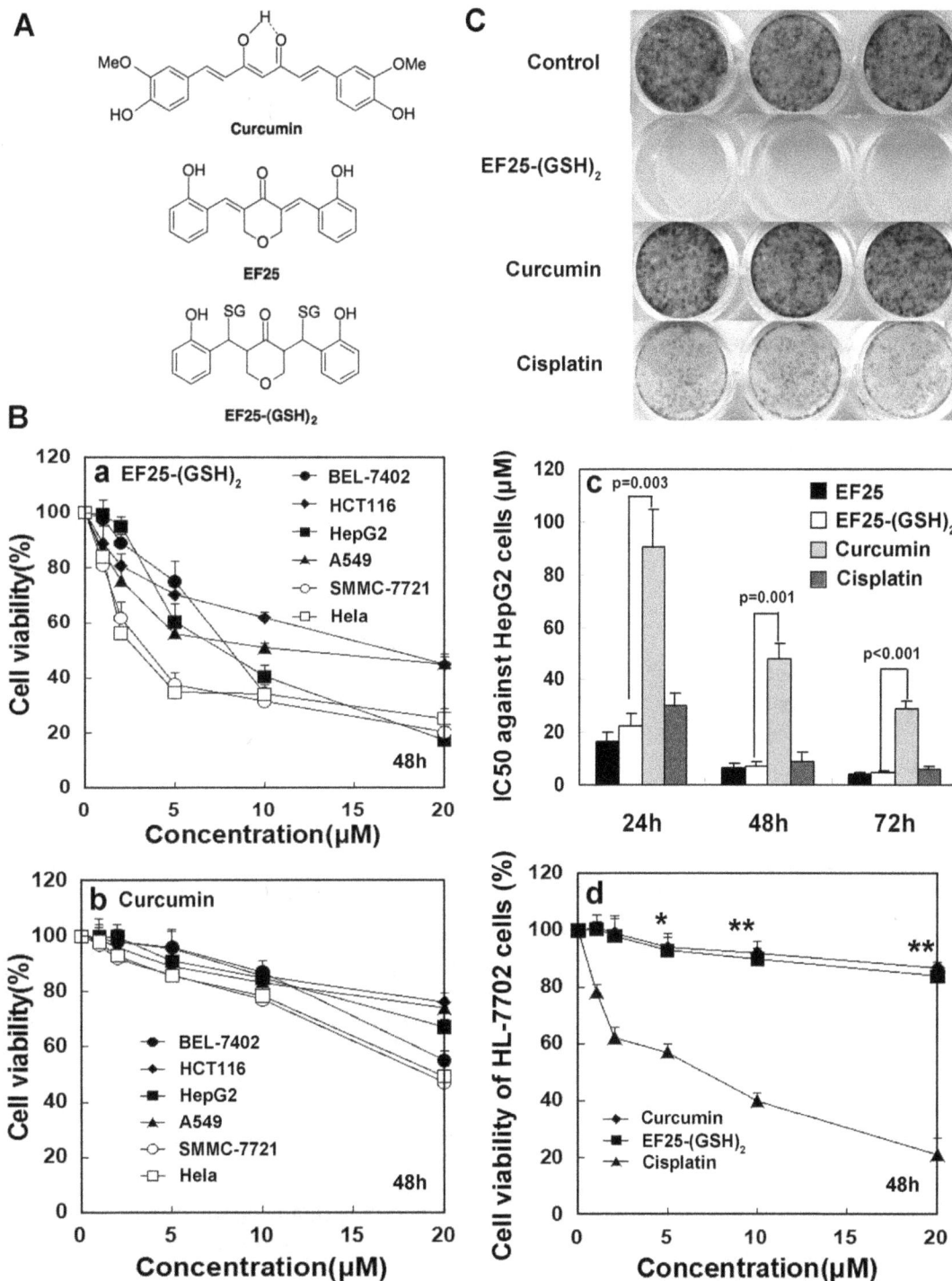

Figure 1. EF25-(GSH)2 inhibited proliferation of tumor cells *in vitro*. (A) The structures of curcumin, EF25 and EF25-(GSH)$_2$. (B) *a and b*, EF25-(GSH)$_2$ showed similar toxicity towards six human tumor cells (BEL-7402, HCT116, HepG2, A549, SMMC-7721 and Hela) (*a*) and the toxicity of curcumin was much lower than that of EF25-(GSH)$_2$ (*b*). *c*, cells were incubated with increasing doses of indicated compounds for 24-, 48-, and 72-h periods and analyzed by MTT assay. The IC$_{50}$ of each agent at each time period was calculated and compared using SPSS. The IC$_{50}$ of EF25-(GSH)$_2$ is much lower than that of curcumin and essentially equivalent to that of cisplatin. *d*, the cytotoxicity of EF25-(GSH)$_2$ to HL-7702 cells was much lower than that of cisplatin and similar to curcumin after 48-hour incubation as determined by MTT assay (*, $p<0.01$, **, $p<0.001$). (C) Cells were incubated with 0.5 μmol/L of the indicated compound for 24 h and subsequently allowed to grow into colonies (2 weeks). EF25-(GSH)$_2$ totally inhibited colony formation leading to clean plates, while curcumin and cisplatin did not. Results are representative of three independent experiments.

libitum access to water and standard mouse chow. 5×10^6 HepG2 cells were injected subcutaneous into the left flank and allowed to form a xenograft. Treatment was initiated when the tumor reached a group mean of 100 mm^3. EF25-(GSH)$_2$ was dissolved in PBS and administrated i.p. daily at a dose of 1.5 mg/kg body weight for 30 days [23,24]. The control group was given the same

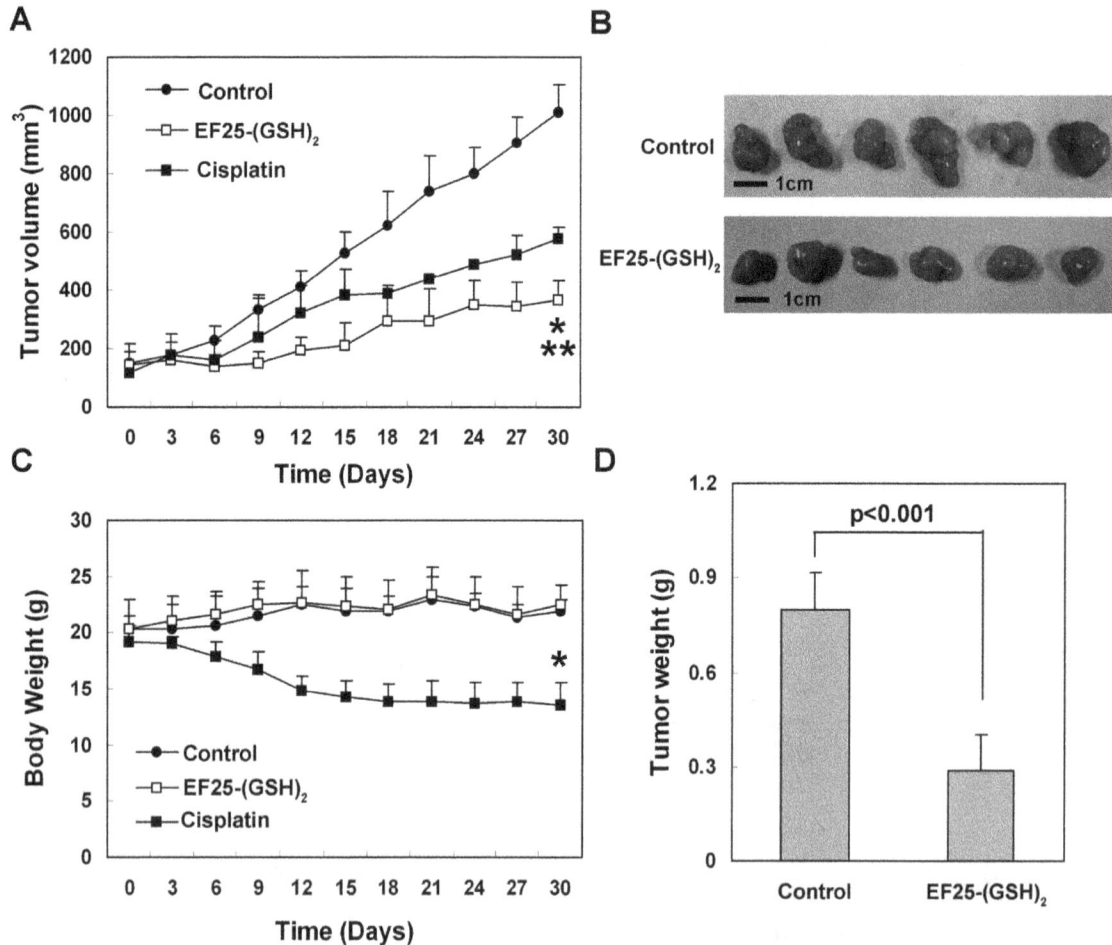

Figure 2. EF25-(GSH)$_2$ suppressed HepG2 xenograft growth *in vivo*. (A) HepG2 cells were injected into the left flank of nude mice and tumors were allowed to grow to a size of about 100 mm^3. Subsequently, EF25-(GSH)$_2$ (dissolved in PBS, 1.5 mg/kg body weight) was injected daily i.p. for 30 d (n = 6). The cisplatin group (dissolved in PBS, 0.5 mg/kg body weight) was injected every other day i.p. (n = 4), and the control group was injected with the same volume of PBS daily i.p. (n = 6). Tumor growth was significantly suppressed in the EF25-(GSH)$_2$-treated group compared to either control (**, p<0.001) or cisplatin-treated group (*, p<0.01). (B) At the end of the treatment, tumor volume in the EF25-(GSH)$_2$-treated group was much smaller than that of the control group. (C) The EF25-(GSH)$_2$-treated group maintained normal weight gain while the cisplatin-treated group suffered a remarkable weight loss throughout the treatment (*, p<0.001). (D) At the end of the treatment, EF25-(GSH)$_2$ treatment resulted in significantly lower tumor weight when compared with control group.

volume of PBS only. Tumor volume was calculated using the formula $V = a^2 \times b/2$, where a and b represent the shorter and longer diameters of the tumor, respectively. At the end of the treatment, the mice were sacrificed under etherization, and the tumors were weighed.

9. Transmission electron microscopy

Treated cells were collected by trypsinization, washed twice with PBS, and then fixed with ice-cold 3% glutaraldehyde in 0.1 mol/L cacodylate buffer at 4°C overnight. Cells were then postfixed in osmium tetroxide and embedded in Polybed resin. Ultrathin sections were double stained with uranyl acetate and lead citrate and examined with a JEM-2100 electron microscope.

10. 4, 6-diamidino-2-phenylindole (DAPI) staining

At the end of the EF25-(GSH)$_2$ treatment, DAPI was added to the medium at a final concentration of 1 μg/mL. After staining with DAPI for 15 min, cell morphology was examined by laser confocal microscopy. Uniformly stained nuclei with clear margins

were regarded as normal, while condensed or fragmented nuclei with strengthened fluorescence were considered apoptotic.

11. Transient transfection

HepG2 cells were seeded in six-well plates and incubated overnight. mCherry-GFP -LC3 was transfected using Lipofectamine 2000 according to the manufacturer's instructions. The transfection mixture was replaced with 10% FBS containing DMEM without antibiotic 6 hours after transfection and incubated for another 24 hours. Cells were then treated with EF25-(GSH)$_2$ for the indicated time. Green (GFP) and red (mCherry) fluorescence was observed under a laser confocal microscope.

12. Knockdown of Atg5 and Beclin-1 expression by lentivirus-delivered shRNA

For lentivirus preparation, HEK293FT cells were transfected with pLKO.1-shRNA and three helper plasmids (pLP1, pLP2 and pLP/VSVG) with Fugene 6 Reagent (Roche). To generate human Atg5-knockdown or Beclin-1-knockdown cells, HepG2 cells were

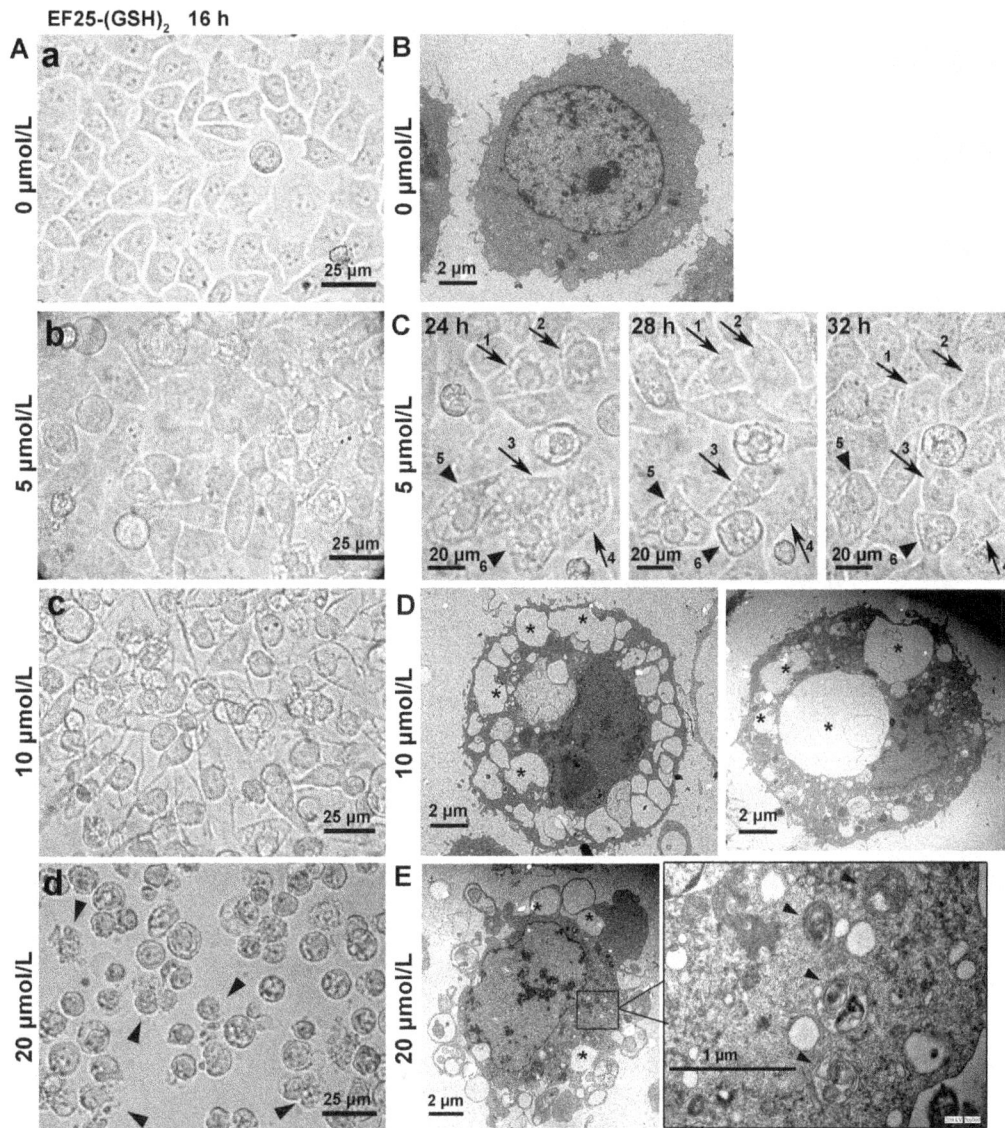

Figure 3. The morphological appearance of EF25-(GSH)₂-treated HepG2 cells. (A) HepG2 cells treated with increasing concentrations of EF25-(GSH)₂ for 16 h were observed under a light microscope and representative images were visualized. EF25-(GSH)₂-treated cells underwent vacuolization, the extent of which varied when treated with different concentrations of EF25-(GSH)₂. At 20 μmol/L, apoptotic-like cell membrane blebbing was observed (arrowheads). (B) A representative transmission electron microscopy (TEM) image of untreated HepG2 cells. (C) In 5 μmol/L EF25-(GSH)₂-treated cells, most vacuolated cells regained normal morphology at 32 h post-treatment (arrows, 1-4) while some did not (arrow heads, 5 and 6). (D) Representative TEM images of cells treated with 10 μmol/L EF25-(GSH)₂ for 16 h. *, large empty vacuoles with varying size. (E) Representative TEM images of cells treated with 20 μmol/L EF25-(GSH)₂ for 16 h. *, large empty vacuoles; arrows, autophagic vacuoles.

transduced with lentivirus expressing shAtg5 or shBeclin-1, respectively, and selected with 2 μg/ml puromycin.

13. Western blot assay

Cell lysates were subjected to SDS-PAGE and blotted onto polyvinylidene difluoride (PVDF) membranes. The membranes were then incubated with the each primary antibody and appropriate secondary antibody. The immunoblots were visualized by a chemiluminescence HRP substrate.

14. Statistical analysis

All values are expressed as the mean±SE. Data were analyzed using two-tailed student's t test. P≤0.05 was considered statistically significant. Statistical analysis was performed using SPSS.

Results

1. EF25-(GSH)₂ inhibited proliferation of tumor cells

The structures of curcumin analogues, EF25 and EF25-(GSH)₂, examined in this study are presented in Figure 1A. We first determined the effect of EF25, EF25-(GSH)₂ and curcumin on cell proliferation of HepG2 cells. Cisplatin, a widely used chemotherapeutic drug, was also examined under the same conditions. EF25-(GSH)₂, which is far more effective than curcumin, showed similar cytotoxicity to cell lines derived from three types of hepatomas (HepG2, SMMC-7721 and BEL-7402) and three other carcinomas (HCT116, A549 and Hela) (Fig. 1B a, b). EF25 and EF25-(GSH)₂ exhibit similar cytotoxicity in a dose- and time-dependent manner, indicating that GSH association does not change the cell-

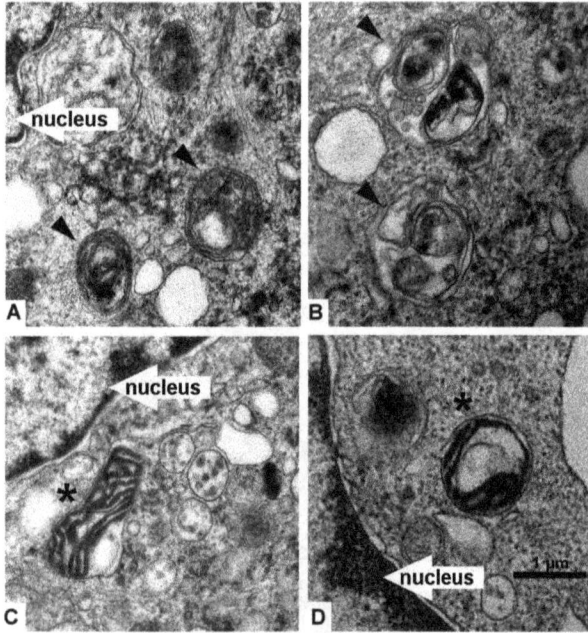

Figure 4. Morphology of autophagosomes in EF25-(GSH)$_2$-treated HepG2 cells. HepG2 cells were treated with 20 μmol/L EF25-(GSH)$_2$ for 16 h and observed under transmission electron microscopy. (A) and (B), multimembranous autophagic vacuoles engulfing cytoplasmic components are indicated with black arrowheads. (C) and (D), autophagic vacuoles containing a mitochondrion are indicated with black asterisk.

kill capacity of the EF25 conjugate. The mechanism of this phenomenon was elucidated in our previous investigation showing that the conjugate is reversible [8]. Thus, the active agent in both cases would appear to be EF25. That the latter showed slightly better activity than EF25-(GSH)$_2$ at 24 h, and that the difference

between them diminished as time prolonged to 72 h (Fig. 1B c), is mostly likely due to differential cell penetration regulated in part by the equilibrium shift from conjugate to free EF25. In effect, EF25-(GSH)$_2$ serves as a pro-drug capable of releasing the active agent EF25 by reversal of the well-known Michael reaction in cells [8]. The cytotxicity of EF25-(GSH)$_2$ to HepG2 cells is much greater than that of curcumin as characterized by its much lower IC$_{50}$ value (7.2 μmol/L at 48 h), which is close to that of cisplatin (9.1 μmol/L at 48 h) (Fig. 1B c). In order to examine if EF25-(GSH)$_2$ can preferentially kill malignant cells, cytotoxicities of the conjugate and cisplatin against immortalized human hepatic cell line HL-7702 were examined at 48 h post-treatment by the MTT assay. The results show that the cytotoxicity of EF25-(GSH)$_2$ to HL-7702 cells was much lower than that of cisplatin (Fig. 1B d).

To examine the long-term effect of EF25-(GSH)$_2$ treatment, the colony formation assay was performed. A quantity of 0.5 μmol/L EF25-(GSH)$_2$ totally inhibited colony formation, while 0.5 μmol/L curcumin had nearly no effect. An 0.5 μmol/L cisplatin treatment also caused a significant reduction in colony number, but was much less efficiently by comparison with EF25-(GSH)$_2$ (Fig. 1C).

2. EF25-(GSH)$_2$ suppresses HepG2 xenograft growth

To assess the antitumor potential of EF25-(GSH)$_2$ *in vivo*, HepG2 xenograft-bearing mice were given EF25-(GSH)$_2$ i.p. daily for 30 days (1.5 mg/kg body weight, PBS as vehicle, n = 6). For comparison, cisplatin was dissolved in PBS and given i.p. every other day at a dose of 0.5 mg/kg body weight (n = 4). Compared with vehicle treatment (n = 6), EF25-(GSH)$_2$ treatment significantly suppressed the growth of tumor volume which was much more efficient than cisplatin treatment (Fig. 2A, B). Notably, while the EF25-(GSH)$_2$-treated group maintained normal weight gain, the cisplatin-treated animals suffered a remarkable weight loss throughout the treatment (Fig. 2C). The tumor weights of EF25-(GSH)$_2$-treated mice were also significantly lower than that of the control group (Fig. 2D). There was no apparent change in liver, kidney and spleen weight in the EF25-(GSH)$_2$-treated group, while

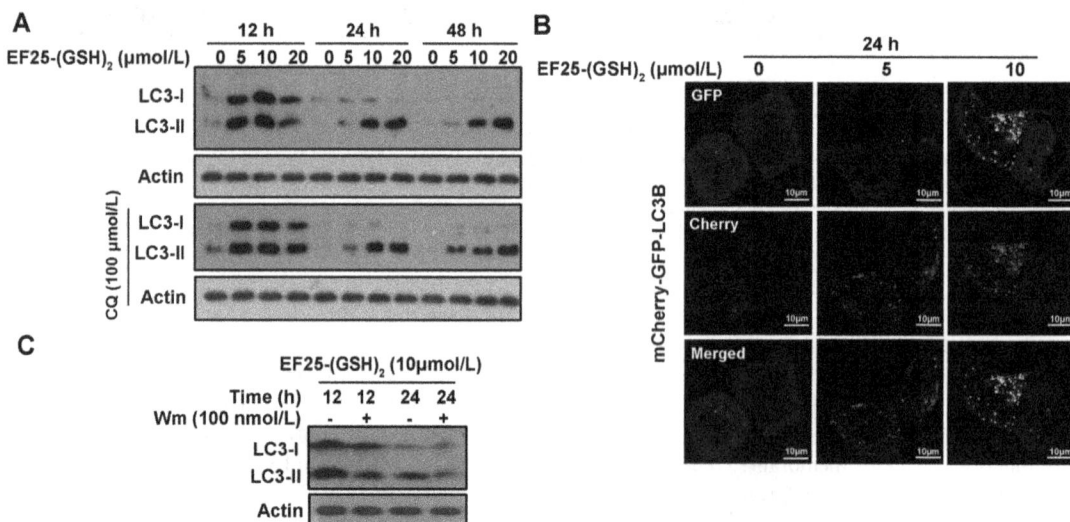

Figure 5. EF25-(GSH)$_2$ induced autophagy in HepG2 cells. (A) Western blot analysis of the LC3B expression in HepG2 cells treated with EF25-(GSH)$_2$ at varying concentrations for 12 to 48 h with or without chloroquine (CQ, 100 μmol/L). (B) The cellular distribution of mCherry-GFP-LC3B in HepG2 cells treated with EF25-(GSH)$_2$ at different concentrations for 24 h was examined under a laser confocal microscope. (C) Lysates from HepG2 cells incubated with 10 μmol/L EF25-(GSH)$_2$ for 12 or 24 h pretreated with or without wortmannin (Wm, 100 nmol/L, pretreated for 2 h) were analyzed by Western blotting for LC3B expression level.

A

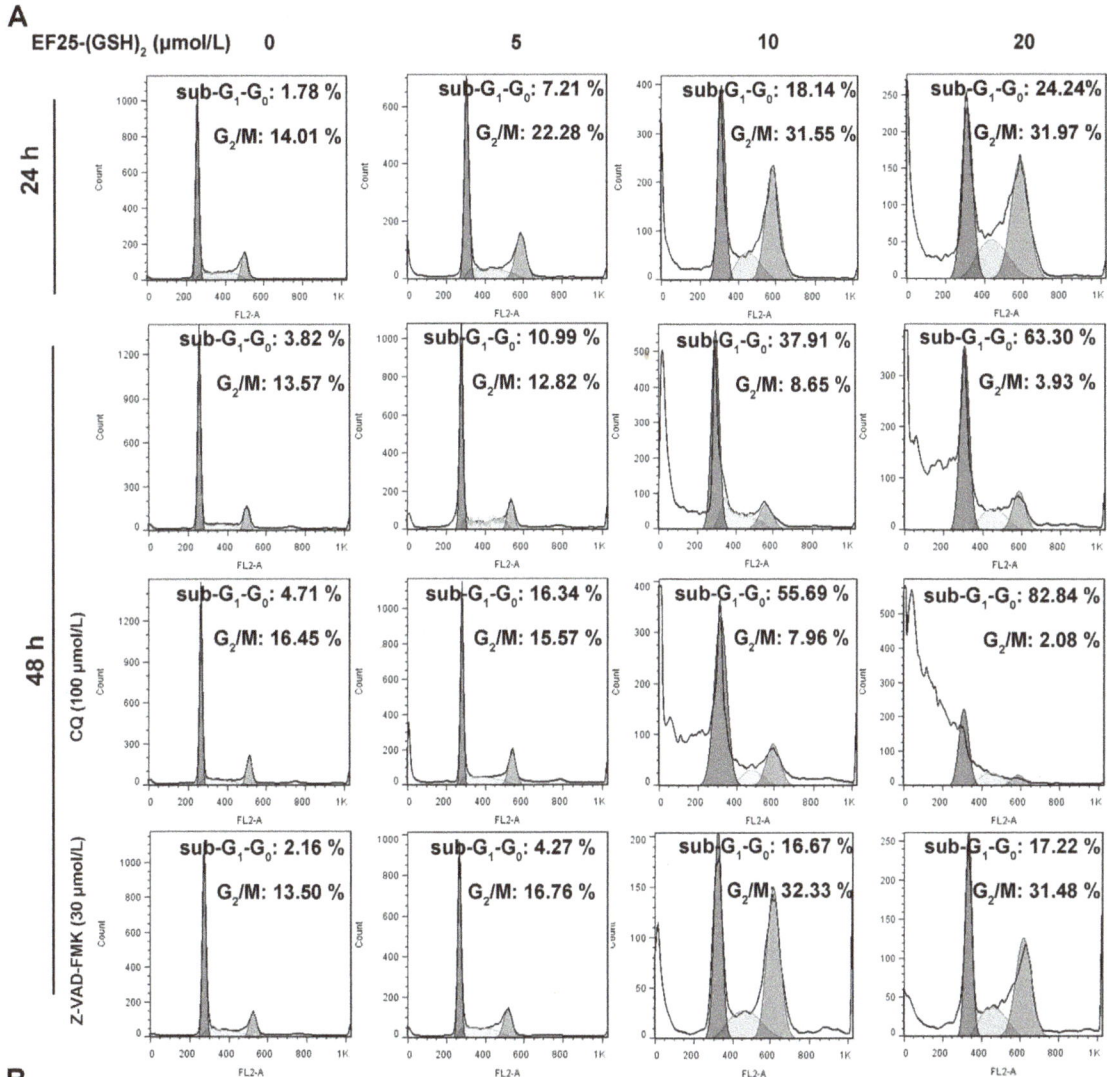

B

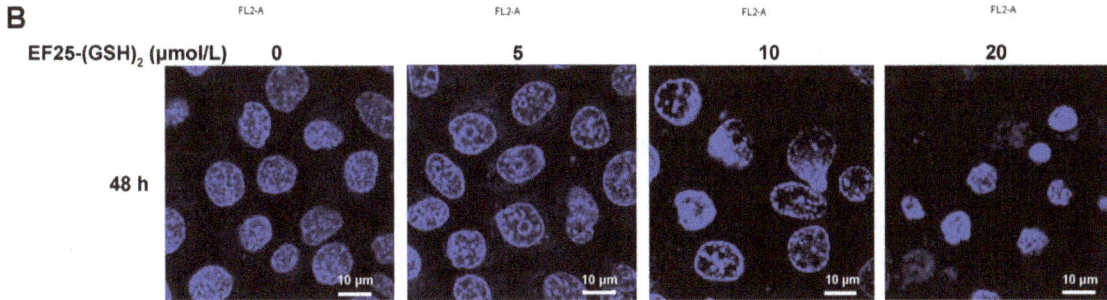

C

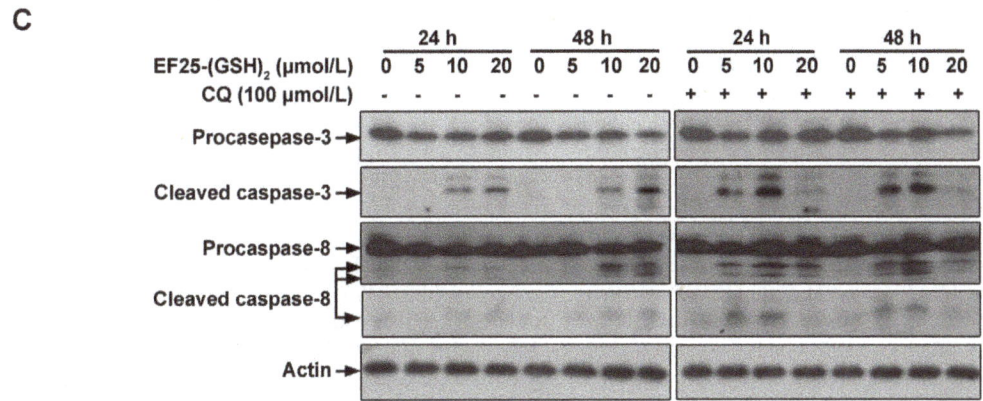

Figure 6. The apoptosis in HepG2 cells triggered by EF25-(GSH)$_2$ in the presence or absence of CQ/Z-VAD-FMK. (A) HepG2 cells were treated with various concentrations of EF25-(GSH)$_2$ for 24 h and 48 h with or without chloroquine (CQ, 100 μmol/L)/Z-VAD-FMK (30 μmol/L, pretreated for 2 h) and then analyzed for DNA content (propidium iodide, PI) and cell cycle distribution. Apoptosis was measured as the percentage of cells containing hupodiploid quantities of DNA (sub-G$_1$-G$_0$ peak). Percentage of cells within the sub-G$_1$-G$_0$ and G$_2$/M stages is shown for each data point. Graphs are representative of data collected from three independent experiments. (B) HepG2 cells incubated with increasing concentrations of EF25-(GSH)$_2$ for 48 h were stained with 4, 6-diamidino-2-phenylindole (DAPI) and examined by laser confocal microscopy. Untreated HepG2 cells showed uniformly stained nuclei, while EF25-(GSH)$_2$-treated cells exhibited chromatin condensation in a concentration-dependent manner. (C) Lysates from HepG2 cells incubated with increasing concentrations of EF25-(GSH)$_2$ for 24 or 48 h with or without chloroquine (CQ, 100 μmol/L) were analyzed by Western blotting for both full length and cleaved caspase-3 and caspase-8 expression levels.

the weight of these organs dropped dramatically in the cisplatin-treated group (data not shown).

3. The morphological appearance of EF25-(GSH)$_2$-treated HepG2 cells

The morphological changes in EF25-(GSH)$_2$-treated cells were observed under a light microscope to observe apparent vacuolization in the cytoplasm. The number of cells that suffered cytoplasmic vacuolization and its extent varied when treated with different concentrations of EF25-(GSH)$_2$, but all reached a maximum at about 16 hours post-treatment (Fig. 3A). When treated with 5 μmol/L EF25-(GSH)$_2$, the cells experienced moderate vacuolization which regained normal morphology after about 8 hours (Fig. 3C). In contrast, most cells exposed to 10 μmol/L EF25-(GSH)$_2$ showed extensive and irreversible vacuolization in the cytoplasm. At 20 μmol/L, EF25-(GSH)$_2$ not only induced massive cytoplasmic vacuolization but also caused apoptotic membrane blebbing (Fig. 3A).

In the cytoplasm of HepG2 cells treated with 10 or 20 μmol/L EF25-(GSH)$_2$ for 16 hours, large vacuoles of varying size were content-free and single membrane bounded, while the small vacuoles resemble autophagic vacuoles (Fig. 3D, E).

4. EF25-(GSH)$_2$ induced autophagy in HepG2 cells

The ultrastructural details of HepG2 cells treated with 20 μmol/L EF25-(GSH)$_2$ for 16 hours were further examined by transmission electron microscopy. Typical multimembrane autophagic vesicles engulfing cytoplasmic components and organelles were identified in the cytoplasm (Fig. 4).

To further confirm whether EF25-(GSH)$_2$ triggered autophagy in HepG2 cells, we examined the expression of the two forms of microtubule-associated protein 1 light chain 3 (LC3). In the process of autophagy, LC3-I residing in the cytosol is modified to LC3-II, which binds to the autophagosome membrane. Thus, the degree of LC3-I to LC3-II conversion correlates to the extent of autophagosome formation [25]. EF25-(GSH)$_2$ treatment obviously increased the expression level of both LC3-I and LC3-II as early as 12 hours post-treatment, but the bands corresponding to LC3-I were weakened and there was no obvious augmentation in the LC3-II expression when EF25-(GSH)$_2$ treatment was prolonged or the dosage was increased, indicating that the lack of conversion of LC3-I to LC3-II may due to incomplete autophagy (Fig. 5A).

The increase in LC3-II expression can be associated with either an enhanced formation of autophagosome or an impaired autophagic degradation [26]. Chloroquine (CQ) is a lysosomal trophic agent that raises the lysosomal pH and, hence, blocks autophagy at the late stages [27]. Accordingly, CQ was used to test if EF25-(GSH)$_2$ can induce complete autophagic flux [28,29]. In cells treated with 5 μmol/L EF25-(GSH)$_2$, the LC3-II showed progressive accumulation in the presence of CQ at 24 h and 48 h. However, at 10 and 20 μmol/L, EF25-(GSH)$_2$-treated samples with and without CQ were indistinguishable with respect to LC3-II expression (Fig. 5A). This data indicates that autophagy flux was

achieved at 5 μmol/L EF25-(GSH)$_2$ but was blocked at 10 and 20 μmol/L.

In addition, we examined the localization of autophagosome-specific protein LC3B in HepG2 cells treated with EF25-(GSH)$_2$ for 24 hours using Cherry-GFP-LC3B plasmid. When autophagy is induced, exogenous LC3 distributes to the membrane of autophagosomes and shows characteristic green (GFP) or red (mCherry) dots. Because GFP is acid-labile, only mCherry red fluorescence can be seen in autophagolysosomes, while the neutral structures display both green and red fluorescence [30]. In untreated cells, mCherry-GFP-LC3B showed a homogeneous distribution, whereas the EF25-(GSH)$_2$-treated cells showed fluorescent dots. At 5 μmol/L, the cells exhibit mostly only red dots, suggestive of autophagic degradation. Meanwhile, at 10 μmol/L, cells expressed double-tagged fusion proteins indicating that autophagic degradation was blocked (Fig. 5B). The data coincide well with the immunoblot analysis of LC3B in the presence of CQ.

5. EF25-(GSH)$_2$ induced G$_2$/M cell cycle arrest and apoptosis in HepG2 cells

Curcumin and its analogs have consistently been reported to induce apoptosis [31,32]. To determine whether EF25-(GSH)$_2$ acts similarly in HepG2 cells, the DNA content of permeabilized PI-stained cells was examined by flow cytometry at 24 h and 48 h post-treatment. The cell cycle analysis showed obvious G$_2$/M cell cycle arrest at 24 h, and the percentage of cells in sub-G$_1$-G$_0$ was greatly augmented at 48 h in a concentration-dependent manner (Fig. 6A).

DAPI staining of the nuclei also indicated that EF25-(GSH)$_2$-treated cells underwent apoptosis, the extent of which was concentration dependent. Untreated HepG2 cells showed uniformly stained nuclei, while nuclei of EF25-(GSH)$_2$-treated cells were condensed or fragmented with strengthened fluorescence (Fig. 6B).

These findings were further confirmed by analysis of the expression level of cleaved caspase-8 and caspase-3, both of which were augmented at 24 h post-treatment and maintained a high level up to 48 h at concentrations of 10 μmol/L and 20 μmol/L, whereas caspase activation was undetectable at 5 μmol/L (Fig. 6C).

6. Wortmannin advanced EF25-(GSH)$_2$ induced cell death in HepG2 cells in the early period

Autophagy modulation is a double edged sword in cancer treatment, possibly due to various cellular settings [33]. To test whether autophagy contributed to or hampered EF25-(GSH)$_2$ promoted HepG2 cell death, an inhibitor of autophagic sequestration (wortmannin (Wm)) was used to block autophagy at the early stages [26]. In the presence of 100 nmol/L Wm, the expression levels of both LC3B I and II types were largely reduced, indicating that Wm was effective in inhibiting EF25-(GSH)$_2$-induced autophagy formation (Fig. 5C). Wm at 100 nmol/L was only slightly toxic to HepG2 cells but clearly promoted the EF25-(GSH)$_2$-inued death process in the first 24 hours as evidenced by earlier cell shrinkage, rounding up (data not shown) and a 7–12%

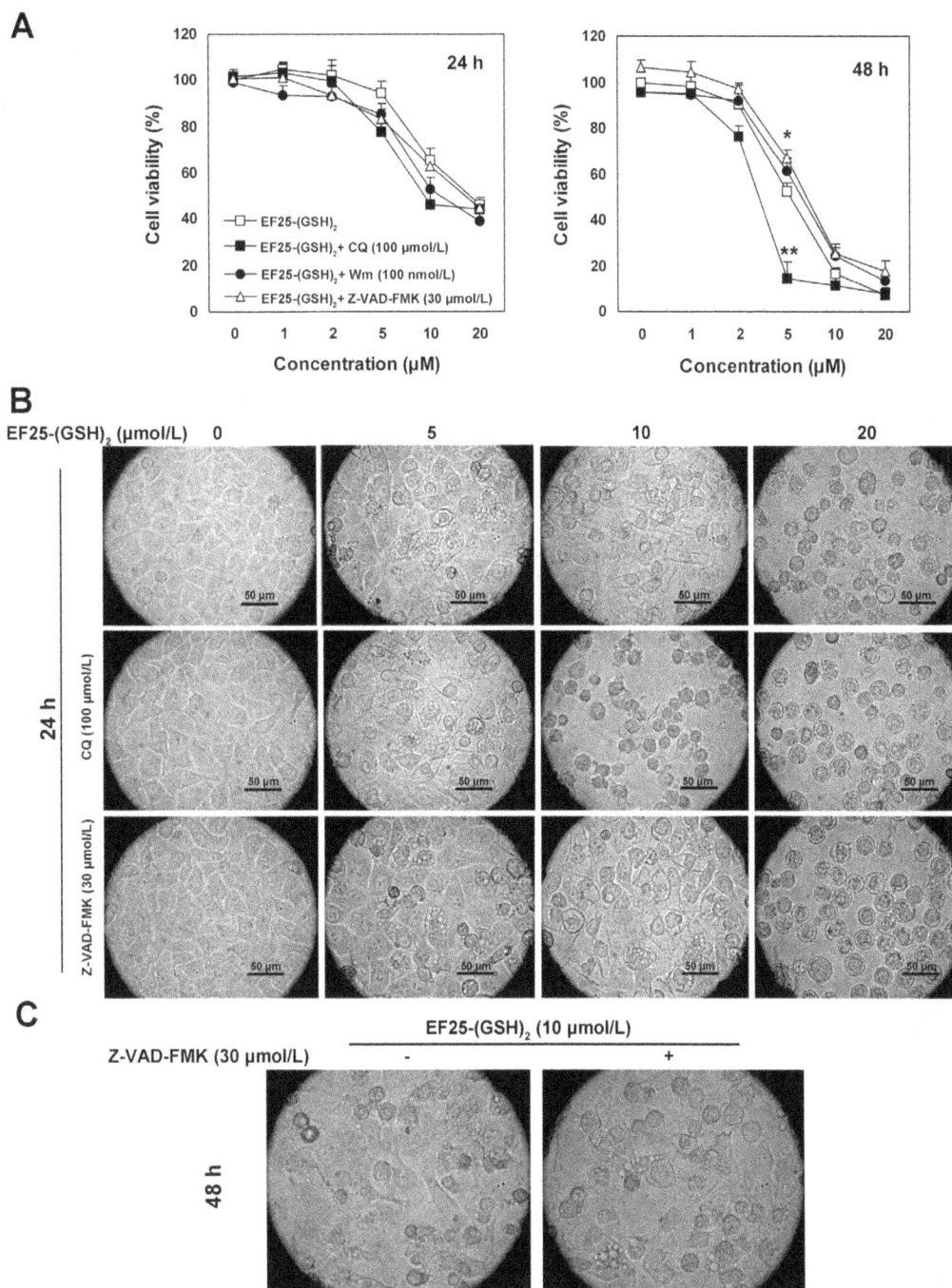

Figure 7. The effect of Wm, CQ and Z-VAD-FMK on the cytotoxicity and morphological changes induced by EF25-(GSH)$_2$ in HepG2 cells. (A) Cell viability was determined by the MTT assay after treatment with increasing concentrations of EF25-(GSH)$_2$ for 24 h or 48 h in the absence or presence of CQ (100 μmol/L)/Wm (100 nmol/L, pretreated for 2 h)/Z-VAD-FMK (30 μmol/L, pretreated for 2 h). *, $p < 0.001$, EF25-(GSH)$_2$ plus Z-VAD-FMK vs. EF25-(GSH)$_2$ alone. **, $p < 0.001$, EF25-(GSH)$_2$ plus CQ vs. EF25-(GSH)$_2$ alone. (B) Representative light microscopic images of HepG2 cells treated with various concentrations of EF25-(GSH)$_2$ for 24 h in the absence or presence of CQ (100 μmol/L)/Z-VAD-FMK (30 μmol/L, pretreated for 2 h). (C) Representative light microscopic images of HepG2 cells treated with 10 μmol/L EF25-(GSH)$_2$ for 48 h in the absence or presence of Z-VAD-FMK (30 μmol/L, pretreated for 2 h).

fall in cell viability examined by the MTT assay. However, as time progressed, the MTT assay at 48 h showed a slight increase rather than a further decrease of cell viability in Wm-pretreated cells. This indicates that Wm treatment advanced cell death only in the early period but had no obvious effect on the ultimate cytotoxicity of EF25-(GSH)$_2$ (Fig. 7A).

7. Knockdown of Atg5 and Beclin-1 expression did not rescue EF25-(GSH)$_2$-treated HepG2 cells

In order to avoid the non-specific effect of Wm, we knocked down the cellular expression of two autophagy essential genes, Atg5 and Beclin-1, separately, using specific small hairpin RNAs (shRNA) delivered by the lentiviral expression system. The cells

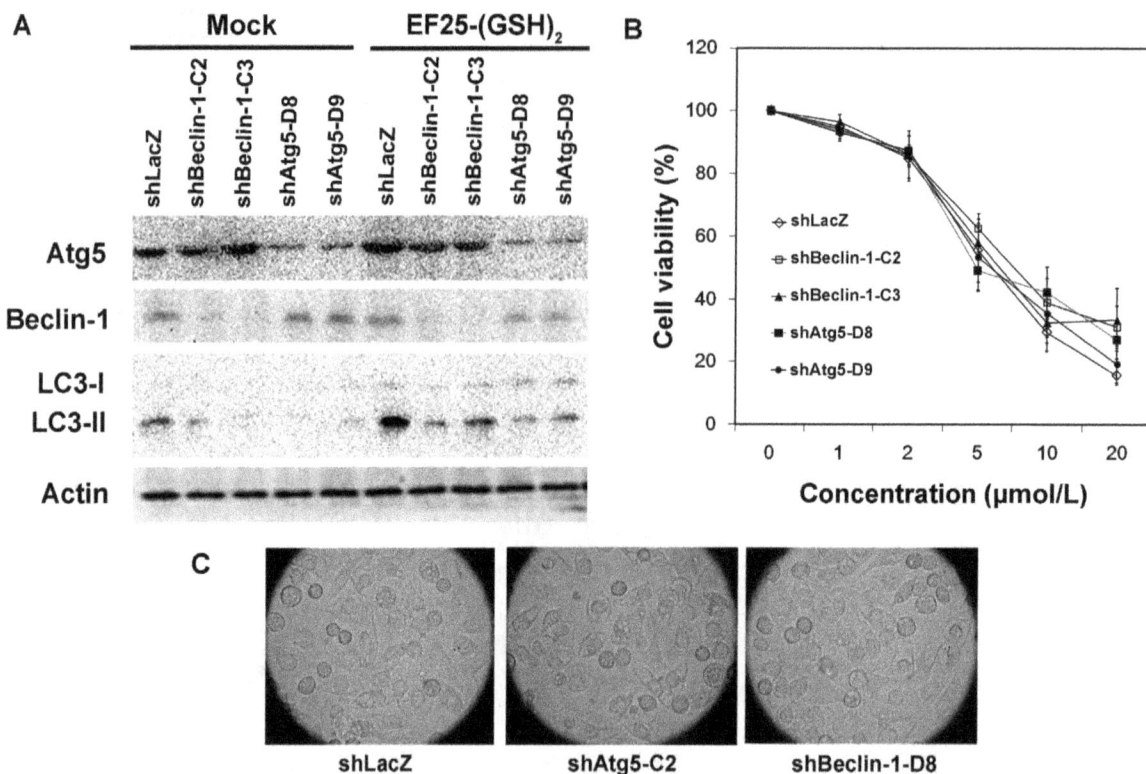

Figure 8. Knockdown of Atg5 and Beclin-1 expression does not rescue EF25-(GSH)$_2$-treated HepG2 cells. (A) HepG2 cells respectively transduced with shLacZ-, shBeclin-1-C2-, shBeclin-1-C3-, shAtg5-D8- and shAtg5-D9-lentivirus were mock-, or treated with 10 µmol/L EF25-(GSH)$_2$ for 24 h. Cells lysates were analyzed by Western blotting with antibodies against Atg5, Beclin-1, LC3 or actin, as indicated. (B) For HepG2 cells respectively transduced with shLacZ-, shBeclin-1-C2-, shBeclin-1-C3-, shAtg5-D8- and shAtg5-D9-lentivirus, cell viability was determined by MTT assay after treatment with increasing concentrations of EF25-(GSH)$_2$ for 48 h. (C) HepG2 cells respectively transduced with shLacZ-, shBeclin-1-C2- and shAtg5-D8-lentivirus were treated with 10 µmol/L EF25-(GSH)$_2$ for 24 h and observed under the light microscope.

were transduced with lentivirus expressing the shRNA targeting LacZ, Atg5 or Becllin 1, and were selected with puromycin. Puromycin-selected cells were then treated with 10 µmol/L EF25-(GSH)$_2$ for 24 h. Atg5- and Beclin-1-knockdown was evident by reduced expression level of Atg5 and Beclin-1, respectively. Furthermore, both Atg5- and Beclin-1-knockdown resulted in the attenuated expression level of LC3II visualized with immunoblotting (Fig. 8A). The MTT assay showed no obvious distinction in cell viability between LacZ-knockdown and Atg5/Beclin-1-knockdown HepG2 cells, which produced similar results with Wm (Fig. 8B). Furthermore, Atg5/Beclin-1-knockdown did not prevent the extensive cytoplasmic vacuolization induced by EF25-(GSH)$_2$, suggesting that this phenomenon is not directly induced by autophagic degradation (Fig. 8C).

8. CQ promoted cytoplasmic vacuolization, apoptosis and cell death induced by EF25-(GSH)$_2$ in HepG2 cells

It has been previously reported that inhibition of autophagy at different stages of the process can lead to distinct results [34,35]. In our study, inhibition of autophagy at an early stage by Wm did not significantly alter either the extent of cytoplasmic vacuolization or the final cell viability at 48 h. However, the late stage inhibitor CQ not only advanced the cell death process but also significantly enhanced cytoplasmic vacuolization, apoptosis and cytotoxicity induced by EF25-(GSH)$_2$. This combination effect of CQ was most dramatic by treatment of EF25-(GSH)$_2$ at 5 µmol/L.

When exposed to 5 µmol/L EF25-(GSH)$_2$ alone, only a small portion of cells was moderately vacuolated, but in the presence of

CQ the majority of cells underwent extensive vacuolization to an extent similar to that caused by 10 µmol/L EF25-(GSH)$_2$ (Fig. 7B). This observation indicates that EF25-(GSH)$_2$-induced autophagy exhibits a cytoprotective role at lower concentration.

The MTT assay showed that CQ enhanced the effectiveness of EF25-(GSH)$_2$ within a 24-h period, continued to 48 h and proved especially clear-cut at the concentration of 5 µmol/L where cell viability dramatically dropped from 52.4% to 14.5% after 48 h treatment (Fig. 7A).

We also found that combining CQ with EF25-(GSH)$_2$ greatly augmented the apoptosis rate evidenced by a large increase in the percentage of cells in the sub-G$_1$-G$_0$ stage in a concentration-dependent manner (Fig. 6A).

In the presence of CQ, the expression level of activated caspase-3 increased at concentrations of 5 µmol/L and 10 µmol/L, but unexpectedly decreased at 20 µmol/L. Similarly, the expression level of cleaved caspase-8 was clearly increased by CQ treatment except at a concentration of 20 µmol/L EF25-(GSH)$_2$ at 48 h (Fig. 6C).

9. Z-VAD-FMK prolonged vacuolization and G2/M cell cycle arrest partially rescues HepG2 cells from EF25-(GSH)2 toxicity

To determine whether caspase activation plays a crucial role in EF25-(GSH)$_2$-induced cytotoxicity, the pan caspase inhibitor Z-VAD-FMK was employed. In the presence of this compound at 48 h post-treatment, cell cycle analysis showed a clear decrease of cells in the sub-G_1-G_0 stage especially at concentrations of 10 (from 37.9% to 16.7%) and 20 μmol/L (from 63.3% to 17.2%) (Fig. 6A). These data indicate that apoptosis induced by EF25-$(GSH)_2$ is primarily caspase- and concentration-dependent and partially caspase-independent to the extent of about 17%.

However, compared to the 21.2% (10 μmol/L) and 46.1% (20 μmol/L) decrease of apoptotic cells in the presence of Z-VAD-FMK at 48 h, only a 6.3% (10 μmol/L) and 19.3% (20 μmol/L) rise in cell viability was observed when pretreated with Z-VAD-FMK as examined by the MTT assay at 48 h (Fig. 7A), indicating the operation of non-apoptotic cell death. The latter was accompanied by prolonged cytoplasmic vacuolization and G_2/M cell cycle arrest.

The extent of cytoplasmic vacuolization was not significantly enhanced in the presence of Z-VAD-FMK (Fig. 7B), but the period of vacuolization was prolonged beyond the 48 h treatment. Cells exposed to 10 μmol/L EF25-$(GSH)_2$ alone avoided vacuolization and begin to shrink at 48 h. In contrast, cells exposed to co-treatment of 10 μmol/L EF25-$(GSH)_2$ and 30 μmol/L Z-VAD-FMK exhibited extensive vacuolization (Fig. 7C).

Cell cycle analysis showed obvious G_2/M cell cycle arrest in the presence of Z-VAD-FMK at 48 h post-treatment, which is similar to what was observed at 24 h post-treatment with EF25-$(GSH)_2$ alone, indicating that Z-VAD-FMK prolonged the status of G_2/M cell cycle arrest induced by the EF25 conjugate (Fig. 6A).

Discussion

Effective and less toxic alternative chemotherapeutic agents against HCC are needed to address the emerging problem of drug resistance and severe side effects [2]. Widely used drugs like cisplatin exhibit no selectivity for malignant cells, while natural compounds like curcumin, which possess a good safety profile, exert inadequate effectiveness [7].

By contrast, our *in vitro* and *in vivo* data show the novel compound EF25-$(GSH)_2$ to exert preferential toxicity toward HCC cells, offering potential as a promising anti-HCC therapeutic agent. In addition, the double GSH conjugation successfully solves the problems of instability and water insolubility which limits the usage of curcumin and its analogues [8].

Basic and clinical studies have clearly established the importance of apoptosis in therapeutic tumor-cell death, but many notable studies have confirmed that other forms of cell death are crucial for effective cancer therapy, and that apoptosis is not the comprehensive answer especially when dealing with the whole tumor instead of isolated tumor cells [36]. We found that the action of EF25-$(GSH)_2$ is complex in terms of which death pathways are involved. In EF25-$(GSH)_2$ treated HepG2 cells, autophagy and apoptosis were detected and extensive cytoplasmic vacuolization was observed. These events do not occur independently, but are closely connected.

The role of autophagy in cancer therapy is complex and depends on the specific cellular setting and treatment scenario. Under some circumstances, autophagy rescues cells under stress conditions and, in this sense, may suppress apoptosis and/or other

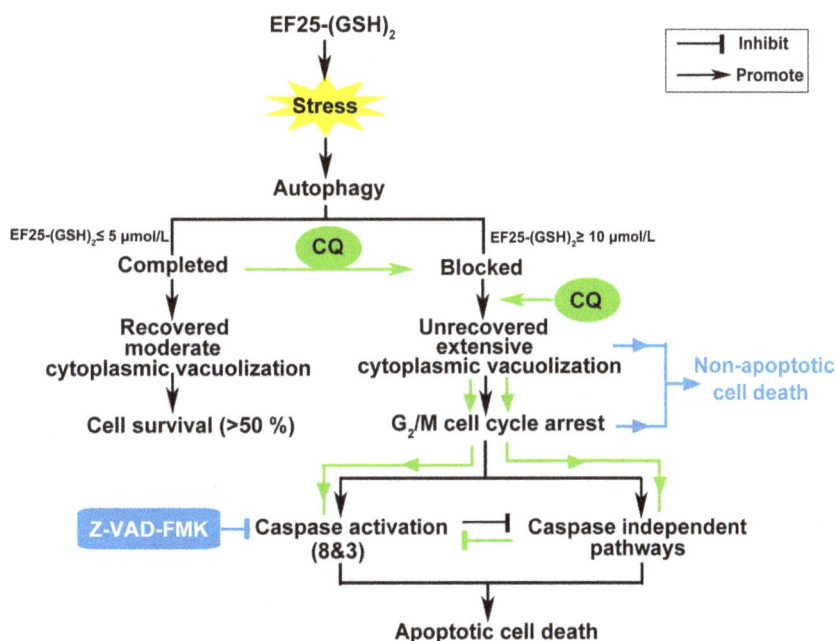

Figure 9. Working model of the mechanisms of EF25-(GSH)₂-induced cell death in HepG2 cells. Stress induced by EF25-(GSH)₂ promotes autophagy in HepG2 cells. When treated with EF25-(GSH)₂ at concentrations of 5 μmol/L or lower, cells experienced full-scale autophagy that displayed moderate cytoplasmic vacuolization, ultimate recovery and partial rescue of cells from the resulting stress. In contrast, the protective autophagy was blocked in cells treated with EF25-(GSH)₂ at concentrations of 10 μmol/L or higher which led to massive cytoplasmic vacuolization. The latter cells arrested in the G₂/M phase succumbed to both caspase-dependent and caspase-independent cell death. EF25-(GSH)₂ treatment alone led mainly to caspase-dependent apoptotic cell death, but also to a significant proportion of caspase-independent apoptosis. The action of EF25-(GSH)₂ could be modulated by CQ (green) and Z-VAD-FMK (blue). Co-treatment of EF25-(GSH)₂ with CQ promoted autophagy blockage and cytoplasmic vacuolization, which then enhanced apoptosis for both caspase-dependent and caspase-independent mechanisms. Co-treatment of EF25-(GSH)₂ with Z-VAD-FMK inhibited caspase activation and subsequently blocked the caspase-dependent apoptotic death route. Thus, cells were trapped by cytoplasmic vacuolization and G₂/M cell cycle arrest, which eventually led to non-apoptotic cell death.

types of cell death. In other scenarios, irreversible self-destruction caused by massive autophagy leads to cell demise [33]. To investigate the exact role of autophagy in chemotherapy, autophagy inhibitors at different stages have been previously employed. Interestingly, the blockade of autophagy at an early or late stage has been reported by some groups to cause different effects. For example, the late stage inhibition by Bafilomycin A1 was found to enhance apoptosis and cell death, whereas inhibition of autophagy at early stages using 3-MA failed to do so [34,35].

Our autophagy inhibitor data using Wm and CQ also show different effects. Inhibition of autophagy at early stages by Wm advanced the cell death process during early phases of EF25-$(GSH)_2$ treatment, but altered the final toxicity insignificantly. In contrast, CQ greatly enhanced cytoplasmic vacuolization, apoptosis and cell death. These data suggest that autophagy does not directly execute cell death through extensive digestion of cellular cytoplasm, but exhibits a cytoprotective role and functions as a fail-safe response to the stressful condition induced by EF25-$(GSH)_2$. In spite of this, protective autophagic degradation is only operative at low concentrations and is blocked by the action of the compound itself at higher and more cytotoxic concentrations.

However, we found that blocked autophagy contributes to cell death induced by EF25-$(GSH)_2$. In EF25-$(GSH)_2$-treated HepG2 cells, autophagy degradation blockage is accompanied by extensive cytoplasmic vacuolization. The latter phenomenon was found in tumor cells under various chemotherapeutic treatments. Although the cells present with a common morphology, various mechanisms were proposed [14,37–39]. Hence, we conclude that accumulation of autophagosomes instead of autophagic degradation promotes the formation of extensive cytoplasmic vacuolization and subsequent cell death. In some effective cancer therapies, impaired autophagy has been observed [40], which may cause metabolic dysfunction and make cells more susceptible to other types of cell death. Notably, preclinical investigations combining the autophagy late stage inhibitor hydroxychloroquine (HCQ) with various chemotherapies has already entered clinical trials [41].

With EF25-$(GSH)_2$ alone, the number of cells within the G_2/M stage was found to be augmented at a 24 h post-treatment and then largely diminished at 48 h when the number of apoptotic cells greatly soared. Non-apoptotic cell death occurs when the process from G_2/M stage arrest to caspase-dependent apoptosis is blocked by Z-VAD-FMK, implying that cells arrested at G_2/M have already reached a "point of no return" in the lethal process and that caspase activation may not be necessary. Notably, this result suggests that for cells failed to undergo apoptosis, EF25-$(GSH)_2$ induced cell death through non-apoptotic mechanisms, although less effectively without the participation of caspase activation.

As expected, activation of both caspase-3 and caspase-8 was enhanced under co-treatment of CQ and 5 μmol/L or 10 μmol/L EF25-$(GSH)_2$. However, caspase activation was undetectable with co-treatment of CQ and 20 μmol/L EF25-$(GSH)_2$, whereupon the apoptosis rate soared, indicating that the apoptosis in this scenario is mainly caspase-independent. Cell cycle analysis in the presence of the pan-caspase inhibitor Z-VAD-FMK suggests that EF25-

$(GSH)_2$ alone causes mainly caspase-dependent apoptosis, but also partially caspase-independent apoptosis.

To sum up, we propose an anti-hepatoma mechanistic model for EF25-$(GSH)_2$ in Figure 9. When treated with EF25-$(GSH)_2$ at a concentration of no more than 5 μmol/L, cells experience successful autophagic degradation. In this case, moderate cytoplasmic vacuolization takes place followed by subsequent recovery, which partially rescues cells from a stressed condition. However, EF25-$(GSH)_2$ at a concentration of 10 μmol/L or higher leads to impaired autophagy during which the autophagic degradation step is blocked and followed by massive cytoplasmic vacuolization. At this point, cells undergo both caspase-dependent and caspase-independent apoptosis. EF25-$(GSH)_2$ treatment alone leads mainly to caspase-dependent apoptosis accompanied by partial caspase-independent apoptosis. Co-treatment with CQ stimulates autophagosome accumulation and cytoplasmic vacuolization, which then promotes both caspase-dependent and caspase-independent apoptosis. Z-VAD-FMK inhibits caspase activation and subsequently blocks the path to apoptotic death. In this case, the status of vacuolization and G_2/M cell cycle arrest is prolonged and eventually leads to non-apoptotic cell death.

In conclusion, our results show that the novel curcumin analog EF25-$(GSH)_2$ has promising potential as a low toxicity chemotherapeutic agent for HCC. Similar to curcumin, the anti-tumor action of EF25-$(GSH)_2$ involved in autophagic, apoptotic and non-apoptotic mechanisms would broaden its application. The combination of EF25-$(GSH)_2$ with chloroquine is suggested to provide a safer and more effective treatment for HCC.

Supporting Information

Figure S1   MS/HR-ESI-MS spectra of EF25-$(GSH)_2$.

Figure S2   Overlay of EF25 (blue) and EF25-$(GSH)_2$ (green) 1H NMR spectra in DMSO-d6. EF25 1H NMR spectrum in DMSO-d6: solvent peak at 2.5 ppm (light yellow); 10.2(s) (OH), 7.9 (=C–H), 6.8–7.3 (aromatic) ppm.

Figure S3   Overlay of EF25 in DMSO-d6 (blue) and EF25-$(GSH)_2$ in D20 (green), buffer pH7, 1H NMR spectra.

Acknowledgments

We thank Dr. Hui Zhong (Academy of Military Medical Sciences, China), Dr. Qinghua Shi (University of Science and Technology of China), Dr. Mian Wu (University of Science and Technology of China) for providing the cell lines and plasmids, Dr. Jun Wang and Mr. Yonglong Zhuang (Anhui University) for technical assistance.

Author Contributions

Conceived and designed the experiments: BH HF. Performed the experiments: TZ LY YB AS BC. Analyzed the data: TZ LY YB AS BC. Contributed reagents/materials/analysis tools: D. Liotta JPS D. Liu YL. Wrote the paper: TZ BH JPS HF.

References

1. Fattovich G, Stroffolini T, Zagni I, Donato F (2004) Hepatocellular carcinoma in cirrhosis: incidence and risk factors. Gastroenterology 127: 35–50.

2. Llovet JM, Bruix J (2008) Novel advancements in the management of hepatocellular carcinoma in 2008. J Hepatol 48: 20–37.

3. Bruix J, Sherman M (2011) Management of hepatocellular carcinoma: an update. Hepatology 53: 1020–1022.

4. Bunchorntavakul C, Hoteit M, Reddy KR (2012) Staging of Hepatocellular Carcinoma. In: N Reau and F. F Poordad, editors. Primary Liver Cancer. New York: Springer Science+Business Media. pp. 161–175.

5. Aoki H, Takada Y, Kondo S, Sawaya R, Aggarwal BB, et al. (2007) Evidence that curcumin suppresses the growth of malignant gliomas in vitro and in vivo through induction of autophagy: role of Akt and extracellular signal-regulated kinase signaling pathways. Mol Pharmacol 72: 29–39.

6. Anand P, Thomas SG, Kunnumakkara AB, Sundaram C, Harikumar KB, et al. (2008) Biological activities of curcumin and its analogues (Congeners) made by man and Mother Nature. Biochem Pharmacol 76: 1590–1611.

7. Steward WP, Gescher AJ (2008) Curcumin in cancer management: recent results of analogue design and clinical studies and desirable future research. Mol Nutr Food Res 52: 1005–1009.

8. Sun A, Lu YJ, Hu H, Shoji M, Liotta DC, et al. (2009) Curcumin analog cytotoxicity against breast cancer cells: exploitation of a redox-dependent mechanism. Bioorg Med Chem Lett 19: 6627–6631.

9. Thomas SL, Zhong D, Zhou W, Malik S, Liotta D, et al. (2008) EF24, a novel curcumin analog, disrupts the microtubule cytoskeleton and inhibits HIF-1. Cell Cycle 7: 2409–2417.

10. Kasinski AL, Du Y, Thomas SL, Zhao J, Sun SY, et al. (2008) Inhibition of IκB Kinase-Nuclear Factor-κB Signaling Pathway by 3,5-Bis(2-flurobenzylidene)piperidin-4-one (EF24), a Novel Monoketone Analog of Curcumin. Mol Pharmacol 74: 654–661.

11. Thomas SL, Zhao J, Li Z, Lou B, Du Y, et al. (2010) Activation of the p38 pathway by a novel monoketone curcumin analog, EF24, suggests a potential combination strategy. Biochem Pharmacol 80: 1309–1316.

12. O'Sullivan-Coyne G, O'Sullivan GC, O'Donovan TR, Piwocka K, McKenna SL (2009) Curcumin induces apoptosis-independent death in oesophageal cancer cells. Br J Cancer 101: 1585–1595.

13. Shinojima N, Yokoyama T, Kondo Y, Kondo S (2007) Roles of the Akt/mTOR/p70S6K and ERK1/2 signaling pathways in curcumin-induced autophagy. Autophagy 3: 635–637.

14. Yoon MJ, Kim EH, Lim JH, Kwon TK, Choi KS (2010) Superoxide anion and proteasomal dysfunction contribute to curcumin-induced paraptosis of malignant breast cancer cells. Free Radic Biol Med 48: 713–726.

15. Adams BK, Ferstl EM, Davis MC, Herold M, Kurtkaya S, et al. (2004) Synthesis and biological evaluation of novel curcumin analogs as anti-cancer and anti-angiogenesis agents. Bioorg Med Chem 12: 3871–3883.

16. Hui IC, Tung EK, Sze KM, Ching YP, Ng IO (2010) Rapamycin and CCI-779 inhibit the mammalian target of rapamycin signalling in hepatocellular carcinoma. Liver international: official journal of the International Association for the Study of the Liver 30: 65–75.

17. Lu B, Ma Y, Wu G, Tong X, Guo H, et al. (2008) Methylation of Tip30 promoter is associated with poor prognosis in human hepatocellular carcinoma. Clinical cancer research 14: 7405–7412.

18. Gao J, Li X, Gu G, Sun B, Cui M, et al. (2011) Efficient synthesis of trisaccharide saponins and their tumor cell killing effects through oncotic necrosis. Bioorg Med Chem Lett 21: 622–627.

19. Tang B, Yu F, Li P, Tong L, Duan X, et al. (2009) A near-infrared neutral pH fluorescent probe for monitoring minor pH changes: imaging in living HepG2 and HL-7702 cells. J Am Chem Soc 131: 3016–3023.

20. Kuck D, Caulfield T, Lyko F, Medina-Franco JL (2010) Nanaomycin A selectively inhibits DNMT3B and reactivates silenced tumor suppressor genes in human cancer cells. Molecular cancer therapeutics 9: 3015–3023.

21. Prause M, Christensen DP, Billestrup N, Mandrup-Poulsen T (2014) JNK1 protects against glucolipotoxicity-mediated beta-cell apoptosis. PLoS one 9: e87067.

22. Lin Y, Peng S, Yu H, Teng H, Cui M (2012) RNAi-mediated downregulation of NOB1 suppresses the growth and colony-formation ability of human ovarian cancer cells. Med Oncol 29: 311–317.

23. Yang CH, Yue J, Sims M, Pfeffer LM (2013) The curcumin analog EF24 targets NF-kappaB and miRNA-21, and has potent anticancer activity in vitro and in vivo. PloS one 8: e71130.

24. Yadav VR, Sahoo K, Roberts PR, Awasthi V (2013) Pharmacologic suppression of inflammation by a diphenyldifluoroketone, EF24, in a rat model of fixed-volume hemorrhage improves survival. The Journal of pharmacology and experimental therapeutics 347: 346–356.

25. Kabeya Y, Mizushima N, Ueno T, Yamamoto A, Kirisako T, et al. (2000) LC3, a mammalian homologue of yeast Apg8p, is localized in autophagosome membranes after processing. EMBO J 19: 5720–5728.

26. Klionsky DJ, Abeliovich H, Agostinis P, Agrawal DK, Aliev G, et al. (2008) Guidelines for the use and interpretation of assays for monitoring autophagy in higher eukaryotes. Autophagy 4: 151–175.

27. Choi M-J, Jung KH, Kim D, Lee H, Zheng H-M, et al. (2011) Anti-cancer effects of a novel compound HS-113 on cell growth, apoptosis, and angiogenesis in human hepatocellular carcinoma cells. Cancer letters 306: 190–196.

28. Steele S, Brunton J, Ziehr B, Taft-Benz S, Moorman N, et al. (2013) Francisella tularensis harvests nutrients derived via ATG5-independent autophagy to support intracellular growth. PLoS Pathog 9: e1003562.

29. Shea FF, Rowell JL, Li Y, Chang TH, Alvarez CE (2012) Mammalian alpha arrestins link activated seven transmembrane receptors to Nedd4 family e3 ubiquitin ligases and interact with beta arrestins. PloS one 7: e50557.

30. Pankiv S, Clausen TH, Lamark T, Brech A, Bruun JA, et al. (2007) p62/SQSTM1 binds directly to Atg8/LC3 to facilitate degradation of ubiquitinated protein aggregates by autophagy. J Biol Chem 282: 24131–24145.

31. Adams BK, Cai J, Armstrong J, Herold M, Lu YJ, et al. (2005) EF24, a novel synthetic curcumin analog, induces apoptosis in cancer cells via a redox-dependent mechanism. Anti-Cancer Drugs 16: 263–275.

32. Selvendiran K, Tong L, Vishwanath S, Bratasz A, Trigg NJ, et al. (2007) EF24 induces G2/M arrest and apoptosis in cisplatin-resistant human ovarian cancer cells by increasing PTEN expression. J Biol Chem 282: 28609–28618.

33. Maiuri MC, Zalckvar E, Kimchi A, Kroemer G (2007) Self-eating and self-killing: crosstalk between autophagy and apoptosis. Nat Rev Mol Cell Biol 8: 741–752.

34. Shingu T, Fujiwara K, Bögler O, Akiyama Y, Moritake K, et al. (2009) Inhibition of autophagy at a late stage enhances imatinib-induced cytotoxicity in human malignant glioma cells. Int J Cancer 124: 1060–1071.

35. Kanzawa T, Germano I, Komata T, Ito H, Kondo Y, et al. (2004) Role of autophagy in temozolomide-induced cytotoxicity for malignant glioma cells. Cell Death Differ 11: 448–457.

36. Okada H, Mak TW (2004) Pathways of apoptotic and non-apoptotic death in tumour cells. Nat Rev Cancer 4: 592–603.

37. Chen TS, Wang XP, Sun L, Wang LX, Xing D, et al. (2008) Taxol induces caspase-independent cytoplasmic vacuolization and cell death through endoplasmic reticulum (ER) swelling in ASTC-a-1 cells. Cancer Lett 270: 164–172.

38. Sy LK, Yan SC, Lok CN, Man RY, Che CM (2008) Timosaponin A-III induces autophagy preceding mitochondria-mediated apoptosis in HeLa cancer cells. Cancer Res 68: 10229–10237.

39. Bhanot H, Young AM, Overmeyer JH, Maltese WA (2010) Induction of nonapoptotic cell death by activated Ras requires inverse regulation of Rac1 and Arf6. Mol Cancer Res 8: 1358–1374.

40. Kyoko O, Yoko S, Katsuyuki I, Haruki S, Yoshihiro S (2011) Induction of an incomplete autophagic response by cancer-preventive geranylgeranoic acid (GGA) in a human hepatoma-derived cell line. Biochem J 440: 63–71.

41. Amaravadi RK, Lippincott-Schwartz J, Yin X-M, Weiss WA, Takebe N, et al. (2011) Principles and current strategies for targeting autophagy for cancer treatment. Clin Cancer Res 17: 654–666.

9

Goosecoid Promotes the Metastasis of Hepatocellular Carcinoma by Modulating the Epithelial-Mesenchymal Transition

Tong-Chun Xue[1,2⑤], Ning-Ling Ge[1,2⑤], Lan Zhang[1,2], Jie-Feng Cui[1,2], Rong-Xin Chen[1,2], Yang You[1,2], Sheng-Long Ye[1,2], Zheng-Gang Ren[1,2*]

1 Liver Cancer Institute, Zhongshan Hospital, Fudan University, Shanghai, P.R. China, 2 Key Laboratory of Carcinogenesis and Cancer Invasion (Fudan University), Ministry of Education, Shanghai, P.R. China

Abstract

The homeobox gene, goosecoid (GSC), is a transcription factor that participates in cell migration during embryonic development. Because cell migration during development has characteristics similar to cell invasion during metastasis, we evaluated the potential role of GSC in the metastasis of hepatocellular carcinoma (HCC). GSC expression in HCC cell lines and tissues was evaluated, and its effects on the migration potential of HCC cells were determined by GSC knock-down and overexpression methods. In addition, the prognostic role of GSC expression in the metastasis of cancer cells in HCC patients was determined. Our data showed that GSC was highly expressed in several HCC cell lines, particularly in a highly metastatic HCC cell line. Overexpression of GSC promoted cell migration and invasion of HCC cells in vitro. Gain-of-function induced the epithelial-mesenchymal transition but not collective cell migration, whereas loss-of-function induced the reverse change. High-level expression of GSC correlated closely with poor survival and lung metastasis in HCC patients; lung metastases showed more upregulated GSC expression than the primary tumor. We conclude that GSC promotes metastasis of HCC potentially through initiating the epithelial-mesenchymal transition. GSC is also a prognostic factor for poor survival and metastasis of HCC, which suggests its potential as a therapeutic target for metastatic HCC.

Editor: Jung Weon Lee, Seoul National University, Republic of Korea

Funding: This study was supported by The National Clinical Key Special Subject of China, The National Natural Science Foundation of China (81172275 and 21272565) and The National Basic Research Program of China (973 Program, 2009CB521700). The funders had no role in study design, data collection and analysis, decision to publish, or preparation of the manuscript.

Competing Interests: The authors have declared that no competing interests exist.

* Email: ren.zhenggang@zs-hospital.sh.cn

⑤ These authors contributed equally to this work.

Introduction

To date, metastasis is still one of the main obstacles to the survival of patients with hepatocellular carcinoma (HCC) [1,2]. Tumor cells have evolved traits that allow them to disseminate and travel systemically, and these characteristics are similar to the migration ability of embryonic cells during development.

Cell migration is an important process during embryonic development [3]. There are two types of migration in embryonic development, which include epithelial-mesenchymal transition (EMT) [4,5] and collective cell migration [6,7]. EMT is characterized as the shift of cell phenotype from epithelial cells to mesenchymal cells, which have increased ability to migrate. The process of EMT is essential for germ layer formation and cell migration in the early vertebrate embryo, particularly during gastrulation [8]. On the other hand, collective cell migration is characterized as movement of groups of cells by membrane ruffling at the free edge only, while cell-cell junctions within the moving cell group remain intact. This process occurs in the developmental context during gastrulation [9] and formation of the neural crest [10]. Similarly, it has been well demonstrated that EMT takes place during the metastasis of tumors. Meanwhile,

collective cell migration also has been shown to play critical roles in invasion and spreading of tumors, such as melanoma. Therefore, the essential genes that control EMT or collective cell migration during embryogenesis may potentially play critical roles in invasion and metastasis of malignancies.

Goosecoid (GSC), a paired-like homeobox gene expressed in the vertebrate organizer, plays critical roles in both gastrulation [11–13] and neural crest development [14]. Therefore, GSC expression is correlated with both the EMT process and collective migration. Accumulated evidence has shown that GSC induces morphogenetic movements during gastrulation and controls cell migration in Xenopus embryos [15], which suggests that the target genes controlled by the GSC DNA-binding protein might include genes involved in intercellular signaling, cell motility, and cell adhesion. In Xenopus embryos, GSC-controlled cell movement affects migration of groups of cells but not of individual cells. However, another report suggested a role for GSC in promoting metastasis of human breast tumors through initiation of EMT [16]. Therefore, the potential role of GSC in other malignancies remains to be uncovered. It has been shown that EMT is correlated closely to the invasion and metastasis of HCC; however, the underlying molecular mechanisms controlling the behavior of

HCC tumor cells remain unclear. The finding that GSC controls the metastasis of breast tumors, which are derived from an epithelial source, has led us to investigate in the potential roles of GSC in migration of HCC cells.

Herein, we evaluated the expression of GSC in HCC cell lines with different metastatic potential. Wound-healing and Matrigel invasion assays were used to evaluate the function of GSC in HCC cell movements. Gain-of-function and knock-down of GSC in HCC were used to further explore the potential mechanism of GSC in this process. The prognostic role of GSC in extra-hepatic metastasis and survival of human HCC after hepatic resection also was evaluated.

Materials and Methods

Cells lines

Human HCC cell lines with elevated lung metastasis potential (namely, MHCC97L, MHCC97H, and HCCLM3) were established at the Liver Cancer Institute of Fudan University. The human HCC cell lines with low metastatic potential that we evaluated were SMMC-7721 (established at Second Military Medical University), Hep3B, and HepG2 (obtained from American Type Culture Collection). L02, an immortalized human liver cell line, was obtained from the Chinese Scientific Academy. These cell lines were cultured in high glucose DMEM (GibcoBRL, Grand Island, NY) supplemented with 10% fetal bovine serum (Hyclone, Logan, UT).

Patients and follow-up

A tissue microarray (TMA) composed of samples from 112 HCC patients was used in this study. These patients were retrieved from a prospectively designed database. Paraffin tissue sections were stained by hematoxylin and eosin, and reviewed by two pathologists according to the WHO histomorphologic criteria. Ninety-four patients were positive for the hepatitis B surface antigen (HBsAg). All patients were classified as Child-Pugh A. The follow-up procedures were carried out as described in our previous study [17]. Ethics approval was obtained from the Zhongshan Hospital research ethics committee, and written informed consent was obtained from each patient.

Quantitative Real Time RT-PCR

Real-time reverse transcription-PCR (RT-PCR) was established using Taqman PCR reagents and ABI PRISM 7700 sequence detection system (Applied Biosystems, Foster, CA) in accordance with the protocol described previously [18]. The primers used for GSC amplification were described previously [16]. The assay was performed in triplicate, and the results were analyzed using Student's t test.

Western blot

Western blotting was performed according to the protocol of Bio-Rad wet transfer using the Bio-Rad Transfer Cell System (Bio-Rad, Ontario, Canada). Mouse anti-human GSC IgG (Abcam, Cambridge, MA) 1:500, rabbit anti-human E-cadherin mAb 1:1000, N-cadherin 1:1000, β-catenin 1:2000, vimentin 1:800 (Cell Signaling Technologies, Danvers, MA), and rabbit anti-human β-actin mAb (Epitomics, Burlingame, CA) 1:1000 were used as primary antibodies in detection. Horseradish peroxidase-conjugated goat anti-rabbit IgG F(ab')2 antibody (Jackson ImmunoResearch, West Grove, PA) at 1:5000 was used as secondary. Photos were analyzed using Image Lab software (Bio-Rad, Ontario, Canada). The relative protein expression levels were normalized to β-actin before comparison.

Lentivirus constructs and cell infection

Full-length human GSC cDNA was subcloned into the LV5-EF1a-GFP/Puro lentivirus vector (GenePharma Corp., Shanghai, China). Viral particles were produced by co-transfection of the shRNA plasmid and the lentiviral packaging plasmid into 293T cells. A corresponding vector containing the GFP gene was used as control. HCC cells were infected with the lentiviral particles, and were selected with 3 mg/mL puromycin (P8833; Sigma-Aldrich). Stably transfected clones were characterized for expression levels of GSC protein using inverted fluorescence microscopy, real time RT-qPCR, and immunoblotting.

RNA interference

Small interfering RNAs (siRNAs) were synthesized to target expression of GSC (GenePharma Corp., Shanghai, China). The coding sequences were as follows: siGSC-158, 5'-GCAUGUU-CAGCAUCGACAATT-3' (position 158 of GSC mRNA); negative control siRNA, 5'-UUC UCC GAA CGU GUC ACG UTT-3'. Tumor cells were seeded at a density of 5×10^4 cells in wells of 24-well plates and cultured overnight. SiRNA (20 pmol) was transfected by use of Lipofectamine2000 according to the manufacturer's protocol (Life Technologies, Grand Island, NY). Cells were harvested at 24 h or 48 h post-transfection.

Measurement of cell proliferation

We measured the proliferation of HepB3-GSC versus HepB3-NC using the Cell Counting Kit-8 (CCK8; Dojindo Molecular Technologies Inc., Kumamoto, Japan) according to the manufacturer's instructions. Cells were counted and stained with Trypan blue staining to determine cell viability; cultures with at least 99% viable cells were used for the CCK8 assay. Briefly, the HCC cell lines were cultured in 96-well culture plates at 3×10^3 cells/well in growth medium for 24, 48, and 72 hours, and then harvested for the CCK8 assay. Results were expressed as the absorbance of each well at 450 nm (OD_{450}) as measured using a microplate spectrophotometer (Multiskan Spectrum, Thermo Fisher Scientific, Waltham, MA, USA). The assay was performed in triplicate.

Wound healing assay

For the scratch assay, cells were grown to confluence in a 6-well plate, and a "wounding" line was scratched into the cell monolayer with a sterile 200-μl pipette tip. The remaining cells were washed twice with culture medium to remove cell debris, and the cultures were incubated at 37°C with 1% serum–containing DMEM culture medium. The width of the wound was measured under a microscope at 0, 24 hours, and 48 hours after the scratch to assess the migration ability of the cells. Wound healing was determined at each time point by calculating the distance migrated relative to the original distance at 0 hour. The assay was performed in triplicate, and results were analyzed using Student's t test.

Matrigel invasion assay

Tumor cell invasion assay was performed as previously [18]. Briefly, using 24-well Transwell chambers, the upper chambers with polycarbonate filters (8-μm pore size; Costar, Acton, MA, USA) were coated with 50 μl of Matrigel (BD Biosciences, San Diego, CA, USA). Cells (1.0×10^3 in 100 μl DMEM) were collected and added to the pre-coated wells. The cells were allowed to invade toward the lower chamber. The cells migrating to the membrane were enumerated with Giemsa staining. The assay was performed three times. Results were analyzed using Student's t test.

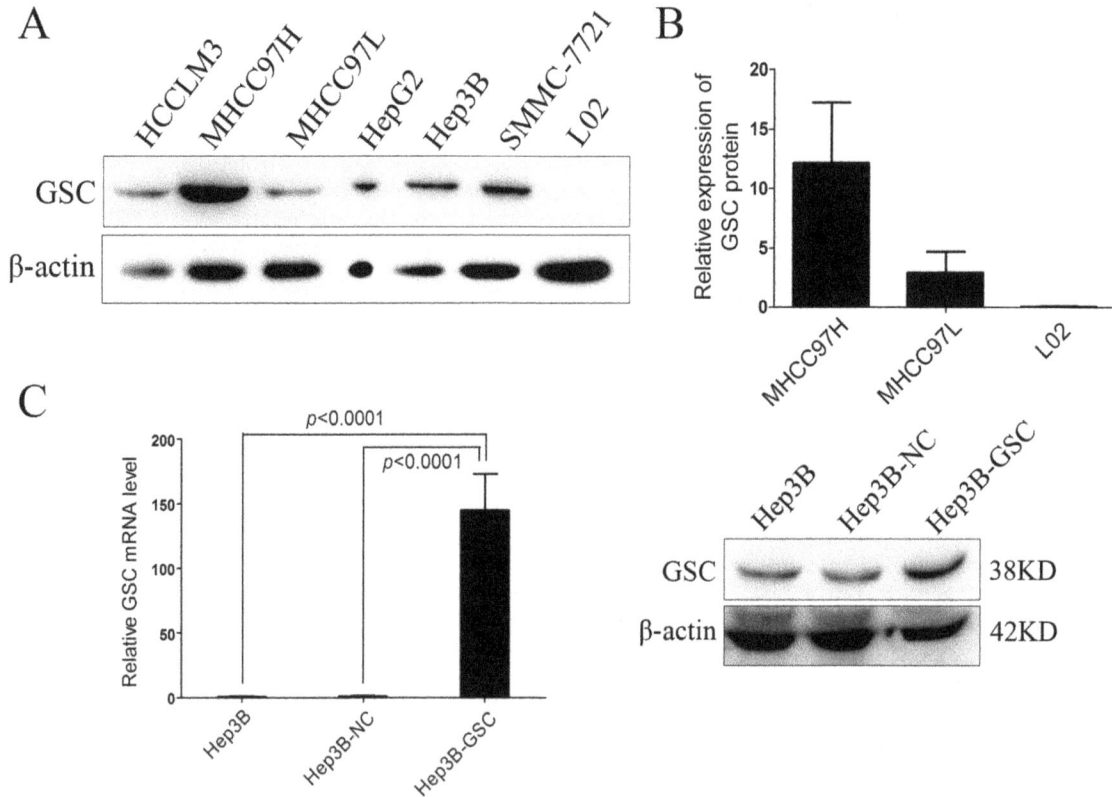

Figure 1. GSC expression in HCC cell lines. (A) Western blot indicates that GSC is abnormally expressed in HCC cell lines, whereas it is not detectable in a normal hepatic cell line. (B) Western blot shows that GSC is strongly expressed in the highly metastatic HCC cell line versus the cell line with low metastatic potential. (C) *GSC* was overexpressed in HCC cells through lentivirus infection. A stable cell line was selected with 3 mg/mL puromycin. Quantitative real-time RT-PCR shows the prominent overexpression of *GSC* in Hep3B cells, which was confirmed by western blot. The data are presented as the mean ± SD of at least three independent experiments.

Fluorescence analysis of collective cell migration

Cell-sheet migration assay was performed based on modification of a previous method [19]. Hep3B-GSC cells and Hep3B-NC cells expressing GFP were cultured in six-well culture plates at 5×10^5 cells/well in growth medium and grown to confluence. The cell monolayer was wounded using a sterile pipet tip (~700 μm in width), and the cells were incubated with 2% serum-containing culture medium. Lines lightly etched with a razor blade on the bottom of the dish provided a reference under the microscope. Dynamic activity of marginal protrusions was visualized every 6 hours by fluorescence microscopy.

Tissue Micro Array (TMA) and immunohistochemistry

The construction of the TMA and the protocol for immunohistochemistry were described previously [20]. Because the lung is the most frequent target organ of HCC metastasis, the TMA was constructed based on whether or not the patients experienced lung metastasis during the long follow-up period post-resection. Tissues from 112 HCC patients were used to generate the TMA, and all tissues were from the primary HCC lesion. Six lung tissue samples from patients who underwent partial pulmonary resection also were included in the TMA. A two-step immunohistochemistry method that included a heat-induced antigen-retrieval procedure was performed as previously described [21]. Mouse anti-human GSC mAb (Abcam, Cambridge, MA, USA) at 1:200 was used as the primary antibody. Normal colon tissue was used as the positive control. Normal liver tissue, a hepatic hemangioma sample, and omission of primary antibody were used as negative controls. Two pathologists read the slides independently, and they were blinded to the study design and the patient data. The immunoassay results were defined by the staining intensity and the percentage of positive tumor cells as described previously [22]. Categories of staining (GSC^{High}, GSC^{Medium}, and GSC^{Low}) were established previously [20].

Statistical analysis

When two groups of cells or animals were compared, analysis was performed using Student's t test. For comparison of multiple groups, a one-way ANOVA was used with Turkey's HSD post-hoc analysis to determine individual group differences. Testing for the homogeneity of variance was performed before the post-hoc analysis. The Pearson Chi-Square test was used to compare qualitative variables in clinical pathology analysis. When expected sample values were below 5, Fisher's exact test was used. Spearman's rank test was used to detect the correlation between variables. Overall survival (OS), relapse-free survival and extra-hepatic metastasis-free survival were determined using the Kaplan-Meier method to describe the survival curves, and the log-rank test was used to compare survival distributions between groups. Univariate and multivariate analyses were based on the Cox Proportional Hazards Regression model. Receiver Operating Characteristic curve (ROC) was used to confirm the predictive accuracy of risk factors. All P values were 2-tailed, and the statistical significance was set at $P < 0.05$. Statistical analyses were performed using SPSS18.0 software (SPSS Inc., Chicago, IL).

Results

Expression of GSC in HCC cell lines

To measure GSC expression in HCC, several HCC cell lines were selected including HCCLM3, MHCC-97H, MHCC-97L, HepG2, Hep3B, SMCC-7721 and an immortalized liver cell line. The HCC cell lines showed upregulated GSC expression compared to the L02 cell line (Figure 1A). In addition, highly metastatic MHCC97H cells had stronger GSC expression than the low metastatic potential MHCC97L cells, which have a genetic background that is similar to MHCC97H (Figure 1B). The Hep3B cell line was chosen for further *in vitro* analyses.

Highly expressed GSC promotes HCC migration and invasiveness

To characterize the role of GSC in HCC, GSC was overexpressed in Hep3B cells by lentivirus infection. Real-time RT-PCR showed the upregulation of *GSC* in Hep3B cells, which was confirmed by the Western blot results (Figure 1C). Results from the wound healing assay indicated that Hep3B cells overexpressing GSC (Hep3B-GSC) migrated faster than the Hep3B-NC (negative control group) at 24 h and 48 h ($P<0.05$) (Figure 2A). Meanwhile, the CCK-8 assay indicated that there was no difference in cell number between the three groups at 48 h ($P>0.05$) (Figure S1). Invasion assay results indicated that the number of Hep3B-GSC cells that migrated through the Matrigel were significantly greater than the number of Hep3B-NC and Hep3B cells at 36 h ($P<0.01$) and 48 h ($P<0.001$) (Figure 2B).

GSC increases the migration potential of HCC cells, which is mediated through EMT

Early research in development indicated that GSC controls cell migration in *Xenopus* embryos, and that GSC-controlled cell movement affects migration of groups of cells [15]. On the other hand, recent research suggested that GSC increased the metastatic potential of breast cancer cells by initiating EMT [16]. The gain-of-function assays suggested the potential role of GSC in HCC metastasis; therefore, we explored whether this phenomenon also occurs in HCC.

In the Hep3B-GSC cell line, expression of E-cadherin was decreased (compared with Hep3B $P<0.001$ and Hep3B-NC $P<0.001$, respectively) and β-catenin was decreased (compared with Hep3B $P=0.004$ and Hep3B-NC $P=0.013$, respectively); whereas N-cadherin was increased (compared with Hep3B $P<0.001$ and Hep3B-NC $P<0.001$, respectively) and vimentin expression was increased (compared with Hep3B $P=0.009$ and Hep3B-NC $P=0.014$, respectively), which is suggestive of EMT (Figure 3A). On the contrary, after knocking-down GSC expression in Hep3B cells, E-cadherin expression increased (compared with Hep3B $P<0.001$ and Hep3B-NC $P<0.001$, respectively); whereas vimentin was strongly decreased (compared with Hep3B $P<0.001$ and Hep3B-NC $P<0.001$, respectively), suggesting that the reverse process, MET, was taking place (Figure 3B). Similar

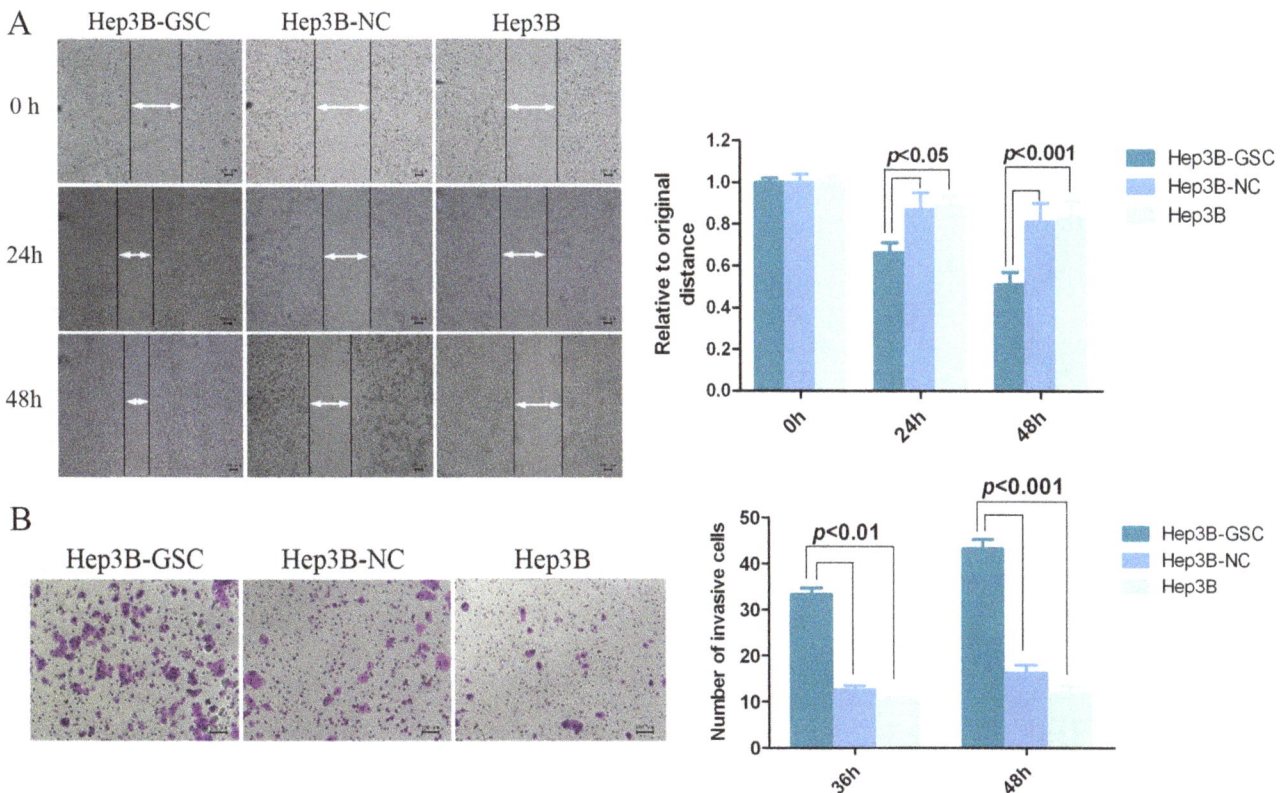

Figure 2. Effects of GSC overexpression on migration of HCC. Hep3B-GSC cells were infected by *GSC* lentivirus and were selected with puromycin. (A) Wound-healing assay shows that Hep3B-GSC cells migrated faster than normal Hep3B or Hep3B cells without treatment after 24 h and 48 h. The cleared area of Hep3B-GSC was less than the controls. (50× original magnification, size bar: 100 μm) Results were analyzed with the Student *t* test. (B) Giemsa staining indicated the number of Hep3B-GSC cells that migrated through Matrigel was higher than Hep3B cells without treatment or treated with negative control (100× original magnification, size bar: 100 μm). The data are presented as the mean ± SD of at least three independent experiments. Results were analyzed using Student's *t* test.

results were observed in the MHCC97H cell line when GSC expression was downregulated (data not shown). Hep3B-GSC cells, which showed decreased E-cadherin expression, also exhibited decreased cell-cell contact during migration and increased disseminating potential. Cell counts confirmed the increased numbers of single or isolated Hep3B-GSC cells versus controls ($P<0.001$) (Figure 3C).

We also evaluated the potential role of GSC in the collective migration of HCC cells. Hep3B-NC cells showed evidence of collective migration as detected by fluorescence microscopy. Furthermore, Hep3B-GSC cells did not have an increase in collective migration ability. In contrast, overexpression of GSC in Hep3B cells induced the migration of individual cells versus groups of cells (Figure 3D).

GSC expression and clinico-pathologic features

To confirm the high expression of GSC in HCC cell lines, immunohistochemistry analysis was performed using tumors and tissue adjacent to tumor. Of 112 tumor tissues, GSC was detected in most cases (105/112). Meanwhile, 55% (62/112) HCC tissues expressed relatively strong GSC staining. However, in only one case was GSC detected in tissue adjacent to tumor. The intra-tumor expression of GSC was significantly stronger than expression in tissue surrounding the tumors.

In the positive control, GSC staining was localized mainly to the nucleus of HCC cells (Figure 4A). The positive nuclear expression in colon tissue, negative expression in normal liver tissue or in hepatic hemangioma indicated the specificity of the anti-GSC monoclonal antibody. Patients were stratified according to GSC staining intensity of tumor samples into three groups. GSC^{High}, GSC^{Medium}, and GSC^{Low} staining was observed in 24, 38, and 50 patients, respectively. There was no significant difference in clinico-pathologic data between the three groups of patients except with respect to lung metastasis ($P=0.009$) (see Table S1), indicating the strong relationship between GSC expression and distant metastasis in HCC.

Higher expression of GSC in lung metastatic foci of HCC

Six tumor samples from lung metastatic foci of HCC were retrieved from the followed-up database. These tumor tissues were confirmed histologically to have metastasized from HCC. As shown in Figure 4B, five tissues were GSC positive, including three tissues with highly expressed GSC. Furthermore, the comparison between two paired lung metastatic foci to primary liver cancer indicated significant upregulation of GSC expression in lung metastatic foci.

Highly expressed GSC is associated with poor survival and lung metastasis in HCC

There was a statistically significant difference in OS ($P=0.002$, log-rank test) and relapse-free survival ($P=0.018$, log-rank test) among the three groups (Figure 5A and 5B). The median OS of group GSC^{High} was significantly shorter than that of group GSC^{Medium} and group GSC^{Low} (26 months versus 45 months and 82 months, respectively).

In group GSC^{High}, the cumulative 1-year, 3-year, and 5-year lung metastasis-free survival were only 50%, 20%, and 20%, respectively, whereas in group GSC^{Low}, the cumulative 1-year, 3-year, and 5-year rates were 76%, 49%, and 45%, respectively. Time to development of lung metastasis for group GSC^{High} was shorter than for group GSC^{Low} ($P=0.008$, log-rank test) (Figure 5C). The median time for developing lung metastasis for group GSC^{High} was significantly shorter than for group GSC^{Low} (25 months versus 78 months).

GSC is an independent prognostic factor for time-to-lung metastasis of HCC

High AFP level, multiple tumor nodules, microvascular invasion, poor tumor differentiation, portal lymphatic invasion, and high GSC expression were all found to be associated with shorter time to lung metastasis by univariate analysis (Table 1). Cox proportional hazards analysis indicated that highly expressed GSC was an independent prognostic factor for shorter time-to-lung metastasis (hazard ratio = 1.842, $P=0.001$) (Table 1). Group GSC^{High} had nearly twice the likelihood of metastasis to lung than group GSC^{Low}. ROC analysis further confirmed the value of GSC as a potential prognostic factor for the occurrence of lung metastasis, with AUC 0.652 (95% CI, 0.550–0.754, $P=0.006$) (Figure 5D).

In addition, univariate analysis showed that high AFP level, microvascular invasion, portal lymphatic invasion, and high GSC expression were associated with worse OS (Table 1). Moreover, Cox analysis indicated that high GSC expression was an independent prognostic factor for worse OS (hazard ratio = 1.685, $P=0.004$) (Table 1).

Discussion

This study is the first to demonstrate that expression of the embryonic gene *GSC* is associated with the metastasis of HCC. First, we determined that GSC was strongly expressed in HCC cell lines, particularly in the highly metastatic HCC cell line. GSC expression in tumors was prominently higher than in peri-tumoral tissue. Overexpression of GSC promoted the migration and invasion ability of HCC cells. Furthermore, GSC expression was correlated closely with extra-hepatic metastasis and poor survival of HCC patients. Importantly, high expression of GSC was shown to be an independent prognostic factor of lung metastasis. These findings suggest the critical role of GSC in metastasis of HCC. Similar to our findings, GSC has been demonstrated to promote metastasis of breast tumors [16]. Therefore, this study further supports the value of GSC as an overexpressed embryonic gene that has a critical role in tumor metastasis in HCC.

In this study, overexpression GSC in HCC cells induced the EMT whereas downregulation GSC inhibited the EMT, suggesting that EMT is one of the potential mechanisms through which GSC promotes metastasis of HCC. Our observation that GSC participates in HCC metastasis through inducing EMT is in concordance with a similar report in breast cancer [16]. On the other hand, HCC-GSC cells showed scattering-type motility whereas control HCC cells exhibited more collective migration, which suggests that highly expressed GSC modifies the migration character of HCC cells from collective cell migration transition to EMT. During embryonic development when neural crest cells separate from their surrounding tissues, their delamination involves partial or complete EMT, then collective migration, which is affected by many positive and negative regulators [23,24]. It has been shown that GSC expression correlates closely with the function of neural crest cells [14]. Thus, the role of GSC and its relationship to type of migration of HCC cells may be modified by positive and negative regulators in the context of HCC. Our future direction is to evaluate the potential regulators that modify GSC function. Hepatocyte growth factor, which plays a critical role in the metastasis of HCC [25,26] has been reported to induce not only scattering but also collective migration of colorectal adenocarcinoma cells [27]. In addition, the TGF-β superfamily,

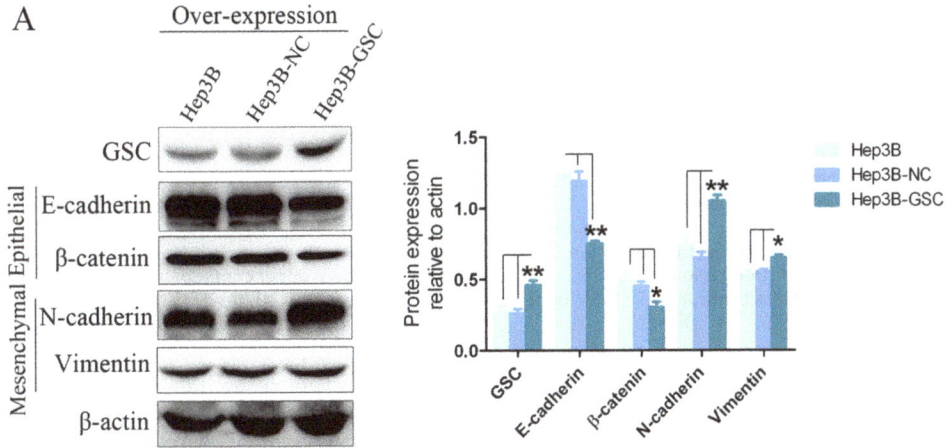

A

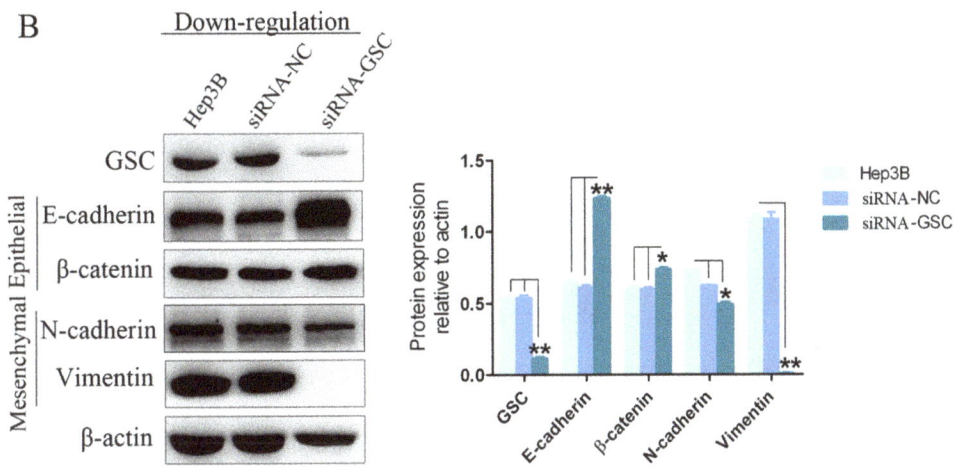

B

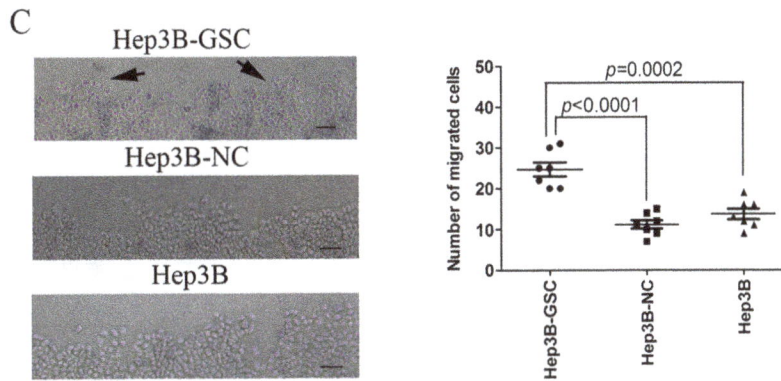

C

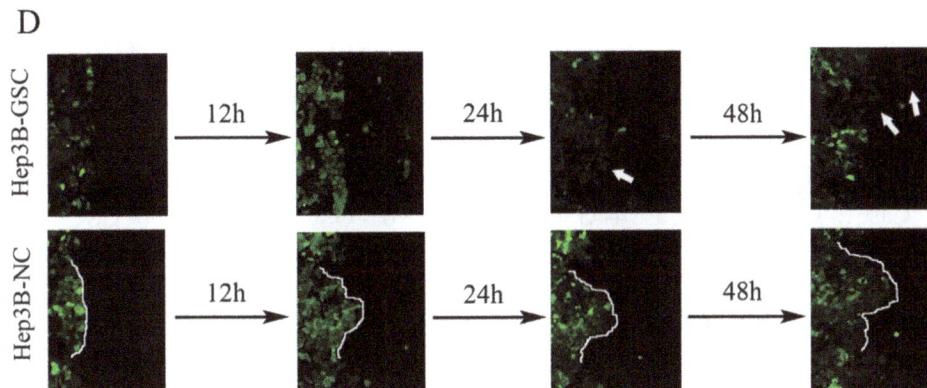

D

Figure 3. GSC induces EMT but not collective cell migration of HCC cells. (A) Ectopic expression of GSC in Hep3B cells induced changes in expression of EMT markers, particularly E-cadherin. The expression of each protein was normalized to β-actin. Results were analyzed using Student's t test. (*, $P<0.05$; **, $P<0.01$) ANOVA analysis also indicated significant differences among the three groups ($P=0.001$ for GSC, $P<0.001$ for E-cadherin, $P=0.004$ for β-catenin, $P<0.001$ for N-cadherin, and $P=0.007$ for vimentin). In addition, post hoc analysis confirmed the significant difference between Hep3B-GSC cells and Hep3B cells without treatment or treated with negative control. (B) Downregulation of GSC in Hep3B cells reversed the changes in expression of EMT markers as detected by Western blot. Results were analyzed using Student's t test. (*, $P<0.05$; **, $P<0.01$) ANOVA analysis also indicated significant differences among the three groups ($P<0.001$ for GSC, $P<0.001$ for E-cadherin, $P<0.001$ for β-catenin, $P<0.001$ for N-cadherin, and $P<0.001$ for vimentin). Furthermore, post-hoc analysis confirmed the significant difference between Hep3B-GSC cells and Hep3B cells without treatment or treated with negative control. (C) The scattering cells (black arrow) in the Hep3B-GSC group were prominently increased compared to the control groups. Continuous counting of seven fields of individual migrating cells showed higher numbers of Hep3B-GSC cells migrating than the Hep3B and the Hep3B-NC groups. (D) Fluorescence micrographs of Hep3B cells expressing GSC or GFP control. Hep3B-GSC cells showed decreased cell-cell contact and strong migration of the individual type (white arrows) under continuous observation. Hep3B-NC cells showed characteristic integrated migration (white contour line). (100× original magnification, size bar: 100 μm).

including TGF-β or the Nodal family of proteins, has been shown to induce the upregulation of GSC in invasive breast cancer cells and during embryonic development [16,28]. Thus, these regulators play potential roles in GSC function in HCC.

Published research has indicated that the upregulation of GSC occurs quite early in multistep cancer progression rather than concurrently with the overt display of the invasive phenotype. For instance, it has been postulated that, in ductal-type breast tumors, GSC primes cells for the expression of aggressive phenotypes [16]. In this study, however, it was the lung metastases that showed the highest expression of GSC. In addition, the paired IHC results confirmed the upregulated expression of GSC in metastatic tissues

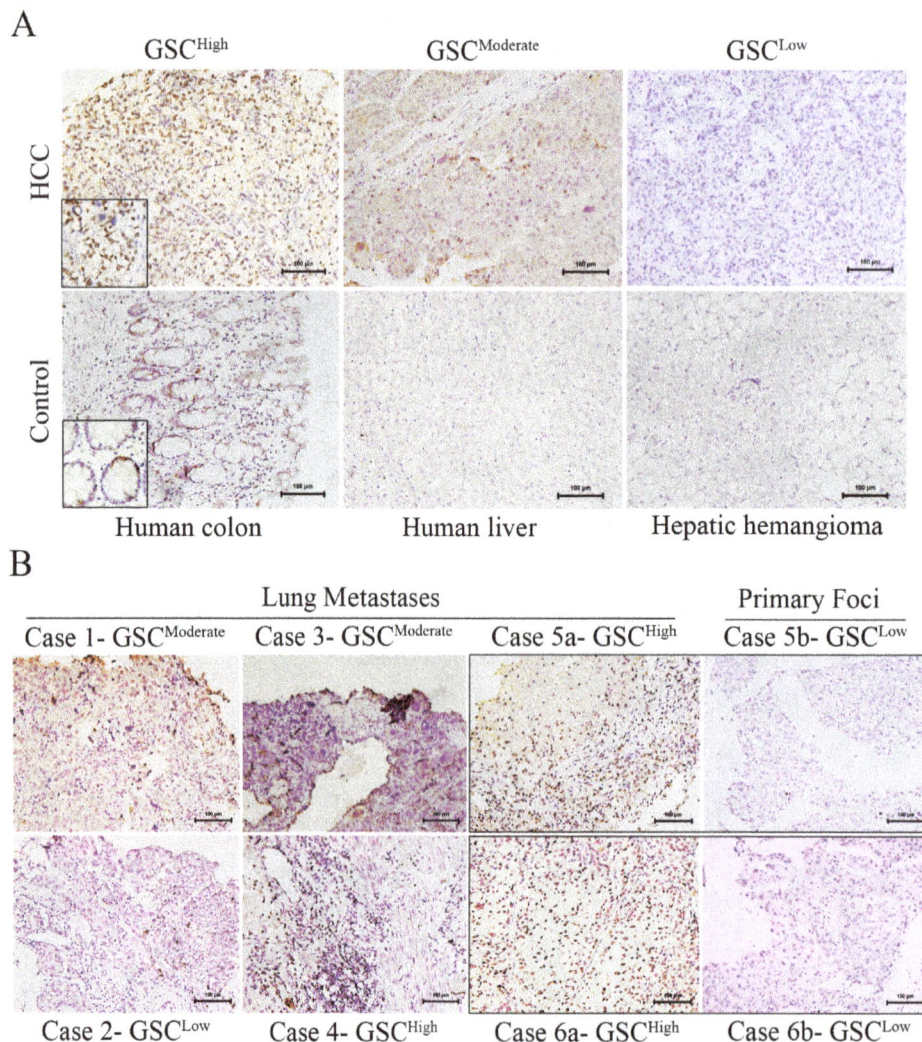

Figure 4. GSC expression in HCC tumor tissues. Immunohistochemistry analysis was performed based on tissue microarray. (A) Top-row shows the staining of GSC from strong to low. Bottom-row shows the controls to confirm the specificity of the GSC antibody. Colon tissue staining was used as the positive control. (B) Six tumor tissues in lung metastases from HCC showed the highly expressed GSC. Comparison of two paired tissues (case 5 and case 6) from lung metastatic cancer and primary foci showed the upregulated GSC expression in lung tissues. (200× original magnification, size bar: 100 μm).

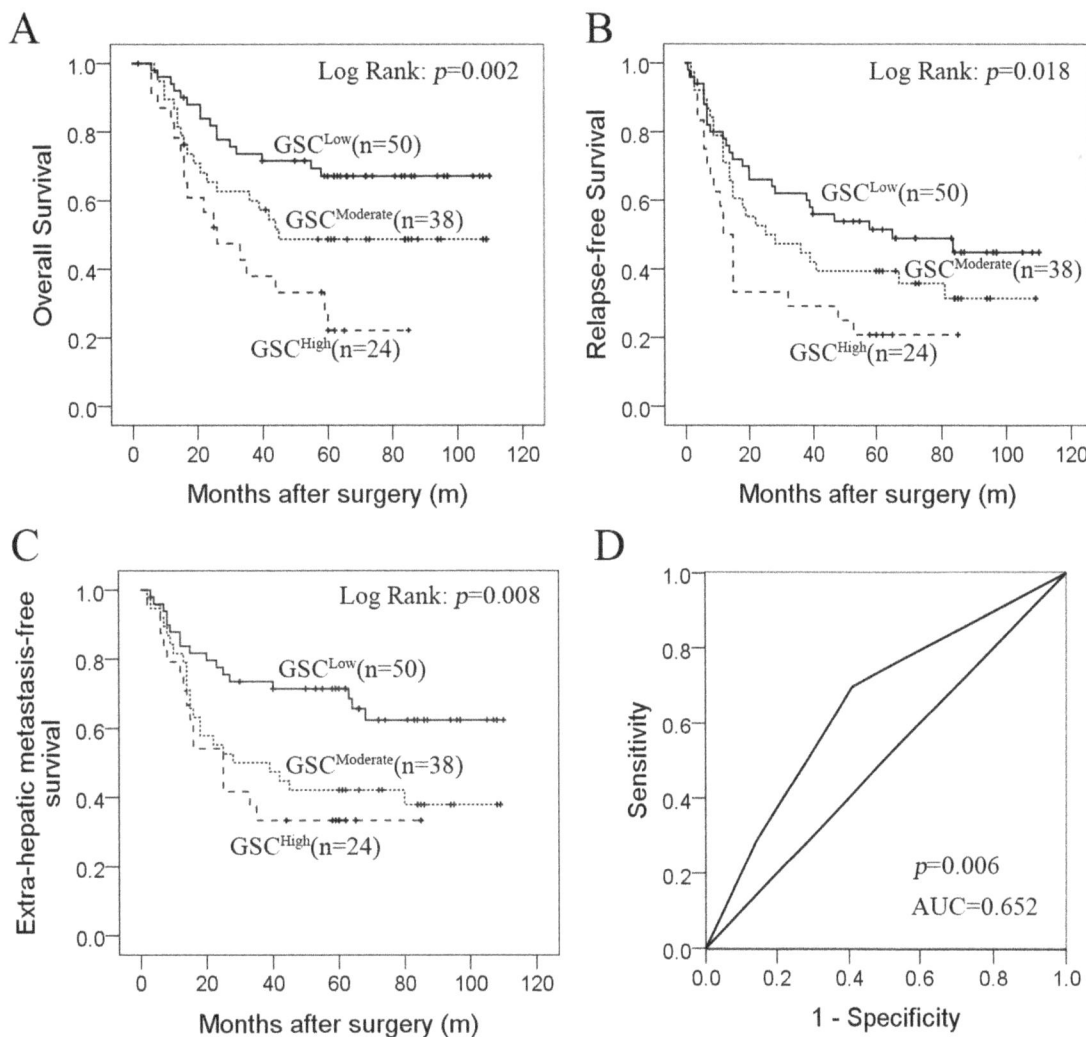

Figure 5. GSC expression correlates with poor survival and lung metastasis in HCC. Immunohistochemistry assay was based on tissue microarray from 112 tumor tissues. (A) Patients with highly expressed GSC had a significantly worse 5-year survival (Kaplan-Meier, log-rank test). (B) Patients with highly expressed GSC had showed early relapse and poor relapse-free survival when compared to other subgroups (Kaplan-Meier, log-rank test). (C) Groups with highly expressed GSC had lower extra-hepatic metastasis-free survival than the group with lower expressed GSC (Kaplan-Meier, log-rank test). (D) Receiver Operating Characteristic (ROC) curve analysis of GSC expression for occurrence of lung metastasis showed areas under the curve (AUC) of >0.5 ($P<0.05$).

compared to the primary foci. Therefore, it is possible that GSC was upregulated during the late metastatic stage in HCC. In addition, GSC is a member of the homeobox gene family and accumulated evidence suggests that deregulated homeobox gene expression may promote oncogenesis. Meanwhile, the abnormal expression of homeobox genes may be the consequence of wrong cellular context in cancer [29]. Therefore, the upregulation of GSC in metastatic lung tissues may the consequence of a deregulated local microenvironment, which deserves further research.

Taken together, findings from the present study indicate that the embryonic gene GSC is abnormally expressed in HCC and its expression is correlated with metastasis. Moreover, GSC potentially promotes metastasis of HCC through EMT rather than via collective cell migration. However, more in-depth studies exploring mechanisms of *GSC*-related cell-cell contact, organization of

the actin cytoskeleton, and cell polarization are needed. Our results suggest GSC is a potential therapeutic target for metastatic HCC.

Supporting Information

Figure S1 Effects of GSC overexpression on proliferation of HCC cells. CCK8 assay was used to evaluate the proliferation of tumor cells at 24 h, 48 h, and 72 h time points. No significant difference was observed among Hep3B-GSC, Hep3B-NC, and Hep3B cells. The data are presented as the mean ± SD of at least three independent experiments. Results were analyzed using Student's *t* test.

Table S1 Clinicopathologic factors and GSC expression in HCC.

Table 1. Univariate and multivariate analysis of factors associated with survival and lung metastasis in HCC patients.

Features	Overall survival				Time-to-lung metastasis			
	Univariate P	Multivariate			Univariate P	Multivariate		
		Hazard		P		Hazard		P
	values	Ratio	95%CI	Value	values	Ratio	95%CI	Value
Age (≤60 vs. >60 years)	0.887			NA	0.917			NA
Gender (male vs. female)	0.403			NA	0.328			NA
HBsAg (positive vs. negative)	0.726			NA	0.273			NA
Cirrhosis (present vs. absent)	0.721			NA	0.539			NA
AFP (≤20 vs. >20 µg/L)	0.008	2.085	1.065–4.084	0.032	0.011			NS
Tumor size (≤5 vs. >5 cm)	0.237			NA	0.278			NA
No. tumor nodules (single vs. multiple)	0.200			NA	0.096	2.066	1.068–3.994	0.031
Tumor capsule (complete vs. none)	0.348			NA	0.136			NA
Microvascular invasion (positive vs. negative)	<0.001	2.690	1.522–4.755	0.001	<0.001	2.343	1.306–4.202	0.004
Tumor differentiation	0.103			NA	0.058	2.363	1.338–4.171	0.003
Portal lymphatic status (yes vs. no)	0.004	3.837	1.552–9.486	0.004	0.003	3.064	1.328–7.073	0.009
GSC level (high vs. medium vs. low)	0.002	1.685	1.187–2.394	0.004	0.008	1.842	1.286–2.639	0.001

Abbreviations: AFP, alpha fetoprotein; ALT, alanine aminotransferase; NA, not adopted; NS, not significant.

Acknowledgments

The established Hep3B-GSC cell line, the GSC lentivirus vector, and the HCC tissue microarrays will be made available to other researchers upon request.

Author Contributions

Conceived and designed the experiments: TCX NLG SLY ZGR. Performed the experiments: TCX LZ JFC RXC YY. Analyzed the data: TCX NLG. Contributed reagents/materials/analysis tools: ZGR. Wrote the paper: TCX.

References

1. Tang ZY, Ye SL, Liu YK, Qin LX, Sun HC, et al. (2004) A decade's studies on metastasis of hepatocellular carcinoma. J Cancer Res Clin Oncol 130: 187–196.
2. Zhou XD (2002) Recurrence and metastasis of hepatocellular carcinoma: progress and prospects. Hepatobiliary Pancreat Dis Int 1: 35–41.
3. Locascio A, Nieto MA (2001) Cell movements during vertebrate development: integrated tissue behaviour versus individual cell migration. Curr Opin Genet Dev 11: 464–469.
4. Thiery JP, Acloque H, Huang RY, Nieto MA (2009) Epithelial-mesenchymal transitions in development and disease. Cell 139: 871–890.
5. Yang J, Weinberg RA (2008) Epithelial-mesenchymal transition: at the crossroads of development and tumor metastasis. Dev Cell 14: 818–829.
6. Friedl P, Gilmour D (2009) Collective cell migration in morphogenesis, regeneration and cancer. Nat Rev Mol Cell Biol 10: 445–457.
7. Friedl P, Hegerfeldt Y, Tusch M (2004) Collective cell migration in morphogenesis and cancer. Int J Dev Biol 48: 441–449.
8. Nakaya Y, Sheng G (2008) Epithelial to mesenchymal transition during gastrulation: an embryological view. Dev Growth Differ 50: 755–766.
9. Chuai M, Hughes D, Weijer CJ (2012) Collective epithelial and mesenchymal cell migration during gastrulation. Curr Genomics 13: 267–277.
10. Carmona-Fontaine C, Matthews HK, Kuriyama S, Moreno M, Dunn GA, et al. (2008) Contact inhibition of locomotion in vivo controls neural crest directional migration. Nature 456: 957–961.
11. Yasuo H, Lemaire P (2001) Role of Goosecoid, Xnot and Wnt antagonists in the maintenance of the notochord genetic programme in Xenopus gastrulae. Development 128: 3783–3793.
12. Blum M, Gaunt SJ, Cho KW, Steinbeisser H, Blumberg B, et al. (1992) Gastrulation in the mouse: the role of the homeobox gene goosecoid. Cell 69: 1097–1106.
13. Luu O, Nagel M, Wacker S, Lemaire P, Winklbauer R (2008) Control of gastrula cell motility by the Goosecoid/Mix.1/Siamois network: basic patterns and paradoxical effects. Dev Dyn 237: 1307–1320.
14. Clouthier DE, Hosoda K, Richardson JA, Williams SC, Yanagisawa H, et al. (1998) Cranial and cardiac neural crest defects in endothelin-A receptor-deficient mice. Development 125: 813–824.
15. Niehrs C, Keller R, Cho KW, De Robertis EM (1993) The homeobox gene goosecoid controls cell migration in Xenopus embryos. Cell 72: 491–503.
16. Hartwell KA, Muir B, Reinhardt F, Carpenter AE, Sgroi DC, et al. (2006) The Spemann organizer gene, Goosecoid, promotes tumor metastasis. Proc Natl Acad Sci U S A 103: 18969–18974.
17. Xue TC, Chen RX, Ren ZG, Zou JH, Tang ZY, et al. (2013) Transmembrane receptor CXCR7 increases the risk of extrahepatic metastasis of relatively well-differentiated hepatocellular carcinoma through upregulation of osteopontin. Oncol Rep 30: 105–110.
18. Xue TC, Chen RX, Han D, Chen J, Xue Q, et al. (2012) Down-regulation of CXCR7 inhibits the growth and lung metastasis of human hepatocellular carcinoma cells with highly metastatic potential. Exp Ther Med 3: 117–123.
19. Farooqui R, Fenteany G (2005) Multiple rows of cells behind an epithelial wound edge extend cryptic lamellipodia to collectively drive cell-sheet movement. J Cell Sci 118: 51–63.
20. Xue TC, Han D, Chen RX, Zou JH, Wang Y, et al. (2011) High expression of CXCR7 combined with Alpha fetoprotein in hepatocellular carcinoma correlates with extra-hepatic metastasis to lung after hepatectomy. Asian Pac J Cancer Prev 12: 657–663.
21. Simon R, Mirlacher M, Sauter G (2010) Immunohistochemical analysis of tissue microarrays. Methods Mol Biol 664: 113–126.
22. Lugli A, Spichtin H, Maurer R, Mirlacher M, Kiefer J, et al. (2005) EphB2 expression across 138 human tumor types in a tissue microarray: high levels of expression in gastrointestinal cancers. Clin Cancer Res 11: 6450–6458.
23. Shoval I, Kalcheim C (2012) Antagonistic activities of Rho and Rac GTPases underlie the transition from neural crest delamination to migration. Dev Dyn 241: 1155–1168.
24. Theveneau E, Mayor R (2012) Neural crest delamination and migration: from epithelium-to-mesenchyme transition to collective cell migration. Dev Biol 366: 34–54.
25. Ogunwobi OO, Liu C (2011) Hepatocyte growth factor upregulation promotes carcinogenesis and epithelial-mesenchymal transition in hepatocellular carcinoma via Akt and COX-2 pathways. Clin Exp Metastasis 28: 721–731.
26. Ozen E, Gozukizil A, Erdal E, Uren A, Bottaro DP, et al. (2012) Heparin inhibits Hepatocyte Growth Factor induced motility and invasion of hepatocellular carcinoma cells through early growth response protein 1. PLoS One 7: e42717.
27. Nabeshima K, Shimao Y, Inoue T, Itoh H, Kataoka H, et al. (1998) Hepatocyte growth factor/scatter factor induces not only scattering but also cohort migration of human colorectal-adenocarcinoma cells. Int J Cancer 78: 750–759.
28. Gritsman K, Talbot WS, Schier AF (2000) Nodal signaling patterns the organizer. Development 127: 921–932.
29. Abate-Shen C (2002) Deregulated homeobox gene expression in cancer: cause or consequence? Nat Rev Cancer 2: 777–785.

10

The Intracellular HBV DNAs as Novel and Sensitive Biomarkers for the Clinical Diagnosis of Occult HBV Infection in HBeAg Negative Hepatocellular Carcinoma in China

Hui Wang[1], Meng Fang[1], Xing Gu[1], Qiang Ji[1], Dongdi Li[2], Shu-Qun Cheng[3], Feng Shen[4], Chun-Fang Gao[1]*

1 Department of Laboratory Medicine, Eastern Hepatobiliary Surgery Hospital, Second Military Medical University, Shanghai, PR China, **2** Research School of Chemistry, The Australian National University, Canberra ACT, Australia, **3** Department of Hepatic Surgery (VI), Eastern Hepatobiliary Surgery Hospital, Second Military Medical University, Shanghai, PR China, **4** Department of Hepatic Surgery (IV), Eastern Hepatobiliary Surgery Hospital, Second Military Medical University, Shanghai, PR China

Abstract

This study aimed to investigate the virological status in liver (both tumor and adjacent non-tumor tissue), the clinical features and the contribution of occult HBV infection (OBI) to postoperative prognosis in HBeAg-negative(−) hepatocellular carcinoma (HCC) patients in China. Using quantitative TaqMan fluorescent real-time PCR assays, HBV covalently closed circular DNA (cccDNA) and total DNA (tDNA) were both quantified in 11 (HBsAg(−)) and 57 (HBsAg-positive(+)) pairs of tumor tissue (TT) and adjacent non-tumor tissue (ANTT) obtained from HBeAg(−) HCC patients who received no antiviral treatment and were negative for anti-HCV before surgical treatment. Of 11 HBsAg(−) patients, 36% were with HBsAb(+) HBeAb(+) HBcAb(+). However, only 9% of the HBsAg(−) patients were HBsAb(−) HBeAb(+) HBcAb(+), which accounted for the majority (93%) in the HBsAg(+) group. TT and ANTT HBV tDNAs in 11 HCC patients with HBsAg (−) and HBeAg (−) were all detectable. HBV cccDNA and tDNA were all lower in the HBsAg(−) group than those in the HBsAg(+) group. By Kaplan-Meier analysis, patients with OBI were associated with a lower risk of cirrhosis and better overall survival (OS). The intracellular HBV DNAs, such as HBV cccDNA and tDNA are valuable biological markers for the diagnosis of occult HBV infection in HCC patients. This would assist the clinical implementation of a more personalized therapy for viral re-activation control and improve the survival rate of OBI patients.

Editor: John Luk, Johnson & Johnson Medical, China

Funding: This study was supported by China National Key Projects for Infectious Disease (No. 2012ZX10002-016); National Natural Science Foundation of China (No. 81271925, No. 81171664); Key Projects of Science and Technology Commission of Shanghai Municipality (No. 10411955200). The funders had no role in study design, data collection and analysis, decision to publish, or preparation of the manuscript.

Competing Interests: The authors have declared that no competing interests exist.

* Email: gaocf1115@163.com

Introduction

Hepatocellular carcinoma (HCC) is the third most common cause of cancer death worldwide [1,2]. The major risk factor for the development of HCC is hepatitis B virus (HBV) infection [3,4]. A peculiar aspect of chronic HBV infection is the persistence of HBV genomes in the absence of serum HBs antigen (HBsAg), so called 'occult' infection. The geographic distribution of occult HBV infection (OBI) is associated with the prevalence of HBV infection and its prevalence is high in HCC populations [5].

OBI can occur not only in individuals with anti-HBs and/or anti-HBc antibodies but also in those who are negative for HBV markers [5,6]. The seronegativity in these OBI patients may be caused by naturally occurring mutants of HBV, which alters either the immunoreactivity of various HBV proteins or the quantity of serum HBsAg [7]. The individuals with OBI usually exhibit lower levels of viremia [8]. A decrease in HBV viral load as well as replication and various relevant mutations have been implicated in the explanation of HBsAg-negative (−) [9]. Several previous

studies have reported the existence of HBV DNA in liver tissues of HBsAg-negative patients [10,11,12,13] and the OBI significantly correlated with cirrhosis in chronic hepatitis C virus (HCV) carriers [14,15,16]. OBI is a worldwide diffused entity, evidence showed that this condition might be potentially oncogenetic [5,17]. However, in those HCC patients with HBsAg and HBeAg negative, the virologic status and the clinical features of OBI are still not thoroughly studied.

HBV covalently closed circular DNA (cccDNA) is an important intermediate in the life cycle of HBV, from which the HBV pregenomic RNA and all HBV messenger RNA transcripts originate [13]. Although the level of HBV replication in those HCC patients with HBsAg and HBeAg negative is low, little is known about the level of HBV covalently closed circular DNA (cccDNA) and total DNA (tDNA) in paired tumor tissues (TT) and adjacent non-tumor tissues (ANTT) in chronic Hepatitits B (CHB) endemic areas, such as China.

We therefore conducted a prospective study. The primary aim was to investigate the virologic status in the liver (both TT and

Table 1. Immunological characteristics of HBeAg-negative HCC patients.

Characteristic	HBsAg (−) and HBeAg (−)	HBsAg (+) and HBeAg (−)	P value
	No. of patients (%)	No. of patients (%)	
HBsAb (+) HBeAb (+) HBcAb (+)	4 (36%)	1 (2%)	P<0.001
HBsAb (+) HBeAb (−) HBcAb (+)	2 (18%)	0	
HBsAb (−) HBeAb (+) HBcAb (+)	1 (9%)	53 (93%)	
HBsAb (−) HBeAb (−) HBcAb (+)	2 (18%)	3 (5%)	
HBsAb (−) HBeAb (−) HBcAb (−)	2 (18%)	0	
Total	11	57	

ANTT) among these HCC patients with HBsAg (−) and HBeAg (−). The second aim was to determine the clinical features and the contribution of occult HBV infection (OBI) to postoperative prognosis for HCC patients with HBsAg (−) and HBeAg (−) in China.

Materials and Methods

Patients and samples

This study included a HBsAg-negative group (n = 11) and a HBsAg-positive (+) group (n = 57) of HCC patients with HBeAg (−) (between March 2007 and May 2009) who received no antiviral treatment and were negative for anti-HCV before surgical resection at the Shanghai Eastern Hepatobiliary Surgery Hospital (EHBH) in Shanghai, China. The study was approved by the Chinese Ethics Committee of Human Resources at the Second Military Medical University. All study participants provided written informed consent.

The inclusion criteria were patients with no evidence of hepatitis C virus (HCV) or hepatitis D virus (HDV) co-infection; no previous antiviral treatment; complete resection of tumor with sufficient safety margin (R0) and histologically proven HCC.

1) The HBsAg-negative group: HBsAg-negative and HBeAg-negative for at least 6 months, undetectable serum HBV DNA.

2) The HBsAg-positive group: HBsAg-positive and HBeAg-negative for at least 6 months.

The exclusion criteria included a history of liver transplantation and other malignancies, tumors of uncertain origin, metastatic liver cancer, autoimmune liver diseases, drug-related liver diseases, alcoholic hepatitis and other causes of chronic liver diseases (such as HCV, HDV, HEV, HIV) diagnosed before enrollment.

Details of patient clinical diagnosis, follow up are included in File S1.

Quantitation of HBV cccDNA and total DNA (tDNA) in tissues

Viral DNAs in frozen tissues were extracted using the QIAamp DNA Mini kit (QIAGEN GmbH, Hilden, Germany). HBV cccDNA and tDNA were detected using real-time polymerase chain reaction (PCR) with TaqMan fluorescent probes (Fosun Diagnostics, Shanghai, China) according to the method described by Bettina et al. with a slight modification [18]. The extracted DNA samples were treated with plasmid DNA-safe ATP-dependent enzyme (Epicentre, Madison, WI). Real-time PCR was performed on an ABI 7500 (Life Technologies Corporation, Foster City, CA) using a 50 μl reaction volume containing 20 ng

of DNA (for cccDNA quantification, a volume equivalent to 20 ng prior to DNase treatment), 2.5 mM $MgCl_2$, 0.5 μM of forward and reverse primers, and a 0.4 μM probe. Forward and reverse primers were F1 and R1 for cccDNA amplification, respectively and F2 and R2 for total intrahepatic HBV DNA amplification, respectively. TaqMan probes were TaqP1 for cccDNA quantification and TaqP2 (Table S1) for total intrahepatic HBV DNA quantification. GAPDH, a single copy housekeeping gene present in human was used in the real-time PCR as a control to estimate the number of cells represented in each PCR reaction. Serial dilutions of genomic DNAs were used as standards to quantitate GAPDH DNA from liver tissues. The results of cccDNA and tDNA were normalized to copies/10^6 cells.

Statistical analysis

All statistical analyses were two sided and performed using SPSS 17.0 for Windows (SPSS Inc., Chicago, IL). A P value of <0.05 was considered as statistically significant. Details are included in File S1.

Results

Immunological characteristics of HCC patients

The immunological characteristics of HBeAg(−) HCC patients are summarized in Table 1. There was significant difference between the HBsAg(−) and the HBsAg(+) group (P<0.001). Of 11 patients in the HBsAg(−) group, 36% were with HBsAb (+) HBeAb (+) HBcAb (+). The patients with HBsAb (+) HBeAb (−) HBcAb (+), HBsAb (−) HBeAb (−) HBcAb (+) and HBsAb (−) HBeAb (−) HBcAb (−) respectively accounted for 18%. However, the percentage of patients with HBsAb (−) HBeAb (+) HBcAb (+) is significantly higher in HBsAg (+) group than in HBsAg (−) one.

In the HBsAg(−) group, there were 6 HBsAb(+) patients (54%) and 5 HBsAb(−) patients (46%), 5 HBeAb(+) patients (46%) and 6 HBeAb(−) patients (54%), and 9 HBcAb(+) patients (82%) and 2 HBcAb(−) patients (18%). However, in the HBsAg(+) group, there were only 1 patients (2%) with HBsAb(+) and 56 patients (98%) with HBsAb(−),54 patients (95%) with HBeAb(+) and 3 patients (5%) with HBeAb(−), and 57 patients (100%) with HBcAb(+).

Intrahepatic HBV DNAs in 11 HCC patients with HBsAg (−) and HBeAg (−) were all detectable

The paired TT/ANTT of HCC patients with HBeAg (−) were stratified into different group (A–E) according to the immunological characteristics, and examined for intracellular HBV cccDNA and tDNA levels (Table 2). Interestingly, in the HBsAg(−) group, all HBV tDNAs were detectable, and 3 TT and 5 ANTT cccDNAs were undetectable. Among the HBsAg(+) group,

Table 2. Quantification of intrahepatic HBV DNAs in HCC patients.

Characteristic	Group	HBsAb	HBeAb	HBcAb	No. of patients (%)	TT ($\log_{10}$ copies/10^6 cells) cccDNA	TT ($\log_{10}$ copies/10^6 cells) HBV tDNA	ANTT ($\log_{10}$ copies/10^6 cells) cccDNA	ANTT ($\log_{10}$ copies/10^6 cells) HBV tDNA	TT ratio (%)	ANTT ratio (%)
HBsAg (−) and HBeAg (−)	A	+	+	+	4 (36%)	3.05±0.53	4.78±1.65	3.29±0.66*	4.83±2.03	11.96±17.09	0.56±0.67
	B	+	−	+	2 (18%)	2.33±0.01	5.62±0.16	2.67±0.56	6.07±0.55	0.05±0.02	0.04±0.01
	C	−	+	+	1 (9%)	1.45	5.59	undetectable	1.64	0.01	undetectable
	D	−	−	+	2 (18%)	6.07*	5.22±5.06	undetectable	2.54±0.15	0.19*	undetectable
	E	−	−	−	2 (18%)	undetectable	2.65±0.01	4.86*	4.81±2.95	undetectable	0.92*
Total					11 (100%)						
HBsAg (+) and HBeAg (−)	A	+	+	+	1 (2%)	3.82	5.17	3.75	6.83	4.45	0.08
	B	+	−	+	0						
	C	−	+	+	53 (93%)	4.57±1.67	6.62±1.42	4.86±1.16	6.95±0.88	2.73±4.45	1.97±2.76
	D	−	−	+	3 (5%)	6.99±0.07*	6.43±3.54	4.70±1.43	6.61±0.61	4.74±4.71*	2.80±3.34
	E	−	−	−	0						
Total					57 (100%)						

Abbreviations: HBV, hepatitis B virus; cccDNA, covalently closed circular DNA; tDNA, total DNA; TT, tumor tissue; ANTT, adjacent non-tumor tissue.

"+" and "−" indicate positive and negative detection.

* indicate the concentration of one sample was undetectable.

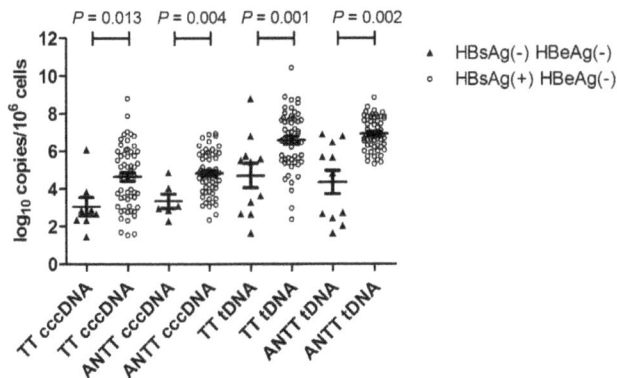

Figure 1. TT/ANTT tDNA and cccDNA are associated with HBsAg status in HBeAg (−) patients.

cccDNA was undetectable in one TT sample. The relationship between serum HBV DNA and cccDNA were shown in Table S2. Both the TT and the ANTT cccDNA made up a smaller portion of the tDNA in the HBsAg(−) group than those in the HBsAg(+) group, other than those patients with HBsAb (+) HBeAb (+) HBcAb (+).

The difference in TT/ANTT HBV cccDNA and tDNA between the HBsAg(−) group and the HBsAg(+) one were shown in Figure 1. The HBV cccDNA was significantly lower in the HBsAg(−) group than in the HBsAg(+) group (TT: 3.05 ± 1.39 vs. 4.64 ± 1.69 $\log_{10}$ copies/10^6 cells, $P = 0.013$; ANTT: 3.35 ± 0.94 vs. 4.83 ± 1.16 $\log_{10}$ copies/10^6 cells, $P = 0.004$). Similarly, the HBV tDNA was also significantly lower in the HBsAg(−) group than in the HBsAg(+) group (TT: 4.70 ± 2.13 vs. 6.59 ± 1.53 $\log_{10}$ copies/10^6 cells, $P = 0.001$; ANTT: 4.34 ± 2.06 vs. 6.93 ± 0.86 $\log_{10}$ copies/10^6 cells, $P = 0.002$). However, no statistical significant difference in TT/ANTT ratios was observed between the HBsAg(−) and the HBsAg(+) group (TT: 6.02 ± 12.87 vs. $2.83 \pm 4.40\%$, $P = 0.509$; ANTT: 0.45 ± 0.55 vs. $1.98 \pm 2.75\%$, $P = 0.180$).

Occult HBV infection was associated with a lower risk of cirrhosis and better overall survival

Eleven Patients with occult HBV infection had higher albumin (ALB), well-differentiated tumors (E-S grades I and II) and a lower risk to develop cirrhosis (Table 3). However, the other demographic and clinicopathologic characteristics were not significantly different between the two groups.

By Kaplan-Meier analysis, although patients with OBI did not differ significantly in overall survival (OS) and disease-free survival (DFS) ($P = 0.173$ and $P = 0.386$, Fig. 2A, 2B), patients with OBI showed lower mortality rates at 1-, 2- and 3-years after resection.

Discussion

HCC is one of the most common cancers worldwide, and its incidence appears to be increasing [1,16]. Most cases of hepatocellular carcinoma (80%) arise in eastern Asia and sub-Saharan Africa, where chronic infection with HBV is the dominant risk factor [1]. However, this malignancy is not only mainly related to an overt (HBsAg positive) HBV infection, but also linked with occult HBV infection (HBsAg negative) [5]. The long-lasting persistence of HBV genomes in the liver (with detectable or undetectable HBV DNA in the serum of individuals testing negative for HBsAg) is termed OBI [17]. Our study based on the quantitative TaqMan fluorescent real-time PCR assay

provides valuable information on the clinical and virological features of HCC patients with both HBsAg and HBeAg negative.

In our study, HBV tDNAs in 11 HCC patients with HBsAg(−) and HBeAg(−) were all detectable in TT or ANTT at the time of surgical resection. There were approximately half of these patients with HBsAb(+) (54%) and with HBeAb(+) (46%), and 82% of patients with HBcAb(+) in the HBsAg(−) and HBeAg(−) group. We confirmed that HBV could persist in liver after the disappearance of HBsAg in individuals with previous exposure to the virus, retaining the serological footprint of HBcAb positivity with such a virologic status [19]. But there were 2 cases with all serological markers negative (HBsAg, HBeAg, HBsAb, HBeAb and HBcAb), in which had detectable HBV tDNA in TT/ANTT. Previous studies have revealed that the HCC patients with OBI who are HBsAg-negative but positive for HBcAb are at risk of HBV reactivation after undergoing chemotherapy or immuno-suppressive therapy [20,21,22]. Thus, it is very important to monitor HBV DNA levels regularly to achieve the early administration of antiviral or antineoplastic drugs before the onset of ALT elevation, however, the optimum testing frequency and noninvasive detection technology of HBV DNA in occult HBV carriers will need additional study.

To clarify the virological characteristics of HBV, we detected the cccDNA levels in cancerous tissues and non-cancerous tissues. cccDNA does not take part in replication directly, because it is maintained as a stable pool inside the hepatocyte nuclei [23]. We found that the levels of cccDNA and tDNA in cancerous tissues and non-cancerous tissues were significantly lower in the HBsAg(−) group than in the HBsAg(+) group. Both TT and ANTT cccDNA made up a smaller portion of the tDNA in the HBsAg-negative group, other than the tumor tissue ratio in the type of HBsAb (+) HBeAb (+) HBcAb (+). It is likely that OBI reactivates with the development of an immunosuppressive status.

Although the cause of OBI reactivation is yet to be understood, it is necessary to consider the following factors: the host's immune surveillance, restored virus, the impact of liver cancer cells and coinfection of other types of HBV. (1) Virus factors: In most cases there is no change in the α determinant that could explain the lack of HBsAg detection [24,25,26]. Although in a few cases (10%) the lack of HBsAg detection is due to infection with mutated viruses unrecognized by available assays (S-escape mutants) [27,28,29], the typical OBI is related to strongly suppressed HBV replication and the cause of HBV suppression is yet to be understood [17]. (2) Host factors: The genetic differences between individuals can lead to different immunological environment. An in vitro study showed that occult viral isolates could fully restore replication, transcription, and protein synthesis abilities once the viruses are taken out of the host liver microenvironment [30]. However, the association between host genomic variation and virus replication suppression needs to be investigated. (3) Coinfection. Because the exclusion criteria in our study included a history of other causes of chronic liver diseases (such as HCV, HDV, HEV, HIV) diagnosed before enrollment, there is no evidence of direct effects of infection of other types of HBV. Further studies are required to determine the characteristics of the reactivated viruses in HBsAg and HBeAg negative but HBsAb(+), HBeAb(+) and HBcAb(+) occult HBV carriers.

In this study, we found that patients with occult HBV infection are less likely to develop cirrhosis and had better overall survival. This observation strongly supported the possible contribution of OBI to the establishment of cirrhosis and the possible direct or indirect role in the development of HCC. In patients with diagnosable/detectable low-grade HBV replication, the virus retains its pro-oncogenic properties [31] [17]. Therefore, the

Table 3. Occult HBV infection was associated with the cirrhosis and E-S grade.

Demographic or Characteristic	HBsAg (+) and HBeAg (−) (n = 57)		HBsAg (−) and HBeAg (−) (n = 11)		P value
	No. of patients	%	No. of patients	%	
Sex					NS(0.360)
Male	48	84	8	73	
Female	9	16	3	27	
Age, years					NS(0.179)
Median	51		58		
Range	34–70		36–75		
AFP, ng/mL					NS(0.065)
Median	119		4		
Range	1.9->1210		1.4->1210		
CEA, ng/mL					NS(0.451)
Median	2.6		2		
Range	0.4–33.7		0.5–7.8		
CA19-9, U/mL					NS(0.779)
Median	26		13		
Range	0.6–295.5		6.7–259.9		
TBIL, μmol/L					NS(0.834)
Median	14		14		
Range	6.4–64.7		8–40.2		
ALB, g/L					0.041
Median	41		44		
Range	34.6–49.9		39.4–49.4		
ALT (IU/L)					NS(0.058)
Median	44		20		
Range	12.8–360.5		5.5–48.1		
GGT, U/L					NS(0.388)
Median	77		55		
Range	23–843		10–355		
Platelet, 10^9/L					NS(0.913)
Median	151		##		
Range	51–382		56–284		
PT (INR)					NS(0.473)
Median	1		1		
Range	0.86–1.9		0.93–1.13		
Creatinine, μmol/L					NS(0.247)

Table 3. Cont.

Demographic or Characteristic	HBsAg (+) and HBeAg (−) (n = 57) No. of patients	%	HBsAg (−) and HBeAg (−) (n = 11) No. of patients	%	P value
Median	70		70		
Range	40–94		50–110		NS(0.075)
Tumor Size, cm					
Median	7.9		5		
Range	2.4–20		1.46–11.3		NS(0.568)
Tumor Number					NS(0.549)
Single	42	74	9	82	
Multiple	15	26	2	18	
Satellite nodules					
Yes	15	26	2	18	
No	41	72	9	82	
Liver cirrhosis					0.008
Yes	47	83	5	46	
No	10	18	6	55	
Tumor capsular invasion					NS(0.272)
Yes	37	65	9	82	
No	20	35	2	18	
Macrovascular invasion					NS(0.257)
Yes	14	25	1	9	
No	43	75	10	91	
E-S grade					0.015
I–II	15	26	7	64	
III–IV	42	74	4	36	
TNM stage					NS(0.219)
I–II	30	53	8	73	
III–IV	27	47	3	27	
Serum HBV DNA (log$_{10}$ IU/mL)					<0.001
Median	4.7		undetectable		
Range	3–7.62		undetectable		
Undetectable	4	7	11	100	
detectable	53	93	0	0	

Abbreviations: NS, not significant; AFP, α-fetoprotein; ALB, albumin; CEA, carcinoembryonic antigen; GGT, γ-glutamyltransferase; TBIL, total bilirubin; ALT, alanine aminotransferase; PT, prothrombin time; E-S grade, Edmonson-Steiner grade; HBV, hepatitis B virus; HBsAg, hepatitis B sruface antigen; HBeAg, hepatitis B e antigen; HCC, hepatocellular carcinoma. Serum HBV DNA of 11 patients with HBsAg (−) and HBeAg (−) were all less than 10^3 IU/mL.

A

B

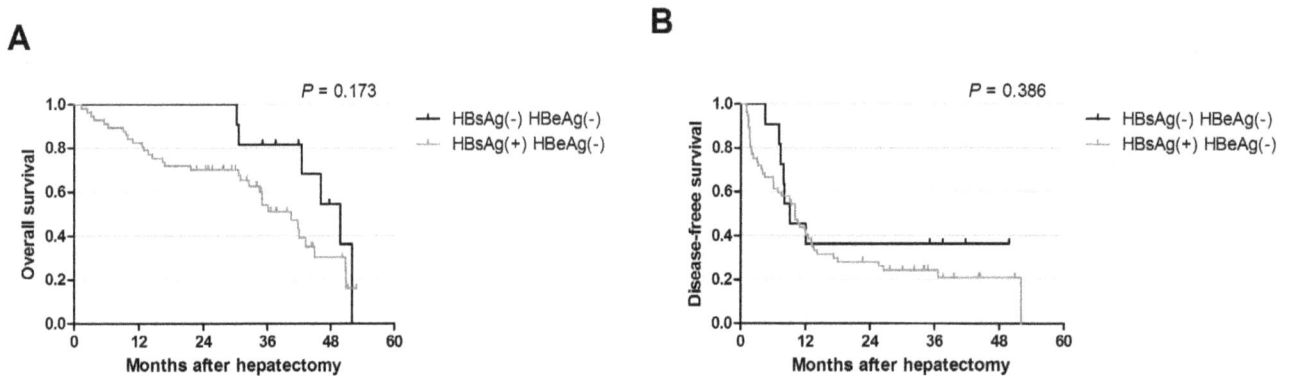

Figure 2. The survival of OBI patients after liver resection. Overall survival curve **A** and disease-free survival curve **B** stratified by HBsAg were constructed using Kaplan-Meier method.

mechanisms leading to HCC in occult HBV carriers seem to be similar to those in overt cases.

Our study has limitations. Firstly, samples were from a single department and the size was limited. In future studies, larger sample size would be preferred in order to validate the findings shown in this study. Besides, studies should continue to functionally characterize viral mutations and the relevant viral genes.

In summary, our findings suggest that the intracellular HBV DNAs, such as HBV cccDNA and tDNA are valuable biological markers for the diagnosis of occult HBV infection in HCC patitents. This would assist the clinical implementation of a more personalized therapy for viral re-activation control and improve the survival rate of OBI patients.

Supporting Information

Table S1 Sequences of primers used in the study for cccDNA and tDNA.

Table S2 Correlations among HBV DNAs in the HBsAg-positive group.

File S1 Supplemental Materials and Methods.

Acknowledgments

The authors thank Prof. Fei-guo Zhou for the clinical interpretation and Dr. Zhi-jun Yang for experimental assistance.

Author Contributions

Conceived and designed the experiments: HW MF XG JC DDL SQC FS CFG. Performed the experiments: HW MF SQC FS CFG. Analyzed the data: HW MF SQC FS CFG. Contributed reagents/materials/analysis tools: HW MF QJ SQC FS CFG. Contributed to the writing of the manuscript: HW MF SQC FS CFG.

References

1. Forner A, Llovet JM, Bruix J (2012) Hepatocellular carcinoma. Lancet 379: 1245–1255.
2. Center MM, Jemal A (2011) International trends in liver cancer incidence rates. Cancer Epidemiol Biomarkers Prev 20: 2362–2368.
3. Pollicino T, Saitta C, Raimondo G (2011) Hepatocellular carcinoma: the point of view of the hepatitis B virus. Carcinogenesis 32: 1122–1132.
4. Nguyen VT, Law MG, Dore GJ (2009) Hepatitis B-related hepatocellular carcinoma: epidemiological characteristics and disease burden. J Viral Hepat 16: 453–463.
5. De Mitri MS, Cassini R, Bernardi M (2010) Hepatitis B virus-related hepatocarcinogenesis: molecular oncogenic potential of clear or occult infections. Eur J Cancer 46: 2178–2186.
6. Brechot C, Thiers V, Kremsdorf D, Nalpas B, Pol S, et al. (2001) Persistent hepatitis B virus infection in subjects without hepatitis B surface antigen: clinically significant or purely "occult". Hepatology 34: 194–203.
7. Saito T, Shinzawa H, Uchida T, Kawamata O, Honma S, et al. (1999) Quantitative DNA analysis of low-level hepatitis B viremia in two patients with serologically negative chronic hepatitis B. J Med Virol 58: 325–331.
8. Rodriguez-Inigo E, Mariscal L, Bartolome J, Castillo I, Navacerrada C, et al. (2003) Distribution of hepatitis B virus in the liver of chronic hepatitis C patients with occult hepatitis B virus infection. J Med Virol 70: 571–580.
9. Gunther S, Fischer L, Pult I, Sterneck M, Will H (1999) Naturally occurring variants of hepatitis B virus. Adv Virus Res 52: 25–137.
10. Brechot C, Pourcel C, Louise A, Rain B, Tiollais P (1980) Presence of integrated hepatitis B virus DNA sequences in cellular DNA of human hepatocellular carcinoma. Nature 286: 533–535.
11. Shafritz DA, Shouval D, Sherman HI, Hadziyannis SJ, Kew MC (1981) Integration of hepatitis B virus DNA into the genome of liver cells in chronic liver disease and hepatocellular carcinoma. Studies in percutaneous liver biopsies and post-mortem tissue specimens. N Engl J Med 305: 1067–1073.
12. Brechot C, Hadchouel M, Scotto J, Fonck M, Potet F, et al. (1981) State of hepatitis B virus DNA in hepatocytes of patients with hepatitis B surface antigen-positive and -negative liver diseases. Proc Natl Acad Sci U S A 78: 3906–3910.
13. Wong DK, Huang FY, Lai CL, Poon RT, Seto WK, et al. (2011) Occult hepatitis B infection and HBV replicative activity in patients with cryptogenic cause of hepatocellular carcinoma. Hepatology 54: 829–836.
14. De Maria N, Colantoni A, Friedlander L, Leandro G, Idilman R, et al. (2000) The impact of previous HBV infection on the course of chronic hepatitis C. Am J Gastroenterol 95: 3529–3536.
15. Sagnelli E, Coppola N, Scolastico C, Mogavero AR, Filippini P, et al. (2001) HCV genotype and "silent" HBV coinfection: two main risk factors for a more severe liver disease. J Med Virol 64: 350–355.
16. Pollicino T, Squadrito G, Cerenzia G, Cacciola I, Raffa G, et al. (2004) Hepatitis B virus maintains its pro-oncogenic properties in the case of occult HBV infection. Gastroenterology 126: 102–110.
17. Raimondo G, Caccamo G, Filomia R, Pollicino T (2013) Occult HBV infection. Semin Immunopathol 35: 39–52.
18. Werle-Lapostolle B, Bowden S, Locarnini S, Wursthorn K, Petersen J, et al. (2004) Persistence of cccDNA during the natural history of chronic hepatitis B and decline during adefovir dipivoxil therapy. Gastroenterology 126: 1750–1758.
19. Raimondo G, Allain JP, Brunetto MR, Buendia MA, Chen DS, et al. (2008) Statements from the Taormina expert meeting on occult hepatitis B virus infection. J Hepatol 49: 652–657.
20. Hui CK, Cheung WW, Zhang HY, Au WY, Yuen YH, et al. (2006) Kinetics and risk of de novo hepatitis B infection in HBsAg-negative patients undergoing cytotoxic chemotherapy. Gastroenterology 131: 59–68.
21. Dervite I, Hober D, Morel P (2001) Acute hepatitis B in a patient with antibodies to hepatitis B surface antigen who was receiving rituximab. N Engl J Med 344: 68–69.

22. Inuzuka T, Ueda Y, Morimura H, Fujii Y, Umeda M, et al. (2014) Reactivation from Occult HBV Carrier Status is Characterized by Low Genetic Heterogeneity with the Wild-type or G1896A Variant Prevalence. J Hepatol.

23. Wong DK, Yuen MF, Poon RT, Yuen JC, Fung J, et al. (2006) Quantification of hepatitis B virus covalently closed circular DNA in patients with hepatocellular carcinoma. J Hepatol 45: 553–559.

24. Blackberg J, Kidd-Ljunggren K (2000) Occult hepatitis B virus after acute self-limited infection persisting for 30 years without sequence variation. J Hepatol 33: 992–997.

25. Jeantet D, Chemin I, Mandrand B, Tran A, Zoulim F, et al. (2004) Cloning and expression of surface antigens from occult chronic hepatitis B virus infections and their recognition by commercial detection assays. J Med Virol 73: 508–515.

26. Wagner AA, Denis F, Weinbreck P, Loustaud V, Autofage F, et al. (2004) Serological pattern 'anti-hepatitis B core alone' in HIV or hepatitis C virus-infected patients is not fully explained by hepatitis B surface antigen mutants. AIDS 18: 569–571.

27. Chemin I, Alain S, Margeridon S, Mrani S, Kay A, et al. (2006) What is really ongoing during occult HBV reactivation. Hepatology 43: 195; author reply 195–196.

28. Alexopoulou A, Baltayiannis G, Jammeh S, Waters J, Dourakis SP, et al. (2004) Hepatitis B surface antigen variant with multiple mutations in the a determinant in an agammaglobulinemic patient. J Clin Microbiol 42: 2861–2865.

29. Jeantet D, Chemin I, Mandrand B, Zoulim F, Trepo C, et al. (2002) Characterization of two hepatitis B virus populations isolated from a hepatitis B surface antigen-negative patient. Hepatology 35: 1215–1224.

30. Pollicino T, Raffa G, Costantino L, Lisa A, Campello C, et al. (2007) Molecular and functional analysis of occult hepatitis B virus isolates from patients with hepatocellular carcinoma. Hepatology 45: 277–285.

31. Chemin I, Trepo C (2005) Clinical impact of occult HBV infections. J Clin Virol 34 Suppl 1: S15–21.

11

Natural History of Malignant Bone Disease in Hepatocellular Carcinoma: Final Results of a Multicenter Bone Metastasis Survey

Daniele Santini[1], Francesco Pantano[1], Ferdinando Riccardi[2], Giovan Giuseppe Di Costanzo[3], Raffaele Addeo[4], Francesco Maria Guida[1], Mariella Spalato Ceruso[1], Sandro Barni[5], Paola Bertocchi[6], Sara Marinelli[7], Paolo Marchetti[8], Antonio Russo[9], Mario Scartozzi[10], Luca Faloppi[10], Matteo Santoni[10], Stefano Cascinu[10], Evaristo Maiello[11], Franco Silvestris[12], Marco Tucci[12], Toni Ibrahim[13], Gianluca Masi[14], Antonio Gnoni[15], Alessandro Comandone[16], Nicola Fazio[17], Alessandro Conti[18], Ilaria Imarisio[19], Salvatore Pisconti[20], Elisa Giommoni[21], Saverio Cinieri[22], Vincenzo Catalano[23], Vincenzo Ostilio Palmieri[24], Giovanni Infante[25], Michele Aieta[26], Antonio Trogu[27], Cosmo Damiano Gadaleta[28], Anna Elisabetta Brunetti[29], Vito Lorusso[29], Nicola Silvestris[29]*

1 Medical Oncology Unit - University Campus Bio-Medico, Rome, Italy, 2 Medical Oncology Unit, Cardarelli Hospital, Naples, Italy, 3 Liver Unit, Cardarelli Hospital, Naples, Italy, 4 Medical Oncology Unit, 'San Giovanni di Dio' Frattamaggiore Hospital, Frattammaggiore, Italy, 5 Medical Oncology Unit, Treviglio-Caravaggio Hospital, Treviglio, Italy, 6 Medical Oncology Unit, Fondazione Poliambulanza, Brescia, Italy, 7 Department of Medical and Surgical Sciences, S.Orsola-Malpighi Hospital, University of Bologna, Bologna, Italy, 8 Department of Medical Oncology, University of Rome La Sapienza, Santa Andrea Hospital, Rome, Italy, 9 Section of Medical Oncology, Department of Surgical, Oncological and Stomatological Disciplines, University of Palermo, Palermo, Italy, 10 Clinica di Oncologia Medica, AOU Ospedali Riuniti-Università Politecnica delle Marche, Ancona, Italy, 11 Medical Oncology Unit – Hospital "Casa Sollievo della Sofferenza", San Giovanni Rotondo, Italy, 12 Department of Biomedical Sciences and Human Oncology, University of Bari Aldo Moro, Bari, Italy, 13 Istituto Scientifico Romagnolo per lo Studio e la Cura dei Tumori (IRST), IRCCS- Osteoncology and Rare Tumors Center, Meldola, Italy, 14 Division of Medical Oncology 2, Azienda Ospedaliero-Universitaria Pisana, Pisa, Italy, 15 Medical Oncology Unit – Hospital of Lecce, Lecce, Italy, 16 Department of Oncology, Gradenigo Hospital and Gruppo Piemontese Sarcomi, Turin, Italy, 17 Unit of Gastrointestinal and Neuroendocrine Tumor, European Institute of Oncology, Milan, Italy, 18 Department of Clinical and Specialist Sciences, Urology, Polytechnic University of the Marche Region, AOU Ospedali Riuniti Umberto I-GM Lancisi and G Salesi, Ancona, Italy, 19 Medical Oncology, Fondazione IRCCS Policlinico S. Matteo, Pavia, Italy, 20 Medical Oncology Unit – S.G. Moscati Hospital ASL TA/1, Taranto, Italy, 21 Medical Oncology Unit – Hospital Careggi, Florence, Italy, 22 Medical Oncology Department & Breast Unit - Hospital of Brindisi and Medical Oncology Department - European Institute of Oncology, Milan, Italy, 23 Medical Oncology, A.O. "Ospedali Riuniti Marche Nord", Presidio S. Salvatore, Pesaro, Italy, 24 Department of Biomedical Sciences and Human Oncology, Clinica Medica "A. Murri", University of Bari, Bari, Italy, 25 U.O. Infectious Disease, P.O. Bisceglie, Bisceglie, Italy, 26 Centro di Riferimento Oncologico della Basilicata IRCCS, Rionero in Vulture, Italy, 27 Medical Oncology unit – Hospital of Aosta, Aosta, Italy, 28 Interventional Radiology Unit with Integrated Section of Translational Medical Oncology – National Cancer Institute "Giovanni Paolo II", Bari, Italy, 29 Medical Oncology Unit – National Cancer Institute "Giovanni Paolo II", Bari, Italy

Abstract

Background: Bone is an uncommon site of metastasis in patients with advanced hepatocellular carcinoma (HCC). Therefore, there are few studies concerning the natural history of bone metastasis in patients with HCC.

Patients and Methods: Data on clinicopathology, survival, skeletal-related events (SREs), and bone-directed therapies for 211 deceased HCC patients with evidence of bone metastasis were statistically analyzed.

Results: The median age was 70 years; 172 patients were male (81.5%). The median overall survival was 19 months. The median time to the onset of bone metastasis was 13 months (22.2% at HCC diagnosis); 64.9% patients had multiple bone metastases. Spine was the most common site of bone metastasis (59.7%). Most of these lesions were osteolytic (82.4%); 88.5% of them were treated with zoledronic acid. At multivariate analysis, only the Child Score was significantly correlated with a shorter time to diagnosis of bone metastases ($p = 0.001$, HR = 1.819). The median survival from bone metastasis was 7 months. At multivariate analysis, HCC etiology ($p = 0.005$), ECOG performance status ($p = 0.002$) and treatment with bisphosphonate ($p = 0.024$) were associated with shorter survival after bone disease occurrence. The site of bone metastasis but not the number of bone lesions was associated with the survival from first skeletal related event (SRE) ($p = 0.021$) and OS ($p = 0.001$).

Conclusions: This study provides a significant improvement in the understanding the natural history of skeletal disease in HCC patients. An early and appropriate management of these patients is dramatically needed in order to avoid subsequent worsening of their quality of life.

Editor: Antonio Moschetta, IRCCS Istituto Oncologico Giovanni Paolo II, Italy

Funding: The authors have no support or funding to report.

Competing Interests: The authors have declared that no competing interests exist.

* Email: n.silvestris@oncologico.bari.it

Introduction

Hepatocellular carcinoma (HCC) is the sixth most prevalent cancer worldwide and the third leading cause of cancer-related death, although its geographical distribution is heterogeneous with the highest incidence in sub-Saharan Africa and Eastern Asia [1]. The choice of its therapy is related to the stage of the disease, severity of the underlying liver disease, and clinical expertise. Unfortunately, two thirds of patients are diagnosed at an advanced stage, when prognosis is poor with 5-year survival rates of less than 20% [2].

HCC is less likely to develop distant metastases, even in the inoperable stage, compared to other solid tumors with the lung as the most common site of localization [3]. Although bone involvement is reported as uncommon in HCC, its incidence has significantly increased in the last decade due to the improvement of overall survival of these patients [4,5]. One recent study considering 342 HCC patients reported skeletal invasion in approximately 25% of extrahepatic metastases [6].

Axial skeleton is the most frequent localization of bone metastases with a prognostic correlation of the time between the primary HCC occurrence and bone metastases detection [7]. They are mainly osteolytic resulting in significant morbidity and reduced quality of life for patients from the associated skeletal-related events (SRE; defined as pathological fracture, the need for radiotherapy or surgery to bone, spinal cord compression, and hypercalcemia) [8]. Radiotherapy is the most common SRE, playing a role in bone pain palliation, mostly for patients whose liver failure can be associated with a reduced patients' opioid tolerance. In most of cases, higher radiotherapy doses are required due to the presence of soft tissue masses in addition to bone involvement [9]. Indeed, few retrospective studies evaluated the use of biphosphonates in HCC-bone metastases [4]. Low doses of sorafenib have been associated to long term progression free survival in some patients [10].

Finally, herein we report the results of the largest multicenter study investigating the natural history (and their clinical management) of bone metastases from HCC.

Patients and Methods

Ethics Statement

This multicentre retrospective observational study has been approved by the Ethics Committee of the coordinator centre (National Cancer Institute of Bari). According to our Ethics Committee, a written consent was not needed. In fact, this is a retrospective observational study considering only died patients whose recruitment in the survey did not influenced their treatment.

Study design

This retrospective, observational multicentre study aimed at defining the natural history of HCC patients with bone metastasis was conducted in 23 Italian hospital centres in which these patients received diagnosis and treatment of disease from January 1993 to May 2013. Data were collected from HCC patients of all ages who received standard treatments in accordance with each own treating physician's practice and were not included neither in clinical trials nor experimental protocols. Moreover, patients had at least one bone metastasis during the course of their disease and died of HCC or HCC-related complications. In details, patients were identified as having bone metastasis if two of the following criteria were satisfied: physician reported bone metastasis; bone metastasis identified by bone scan; record of radiotherapy to bone as a palliative therapy; identification of bone metastasis by other imaging assessment (e.g. standard x-rays, computed tomography scans, or magnetic resonance imaging of the skeleton). Data were collected throughout the disease course and during all cancer treatments, including surgery, radiation therapy, locaregional therapies, chemotherapy, and biological therapies. Variables assessed included age, sex, aetiology, grading, Child score at diagnosis, presence and type of locoregional treatment, the median value of Alpha-fetoprotein (AFP) at diagnosis, number and sites of bone metastasis, visceral metastases, ECOG performance status (PS) at the moment of bone metastases diagnosis, time to appearance of bone metastasis, times to first and subsequent SREs (from diagnosis of bone metastasis), SRE types, survival after bone metastases diagnosis and after first SRE, systemic therapy with Sorafenib and type and time of bisphosphonate therapy.

Statistical analysis

Descriptive statistics were used for patient demographics and incidence of SREs. All survival intervals were determined by the Kaplan-Meier method. The differences in survival according to clinical parameters or treatment were evaluated by the log-rank test and described by the Kaplan–Meier method unless otherwise specified. In the univariate model, all the clinical variables were evaluated as predictors for shorter time to bone metastasis, shorter time from bone metastases to SRE and shorter time from bone metastases to death. Patients who did not have a recorded date for a specific event were censored at the date of death. Finally, the Cox proportional hazards model was applied to the multivariate survival analysis. All the significant variables in the univariate model were used to build the multivariate model of survival, and median values were derived from whole-month values rather than fractions. SPSS software (version 20.00; SPSS, Chicago, IL) was used for statistical analysis. A p value<0.05 was considered statistically significant.

Table 1. Baseline characteristics.

Baseline characteristics (Total N = 211)	Frequency (pts/total applicable)	P (%)
Age		
<70 Years	111/205	54.1
>70 Years	94/205	45.9
Gender		
Male	172/211	81.5
Female	39/211	18.5
Aetiology		
HBV-related	35/211	16.5
HCV-related	110/211	52.1
Alcohol-related **cirrosi**	20/211	9.4
Other	46/211	21.8
Grading		
G1	28/98	28.6
G2	30/98	30.6
G3	40/98	40.8
Locoregional Treatment		
No	149/211	70.6
Yes	62/211	29.4
Type of locoregional Treatment		
Surgery	50/149	33.5
Interventional Radiology	89/149	66.5
Type of interventional Radiology		
RFA	23/89	25.8
TACE	57/89	64.0
PEI	9/89	10.1
CHILD Score		
A	133/191	69.8
B	42/191	22.0
C	16/191	8.4
Visceral Metastasis		
Yes	151/211	71.6
No	60/211	28.4
AFP (cut-off value of 200 ng/mL at diagnosis)		
<200 ng/ml	97/149	65.1
>200 ng/ml	52/149	34.9
AFP (median value at diagnosis)		
<43 ng\ml	75/149	50.4
>43 ng/ml	74/149	49.6
Sorafenib Treatment		
Yes	132/211	62.6
No	79/211	37.4

Abbreviations: n, number; pts, patients; HBV, Hepatitis B virus; HCV, Hepatitis C virus.

Results

Patient characteristics

We retrospectively enrolled 211 patients died from HCC with bone metastasis. Of them, 172 patients were male (81.5%). The median age was 70 years (SD +/−9). Tumor etiology of HCC was HBV related in 35/211 (16.5%) patients, HCV related in 110/211 (52.1%) patients, alcohol related in 20/211 (9.4%) patients and other causes-related in 46/211 (21.8%) patients. The subgroup

Table 2. Skeletal metastases.

Skeletal metastases (total n = 211)	Frequency (pts)	Percentage (%)
ECOG PS (at time of Bone Metastasis)		
0	51/194	26.3
1	78/194	40.2
2	50/194	25.8
3	15/194	7.7
Bone Metastasis at diagnosis		
Yes (synchronous)	161/207	77.8
No (metachronous)	46/207	22.2
Bone Lesion Type		
Osteolytic	169/205	82.4
Osteoblastic	16/205	7.8
Mixed	20/205	9.8
Number of Bone Metastasis		
1	74/211	35.1
>1	137/211	64.9
Bone Metastasis Localization		
Spine	126/211	59.7
Long Bones	41/211	19.4
Hip	74/211	35.1
Other Sites	61/211	28.9
Total SRE Number		
0	84/211	39.9
1	127/211	60.1
2	40/211	18.9
3	6/211	2.8
First SRE Type		
Pathological Fracture	31/127	24.4
Hypercalcemia	7/127	5.5
Spinal Cord Compression	12/127	9.4
Surgery to Bone	7\127	5.5
Radiation to Bone	70/127	55.1
Second SRE Type		
Pathological Fracture	5/40	12.5
Hypercalcemia	6/40	15
Spinal Cord Compression	5/40	12.5
Surgery to Bone	5/40	12.5
Radiation to Bone	19/40	47.5
Third SRE Type		
Pathological Fracture	0/6	0.0
Hypercalcemia	0/6	0.0
Spinal Cord Compression	0/6	0.0
Surgery to Bone	2/6	33.4
Radiation to Bone	4/6	66.6
Biphosphonate Treatment	105/211	49.7
Zoledronic Acid	93/105	88.5
Pamidronate	6/105	5.6
Other	7/105	6.6

Table 3. Predictive factors of onset of bone metastasis.

VARIABLES	MEDIAN TIME (MONTHS)	p VALUE (uni variate)	p VALUE (multivariate)	HAZARD RATIO (HR)
Age		0.604		
<70 Years	12.0 (9.37–14.63)			
>70 Years	16.0 (11.11–20.89)			
Gender		0.807		
Male	15.0 (11.77–18.24)			
Female	12.0 (9.13–14.87)			
Aetiology		0.715		
HBV-related	12.0 (3.84–20.16)			
HCV-related	14.0 (10.35–17.65)			
Alcohol-related cirrhosis	15.0 (9.91–20.09)			
Other	8.0 (5.37–10.63)			
Grading		0.254		
G1	24.0 (12.04–35.96)			
G2	19.0 (12.11.25.90)			
G3	10.0 (2.70–17.30)			
Locoregional Treatment		0.360		
No	14.0 (6.43–21.57)			
Yes	14.0 (10.96–17.04)			
Type of locoregional Treatment		*0.037*	0.988	0.994
Surgery	10.0 (8.41–11.59)			
Interventional Radiology	17.0 (10.83–23.17)			
Type of interventional Radiology		0.716		
RFA	12.0 (2.61–21.39)			
TACE	16.0 (10.35–21.65)			
PEI	24.0 (11.53–36.47)			
CHILD Score (at time of Bone Metastasis)		*0.000*	*0.001*	*1.819*
A	16.0 (10.40–21.60)			
B	12.0 (9.32–14.68)			
C	7.0 (4.93–9.07)			
AFP (at diagnosis)		*0.040*	0.157	1.346
<43 ng\ml	17.0 (12.40–21.61)			
>43 ng/ml	12.0 (8.47–15.53)			
Bone Lesion Type		0.932		
Osteolytic	14.0 (11.27–16.73)			
Ostroblastic	16.0 (0.00–37.69)			
Mixed	14.0 (3.82–24.18)			

Abbreviations: CI, Confidence Interval; AFP, Alpha-fetoprotein; RFA, radiofrequency ablation; TACE, Transcatheter arterial chemoembolization; PEI, percutaneous ethanol injection.

with Child A was the largest (69.8%) patients, followed by the subgroup with Child B (22.0%) and Child C (8.2%) patients. The majority of patients (132/211; 62.6%) was treated with Sorafenib. The remaining baseline characteristics as grading, presence and type of locoregional treatment, presence of visceral metastases and the median value of AFP at diagnosis were summarized in Table 1.

Skeletal metastases

The ECOG PS at the moment of bone metastasis diagnosis was 0 for 51/194 patients (26.3%), 1 for 78/194 (40.2%), 2 for 50/194 (25.8%), 3 for 15/194 (7.7%) and unknown in 17 patients (8%). One hundred and sixty one patients (77.8%) developed bone metastasis after HCC diagnosis while 46 patients (22.2%) showed bone metastasis at the time of HCC diagnosis; 137 of 211 patients (64.9%) had multiple bone metastases and the remaining 74/211

Table 4. Predictive factors of survival after bone metastases diagnosis.

VARIABLES	MEDIAN TIME (MONTHS)	p VALUE (uni variate)	p VALUE (multivariate)	HAZARD RATIO (HR)
Age		0.349		
<70 Years	7.0 (5.83–8.18)			
>70 Years	6.0 (4.35–7.65)			
Gender		0.612		
Male	6.0 (5.07–6.93)			
Female	9.0 (7.33–10.67)			
Aetiology		*0.003*	*0.005*	*0.785*
HBV-related	4.0 (2.18–5.82)			
HCV-related	7.0 (5.61–8.39)			
Alcohol-related cirrhosis	9.0 (4.73–13.27)			
Other	8.0 (5.10–10.90)			
Grading		0.866		
G1	5.0 (3.38–6.62)			
G2	6.0 (3.74–8.26)			
G3	6.0 (4.04–7.96)			
Locoregional Treatment		0.104		
No	6.0 (4.93–7.07)			
Yes	7.0 (5.97–8.03)			
Type of locoregional Treatment		0.644		
Surgery	8.0 (6.23–9.77)			
Interventional Radiology	7.0 (5.72–8.28)			
Type of interventional Radiology		0.366		
RFA	7.0 (4.76–9.24)			
TACE	7.0 (5.25–8.76)			
PEI	7.0 (0.00–19.47)			
CHILD Score (at time of Bone Metastasis)		0.245		
A	6.0 (4.95–7.06)			
B	6.0 (3.93–8.07)			
C	9.0 (5.08–12.92)			
AFP (at diagnosis)		0.549		
<43 ng\ml	7.0 (5.22–8.78)			
>43 ng/ml	7.0 (5.93–8.07)			
Visceral Metastasis		0.615		
Yes	7.0 (4.14–9.86)			
No	7.0 (6.03–7.97)			
ECOG PS (at time of Bone Metastasis)		*0.002*	*0.002*	*1.341*
0	8.0 (5.28–10.72)			
1	8.0 (6.75–9.25)			
2	6.0 (4.85–7.15)			
3	4.0 (0.33–7.67)			
Bone Lesion Type		0.608		
Osteolytic	7.0 (6.05–7.95)			
Ostroblastic	9.0 (7.70–10.30)			
Mixed	7.0 (4.16–9.84)			
Bone metastasis - Spine		*0.006*	0.075	1.339
No	9.0 (7.34–10.66)			

Table 4. Cont.

VARIABLES	MEDIAN TIME (MONTHS)	p VALUE (uni variate)	p VALUE (multivariate)	HAZARD RATIO (HR)
Yes	6.0 (5.05–6.95)			
Bone Metastasis - Long Bones		0.806		
No	7.0 (6.11–7.89)			
Yes	6.0 (2.48–9.52)			
Bone Metastasis - Hip		0.428		
No	7.0 (5.95–8.05)			
Yes	6.0 (3.65–8.35)			
Bone Metastasis - Other		0.941		
No	7.0 (5.86–8.14)			
Yes	7.0 (5.60–8.40)			
First SRE Type		0.268		
Pathologica Fracture	7.0 (3.90–10.10)			
Hypercalcemia	9.0 (7.83–10–17)			
Spinal Cord Compression	4.0 (0.00–9.09)			
Surgery to Bone	9.0 (7.83–10.17)			
Radiation to Bone	8.0 (6.55–9.45)			
Biphosphonate Treatment		0.001	0.024	0.699
No	5.0 (3.58–6.42)			
Yes	8.0 (6.78–9.23)			

patients (35.1%) showed single lesion. Spine were the most common site of bone metastasis (126/211; 59.7%) followed by hip (74/211; 35.1%) and long bones (41/211; 19.4%) and are consistent with previous reports. Osteolytic lesions (169/205; 82.4%) were far more prevalent in this group than the mixed ones (20/205; 9.8%) and osteoblastic lesions (16/205; 7.8%). More than half of the patients (127/211; 60.1%) experienced at least one SRE while, two and three SREs have been reported in 18.9% (40/211) and 2.8% (6/211) of patients, respectively (Table 2). Considering only the first SRE, radiotherapy to bone is the most common (70/127 patients; 55.1%), followed by pathologic fracture (31/127; 24.4%), spinal cord compression (12/127; 9.4%), surgery to bone (7/127; 5.5%) and hypercalcemia (7/127; 5.5%) while for second and third SRE, radiotherapy to bone also had the greater incidence with 47.5% (19/40) and 66.6% (4/6) respectively. Equally, considering all the different SREs, radiotherapy to bone is the most common SRE (53.7% of all events), followed by pathologic fracture (20.8%), spinal cord compression (9.8%), surgery to bone (8%) and hypercalcemia (7.5%). Among the 211 patients with bone metastasis, 105/211 (49.7%) patients received therapy with bisphosphonate: 93 patients (88.5%) were treated with Zoledronic Acid, 6 patients (5.6%) with Pamidronate and 7 patients (6.6%) with other agents, respectively. No patient developed osteonecrosis of the jaw (ONJ) (Table 2).

Predictive factors of onset of bone metastasis

The median time to the onset of bone metastasis was 13 months (CI 95% 9.29–16.71 months). At univariate analysis (Table 3), the median time to the onset of skeletal disease was significantly shorter according to type of locoregional treatment (17 months for interventional radiology vs. 10 months for surgery; CI 95% 8.41–11.58 and 10.82–23.17, respectively; $p = 0.037$), Child Score ($p < 0.001$) and in patients with higher median AFP at diagnosis ($p = 0.040$). At multivariate analysis, only the Child Score was confirmed and independently correlated with a shorter time to diagnosis of bone metastases (Table 3) ($p = 0.001$; HR: 1.819).

Predictive factors of survival after bone metastases diagnosis

The median survival from the diagnosis of bone metastasis was 7 months (CI 95% 5.36–8.64 months). The univariate analysis, reported in Table 4, demonstrates that the median survival after diagnosis of bone metastases was significantly shorter according to HCC etiology (4 months for HBV, 7 months for HCV, 9 months for alcohol related and 8 months for other causes; CI 95% 2.18–5.81, 5.61–8.38, 4.73–13.26 and 5.10–10.89 months, respectively; $p = 0.003$), ECOG PS ($p = 0.002$), in patients with bone metastasis localized to spine ($p = 0.006$) and did not receive any bisphosphonate treatment ($p = 0.001$). Notably, at multivariate analysis (Table 4) all these parameters were confirmed and independently correlated with a shorter survival after bone disease occurrence ($p = 0.005$ with HR: 0.785 for etiology; $p = 0.002$ with HR: 1.341 for ECOG PS and $p = 0.024$ with HR: 0.669 for bisphosphonate treatment, respectively), excluding bone metastasis to spine ($p = 0.075$ with HR: 1.339).

Table 5. Predictive factors of survival after HCC diagnosis.

VARIABLES	MEDIAN TIME [MONTHS (95% C.I.)]	p VALUE (univariate)	p VALUE (multivariate)	HAZARD RATIO (HR)
Age		0.818		
<70 Years	18.0 (14.45–21.55)			
>70 Years	20.0 (16.77–23.23)			
Gender		0.589		
Male	19.0 (14.06–23.94)			
Female	19.0 (15.48–22.52)			
Aetiology		0.077		
HBV-related	15.0 (11.18–18.82)			
HCV-related	24.0 (20.49–27.51)			
Alcohol-related cirrhosis	16.0 (4.27–27.73)			
Other	13.0 (9.00–17.01)			
Grading		0.019	0.137	1.250
G1	27.0 (12.31–41.69)			
G2	26.0 (22.50–29.50)			
G3	12.0 (9.52–14.48)			
Locoregional Treatment		0.000	0.000	0.265
No	8.0 (4.43–11.57)			
Yes	24.0 (22.59–25.41)			
Type of locoregional Treatment		0.594		
Surgery	21.0 (16.36–25.64)			
Interventional Radiology	24.0 (21.94–26.06)			
Type of interventional Radiology		0.180		
RFA	26.0 (17.03–34.97)			
TACE	24.0 (20.62–27.38)			
PEI	29.0 (12.37–45.63)			
CHILD Score (at time of Bone Metastasis)		0.001	0.049	1.572
A	21.0 (15.75–26.25)			
B	18.0 (14.91–21.10)			
C	16.0 (14.06–17.95)			
AFP (at diagnosis)		0.419		
<43 ng\ml	18.0 (12.03–23.97)			
>43 ng/ml	19.0 (14.36–23.64)			
Visceral Metastasis		0.091		
Yes	24.0 (19.85–28.15)			
No	18.0 (15.29–20.71)			
Bone metastasis - Spine		0.018	0.001	2.281
No	21.0 (16.87–25.13)			
Yes	19.0 (15.26–22.74)			
Bone Metastasis - Long Bones		0.639		
No	19.0 (15.65–22.35)			
Yes	21.0 (9.59–32.41)			
Bone Metastasis - Hip		0.840		
No	23.0 (20.29–25.71)			
Yes	15.0 (11.87–18.13)			
Bone Metastasis - Other		0.718		
No	19.0 (15.21–22.79)			
Yes	19.0 (11.00–27.00)			

Table 5. Cont.

VARIABLES	MEDIAN TIME [MONTHS (95% C.I.)]	p VALUE (univariate)	p VALUE (multivariate)	HAZARD RATIO (HR)
First SRE Type		0.742		
Pathologica Fracture	21.0 (16.68–25.32)			
Hypercalcemia	19.0 (11.3–26.70)			
Spinal Cord Compression	24.0 (9.97–38.03)			
Surgery to Bone	18.0 (0.00–38.53)			
Radiation to Bone	18.0 (12.86–23.14)			
Biphosphonate Treatment		0.529		
No	18.0 (12.64–23.36)			
Yes	19.0 (16.35–21.65)			

Predictive factors of survival after HCC diagnosis

Considering all patients included in this study (N = 211) the median overall survival time from diagnosis of HCC was 19 months (CI 95%, 15.62–22.38) while the median survival from the start of Sorafenib was 9 months (CI 95%, 7.44–10.56 months) and median time to progression was 5 months (CI 95%: 3.70–6.30 months). The univariate analysis, reported in Table 5, demonstrates that the median overall survival was significantly correlated to Grading ($p = 0.019$), Child score at diagnosis ($p = 0.001$), presence of bone metastasis localized to spine ($p = 0.018$) and absence of any locoregional treatment ($p < 0.001$). At multivariate analysis, absence of locoregional treatment ($p < 0.001$; HR: 0.265), Child score at diagnosis ($p = 0.049$; HR: 1.572) and presence of bone metastasis to spine ($p = 0.001$; HR = 2.281) were confirmed and independently correlated with a shorter overall survival (Table 5).

Skeletal outcomes and SREs in the overall population

The median number of SREs experienced by patients was one (range 0–3). Median survival after development of the first SRE was 8 months (CI 95% 7.17–8.20 months). The univariate analysis, reported in Table 6, demonstrates that the median survival after development of the first SRE was significantly shorter according to the type of first SRE (2 months for spinal cord compression, 3 months for surgery to bone, 4 months for pathological fracture, 5 months for hypercalcemia and for radiation to bone; CI 95%: 0.32–3.67, 0.00–7.80, 2.24–5.75, 0.00–10.13 and 3.79–6.20 months respectively; $p = 0.024$) and in patients that did not receive any locoregional treatment ($p < 0.001$), bisphosphonate therapy ($p = 0.001$) and with presence of bone metastasis localized to spine ($p = 0.027$). At multivariate analysis, locoregional treatment and presence of bone metastasis localizated to spine were confirmed and independently correlated with a shorter survival after development of the first SRE ($p = 0.030$; HR: 4.709 and $p < 0.001$; HR: 12.280, respectively) (Table 6). The median time to first SRE after confirmed diagnosis of bone metastasis was 3 months (CI 95%, 2.27–3.73 months), indicative of the severity of bone metastasis in HCC. The median time to second SRE was 6 months and to third SRE was 9 months. At univariate analysis (Table 7), the median time to first SRE after confirmed diagnosis of bone metastasis was significantly shorter

according to Child Score ($p < 0.001$), ECOG PS ($p = 0.014$) and in patients with presence of bone metastasis localized to Spine ($p = 0.021$) and in other site excluding hip, long bones and the same spine ($p = 0.021$). At multivariate analysis, only bone metastasis localized in other site which are not spine, hip and long bones were confirmed and independently correlated with a shorter time to first SRE after confirmed diagnosis of bone metastasis ($p = 0.025$; HR: 0.570). All data described are reported in Table 7.

Skeletal outcomes and SREs according to time of bone metastases appearance

The entire population was divided in three subpopulations (synchronous bone metastases, metachronous bone metastases and patients with only bone metastases) and each subgroups was characterised for the following parameters: clinical, pathological and bone metastases characteristics, SREs and skeletal outcomes.

The three groups were homogeneous for age, gender, visceral metastases, type, site and number of bone lesions and type and number of SRE. Interestingly, median survival after bone metastases diagnosis resulted the same (7 months) in the three groups of patients, indicative of the poor prognosis strictly related to the presence of bone disease in HCC patients.

Discussion

Bone is an uncommon site of metastasis in HCC, with the incidence ranging from 3% to 20% [11–14]. Anyway bone involvement in patients with HCC is increased in the last decades probably due to the longer survival of HCC patients related to recent progresses made both in the diagnosis and treatment of the disease [14,15]. Some retrospective studies with a limited number of patients have described the characteristics of bone metastasis from HCC [11–16]. To our knowledge, this study is the recent largest multicentre survey investigating the natural history of metastatic bone disease in patients with HCC. Approximately less than one third presented bone metastasis at the time of initial HCC diagnosis, whereas the others developed bone metastasis during disease progression. Interestingly, median survival after

Table 6. Predictive factors of survival after the development of the first SRE.

VARIABLES	MEDIAN TIME [MONTHS- (95% C.I.)]	p VALUE (univariate)	p VALUE (multivariate)	HAZARD RATIO (HR)
Age		0.872		
<70 Years	2.0 (0.63–3.37)			
>70 Years	2.0 (0.34–3.66)			
SEX		0.799		
Male	1.0 (0.00–2.21)			
Female	3.0 (1.67–4.32)			
Aetiology		0.339		
HBV-related	0.0 (0.00–0.00)			
HCV-related	3.0 (1.51– (4.49)			
Alcohol-related cirrhosis	2.0 (0.93–3.07)			
Other	0.0 (0.00–0.00)			
Grading		0.847		
G1	3.0 (0.06–5.94)			
G2	2.0 (0.00–5.96)			
G3	1.0 (0.00–2.16)			
Locoregional Treatment		*0.000*	*0.030*	*0.575*
No	0.0 (0.00–0.00)			
Yes	3.0 (1.91–4.10)			
Type of locoregional Treatment		0.330		
Surgery	4.0 (2.90–5.10)			
Interventional Radiology	2.0 (0.51–3.50)			
Type of interventional Radiology		0.089		
RFA	3.0 (1.21–4.79)			
TACE	2.0 (2.32–5.80)			
PEI	1.0 (0.00–10.70)			
CHILD Score (at time of Bone Metastasis)		0.509		
A	1.0 (0.00–3.49)			
B	3.0 (2.26–3.74)			
C	4.0 (2.06–5.95)			
AFP (median value at diagnosis)		0.186		
<43 ng\ml	3.0 (1.80–4.20)			
>43 ng/ml	1.0 (0.70–3.10)			
Visceral Metastasis		0.119		
Yes	1.0 (0.00–1.94)			
No	2.0 (1.06–2.95)			
ECOG PS (at time of Bone Metastasis)		0.115		
0	1.0 (0.00–3.34)			
1	3.0 (1.65–4.35)			
2	2.0 (0.00–4.31)			
3	0.0 (0.00–0.00)			
Bone Lesion Type		0.362		
Osteolytic	2.0 (0.44–3.57)			
Ostroblastic	2.0 (0.88–3.12)			
Mixed	2.0 (0.00–4.11)			
Bone metastasis - Spine		*0.027*	*0.000*	*2.049*
No	3.0 (1.30–4.70)			
Yes	1.0 (0.00–2.00)			

Table 6. Cont.

VARIABLES	MEDIAN TIME [MONTHS- (95% C.I.)]	p VALUE (univariate)	p VALUE (multivariate)	HAZARD RATIO (HR)
Bone Metastasis - Long Bones		0.191		
No	1.0 (0.00–2.16)			
Yes	4.0 (2.73–5.27)			
Bone Metastasis - Hip		0.382		
No	2.0 (0.84–3.16)			
Yes	2.0 (0.00–4.19)			
Bone Metastasis - Other		0.154		
No	3.0 (2.19–3.81)			
Yes	0.0 (0.00–0.00)			
First SRE Type		0.024	0.239	0.935
Pathologica Fracture	4.0 (2.24–5.76)			
Hypercalcemia	5.0 (0.00–10.13)			
Spinal Cord Compression	2.0 (0.33–3.67)			
Surgery to Bone	3.0 (0.00–7.80)			
Radiation to Bone	5.0 (3.80–6.20)			
Biphosphonate Treatment		0.001	0.727	0.931
No	0.0 (0.00–0.00)			
Yes	4.0 (2.99–5.02)			

bone metastases diagnosis resulted the same in both groups (7 months). Moreover, these two populations of bone metastatic HCC patients did not show any significant difference in terms of clinical, pathological and bone metastases characteristics, SREs and skeletal outcomes. The lack of differences could be indicative of the poor prognosis associated with the presence of bone disease in HCC patients. Among all the clinical and pathological parameters predicting the appearance of metastasis, only the Child Score resulted independently correlated early bone progression. This is the first report that indicates the Child Score not only as a predictor of overall survival, but also of a greater tendency to bone metastatization and biological osteotropism of HCC. The most common site (spine) and type (osteolytic) of bone metastasis are consistent with previous smaller reports and were confirmed in this study [14,16]. Moreover, we found in the multivariate analysis that the localization of bone metastasis to spine is correlated with a shorter survival after development of first SRE and, in addition, a shorter overall survival from HCC diagnosis. This is quite different from the analysis of other bone metastasic hystotypes and from the previous reports in HCC [17]. Thus, we have found that the site of metastasis is correlated with survival, whereas the number of bone lesions do not.

Prospective data on the efficacy of bisphosphonates in bone metastatic HCC are lacking in literature [18]. This study revealed also that the bisphosphonate treatment impact on survival from the diagnosis of bone metastasis but, surprisingly, not on time to first SRE. It is possible that this result may be influeced by a selection bias exposed in the limitations of this study. Limitations of this study include its retrospective design and inclusion of an unselected heterogeneous cohort of patients with all types of aetiologic variants of HCC, liver function variants (Child score) as

well as only approximately more than half of patients have been treated with Sorafenib. However, the types of patients included in this study represent the typical scenario of a real clinical practice. Another limitation is the heterogeneity of standardized methods used for detecting bone metastases, with each methodology having its own limit of detection. In summary, the results presented in this multicenter survey represent a significant improvement in the understanding the natural history of skeletal disease in HCC patients. In particular, we showed that the presence of bone metastases should always be considered in patients with a worst Child Score, even in the absence of clear symptoms, due to associated greater biological osteotropism. Second, the site of bone metastasis but not the number of the lesions is an important prognostic factor of survival from first SRE and, surprisingly, of overall survival. With impact on clinical practice, our results showed also that the use of bisphosphonates has an impact on survival from the diagnosis of bone metastasis in this population and, even if the study was unpowered to demonstrate that, bisphosphonates therapy should be considered.

The major limitation of this study is the absence of the control group. In fact, this study was designed as a retrospective observational study, aimed to describe only the natural history of HCC patients with bone metastases.

Finally, we found a significantly longer median survival after bone metastases diagnosis (7 months) compared to previous reports [14,17]. This is extremely important since longer survival means augmented risk of SRE e subsequent worsening in quality of life (QOL).

Table 7. Predictive factors of onset of first SRE.

VARIABLES	MEDIAN TIME [MONTHS (95% C.I.)]	p VALUE (univariate)	p VALUE (multivariate)	HAZARD RATIO (HR)
Age		0.670		
<70 Years	8.0 (7.11–8.89)			
>70 Years	7.0 (5.33–8.67)			
Gender		0.403		
Male	8.0 (6.70–9.30)			
Female	8.0 (6.91–9.09)			
Aetiology		0.095		
HBV-related	8.0 (5.72–10.28)			
HCV-related	8.0 (7.11–8.89)			
Alcohol-related cirrhosis	7.0 (4.46–9.54)			
Other	11.0 (6.23–15.77)			
Grading		0.907		
G1	7.0 (4.29–9.71)			
G2	11.0 (4.78–17.22)			
G3	9.0 (6.85–11.15)			
Locoregional Treatment		0.239		
No	10.0 (5.61–14.39)			
Yes	7.0 (6.27–7.73)			
Type of locoregional Treatment		0.717		
Surgery	7.0 (5.63–8.37)			
Interventional Radiology	8.0 (7.19–8.81)			
Type of interventional Radiology		0.378		
RFA	8.0 (6.07–9.94)			
TACE	7.0 (6.10–7.90)			
PEI	14.0 (6.27–21.74)			
CHILD Score (At time of bone metastasis)		*0.000*	0.369	1.138
A	9.0 (6.24–11.76)			
B	8.0 (6.94–9.07)			
C	6.0 (4.96–7.04)			
AFP (median value atdiagnosis)		0.297		
<43 ng\ml	9.0 (6.78–11.22)			
>43 ng/ml	7.0 (6.37–7.63)			
Visceral Metastasis		0.073		
Yes	7.0 (6.24–7.76)			
No	12.0 (9.53–14.47)			
ECOG PS (at time of Bone Metastasis)		*0.014*	0.297	1.133
0	12.0 (9.24–14.76)			
1	8.0 (7.06–8.94)			
2	7.0 (5.75–8.26)			
3	7.0 (3.02–10.98)			
Bone Lesion Type		0.895		
Osteolytic	8.0 (7.04–8.96)			
Ostroblastic	9.0 (5.88–12.12)			
Mixed	8.0 (7.00–9.00)			
Bone metastasis - Spine		*0.021*	0.767	1.062
No	10.0 (7.93–12.07)			
Yes	7.0 (6.27–7.74)			
Bone Metastasis - Long Bones		0.422		
No	8.0 (7.11–8.89)			

Table 7. Cont.

VARIABLES	MEDIAN TIME [MONTHS (95% C.I.)]	p VALUE (univariate)	p VALUE (multivariate)	HAZARD RATIO (HR)
Yes	8.0 (5.74–10.26)			
Bone Metastasis - Hip		0.101		
No	7.0 (6.24–7.77)			
Yes	9.0 (6.21–11.79)			
Bone Metastasis - Other		*0.021*	*0.025*	*0.570*
No	7.0 (6.14–7.86)			
Yes	12.0 (8.38–15.62)			
Biphosphonate Treatment		0.578		
No	4.0 (1.38–6.62)			
Yes	7.0 (5.99–8.01)			
Sorafenib Treatment		0.650		
No	3.0 (0.00–7.83)			
Yes	6.0 (4.65–7.35)			

Author Contributions

Conceived and designed the experiments: DS FP NS. Performed the experiments: FR GGDC RA FMG MSC SB PB SM PM AR M. Scartozzi LF M. Santoni EM FS MT TI GM AG A. Comandone NF A. Conti II SP EG S. Cinieri S. Cascinu VC VOP GI MA CDG AT VL AEB. Analyzed the data: DS FP FR NS. Contributed reagents/materials/analysis tools: FR GGDC RA FMG MSC SB PB SM PM AR M. Scartozzi LF M. Santoni EM FS MT TI GM AG A. Comandone NF A. Conti II SP EG S. Cinieri VC VOP GI MA AT VL AEB. Contributed to the writing of the manuscript: DS NS.

References

1. El-Serag HB (2012) Epidemiology of viral hepatitis and hepatocellular carcinoma. Gastroenterology 142: 1264–1273.
2. Lin S, Hoffmann K, Schemmer P (2012) Treatment of hepatocellular carcinoma: a systematic review. Liver Cancer 1: 144–158.
3. Kanda M, Tateishi R, Yoshida H, Sato T, Masuzaki R, et al. (2008) Extrahepatic metastasis of hepatocellular carcinoma: incidence and risk factors. Liver Int 28: 1256–1263.
4. Si MS, Amersi F, Golish SR, Ortiz JA, Zaky J, et al. (2003) Prevalence of metastases in hepatocellular carcinoma: risk factors and impact on survival. Ann Surg 69: 879–885.
5. Cho HS, Oh JH, Han I, Kim HS (2009) Survival of patients with skeletal metastases from hepatocellular carcinoma after surgical management. J Bone Joint Surg 91: 1505–1512.
6. Uchino K, Tateishi R, Schiina S, Kanda M, Masuzaki R, et al. (2011) Hepatocellular carcinoma with extrahepatic disease: clinical features and prognostic factors. Cancer 117: 4475–4483.
7. Natsuizaka M, Omura T, Akaika T, Kuwata Y, Yamazaki K, et al. (2005) Clinical features of hepatocellular carcinoma with extrahepatic metastases. J Gastroenterol Hepatol 20: 1781–1787.
8. Longo V, Brunetti O, D'Oronzo S, Ostuni C, Gatti P, et al. (2013) Bone metastases in hepatocellular carcinoma: an emerging issue. Cancer Metastasis Rev [Epub ahead of print].
9. Seong J, Koom WS, Park HC (2005) Radiotherapy for painful bone metastases from hepatocellular carcinoma. Liver Int 25: 261–265.
10. Du J, Qian X, Liu B (2013) Long-term progression-free survival in a case of hepatocellular carcinoma with vertebral metastasis treated with a reduced dose of sorafenib: case report and review of the literature. Oncol Letters 5: 381–385.
11. The Liver Cancer Study Group of Japan (1987) Primary liver cancer in Japan: Sixth report. Cancer 60: 1400–1411.
12. Okazaki N, Yoshino M, Yoshida T, Hirohashi S, Kishi K, et al. (1985) Bone metastasis in hepatocellular carcinoma. Cancer 55: 1991–1994.
13. Lee YT, Geer DA (1987) Primary liver cancer: pattern of metastasis. J Surg Oncol 36: 26–31.
14. Fukutomi M, Yokota M, Chuman H, Harada H, Zaitsu Y, et al. (2001) Increased incidence of bone metastasis in hepatocellular carcinoma. Eur J Gastroenterol Hepatol 13: 1083–1088.
15. Ahmad Z, Nisa AU, Uddin Z, Azad NS (2007) Unusual metastases of hepatocellular carcinoma (HCC) to bone and soft tissues of lower limb. J Coll Physicians Surg Pak 17: 222–223.
16. Kim S, Chun M, Wang H, Cho S, Oh YT, et al. (2007) Bone Metastasis from Primary Hepatocellular Carcinoma: Characteristics of Soft Tissue Formation. Cancer Res Treat 39: 104–108.
17. Cho HS, Oh JH, Han I, Kim HS (2009) Survival of patients with skeletal metastases from hepatocellular carcinoma after surgical management. J Bone Joint Surg Br 91: 1505–1512.
18. Montella L, Addeo R, Palmieri G, Caraglia M, Cennamo G, et al. (2010) Zoledronic acid in the treatment of bone metastases by hepatocellular carcinoma: a case series. Cancer Chemother Pharmacol 65: 1137–1143.

12

Risk of Primary Liver Cancer Associated with Gallstones and Cholecystectomy

Yanqiong Liu, Yu He, Taijie Li, Li Xie, Jian Wang, Xue Qin, Shan Li*

Department of Clinical Laboratory, First Affiliated Hospital of Guangxi Medical University, Nanning, Guangxi Zhuang Autonomous Region, China

Abstract

Background: Recent epidemiological evidence points to an association between gallstones or cholecystectomy and the incidence risk of liver cancer, but the results are inconsistent. We present a meta-analysis of observational studies to explore this association.

Methods: We identified studies by a literature search of PubMed, EMBASE, Cochrane Central Register of Controlled Trials, and relevant conference proceedings up to March 2014. A random-effects model was used to generate pooled multivariable adjusted odds ratios (ORs) and 95% confidence intervals (CIs). Between-study heterogeneity was assessed using Cochran's Q statistic and the I^2.

Results: Fifteen studies (five case-control and 10 cohort studies) were included in this analysis. There were 4,487,662 subjects in total, 17,945 diagnoses of liver cancer, 328,420 exposed to gallstones, and 884,507 exposed to cholecystectomy. Pooled results indicated a significant increased risk of liver cancer in patients with a history of gallstones (OR = 2.54; 95% CI, 1.71–3.79; $n = 11$ studies), as well as cholecystectomy (OR = 1.62; 95% CI, 1.29–2.02; $n = 12$ studies), but there was considerable heterogeneity among these studies. The effects estimates did not vary markedly when stratified by gender, study design, study region, and study quality. The multivariate meta-regression analysis suggested that study region and study quality appeared to explain the heterogeneity observed in the cholecystectomy analysis.

Conclusions: Our results suggest that individuals with a history of gallstones and cholecystectomy may have an increased risk of liver cancer.

Editor: Balraj Mittal, Sanjay Gandhi Medical Institute, India

Funding: The authors have no support or funding to report.

Competing Interests: The authors have declared that no competing interests exist.

* Email: lis8858@126.com

Introduction

Primary liver cancer mainly includes hepatocellular carcinoma (HCC), which originates in liver cells, and intrahepatic cholangiocarcinoma (ICC), which arises from the intrahepatic bile duct [1]. The worldwide burden of primary liver cancer for 2012 was estimated at 782,000 new cancer cases [2]. It ranks as the fifth most common incident cancer in men and the ninth in women [2]. Owing to its poor prognosis, it is the second commonest cause of death from cancer worldwide [2]. The above data highlight the importance of a better understanding of risk factors related to liver cancer development. However, the etiology of this disease remains largely elusive, apart from known relationships with hepatitis B or C virus infection, alcohol, aflatoxins, liver cirrhosis, and diabetes [3,4].

It has been hypothesized that gallstones (i.e., cholelithiasis) and cholecystectomy are associated with an increased risk of several cancers, especially the risk of rectal cancer [5], pancreatic cancer [6], and colorectal cancer [7,8]. Gallstones are known to induce biliary inflammation, and cholecystectomy is typically followed by dilation of the common bile ducts and elevated bile duct pressure, which also results in chronic inflammation [9]. The link between chronic inflammation and cancer is well established [10]. It has also been proposed that gallstones and cholecystectomy result in the accumulation of bile and secondary bile acids, in particular, deoxycholic acid [11–15], and that bile acids can act as carcinogens [16].

Several epidemiological studies have investigated the association between gallstones, cholecystectomy, and liver cancer [17–31]. However, the existing results are controversial. Most studies have reported a positive relationship between gallstones and liver cancer [17–19,21,22,24,26,27,29,30], but one failed to demonstrate a significant association [23]. With regard to cholecystectomy, several studies suggested a significant increased risk of liver cancer [18,20,24,25,27,28,31], whereas others demonstrated a nonsignificant adverse effect [17,19,21,26,29].

No meta-analysis has previously been published on the relationship between gallstones or cholecystectomy and the incidence risk of liver cancer. The aim of this detailed meta-analysis was to summarize the association between cholecystectomy, gallstones, and the risk of developing liver cancer in observational studies. A better understanding of these relationships may highlight the need to consider additional intervention methods in this area.

Methods

This study complies with the guidelines of the PRISMA (Preferred Reporting Items for Systematic Reviews and Meta-Analyses) checklist and flow diagram [32] (Checklist S1).

Data sources and search strategy

We searched PubMed, EMBASE, and Cochrane Central Register of Controlled Trials (CENTRAL) in the Cochrane Library for all relevant articles on the risk of liver cancer in patients with history of gallstones or cholecystectomy. The search was performed in each database from time of inception until March 12, 2014 by two independent investigators (Y.L. and S.L.). Medical subject heading terms and keywords used in the search included "cholecystectomy", "gallbladder surgery", "gallstones", "gallstone", "cholelithiasis", "cholecystolithiasis", "choledocholithiasis" combined with "HCC", "hepatocellular carcinoma", "liver cancer", "liver tumors", "liver neoplasms", "hepatic carcinoma". No language restrictions were imposed. We also reviewed the abstracts submitted to major gastroenterology and hepatology conferences (annual meeting of the *American College of Gastroenterology, American Association for the Study of Liver Diseases, Digestive Diseases Week; World Congress of the International Hepato-Pancreato-Biliary Association*) between 2009 and 2013. The reference lists in all identified articles were checked for further relevant articles.

Eligibility criteria and study selection

Studies considered in this meta-analysis met all the following inclusion criteria: (1) cohort or case-control; (2) focus of the study was a history of gallstones or cholecystectomy; (3) end point was liver cancer incidence; (4) provided multivariate-adjusted relative risks, with corresponding 95% confidence intervals (CIs) for events associated with gallstones or cholecystectomy vs. controls, at least adjusted for three of eight factors (hepatitis B or C virus infection, smoking, alcohol, cirrhosis, diabetes, body mass index, age, gender). Primary exclusion criteria were cross-sectional studies, literature reviews, commentaries, editorials, and case reports. Studies were also excluded where adjusted relative risks and/or CIs had not been provided, or they did not fulfill the inclusion criteria. When there were multiple studies of the same population, only data from the most recent comprehensive report was included. Two authors (Y.L. and Y.H.) independently evaluated all records by title and abstract and subsequently retrieved and assessed, in detail, the full text of any potentially relevant articles using the above eligibility criteria. Disagreements regarding eligibility were resolved through discussion and by referencing the original report.

Data abstraction and quality assessment

Data were independently abstracted onto a standardized form by two investigators (T.L. and L.X.). Disagreements were resolved through consensus, referring back to the original article. The following data were collected from each study: first author's name, year of publication, country of the population studied, mean age, study duration, number of patients with gallstones or cholecystectomy studied, number of incident cases of liver cancer, adjustment factors, and multivariable adjusted relative risk estimates and their 95% CIs (relative risk [RR] for cohort studies, odds ratios [OR] for case-control studies, or standardized incidence rates [SIR] for

studies comparing the rates of observed to expected cases). Because the liver cancer incidence is low ($\leq 10\%$) and the estimated effects are small, odds ratios (ORs) can be considered close approximations of risk ratios [33].

The methodological quality of the case-control and cohort studies was initially assessed independently by two authors using the Newcastle-Ottawa scale (NOS) [34] (X.Q. and S.L.). Disagreements were resolved through discussion with an additional adjudicator (J.W.) who was completely blinded to the study until a consensus was reached. Observational studies were scored across three categories and allocated a maximum of 9 points: selection (up to 4 points), comparability (up to 2 points), and outcome (up to 3 points). The overall study quality was arbitrarily defined as poor (score 0–3), fair (score 4–6), or good (score 7–9).

Outcomes assessed

The primary analysis focused on assessing the risk of liver cancer in patients with a history of gallstones, and risk of liver cancer in patients with a history of cholecystectomy. Additionally, based on information available from individual studies, we assessed sex-specific differences in risk estimates.

Data synthesis and statistical analysis

We used the random-effects model described by DerSimonian and Laird [35] to calculate summary ORs and 95% CIs. Heterogeneity was first tested by Cochran's Q test, and a P-value <0.10 was considered suggestive of significant heterogeneity [36]. To estimate the proportion of total variation across the studies that was due to study-related factors rather than chance, the I^2 statistic was calculated [37]. An I^2 less than 30% was considered as low, 30%–60% as moderate, 60%–75% as substantial, and more than 75% as considerable [38].

To explore sources of heterogeneity between the combined studies, we performed subgroup analyses based on study design (case-control vs. cohort), study location (Asian, Europe, and the U.S.), and study quality (good vs. fair, and poor). In addition, a restricted maximum likelihood-based random-effects meta-regression analysis was performed to assess heterogeneity associated with the aforementioned factors [39].

Sensitivity analyses were conducted to assess the robustness of the results by sequential omission of individual studies [40]. Publication bias was assessed graphically using a funnel plot and quantitatively using Egger's regression asymmetry tests [41]. A 2-tailed P-value less than 0.05 was considered statistically significant for all analyses except for the Cochran's Q test. All analyses were performed using STATA, version 12.0 (StataCorp, College Station, TX, USA).

Results

Study selection, study characteristics, and quality

Fig. 1 summarizes the process of study identification, exclusion, and inclusion. Table S1 shows the list of excluded studies from the full text studies review. At least 15 studies fulfilled all inclusion criteria and were included in the meta-analysis [17–31]. Fourteen articles were published in full [17,18,20–31], and one was in abstract form [19]. There were five case control studies [18,22,23,26,27] and 10 cohort studies [17,19–21,24,25,28–31]. Individual study characteristics are outlined in Table 1. Included articles were published in the period 1993–2014. There was a total study population of 4,487,662 individuals, 17,945 of whom had been diagnosed with liver cancer, with 328,420 exposed to gallstones and 884,507 exposed to cholecystectomy. The majority of the studies ($n = 8$) were conducted in European populations

[23–26,28–31]. Three studies were performed in a North American population [18,19,27], and four studies were conducted in an Asian population [17,20–22]. Thirteen studies were population based [17–22,24–27,29–31], and two were hospital based [23,28]. Of the included studies, 11 reported an association between gallstones and the risk of liver cancer [17–19,21–24,26,27,29,30]. Twelve studies reported an association between cholecystectomy and the risk of liver cancer [17–21,24–29,31].

Table 1 summarizes the methodological quality of all studies, and additional data are given in Table S2. According to the Newcastle-Ottawa scale, most studies were fair (scale of 4–6) to good (scale of 7–9) quality, except the abstract identified from the conference proceedings [19].

Risk of gallstones in the incidence of liver cancer

Eleven studies [17–19,21–24,26,27,29,30] reported 7,453 liver cancer events in 328,420 patients with gallstones. The multivariate-adjusted ORs for incident liver cancer with gallstones vs. controls for each study and all studies combined are presented in Fig. 2. The liver cancer incidence was increased in patients with gallstones, with an OR of 2.54 (95% CI, 1.71–3.79) but with considerable heterogeneity ($I^2 = 97.8\%$; $P<0.001$).

Some studies [17,22,24] provided separate estimates of the OR for liver cancer in male and female gallstone patients. An increased risk of liver cancer in patients with gallstones was seen in females (three studies; adjusted OR, 3.29; 95% CI, 1.02–10.62), as well as in males (three studies; adjusted OR, 2.84; 95% CI, 1.44–5.61), with significant evidence of heterogeneity in both subsets (Table 2).

We then conducted further subgroup meta-analysis according to study design, study location, and study quality (Table 2). No substantial differences in the summary ORs were found between case-control and cohort studies, good and fair/poor quality studies, as well as studies conducted in Asia and Western country. All of these analyses were with considerable heterogeneity.

We also conducted a meta-regression analysis to investigate the impact of heterogeneous factors on the OR estimates. The study design, study location, and study quality were chosen as the potential heterogeneous factors. In multivariate meta-regression analysis, none of these factors were significant ($P = 0.200$ for study design; $P = 0.892$ for study location; $P = 0.905$ for study quality). The meta-regression analysis indicated that study design, study location, and study quality might not be major sources contributing to the heterogeneity presented in the overall analyses.

We observed no evidence of overly influential studies in sensitivity analyses based on repeatedly computing the pooled ORs, omitting one study at a time. The pooled ORs ranged from 2.13 (1.68–2.70) when the study by Welzel et al. [27] was excluded, to 2.75 (1.81–4.16) when the study by Tavani et al. [23] was excluded.

In the publication bias assessment, the inverted funnel plot appeared to be symmetric (Fig. 3A). The P value for the Egger test was 0.847, suggesting a very low probability of publication bias.

Risk of cholecystectomy in the incidence of liver cancer

Twelve eligible studies [17–21,24–29,31] were included in the analysis of the potential role of cholecystectomy in the risk of liver cancer. These included 884,507 patients with a history of cholecystectomy and 3,687 liver cancer outcome events. Meta-analysis of these 12 studies showed that compared to individuals without a history of cholecystectomy, those who had their gallbladder removed had a 62% greater risk of liver cancer (OR = 1.62, 95% CI, 1.29–2.02), with considerable heterogeneity among studies; test for heterogeneity ($P<0.001$, $I^2 = 91.0\%$) (Fig. 4).

Four studies reported sex-specific risk estimates of liver cancer [17,20,24,25]. No difference was observed in the risk of liver cancer between males (OR = 1.70; 95% CI, 1.05–2.75) and females (OR = 1.68; 95% CI, 1.00–2.82) with a history of cholecystectomy. There was considerable heterogeneity observed in both analyses (Table 2).

When stratifying the data into subgroups based on study design, study location and study quality (Table 2), we found a significant association between cholecystectomy and risk of liver cancer

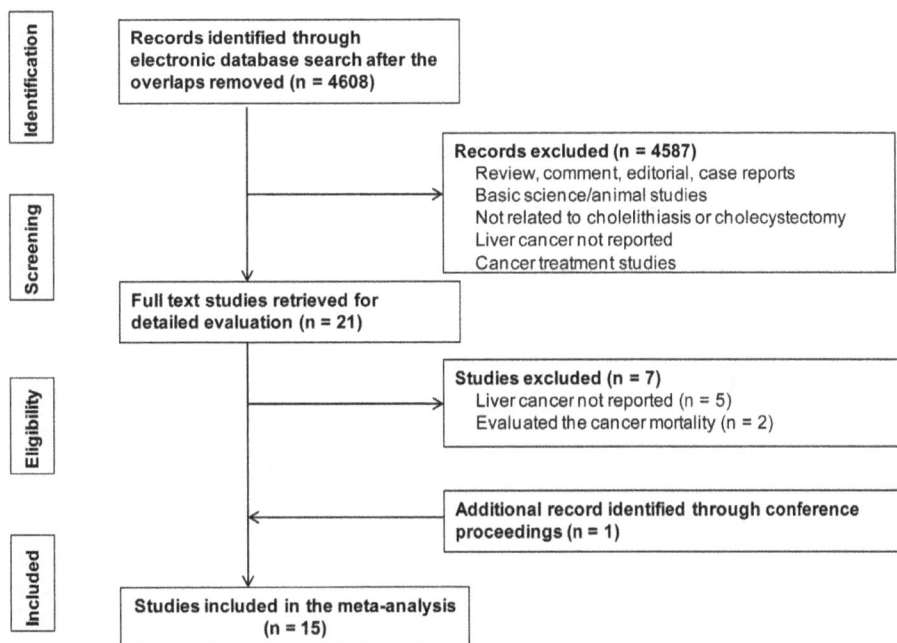

Figure 1. Flow chart depicts the selection of eligible studies.

Table 1. Characteristics of included studies on the association of gallstones, cholecystectomy and risk of liver cancer.

Study	Year	Country	Study design	Setting	Average age, years	Period of observation	Exposure	Number of Exposure	Total LC cases	All subjects Total	Adjustment factors	QS
Vogtmann et al. [17]												
SWHS cohort#	2014	China	Cohort	PB	54.2	2000–2010	Gallstones	8161	160	73209	1–12	7
							Cholecystectomy	3151				
SMHS cohort$	2014	China	Cohort	PB	57.4	2002–2010	Gallstones	4614	252	61337	1–11	7
							Cholecystectomy	1684				
Nogueira, et al. [18]	2014	US	Case control	PB	76.5	1992–2005	Gallstones	15097	10219	1,238,390	7, 13	6
							Cholecystectomy	9109				
Nogueira, et al. [19]	2013	US	Cohort	PB	NR	NR	Gallstones	30,674	414	487,207	1, 2, 4, 5, 9, 10, 14–16	2
							Cholecystectomy	25,457				
Kao, et al. [20]	2013	China	Cohort	PB	66.0	1996–2008	Cholecystectomy	2590	67	1,002,590	1, 14	7
Chen, et al. [21]	2013	China	Cohort	PB	55.0	2000–2010	Gallstones	15545	791	77,725	1, 7, 12, 14, 17–20	7
							Cholecystectomy	5850				
Chang, et al. [22]	2013	China	Case control	PB	NR	2004–2008	Gallstones	1484	2978	14890	1, 7, 8, 14, 18, 19, 20	8
Tavani, et al. [23]	2012	Italy and Switzerland	Case control	HB	60	1982–2009	Gallstones	206	684	2640	1, 2–5, 14, 21–25	6
Nordenstedt, et al. [24]	2012	Sweden	Cohort	PB	59.9	1965–2008	Gallstones	192,960	170	538211	1, 13, 14	6
							Cholecystectomy	345,251				
Lagergren, et al. [25]	2011	Sweden	Cohort	PB	52.0	1965–2008	cholecystectomy	345,251	333	345,251	1, 13, 14	6
Welzel, et al. [26]	2007	Denmark	Case control	PB	NR	1978–1991	Gallstones	35	764	3820	1, 14, 21	7
							Cholecystectomy	25				
Welzel, et al. [27]	2007	US	Case control	PB	79.0	1993–1999	Gallstones	4445	535	103317	1, 14, 15, 26, 27	6
							Cholecystectomy	1690				
Goldacre, et al. [28]	2005	UK	Cohort	HB	15–84	1963–1999	Cholecystectomy	39,254	344	374067	1, 13, 14, 26	6
Chow, et al. [29]	1999	Denmark	Cohort	PB	61.0	1977–1993	Gallstones	17715	82	60176	1, 13, 14	5
							Cholecystectomy	42461				
Johansen, et al. [30]	1996	Denmark	Cohort	PB	60.0	1977–1992	Gallstones	42,098	56	42,098	1, 13, 14	5
Ekbom, et al. [31]	1993	Sweden	Cohort	PB	NR	1965–1987	Cholecystectomy	62,734	96	62,734	1, 13, 14	5

Abbreviations: PB, population based; HB, hospital based; LC, liver cancer; CI, confidence interval; QS: quality score; NR, not report.

#Shanghai Women'sHealth Study (SWHS) (1996–2010).

$Shanghai Men's Health Study (SMHS) (2002–2010).

Adjustment factors: 1 age, 2 BMI, 3 education, 4 smoking status, 5 alcohol consumption, 6 family history of liver cancer, 7 history of diabetes, 8 history of hepatitis/chronic liver disease, 9 physical activity, 10 total energy intake, 11, income, 12 menopausal status, 13 calendar years, 14 gender, 15 race, 16 non-steroidal anti-inflammatory drugs intake, 17 perlipidemia, 18 hepatitis B virus infection, 19 hepatitis C virus infection, 20 cirrhosis, 21 time of diagnosis, 22, chronic pancreatitis, 23 study center, 24 year of interview, 25 study period, 26 geographic region, 27, state buy-in status.

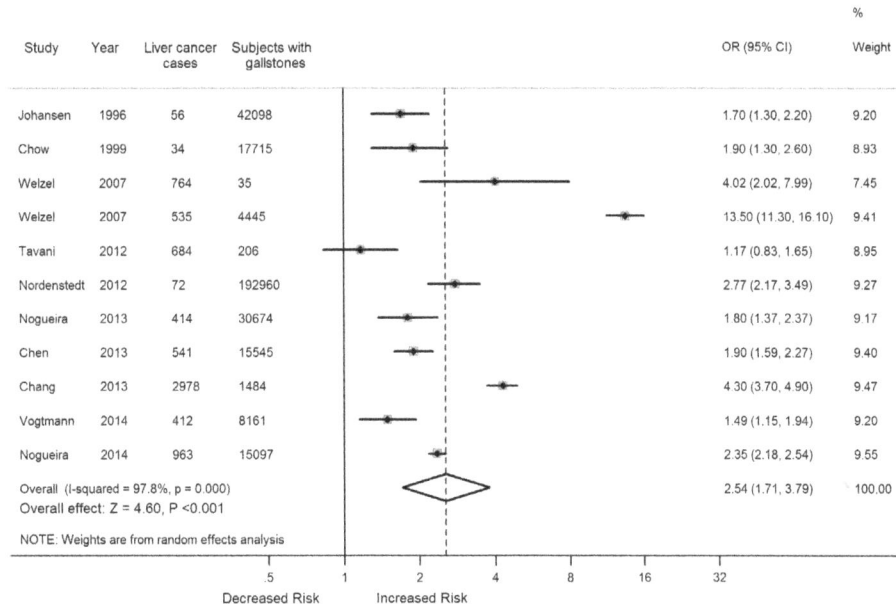

Figure 2. Forest plot of the association between gallstones and risk of liver cancer.

among cohort studies (OR = 1.47) and studies conducted in Europe (OR = 1.30). On restricting analysis to high-quality studies (≥7 scores), we observed a similar association between cholecystectomy and risk of liver cancer (OR = 1.29; 95% CI, 1.21–1.37). However, a non-significant increased risk of liver cancer in patient with cholecystectomy was observed in case-control studies (OR = 2.23; 95% CI, 0.73–6.79), studies conducted in America (OR = 2.14; 95% CI, 0.78–5.88) and in Asia (OR = 1.76; 95% CI, 0.86–3.57).

We then conducted a meta-regression analysis to investigate the impact of study design, study location, and study quality on the estimated ORs. In multivariate meta-regression analysis, study region and study quality were significant factors ($P = 0.039$ and $P = 0.008$, respectively), with these two variables explaining most between-study variability.

In sensitivity analyses, the pooled OR remained significantly increased when studies were excluded one at a time, with the pooled OR ranging from 1.44 (1.22–1.70) when the study by Welzel et al. [26] was excluded, to 1.67 (1.31–2.12) when the study by Chen et al. [21] was excluded.

The shape of the funnel plots for studies on the association between cholecystectomy and liver cancer risk seemed somewhat asymmetrical. However, the P-value of Egger's regression test ($P = 0.581$) was more than 0.05, indicating no statistical evidence of publication bias (Fig. 3B).

Discussion

To the best of our knowledge, this is the first comprehensive meta-analysis of observational studies to investigate the risk of liver cancer in gallstone patients and cholecystectomy patients. The results of the present meta-analysis of 15 studies point to significant evidence for an increased risk of liver cancer among gallstone patients as compared to those without gallstones (OR = 2.54). In the current study, cholecystectomy was associated with a 62% excess risk of liver cancer. The association persisted across a broad range of sensitivity analyses. Further, the significant association was observed in both women and men. However, there was considerable heterogeneity among most analyses.

There is a long-standing debate about the risk of cancer in patients who have gallstones and undergo cholecystectomy. Several review studies have discussed the potential risk of gallstones or cholecystectomy in various tumors, such as colorectal [42] and colonic adenomas [43], and in several types of cancer, such as colorectal [5,7,8], pancreatic [6], esophageal, and gastric [44]. In 1993, Giovannucci et al. found a 34% increased risk of colorectal cancer following cholecystectomy based on combined results from 33 case-control studies [8]. In addition, an analysis by Lin et al. of 18 studies found that cholecystectomy was associated with a 23% excess risk of pancreatic cancer [6]. In contrast, other studies found no effect of cholecystectomy on the risk of colorectal adenoma [42], esophageal and gastric cancer [44], rectal cancer [7] and colonic adenoma [43]. However, Chiong et al. reported a statistically significant risk of rectal cancer (OR = 1.33) [5] and colonic adenoma (OR = 2.26) [43] if gallstones were present. To date, several epidemiological studies have investigated the relationship between gallstones, cholecystectomy, and the risk of liver cancer, but no definitive conclusions have been drawn. The results of our comprehensive meta-analysis of 15 studies, which included 4,487,662 participants and 17,945 liver cancer cases, suggest that gallstones and cholecystectomy might be important contributors to the risk of liver cancer. An understanding of the clinicopathological development of liver cancer is essential for effective screening.

The pathophysiology of tumorigenesis associated with gallstones and after cholecystectomy has yet to be elucidated. One potential mechanism may involve chronic inflammation. Gallstones may induce biliary inflammation, and cholecystectomy is typically followed by dilation of the common bile ducts and elevated bile duct pressure [9], both of which might cause chronic inflammation. The link between chronic inflammation and cancer is well established. In the microenvironment, chronic inflammation can stimulate the release of cytokines, chemokines, growth factors, reactive oxygen species, and reactive nitrogen intermediates, all of which are important constituents of the local environment of tumors [10]. Inflammatory responses also play decisive roles in the cancer development, including initiation, promotion, invasion,

Table 2. Subgroup analysis of odds ratios for the association between gallstones, cholecystectomy and the risk of liver cancer.

Study characteristics	No. of studies	Odds ratios (95% CI)	P_{OR} value	Heterogeneity	
				I^2 (%)	P value
Gallstones	11	2.54 (1.71, 3.79)	<0.001	97.8	<0.001
Study Design					
Case-control studies	5	3.66 (1.75, 7.64)	0.001	98.8	<0.001
Cohort studies	6	1.90 (1.60, 2.25)	<0.001	63.8	0.017
Study Location					
Studies in America	3	3.86 (1.15, 12.91)	0.029	99.4	<0.001
Studies in Europe	5	2.02 (1.42, 2.86)	<0.001	81.9	<0.001
Studies in Asia	3	2.31 (1.19, 4.50)	0.013	97.4	<0.001
studies quality					
Good (≥7 scores)	4	2.58 (1.44, 4.62)	0.001	96.1	<0.001
Fair and poor (<7 scores)	7	2.51 (1.37, 4.60)	0.003	98.4	<0.001
Gender					
Males	3	2.84 (1.44, 5.61)	0.003	93.8	<0.001
Females	3	3.29 (1.02, 10.62)	0.046	97.9	<0.001
Cholecystectomy	12	1.62 (1.29, 2.02)	<0.001	91.0	<0.001
Study Design					
Case-control studies	3	2.23 (0.73, 6.79)	0.159	97.0	<0.001
Cohort studies	9	1.47 (1.19, 1.81)	<0.001	85.0	<0.001
Study Location					
Studies in America	3	2.14 (0.78, 5.88)	0.140	97.0	<0.001
Studies in Europe	6	1.30 (1.20, 1.41)	<0.001	0.0	0.794
Studies in Asia	3	1.76 (0.86, 3.57)	0.120	94.2	<0.001
studies quality					
Good (≥7 scores)	4	1.29 (1.21, 1.37)	0.019	95.4	<0.001
Fair and poor (<7 scores)	8	2.32 (1.15, 4.69)	<0.001	0.0	0.911
Gender					
Males	4	1.70 (1.05, 2.75)	0.031	90.4	<0.001
Females	4	1.68 (1.00, 2.82)	0.049	91.9	<0.001

and metastasis [45]. Conversely, tumor-related inflammation contributes to further production of reactive oxygen species, reactive nitrogen intermediates, and cytokines [10]. Another hypothesis for the pathophysiology of tumorigenesis associated with gallstones is that removal of the gallbladder results in the accumulation of bile, and secondary bile acids, in particular deoxycholic acid [11–13], with the bile acids acting as carcinogens

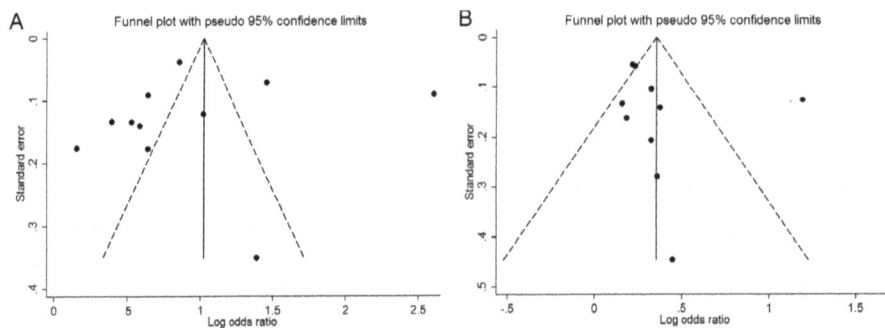

Figure 3. Funnel plot analysis to detect publication bias. A Funnel plot for studies evaluating the association between gallstones and liver cancer risk; B Funnel plot for studies evaluating the association between cholecystectomy and liver cancer risk.

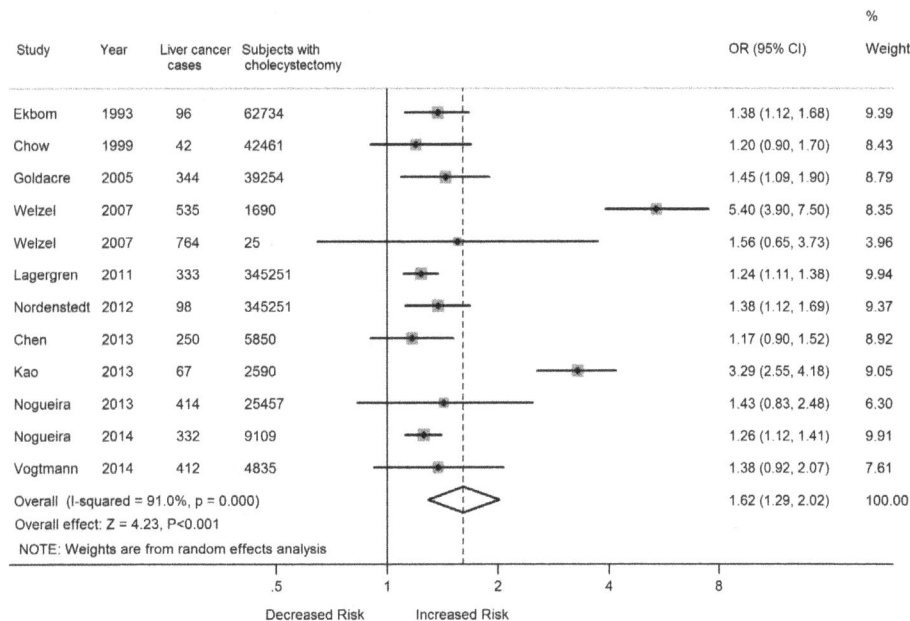

Study	Year	Liver cancer cases	Subjects with cholecystectomy	OR (95% CI)	% Weight
Ekbom	1993	96	62734	1.38 (1.12, 1.68)	9.39
Chow	1999	42	42461	1.20 (0.90, 1.70)	8.43
Goldacre	2005	344	39254	1.45 (1.09, 1.90)	8.79
Welzel	2007	535	1690	5.40 (3.90, 7.50)	8.35
Welzel	2007	764	25	1.56 (0.65, 3.73)	3.96
Lagergren	2011	333	345251	1.24 (1.11, 1.38)	9.94
Nordenstedt	2012	98	345251	1.38 (1.12, 1.69)	9.37
Chen	2013	250	5850	1.17 (0.90, 1.52)	8.92
Kao	2013	67	2590	3.29 (2.55, 4.18)	9.05
Nogueira	2013	414	25457	1.43 (0.83, 2.48)	6.30
Nogueira	2014	332	9109	1.26 (1.12, 1.41)	9.91
Vogtmann	2014	412	4835	1.38 (0.92, 2.07)	7.61
Overall (I-squared = 91.0%, p = 0.000)				1.62 (1.29, 2.02)	100.00
Overall effect: Z = 4.23, P<0.001					
NOTE: Weights are from random effects analysis					

Decreased Risk   Increased Risk

Figure 4. Forest plot of the association between cholecystectomy and risk of liver cancer.

[16]. Gallstones are thought to block the flow of bile through the cystic duct.

Heterogeneity is a potential problem when interpreting the results of all meta-analyses, and finding the sources of heterogeneity is one of the most important goals of any meta-analysis [46]. In our meta-analysis, considerable heterogeneity was observed in most of the analyses. To investigate the sources of heterogeneity, we performed subgroup and meta-regression analyses. In the gallstone studies, despite stratifying the data into subgroups based on study design, study location, study quality, and gender, significant heterogeneity was still detected. The multivariate meta-regression analysis also suggested that none of these variables could explain the heterogeneity observed in the overall analysis. With respect to cholecystectomy, subgroup analyses by study design, study location, and study quality indicated that heterogeneity still existed in the case-control studies, cohort studies, U.S. studies, Asian studies, and high-quality score studies. There was little evidence of heterogeneity in the subgroup analyses of studies in Europe $(P = 0.794, I^2 = 0.0\%)$ and low-quality studies $(P = 0.911, I^2 = 0.0\%)$. To further investigate the heterogeneity, multivariate meta-regression analyses were performed. Meta-regression analysis of the data showed that the study region and study quality might substantially influence the initial heterogeneity. When these two parameters were considered together, the results indicated that the U.S. and Asian studies might be a major source of the heterogeneity in the cholecystectomy data.

The presence of heterogeneity in study design, population characteristics, sample size, information collection methods (e.g., questionnaires or medical records), definition of exposure, assessment of outcome, period of observation, and duration of study follow-up is not surprising. For example, in the 15 studies included in the present meta-analysis, the period of observation was from 1963 to 2010. The older studies [23,25,28–30] did not seem to be adequately powered to detect a significant difference in liver cancer incidence following gallstones and cholecystectomy, with a low risk ratio reported in these studies. The period of observation of these studies was up to 36 years (from 1963 to 1999). As the most important etiology of primary liver cancer is

hepatitis B or C virus infection, we suspect that the low risk ratio may be due to the exclusion of hepatitis C virus infection in the older studies. We suspect that the low risk ratio may be due to without exclusion of hepatitis C virus infection. Thus, pooled effect estimates based on heterogeneous data should be interpreted with caution.

Our study has several strengths. First, our meta-analysis included 15 studies, involving 4,487,662 participants and 17,945 liver cancer cases. The large sample size afforded increased statistical power. We were also able to carry out multiple subgroup analyses and evaluate heterogeneity and the presence of publication bias. Moreover, the present meta-analysis included an approved quality evaluation system. Thus, it minimized potential bias. Further, the likelihood of important selection or publication bias in our meta-analysis is small.

However, several limitations should be acknowledged when interpreting our findings. First, there was significant evidence of considerable heterogeneity among almost all the analyses, despite stratifying the data into subgroups based on several variables. Second, all studies included in our analysis were observational studies, which have inherent limitations. Therefore, confounding factors and bias might have distorted the results [47]. In particular, in the case-control studies, we cannot rule out the possibility of recall bias. Third, as shown in Table 1, the number and content of the adjusted confounders differed between studies. The established risk factors for liver cancer include hepatitis B/C virus infection, contamination of foodstuff with aflatoxins, smoking, alcohol, liver cirrhosis, and diabetes [3,4]. Most studies [17,19–31] adjusted for age and gender using multivariate statistical models. Some studies [17,19,21–23] adjusted for smoking, alcohol, liver cirrhosis, diabetes, and family history of liver cancer. Only a few studies [21,22] adjusted for hepatitis B or C virus infection. The effects of gallstones and cholecystectomy on the risk of liver cancer may be overestimated if other risk factors for liver cancer are imprecisely measured. However, researchers do not always consider the same factors to be potential confounders. It is also almost impossible to obtain and analyze effects estimates extracted from homogeneous models. We believe that selecting the most multivariable-adjusted effects estimates in our meta-analysis minimized the effects of residual confounding. Fourth, publication bias is a problem when interpreting our results. Negative studies are less likely to be published in indexed journals, leading to potential publication bias. We saw no evidence of such publication bias in the Egger's linear regression test, but the funnel plot seemed asymmetrical. However, according to the *Cochrane Handbook for Systematic Reviews of Interventions*, Egger's teat typically has low power. Thus, even when they do not provide evidence of funnel plot asymmetry, bias, including publication bias, cannot be excluded. Thus, publication bias remains one possible alternative explanation for our positive finding of an association between gallstones and cholecystectomy and an increased risk of liver cancer.

In conclusion, although this meta-analysis has some limitations, particularly the heterogeneity of the studies, the results suggest that a history of gallstones and cholecystectomy is associated with an increased risk of liver cancer. This issue would probably be best addressed using well-designed prospective studies with adequate exposure measurements, accurate case definition, and careful adjustment for major confounders.

Supporting Information

Table S1   References for studies excluded from the full text studies review.

Table S2   Newcastle–Ottawa scale for assessment of study quality. A case control studies; B cohort studies.

Checklist S1   PRISMA check list.

Acknowledgments

We thank *Scribendi.com* for its linguistic assistance during the preparation of this manuscript.

Author Contributions

Conceived and designed the experiments: YL YH XQ SL. Performed the experiments: YL LX TL. Analyzed the data: YL YH. Contributed reagents/materials/analysis tools: JW. Contributed to the writing of the manuscript: YL YH.

References

1. Ahmed I, Lobo DN (2009) Malignant tumours of the liver. Surgery 27: 30–37.
2. Ferlay J, Soerjomataram I, Ervik M, Dikshit R, Eser S, et al (2013) GLOBOCAN 2012 v1.0, Cancer Incidence and Mortality Worldwide: IARC CancerBase No. 11 [Internet]. Lyon, France: International Agency for Research on Cancer. Available: http://globocan.iarc.fr Accessed 2014 March 15.
3. Chuang SC, La Vecchia C, Boffetta P (2009) Liver cancer: Descriptive epidemiology and risk factors other than HBV and HCV infection. Cancer Letters 286: 9–14.
4. Ha NB, Ha NB, Ahmed A, Ayoub W, Daugherty TJ, et al. (2012) Risk factors for hepatocellular carcinoma in patients with chronic liver disease: a case-control study. Cancer Causes Control 23: 455–462.
5. Chiong C, Cox MR, Eslick GD (2012) Gallstone disease is associated with rectal cancer: a meta-analysis. Scandinavian Journal of Gastroenterology 47: 553–564.
6. Lin G, Zeng Z, Wang X, Wu Z, Wang J, et al. (2012) Cholecystectomy and risk of pancreatic cancer: a meta-analysis of observational studies. Cancer Causes Control 23: 59–67.
7. Reid FD, Mercer PM, harrison M, Bates T (1996) Cholecystectomy as a risk factor for colorectal cancer: a meta-analysis. Scand J Gastroenterol 31: 160–169.
8. Giovannucci E, Colditz GA, Stampfer MJ (1993) A meta-analysis of cholecystectomy and risk of colorectal cancer. Gastroenterology 105: 130–141.
9. Chung SC, Leung JW, Li AK (1990) Bile duct size after cholecystectomy: an endoscopic retrograde cholangiopancreatographic study. Br J Surg 77: 534–535.
10. Mantovani A, Allavena P, Sica A, Balkwill F (2008) Cancer-related inflammation. Nature 454: 436–444.
11. Jaunoo SS, Mohandas S, Almond LM (2010) Postcholecystectomy syndrome (PCS). Int J Surg 8: 15–17.
12. Malagelada JR, Go VL, Summerskill WH, Gamble WS (1973) Bile acid secretion and biliary bile acid composition altered by cholecystectomy. Am J Dig Dis 18: 455–459.
13. Pomare EW, Heaton KW (1973) The effect of cholecystectomy on bile salt metabolism. Gut 14: 753–762.
14. Pomare EW, Heaton KW (1973) Bile salt metabolism in patients with gallstones in functioning gallbladders. Gut 14: 885–890.
15. Berr F, Pratschke E, Fischer S, Paumgartner G (1992) Disorders of bile acid metabolism in cholesterol gallstone disease. J Clin Invest 90: 859–868.
16. Perez MJ, Briz O (2009) Bile-acid-induced cell injury and protection. World J Gastroenterol 15: 1677–1689.
17. Vogtmann E, Shu XO, Li HL, Chow WH, Yang G, et al. (2014) Cholelithiasis and the risk of liver cancer: results from cohort studies of 134 546 Chinese men and women. J Epidemiol Community Health.
18. Nogueira L, Freedman ND, Engels EA, Warren JL, Castro F, et al. (2014) Gallstones, cholecystectomy, and risk of digestive system cancers. Am J Epidemiol 179: 731–739.
19. Nogueira L, Cross A, Freedman N, Lai G, Castro F, et al. (2013) Gallstones, cholecystectomy, and risk of digestive system cancers. Cancer Research 73.
20. Kao WY, Hwang CY, Su CW, Chang YT, Luo JC, et al. (2013) Risk of hepatobiliary cancer after cholecystectomy: a nationwide cohort study. J Gastrointest Surg 17: 345–351.
21. Chen YK, Yeh JH, Lin CL, Peng CL, Sung FC, et al. (2013) Cancer risk in patients with cholelithiasis and after cholecystectomy: a nationwide cohort study. J Gastroenterol.
22. Chang JS, Tsai CR, Chen LT (2013) Medical risk factors associated with cholangiocarcinoma in Taiwan: a population-based case-control study. PLoS One 8: e69981.
23. Tavani A, Rosato V, Di Palma F, Bosetti C, Talamini R, et al. (2012) History of cholelithiasis and cancer risk in a network of case-control studies. Ann Oncol 23: 2173–2178.
24. Nordenstedt H, Mattsson F, El-Serag H, Lagergren J (2012) Gallstones and cholecystectomy in relation to risk of intra-and extrahepatic cholangiocarcinoma. British Journal of Cancer 106: 1011–1015.
25. Lagergren J, Mattsson F, El-Serag H, Nordenstedt H (2011) Increased risk of hepatocellular carcinoma after cholecystectomy. Br J Cancer 105: 154–156.
26. Welzel TM, Mellemkjaer L, Gloria G, Sakoda LC, Hsing AW, et al. (2007) Risk factors for intrahepatic cholangiocarcinoma in a low-risk population: a nationwide case-control study. Int J Cancer 120: 638–641.
27. Welzel TM, Graubard BI, El-Serag HB, Shaib YH, Hsing AW, et al. (2007) Risk factors for intrahepatic and extrahepatic cholangiocarcinoma in the United States: a population-based case-control study. Clin Gastroenterol Hepatol 5: 1221–1228.
28. Goldacre MJ, Abisgold JD, Seagroatt V, Yeates D (2005) Cancer after cholecystectomy: record-linkage cohort study. Br J Cancer 92: 1307–1309.
29. Chow WH, Johansen C, Gridley G, Mellemkjaer L, Olsen JH, et al. (1999) Gallstones, cholecystectomy and risk of cancers of the liver, biliary tract and pancreas. Br J Cancer 79: 640–644.
30. Johansen C, Chow WH, Jorgensen T, Mellemkjaer L, Engholm G, et al. (1996) Risk of colorectal cancer and other cancers in patients with gall stones. Gut 39: 439–443.
31. Ekbom A, Hsieh CC, Yuen J, Trichopoulos D, McLaughlin JK, et al. (1993) Risk of extrahepatic bileduct cancer after cholecystectomy. Lancet 342: 1262–1265.
32. Moher D, Liberati A, Tetzlaff J, Altman DG, Group P (2009) Preferred reporting items for systematic reviews and meta-analyses: the PRISMA statement. BMJ 339: b2535.
33. Zhang J, Yu KF (1998) What's the relative risk? A method of correcting the odds ratio in cohort studies of common outcomes. JAMA 280: 1690–1691.
34. Wells GA, Shea B, O'Connell D, Peterson J, Welch V, et al. (2009) The Newcastle-Ottawa Scale (NOS) for assessing the quality of nonrandomised studies in meta-analyses. Ottawa: Ottawa Hospital Research Institute.
35. DerSimonian R, Laird N (1986) Meta-analysis in clinical trials. Control Clin Trials 7: 177–188.
36. Higgins JP, Thompson SG, Deeks JJ, Altman DG (2003) Measuring inconsistency in meta-analyses. BMJ 327: 557–560.
37. Higgins JP and Thompson SG (2002) Quantifying heterogeneity in a meta-analysis. Stat Med 21: 1539–1558.
38. Guyatt GH, Oxman AD, Kunz R, Woodcock J, Brozek J, et al. (2011) GRADE guidelines: 7. Rating the quality of evidence–inconsistency. J Clin Epidemiol 64: 1294–1302.
39. Berkey CS, Hoaglin DC, Mosteller F, Colditz GA (1995) A random-effects regression model for meta-analysis. Stat Med 14: 395–411.
40. Copas J, Shi JQ (2000) Meta-analysis, funnel plots and sensitivity analysis. Biostatistics 1: 247–262.
41. Egger M, Davey Smith G, Schneider M, Minder C (1997) Bias in meta-analysis detected by a simple, graphical test. BMJ 315: 629–634.

42. Zhao C, Ge Z, Wang Y, Qian J (2012) Meta-analysis of observational studies on cholecystectomy and the risk of colorectal adenoma. Eur J Gastroenterol Hepatol 24: 375–381.

43. Chiong C, Cox MR, Eslick GD (2012) Gallstones are associated with colonic adenoma: a meta-analysis. World J Surg 36: 2202–2209.

44. Ge Z, Zhao C, Wang Y, Qian J (2012) Cholecystectomy and the risk of esophageal and gastric cancer. Saudi Med J 33: 1073–1079.

45. Grivennikov SI, Greten FR, Karin M (2010) Immunity, inflammation, and cancer. Cell 140: 883–899.

46. Ioannidis JP, Patsopoulos NA, Evangelou E (2007) Uncertainty in heterogeneity estimates in meta-analyses. BMJ 335: 914–916.

47. Grimes DA, Schulz KF (2002) Bias and causal associations in observational research. Lancet 359: 248–252.

13

Large Variations in Risk of Hepatocellular Carcinoma and Mortality in Treatment Naïve Hepatitis B Patients

Maja Thiele[1]*, Lise Lotte Gluud[2], Annette Dam Fialla[1], Emilie Kirstine Dahl[1], Aleksander Krag[1]

1 Department of Gastroenterology and Hepatology, Odense University Hospital, Odense, Denmark, **2** Gastrounit, Medical Division, Copenhagen University Hospital, Hvidovre, Denmark

Abstract

Background: The complications to chronic hepatitis B (HBV) include incidence of hepatocellular carcinoma (HCC) and mortality. The risk of these complications may vary in different patient groups.

Aim: To estimate the incidence and predictors of HCC and in untreated HBV patients.

Methods: Systematic review with random effects meta-analyses of randomized controlled trials and observational studies. Results are expressed as annual incidence (events per 100 person-years) with 95% confidence intervals. Subgroup and sensitivity analyses of patient and study characteristics were performed to identify common risk factors.

Results: We included 68 trials and studies with a total of 27,584 patients (264,919 person-years). In total, 1,285 of 26,687 (5%) patients developed HCC and 730 of 12,511 (6%) patients died. The annual incidence was 0.88 (95% CI, 0.76–0.99) for HCC and 1.26 (95% CI, 1.01–1.51) for mortality. Patients with cirrhosis had a higher risk of HCC (incidence 3.16; 95% CI, 2.58–3.74) than patients without cirrhosis (0.10; 95% CI, 0.02–0.18). The risk of dying was also higher for patients with than patients without cirrhosis (4.89; 95% CI, 3.16–6.63; and 0.11; 95% CI, 0.09–0.14). The risk of developing HCC increased with HCV coinfection, older age and inflammatory activity. The country of origin did not clearly predict HCC or mortality estimates.

Conclusions: Cirrhosis was the strongest predictor of HCC incidence and mortality. Patients with HBV cirrhosis have a 31-fold increased risk of HCC and a 44-fold increased mortality compared to non-cirrhotic patients. The low incidence rates should be taken into account when considering HCC screening in non-cirrhotic patients.

Trial Registration: Prospero CRD42013004764

Editor: Isabelle A. Chemin, CRCL-INSERM, France

Funding: MT has received a working grant from University of Southern Denmark (www.sdu.dk). The funders had no role in study design, data collection and analysis, decision to publish, or preparation of the manuscript. No other authors received specific funding for this work.

Competing Interests: The author Lise Lotte Gluud is a PLOS ONE Editorial Board member. This does not alter the authors' adherence to PLOS ONE Editorial policies and criteria.

* Email: maja.thiele@rsyd.dk

Introduction

Chronic hepatitis B virus (HBV) affects several hundred million people worldwide. Complications include hepatocellular carcinoma (HCC) and death from liver failure. Antiviral therapies have improved the management of HBV, but treatment is costly and associated with adverse events. As a result several patients with HBV remain untreated [1].

Guidelines recommend HCC screening in patients with HBV, but the validity of the underlying evidence is questionable. Additionally, screening is expensive and has been difficult to implement [2]. Based on cost-benefit analyses, screening is recommended if the annual incidence exceeds 0.2 per 100 patient-years [3]. Incidence estimates for subgroups can help identify high risk patients that may benefit from screening.

Previous studies have evaluated the prognosis of untreated HBV based on central registries [4,5]. This design may underestimate event rates due to inaccurate registration. Discrepancies in the results of cohort studies from Asia, Europe and North America [4,6–8] may reflect differences in study populations such as degree of fibrosis, hepatitis B envelope antigen (HBeAg) positivity, gender, age, disease activity, ethnicity, genotypes and coinfections with hepatitis C (HCV), hepatitis D (HDV) and human immunodeficiency virus (HIV) [9]. Unlike central registries, randomised controlled trials (RCTs) and observational studies include standardised registration and follow up. Several trials and studies on HBV include an untreated control group. We therefore conducted a systematic review to evaluate the incidence of HCC and mortality and the potential influence of patient and study characteristics in untreated patients with HBV, based on analyses of RCTs and observational studies.

Methods

The review is based on a registered protocol (Prospero ID CRD42013004764) and follows the MOOSE guidelines and the Cochrane Handbook for Systematic Reviews [10,11].

Data Sources and Searches

Electronic and manual searches were combined (Checklist S1). The last search update was September 2013.

Study Selection

RCTs and observational studies (prospective cohort and case-control studies) on patients with chronic HBV were eligible for inclusion. Data on untreated patients (patients allocated to placebo or no intervention) were included. The primary outcomes were HCC incidence and all-cause mortality. The secondary outcome was HCC related mortality. To minimize detection and ascertainment bias, studies assembling outcome data from central registries were excluded. All outcomes were assessed after at least 12 months of follow up to exclude prevalent HCC.

Data Extraction

Three authors independently extracted data (MT, ADF, ED). In case of discrepancies, a fourth author was contacted (AK). Extracted data (Datasheet S1) included characteristics of patients (cirrhosis, gender, age, HBeAg positivity, coinfections, Hepatitis B virus DNA (HBV-DNA), alanine aminotransferase (ALT) and HBV genotype) and trials (design, country of origin, duration of follow up, HCC screening and risk of bias).

Quality Assessment

The assessment of bias followed the Critical Appraisal Tool from the Center for Evidence Based Medicine [12]. For each study, we evaluated whether patients were assembled at a common point in the course of their disease, whether the follow up data were complete, whether outcome criteria were either objective or applied in a blind fashion, how likely the outcomes were over time and precision of the prognostic estimates.

Data Synthesis and Analysis

The analyses were performed in Stata version 13 (Statacorp, TX, USA). Incidence estimates (with the corresponding standard errors) were calculated based on the event rates in relation to the duration of follow up (number of person years). Random effects model meta-analyses were performed with results expressed as annual incidence (number of events per 100 person-years) and 95% confidence intervals (CI). I^2 was calculated as a marker of heterogeneity. I^2 values above 50% were considered as important heterogeneity.

The subgroup analyses evaluated the influence of risk factors related to patient and trial characteristics (cirrhosis, HBeAg status, coinfections, gender, age, HBV-DNA, ALT, genotype, HCC screening, study design and country of origin). We used Eggers test for funnel plot asymmetry to test for small study effects. We also performed a post-hoc subgroup analyses that combined cirrhosis and country of origin. The analysis estimated the incidence of HCC and mortality of patients with or without cirrhosis stratified by the geographical region (Asia or Europe).

Due to high heterogeneity post-hoc meta-regression analyses were performed to test for study-level covariates. The covariates included in the meta-regression were proportion with cirrhosis, HBeAg positivity, male gender, mean age, proportion with elevated HBV-DNA, proportion with elevated ALT, HCC screening, study design and study region. Post-hoc investigations on the influence of each individual study on the results of meta-analyses were also performed.

Results

Search Results and Characteristics of Included Studies

The initial searches identified 28,680 potentially eligible references (Figure 1). Sixty-eight of these references referred to studies that fulfilled our inclusion criteria (7 RCTs [13–19], 49 prospective cohort studies [20–68] and 12 case-control studies [69–80]).

HCC screening was performed in 50 studies (three RCTs and 43 observational studies). The quality of the included studies was high with regards to objectiveness of the outcome criteria and the likelihood of outcomes over time. The precision of the outcome estimate was low with a standard deviation of the mean follow up period above 50% in fifteen studies and a standard deviation of 25–50% in 30 studies. Most studies included patients at different time points in the course of the disease. The completeness of follow-up data was sufficiently reported in 13 studies (Table 1).

Characteristics of Included Patients

Our analyses included 27,584 patients and 264,919 person-years. The minimum duration of follow up was 2.0 years and the maximum duration of follow up was 16.5 years (Table S1). The studies were performed in Asia (23,537 patients; $n = 35$ studies), Europe (2,401 patients; $n = 29$ studies) and North America (1,646 patients, $n = 4$ studies). Disease severity ranged from asymptomatic carriers to decompensated cirrhosis. In twenty-eight studies all included patients had cirrhosis at baseline. In 11 studies, all included patients were non-cirrhotic. In the studies that reported the proportion of patients with cirrhosis at inclusion, the median proportion of patients with cirrhosis at baseline was 41%. In total, 3,382 of 23,097 patients (15%) were cirrhotic. Outcome data was available for 3,673 patients with cirrhosis and 16,949 patients without cirrhosis (Table S2). For the remainder of patients, data on cirrhosis status could not be extracted. Most patients were men (range 24–100%). The mean age ranged from 26 to 65 years. Six studies only included HBeAg-positive patients and 11 only included HBeAg-negative patients. In total, 726 of 1,290 (56%) patients spontaneously cleared HBeAg during the study. HCV coinfection was present in 326 patients ($n = 14$ studies) and 437 had HDV coinfection ($n = 10$ studies). None of the studies included HIV-positive patients.

Incidence of HCC

Data on the incidence of HCC were gathered from 57 studies. HCC was diagnosed in 1,285 of 26,687 patients (5%). Random effects meta-analysis showed that the annual incidence of HCC was 0.88 (95% CI 0.76–0.99, $I^2 = 94\%$, Figure 2) per 100 person-years. The incidence of HCC varied considerably in different subgroups (Table 2). In 33 studies, 605 of 2,660 patients (23%) with cirrhosis developed HCC (Figure 3). Five studies found that 71 of 8,471 patients (1%) without cirrhosis developed HCC. In subgroup meta-analyses, the incidence of HCC among patients with cirrhosis was 3.16 (95% CI 2.58–3.74, $I^2 = 82\%$), which was 31-fold higher than among patients without cirrhosis (0.10, 95% CI 0.02–0.18, $I^2 = 90\%$). HCV coinfection (reported in 9 studies)

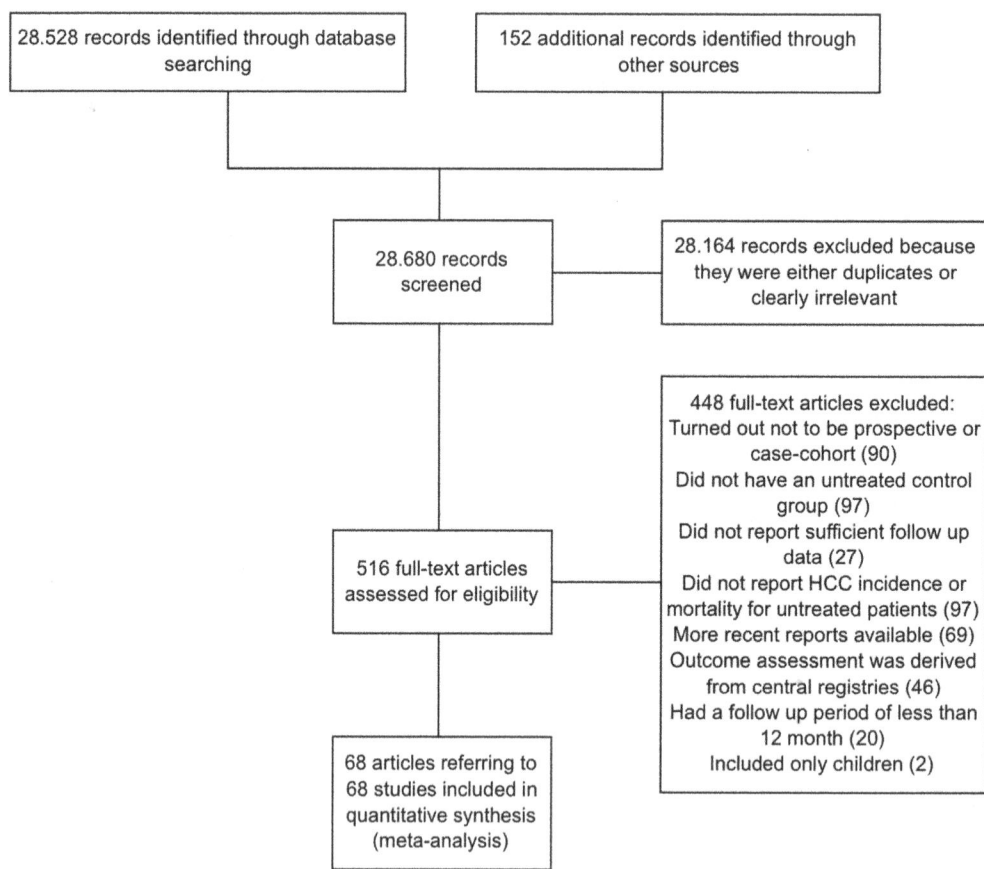

Figure 1. Trial flow diagram.

lead to a 4-fold increase in the risk of HCC (3.73, 95% CI 1.59–5.86, $I^2 = 78$%). Age and the proportion of patients with elevated ALT also predicted the incidence of HCC. Gender, HBeAg-status and HBV-DNA did not seem to be related to HCC incidence. The data did not allow for an assessment of the influence of HDV coinfection or genotype.

The incidence of HCC was higher in studies with systematic HCC screening (1.34, 95% CI 1.14–1.53) than in studies without screening (0.63, 95% CI 0.42–0.83). The annual incidence of

Table 1. Bias assessment.

Bias domains	Number of trials with low risk of bias	Number of trials with uncertain risk of bias	Number of trials with high risk of bias
Were patients assembled at a common point in the course of their disease?[1]	9	17	42
Were the follow up data complete?[2]	13	55	0
Were outcome criteria either objective or applied in a blind fashion?[3]	68	0	0
How likely are the outcomes over time?[4]	68	0	0
How precise are the prognostic estimates?[5]	15	30	23

[1]Low risk of bias if all patients are assembled at a common time point in the course of their disease. Unknown risk of bias if relevant information for assessment of bias can not be assembled. High risk of bias if patients are assembled at different time points in the course of their disease.
[2]Low risk of bias if all patients are acounted for and losses to follow up not likely to affect the outcome estimate. Uncertain risk of bias if data on losses to follow up are missing/not accounted for. High risk of bias if losses to follow up are likely to affect outcome estimate.
[3]All trials low risk of bias as HCC and/or mortality are objective outcome measures.
[4]All trials low risk of bias as the review only included studies with adequate follow up period (>1 year).
[5]Low risk of bias if standard deviation of follow up <25% of the mean follow up. Uncertain risk of bias if standard deviation of follow up is 25–50% of the mean follow up. High risk of bias is standard deviation of follow up is >50% of the mean follow up.

HCC was 1.95 (95% CI 1.16–2.75) in RCTs, 0.76 (95% CI 0.63–0.88) in prospective cohorts and 1.30 (95% CI 0.81–1.79) in case-control series.

European studies had a three-fold higher annual incidence than Asian studies (2.09, 95% CI 1.56–2.62 and 0.75, 95% CI 0.62–0.88, respectively). The median proportion of patients with cirrhosis at inclusion was 30% for Asian studies compared to 100% for European studies. All patients had cirrhosis at baseline in 16 of 29 European studies (55%) and only 12 of 35 Asian studies (34%). The HCC incidence in patients with cirrhosis did not differ between the two regions (Europe 3.35, 95% CI 2.31–4.39; Asia 3.06, 95% CI 2.24–3.87). There was insufficient data to assess HCC in European non-cirrhotic patients.

In the primary meta-analysis and most of the subgroup analyses (except RCTs and in studies including a high proportion of patients with elevated ALT) we found evidence of heterogeneity ($I^2 > 50\%$). Evidence of small study effects (Egger's test $P < 0.05$) was found in all subgroups except for patients without cirrhosis, females, HBe-Ag negative patients, studies including patients with low HBV-DNA, studies including a high proportion of patients with elevated ALT, RCTs and studies performed in North America).

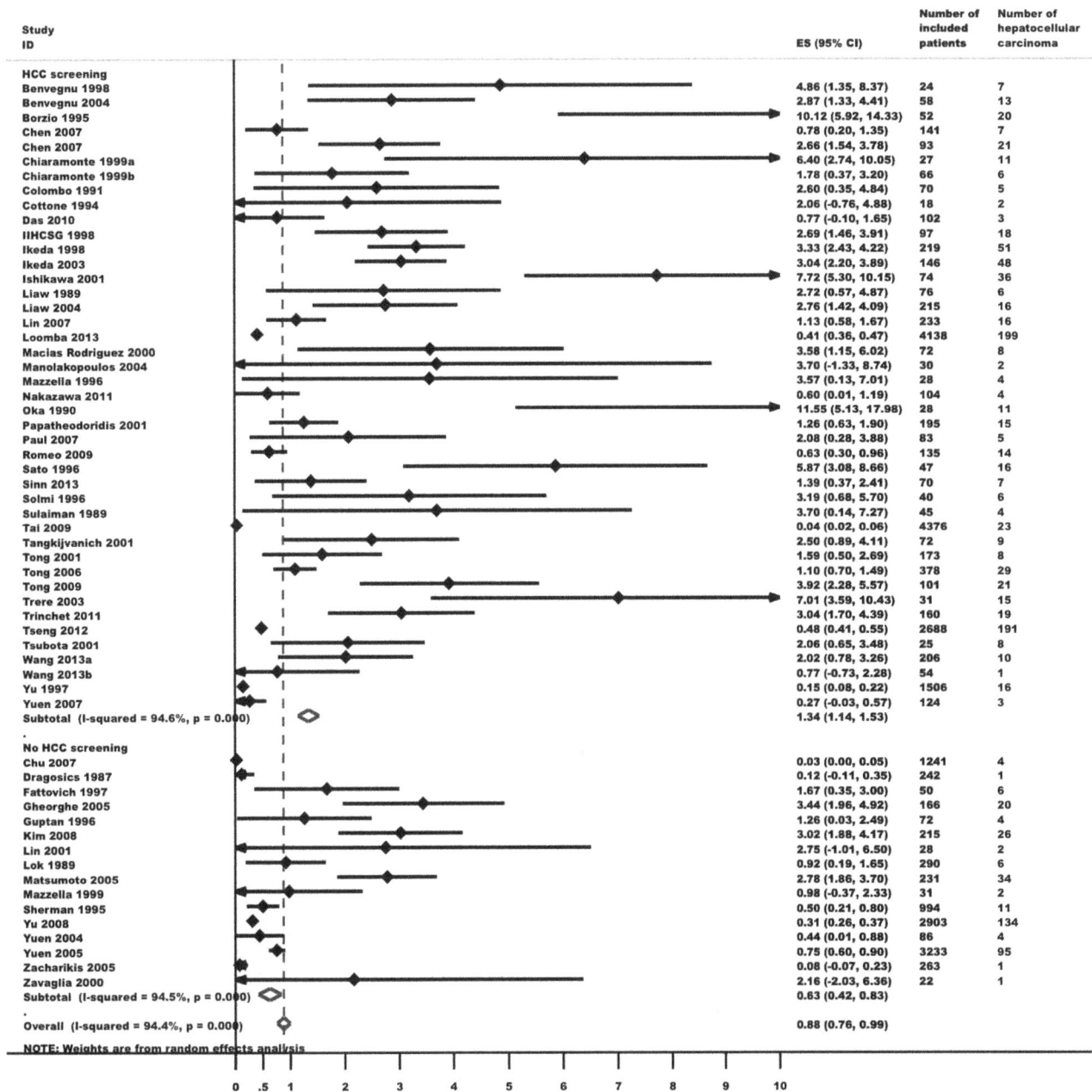

Study ID	ES (95% CI)	Number of included patients	Number of hepatocellular carcinoma
HCC screening			
Benvegnu 1998	4.86 (1.35, 8.37)	24	7
Benvegnu 2004	2.87 (1.33, 4.41)	58	13
Borzio 1995	10.12 (5.92, 14.33)	52	20
Chen 2007	0.78 (0.20, 1.35)	141	7
Chen 2007	2.66 (1.54, 3.78)	93	21
Chiaramonte 1999a	6.40 (2.74, 10.05)	27	11
Chiaramonte 1999b	1.78 (0.37, 3.20)	66	6
Colombo 1991	2.60 (0.35, 4.84)	70	5
Cottone 1994	2.06 (-0.76, 4.88)	18	2
Das 2010	0.77 (-0.10, 1.65)	102	3
IIHCSG 1998	2.69 (1.46, 3.91)	97	18
Ikeda 1998	3.33 (2.43, 4.22)	219	51
Ikeda 2003	3.04 (2.20, 3.89)	146	48
Ishikawa 2001	7.72 (5.30, 10.15)	74	36
Liaw 1989	2.72 (0.57, 4.87)	76	6
Liaw 2004	2.76 (1.42, 4.09)	215	16
Lin 2007	1.13 (0.58, 1.67)	233	16
Loomba 2013	0.41 (0.36, 0.47)	4138	199
Macias Rodriguez 2000	3.58 (1.15, 6.02)	72	8
Manolakopoulos 2004	3.70 (-1.33, 8.74)	30	2
Mazzella 1996	3.57 (0.13, 7.01)	28	4
Nakazawa 2011	0.60 (0.01, 1.19)	104	4
Oka 1990	11.55 (5.13, 17.98)	28	11
Papatheodoridis 2001	1.26 (0.63, 1.90)	195	15
Paul 2007	2.08 (0.28, 3.88)	83	5
Romeo 2009	0.63 (0.30, 0.96)	135	14
Sato 1996	5.87 (3.08, 8.66)	47	16
Sinn 2013	1.39 (0.37, 2.41)	70	7
Solmi 1996	3.19 (0.68, 5.70)	40	6
Sulaiman 1989	3.70 (0.14, 7.27)	45	4
Tai 2009	0.04 (0.02, 0.06)	4376	23
Tangkijvanich 2001	2.50 (0.89, 4.11)	72	9
Tong 2001	1.59 (0.50, 2.69)	173	8
Tong 2006	1.10 (0.70, 1.49)	378	29
Tong 2009	3.92 (2.28, 5.57)	101	21
Trere 2003	7.01 (3.59, 10.43)	31	15
Trinchet 2011	3.04 (1.70, 4.39)	160	19
Tseng 2012	0.48 (0.41, 0.55)	2688	191
Tsubota 2001	2.06 (0.65, 3.48)	25	8
Wang 2013a	2.02 (0.78, 3.26)	206	10
Wang 2013b	0.77 (-0.73, 2.28)	54	1
Yu 1997	0.15 (0.08, 0.22)	1506	16
Yuen 2007	0.27 (-0.03, 0.57)	124	3
Subtotal (I-squared = 94.6%, p = 0.000)	1.34 (1.14, 1.53)		
No HCC screening			
Chu 2007	0.03 (0.00, 0.05)	1241	4
Dragosics 1987	0.12 (-0.11, 0.35)	242	1
Fattovich 1997	1.67 (0.35, 3.00)	50	6
Gheorghe 2005	3.44 (1.96, 4.92)	166	20
Guptan 1996	1.26 (0.03, 2.49)	72	4
Kim 2008	3.02 (1.88, 4.17)	215	26
Lin 2001	2.75 (-1.01, 6.50)	28	2
Lok 1989	0.92 (0.19, 1.65)	290	6
Matsumoto 2005	2.78 (1.86, 3.70)	231	34
Mazzella 1999	0.98 (-0.37, 2.33)	31	2
Sherman 1995	0.50 (0.21, 0.80)	994	11
Yu 2008	0.31 (0.26, 0.37)	2903	134
Yuen 2004	0.44 (0.01, 0.88)	86	4
Yuen 2005	0.75 (0.60, 0.90)	3233	95
Zacharikis 2005	0.08 (-0.07, 0.23)	263	1
Zavaglia 2000	2.16 (-2.03, 6.36)	22	1
Subtotal (I-squared = 94.5%, p = 0.000)	0.63 (0.42, 0.83)		
Overall (I-squared = 94.4%, p = 0.000)	0.88 (0.76, 0.99)		

NOTE: Weights are from random effects analysis

Figure 2. Annual incidence of hepatocellular carcinoma in untreated hepatitis B patients (events per 100 person-year). Random effects meta-analysis with subgroups according to HCC screening.

Table 2. Annual Hepatocellular Carcinoma Incidence and Mortality Rates in Chronic Hepatitis B Patients.

Variable	HCC incidence[1]	95% CI	Mortality[1]	95% CI
Overall	0.88	0.76–0.99	1.26	1.01–1.51
Cirrhosis	3.16	2.58–3.74	4.89	3.16–6.63
Non-cirrhosis	0.10	0.02–0.18	0.11	0.09–0.14
HCC mortality	NA		0.34	0.22–0.45
HBeAg positive	1.47	0.40–2.55	NA	
HBeAg negative	0.72	0.21–1.23	NA	
HCV coinfection	3.73	1.59–5.86	NA	
Male	0.63	0.40–0.86	NA	
Female	0.29	0.04–0.53	NA	
Mean age >50 years	3.92	2.72–5.11	NA	
Mean age <50 years	0.82	0.69–0.95	1.69	1.28–2.10
Elevated HBV-DNA[2]	1.50	1.12–1.88	2.37	1.18–3.56
No HBV-DNA[3]	2.14	0.04–4.25	2.90	1.32–4.49
Elevated ALT[2]	1.86	1.30–2.42	2.78	1.51–4.05
Normal ALT[3]	0.32	0.21–0.43	0.30	0.12–0.49
HCC screening	1.34	1.14–1.53	1.48	1.11–1.84
No HCC screening	0.63	0.42–0.83	1.50	0.98–2.01
Randomized trials	1.95	1.16–2.75	1.57	0.00–3.53
Prospective cohorts	0.76	0.63–0.88	1.15	0.90–1.39
Case-control series	1.30	0.81–1.79	7.30	2.22–12.38
Asia	0.75	0.62–0.88	0.91	0.61–1.20
Europe	2.09	1.56–2.62	2.49	1.60–3.39
North America	1.41	0.60–2.22	NA	

[1]Number of HCC or deaths per 100 person-year. Meta-analysis using a random effects model with incidence as the study effect size and standard error of the incidence as study effect variation.
[2]Studies including >50% of patients with elevated HBV-DNA/ALT.
[3]Studies including >50% of patients with unmeasurable HBV-DNA/normal ALT.
ALT, alanine aminotransferase; CI, confidence interval; HBeAg, hepatitis B envelope antigen; HBV-DNA, hepatitis B virus DNA; HCC, hepatocellular carcinoma; HCV, chronic hepatitis C; NA, not analyzed/not enough data for analysis.

Univariate metaregression analyses of study-level covariates showed that the overall annual incidence estimate was predicted by proportion with cirrhosis (coefficient = 0.024, P<0.001), mean age (coefficient = 0.100, P = 0.001), proportion with inflammatory activity (coefficient = 0.014, P = 0.013) and whether HCC screening was performed (coefficient = 1.050, P = 0.037). None of the variables were significant predictors of the incidence estimate in multivariate metaregression. Analysing the effect of each individual study on the overall incidence estimate revealed that exclusion of either one of two studies would increase the estimate outside its 95% upper CI (Figure S1). Both were prospective cohort studies on several thousand asymptomatic HBsAg carriers [54,64].

Mortality

Thirty studies reported mortality. In total, 730 of 12,511 patients (6%) died (Table 2). Random effects meta-analysis showed that the risk of death (annual mortality per 100 person years) was 1.26 (95% CI 1.01–1.51, I^2 = 94%, Figure 4). Twelve studies reported mortality in patients with cirrhosis, in which 266 of 951 patients (28%) with cirrhosis died. Three studies on patients without cirrhosis reported that 69 of 4,572 died (2%). Subgroup analyses confirmed that patients with cirrhosis had a higher mortality (4.89, 95% CI 3.16–6.63, I^2 = 91%) than patients without cirrhosis (0.11, 95% CI 0.09–0.14, I^2 = 0%). Mortality was higher in studies including a high proportion of patients with inflammatory activity (2.78, 95% CI 1.51–4.05) than in studies with a low proportion of these patients (0.30, 95% CI 0.12–0.49). The mortality did not appear to depend on the proportion of included patients with elevated HBV-DNA.

HCC screening had no influence on the annual mortality per 100 person years. Mortality was higher in case-control series (7.30, 95% CI 2.22–12.38) than in prospective cohorts (1.15, 95% CI 0.90–1.39), but not RCTs (1.57, 95% CI 0.00–3.53). The very high mortality in case-control series was largely carried by a study on patients with decompensated cirrhosis [74]. European studies had higher mortality (2.49, 95% CI 1.60–3.39) than Asian studies (0.91, 95% CI 0.61–1.20). The geographical heterogeneity was evaluated in a post-hoc analysis considering the higher proportion of patients with cirrhosis at inclusion in European studies. Although mortality in patients with cirrhosis seemed higher in European than in Asian studies (9.45, 95% CI 4.11–14.78 versus 3.17, 95% CI 1.59–4.74) the difference in mortality was not significant (test for subgroup differences P>0.05). The high mortality in European studies was primarily due to a study on patients with decompensated cirrhosis and elevated transaminases

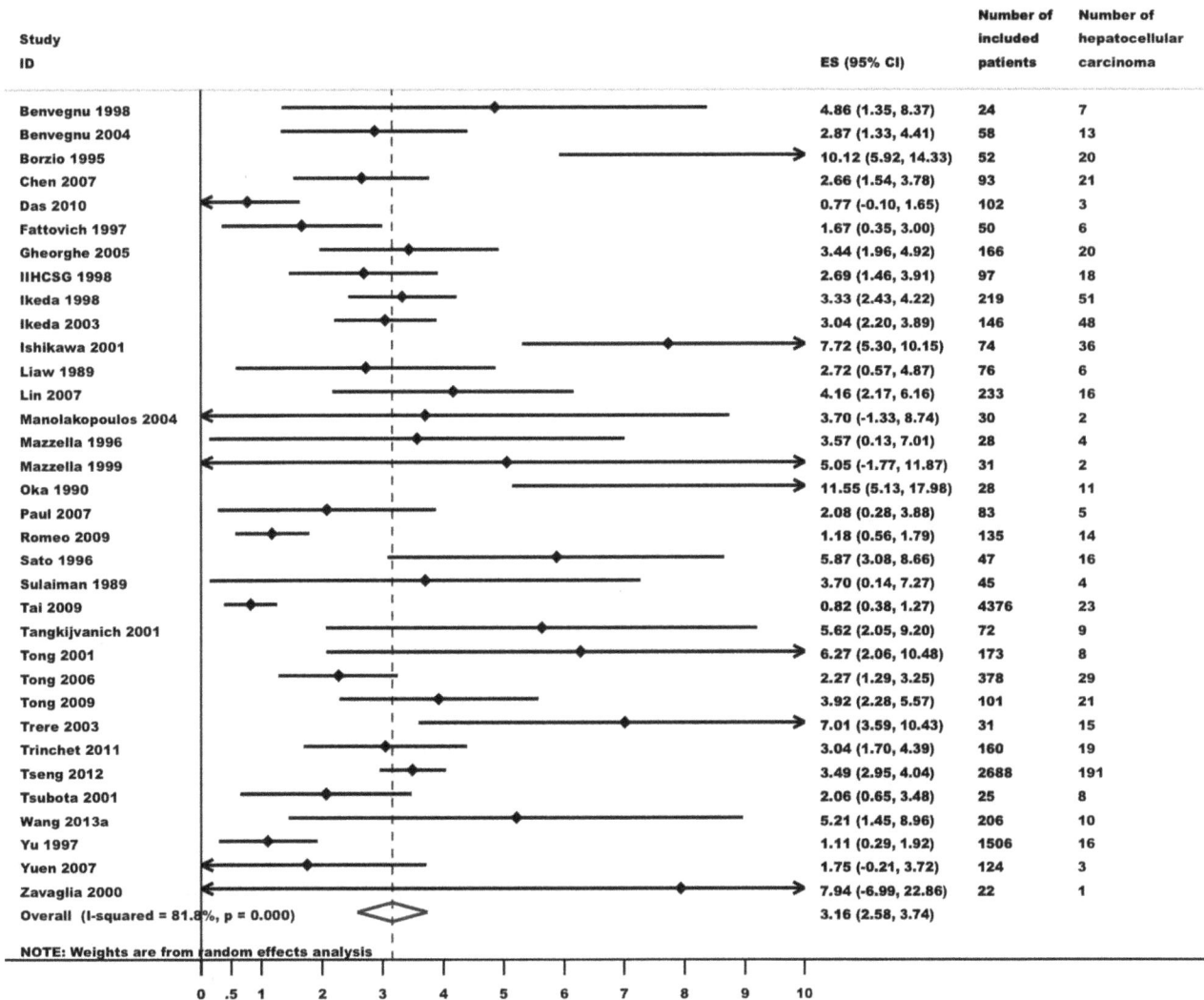

Study ID	ES (95% CI)	Number of included patients	Number of hepatocellular carcinoma
Benvegnu 1998	4.86 (1.35, 8.37)	24	7
Benvegnu 2004	2.87 (1.33, 4.41)	58	13
Borzio 1995	10.12 (5.92, 14.33)	52	20
Chen 2007	2.66 (1.54, 3.78)	93	21
Das 2010	0.77 (-0.10, 1.65)	102	3
Fattovich 1997	1.67 (0.35, 3.00)	50	6
Gheorghe 2005	3.44 (1.96, 4.92)	166	20
IIHCSG 1998	2.69 (1.46, 3.91)	97	18
Ikeda 1998	3.33 (2.43, 4.22)	219	51
Ikeda 2003	3.04 (2.20, 3.89)	146	48
Ishikawa 2001	7.72 (5.30, 10.15)	74	36
Liaw 1989	2.72 (0.57, 4.87)	76	6
Lin 2007	4.16 (2.17, 6.16)	233	16
Manolakopoulos 2004	3.70 (-1.33, 8.74)	30	2
Mazzella 1996	3.57 (0.13, 7.01)	28	4
Mazzella 1999	5.05 (-1.77, 11.87)	31	2
Oka 1990	11.55 (5.13, 17.98)	28	11
Paul 2007	2.08 (0.28, 3.88)	83	5
Romeo 2009	1.18 (0.56, 1.79)	135	14
Sato 1996	5.87 (3.08, 8.66)	47	16
Sulaiman 1989	3.70 (0.14, 7.27)	45	4
Tai 2009	0.82 (0.38, 1.27)	4376	23
Tangkijvanich 2001	5.62 (2.05, 9.20)	72	9
Tong 2001	6.27 (2.06, 10.48)	173	8
Tong 2006	2.27 (1.29, 3.25)	378	29
Tong 2009	3.92 (2.28, 5.57)	101	21
Trere 2003	7.01 (3.59, 10.43)	31	15
Trinchet 2011	3.04 (1.70, 4.39)	160	19
Tseng 2012	3.49 (2.95, 4.04)	2688	191
Tsubota 2001	2.06 (0.65, 3.48)	25	8
Wang 2013a	5.21 (1.45, 8.96)	206	10
Yu 1997	1.11 (0.29, 1.92)	1506	16
Yuen 2007	1.75 (-0.21, 3.72)	124	3
Zavaglia 2000	7.94 (-6.99, 22.86)	22	1
Overall (I-squared = 81.8%, p = 0.000)	3.16 (2.58, 3.74)		

NOTE: Weights are from random effects analysis

Figure 3. Annual incidence of hepatocellular carcinoma in untreated hepatitis B patients with cirrhosis (events per 100 person-year). Random effects meta-analysis.

[74]. There was not enough data on mortality in European non-cirrhotic patients to allow for a post-hoc analysis on differences in non-cirrhotic mortality.

In all subgroup analyses except patients without cirrhosis there was evidence of heterogeneity with I^2 values above 50%. Evidence of small study effects (Egger's test $P<0.05$) was present in most analyses except trials including a high proportion of patients with normal ALT, trials including a high proportion of patients with low HBV-DNA and RCTs.

Analysing the effect of each individual study on the overall mortality estimate revealed that the estimate would increase beyond its 95% upper CI if either one of two large studies on asymptomatic carriers were excluded (Figure S2) [49,64].

Twenty-one studies reported HCC related mortality (190 of 7,641 patients; 3%). The risk of HCC related mortality was 0.34 per 100 person years (95% CI 0.22–0.45). There was considerable heterogeneity ($I^2 = 74\%$) and clear evidence of small study effects (Egger's test $P<0.001$).

Discussion

This systematic review includes data from 68 studies and more than 27,000 patients. Overall, the risk of developing HCC and mortality was high. The large number of patients and studies allowed for adequate statistical power in subgroup analyses. The subgroup analyses led to the identification of several high risk groups. In particular, the risk of HCC was 31-fold higher if patients had cirrhosis. Likewise, cirrhosis was associated with a 44-fold increase in mortality. Inflammatory activity also predicted a higher risk of HCC and mortality. The risk of HCC was higher if HCC screening was applied suggesting that cases of HCC may have been overlooked in studies without systematic screening. Other predictors of a higher risk of HCC included HCV coinfection and older age.

Guidelines recommend HCC screening in patients with HBV. However, screening is expensive and implementation is difficult. The identification of high risk groups may help identify the groups with the highest benefit of screening. Based on cost-benefit analyses, screening is recommended if the annual incidence

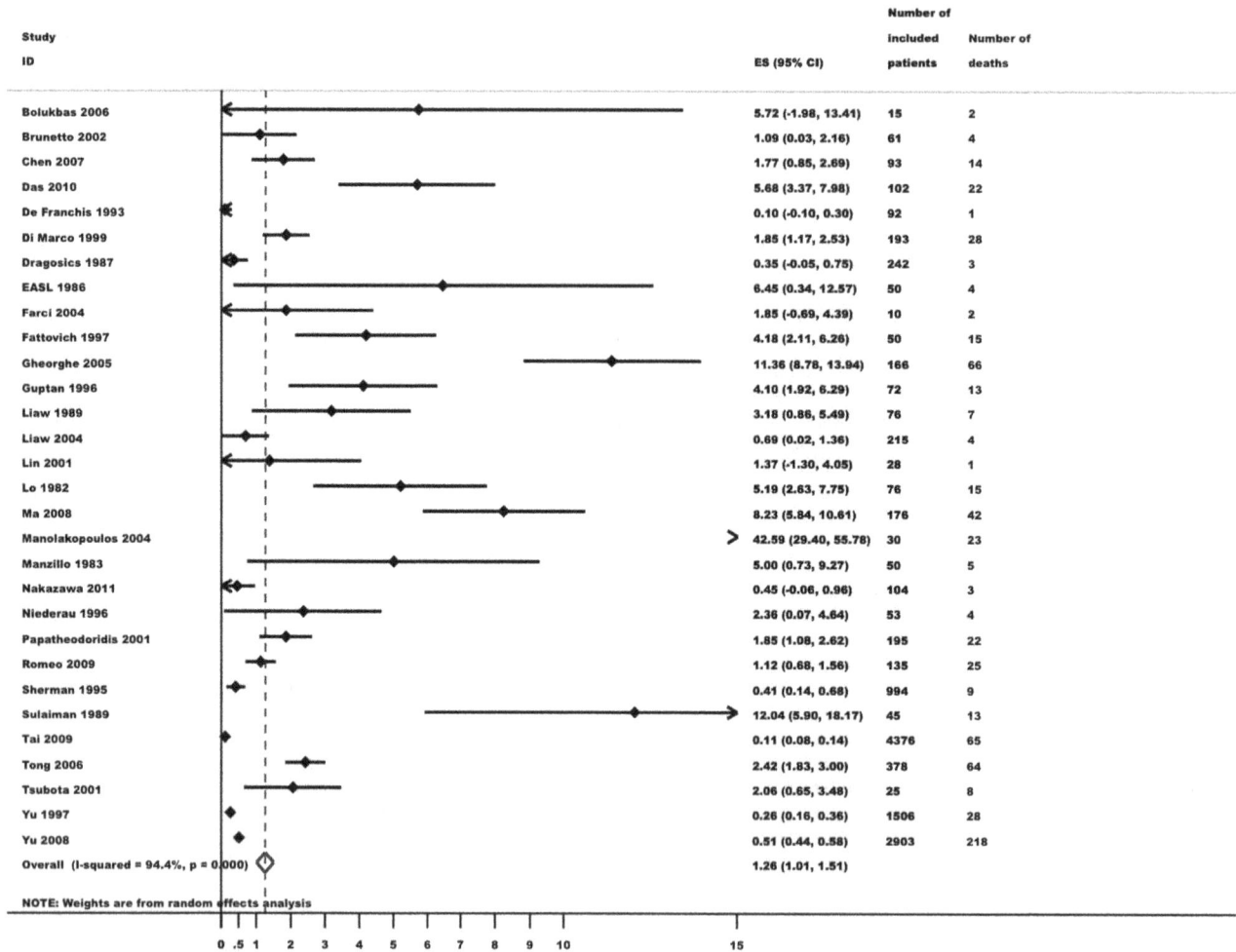

Study ID	ES (95% CI)	Number of included patients	Number of deaths
Bolukbas 2006	5.72 (-1.98, 13.41)	15	2
Brunetto 2002	1.09 (0.03, 2.16)	61	4
Chen 2007	1.77 (0.85, 2.69)	93	14
Das 2010	5.68 (3.37, 7.98)	102	22
De Franchis 1993	0.10 (-0.10, 0.30)	92	1
Di Marco 1999	1.85 (1.17, 2.53)	193	28
Dragosics 1987	0.35 (-0.05, 0.75)	242	3
EASL 1986	6.45 (0.34, 12.57)	50	4
Farci 2004	1.85 (-0.69, 4.39)	10	2
Fattovich 1997	4.18 (2.11, 6.26)	50	15
Gheorghe 2005	11.36 (8.78, 13.94)	166	66
Guptan 1996	4.10 (1.92, 6.29)	72	13
Liaw 1989	3.18 (0.86, 5.49)	76	7
Liaw 2004	0.69 (0.02, 1.36)	215	4
Lin 2001	1.37 (-1.30, 4.05)	28	1
Lo 1982	5.19 (2.63, 7.75)	76	15
Ma 2008	8.23 (5.84, 10.61)	176	42
Manolakopoulos 2004	42.59 (29.40, 55.78)	30	23
Manzillo 1983	5.00 (0.73, 9.27)	50	5
Nakazawa 2011	0.45 (-0.06, 0.96)	104	3
Niederau 1996	2.36 (0.07, 4.64)	53	4
Papatheodoridis 2001	1.85 (1.08, 2.62)	195	22
Romeo 2009	1.12 (0.68, 1.56)	135	25
Sherman 1995	0.41 (0.14, 0.68)	994	9
Sulaiman 1989	12.04 (5.90, 18.17)	45	13
Tai 2009	0.11 (0.08, 0.14)	4376	65
Tong 2006	2.42 (1.83, 3.00)	378	64
Tsubota 2001	2.06 (0.65, 3.48)	25	8
Yu 1997	0.26 (0.16, 0.36)	1506	28
Yu 2008	0.51 (0.44, 0.58)	2903	218
Overall (I-squared = 94.4%, p = 0.000)	1.26 (1.01, 1.51)		

NOTE: Weights are from random effects analysis

Figure 4. Annual mortality (events per 100 person-year) in untreated hepatitis B patients. Random effects meta-analysis.

exceeds 0.2 per 100 person-years [3]. In our overall analysis, the annual incidence of HCC was 0.88 per 100 person years. For patients without cirrhosis, the incidence was only 0.10. Accordingly, cost of screening HBV patients without cirrhosis may outweigh the benefits. Additionally, it is important to balance potential benefits with potential harms of screening [81]. Our results indicate that the lowest HCC incidence can be found in young, asymptomatic carriers without hepatic inflammation. The negative consequences (such as false positive findings) of screening may be too high for this patient group [82]. It was however not within the scope of the review to suggest a prognostic algorithm for HCC or mortality including several risk factors, as this would only be possible from a meta-analysis with individual patient data.

Improved detection of HCC does not guarantee reduced cancer specific mortality. In our analysis, despite that studies with systematic HCC screening had a higher HCC incidence than studies without screening, screening studies did not have lower mortality. Our results do however not allow for an analysis of the impact of HCC screening on patient harm, costs or mortality.

In agreement with previous evidence, we found that the level of inflammation is an important predictor of clinical outcomes in HBV [83,84]. We were able to analyse the influence of cirrhosis, HBeAg status and HCV coinfection, gender, age and markers of disease activity, but not other known predictors such as HDV and

HIV coinfection, genotype, alcohol, diabetes or smoking [85,86]. Additional evidence is needed to determine the influence of these factors.

In most analyses we found evidence of small study effects and high heterogeneity. One of the reasons for this finding is that small studies included a high proportion of patients with cirrhosis. The larger studies mostly included asymptomatic HBsAg carriers. Additionally, our bias assessment revealed that most studies included patients at different time points in the disease, leading to heterogeneous patient populations. Likewise, the heterogeneity of the included studies may be a reflection of the heterogeneous population of chronic HBV infected patients worldwide, thus making statistical heterogeneity difficult to avoid.

We found considerable geographical differences in incidence of HCC and mortality. These differences were caused by a much larger number of European studies including only patients with cirrhosis, compared to Asian studies. However, HCC incidence and mortality in patients with cirrhosis was similar in European and Asian studies, thus supporting our conclusion that cirrhosis was the strongest predictor of HCC and mortality. One may speculate whether the large number studies including only patients with cirrhosis would skew the results of our analyses towards a higher overall HCC incidence and mortality. However, since the studies with the largest number of included patients were mostly in non-cirrhotic patients, only 15% of the total study population had cirrhosis at baseline.

In conclusion, the combined evidence stresses the importance of risk stratification in HBV. The HCC incidence and mortality depends on a number of patient characteristics. In non-cirrhotic patients without inflammatory activity HCC screening could be futile due to the low incidence, whereas efforts should be made to detect HCC in at-risk patients with cirrhosis, HCV coinfection, old age and inflammatory activity.

Supporting Information

Figure S1 Analysis of the influence of a single study on the overall estimate in the meta-analysis, HCC incidence.

Figure S2 Analysis of the influence of a single study on the overall estimate in the meta-analysis, mortality.

Table S1 Supplementary table, trial characteristics.

Table S2 Supplementary table, HCC incidence and mortality in included studies.

Checklist S1 MOOSE checklist.

Datasheet S1 Data extraction sheet.

Acknowledgments

We wish to extend our sincerest gratitude to doctors Sheng-Nan Lu, Henry Lik-Yuen Chan, Takahide Nakazawa, C. J. Chen, Veysel Tahan, Man-Fung Yuen, Seung Up Kim, Yi-Cheng Chen and Tim Harrison, who kindly responded to our requests for additional information.

Author Contributions

Conceived and designed the experiments: MT LLG AK. Performed the experiments: MT ADF EKD. Analyzed the data: MT LLG. Contributed to the writing of the manuscript: MT LLG AK EKD ADF.

References

1. WHO (2009) Position Paper on Hepatitis B Vaccines. WHO Weekly Epidemiological Report 84: 405–420.
2. Wong CR, Garcia RT, Trinh HN, Lam KD, Ha NB, et al. (2009) Adherence to screening for hepatocellular carcinoma among patients with cirrhosis or chronic hepatitis B in a community setting. Dig Dis Sci 54: 2712–2721.
3. Bruix J, Sherman M (2010) AASLD Practice Guideline. Management of Hepatocellular Carcinoma. Hepatology: 1–35.
4. Beasley RP, Lin CC, Hwang LY, Chien CS (1981) Hepatocellular Carcinoma and Hepatitis B Virus: A Prospective Study of 22 707 Men in Taiwan. The Lancet 318: 1129–1133.
5. Manno M, Cammà C, Schepis F, Bassi F, Gelmini R, et al. (2004) Natural history of chronic HBV carriers in northern Italy: Morbidity and mortality after 30 years. Gastroenterology 127: 756–763.
6. McMahon BJ, Holck P, Bulkow L, Snowball M (2001) Serologic and Clinical Outcomes of 1536 Alaska Natives Chronically Infected with Hepatitis B Virus. Annals of Internal Medicine 135: 759–768.
7. Fattovich G, Giustina G, Schalm SW, Hadziyannis S, Sanchez-Tapias J, et al. (1995) Occurrence of hepatocellular carcinoma and decompensation in western European patients with cirrhosis type B. The EUROHEP Study Group on Hepatitis B Virus and Cirrhosis. Hepatology 21: 77–82.
8. Chen CJ, Yang HI (2011) Natural history of chronic hepatitis B REVEALed. Journal of Gastroenterology and Hepatology 26: 628–638.
9. Fattovich G, Bortolotti F, Donato F (2008) Natural history of chronic hepatitis B: Special emphasis on disease progression and prognostic factors. Journal of Hepatology 48: 335–352.
10. Stroup DF, Berlin JA, Morton SC, Olkin I, Williamson GD, et al. (2000) Meta-analysis of observational studies in epidemiology: a proposal for reporting. Meta-analysis Of Observational Studies in Epidemiology (MOOSE) group. JAMA 283: 2008–2012.
11. Higgins JP, Green S, editors (2011) Cochrane Handbook for Systematic Reviews of Interventions. Version 5.1.0 [updated March 2011]: The Cochrane Collaboration.
12. Center for Evidence Based Medicine (2013) Critical Appraisal Tools. Available: http://www.cebm.net/index.aspx?o=1157.
13. Trinchet JC, Chaffaut C, Bourcier V, Degos F, Henrion J, et al. (2011) Ultrasonographic surveillance of hepatocellular carcinoma in cirrhosis: A randomized trial comparing 3- and 6-month periodicities. Hepatology 54: 1987–1997.
14. Wang JH, Chang KC, Kee KM, Chen PF, Yen YH, et al. (2013) Hepatocellular carcinoma surveillance at 4- vs. 12-month intervals for patients with chronic viral hepatitis: a randomized study in community. American Journal of Gastroenterology 108: 416–424.
15. Farci P, Roskams T, Chessa L, Peddis G, Mazzoleni AP, et al. (2004) Long-term benefit of interferon α therapy of chronic hepatitis D: regression of advanced hepatic fibrosis. Gastroenterology 126: 1740–1749.
16. Liaw YF, Sung JJY, Chow WC, Farrell G, Lee CZ, et al. (2004) Lamivudine for Patients with Chronic Hepatitis B and Advanced Liver Disease. New England Journal of Medicine 351: 1521–1531.
17. Mazzella G, Saracco G, Festi D, Rosina F, Marchetto S, et al. (1999) Long-term results with interferon therapy in chronic type B hepatitis: a prospective randomized trial. Am J Gastroenterol 94: 2246–2250.
18. EASL ATGo (1986) Steroids in chronic B-hepatitis. A randomized, double-blind, multinational trial on the effect of low-dose, long-term treatment on survival. A trial group of the European Association for the Study of the Liver. Liver 6: 227–232.
19. Zavaglia C, Severini R, Tinelli C, Franzone JS, Airoldi A, et al. (2000) A randomized, controlled study of thymosin-alpha1 therapy in patients with anti-HBe, HBV-DNA-positive chronic hepatitis B. Dig Dis Sci 45: 690–696.
20. Benvegnù L, Chemello L, Noventa F, Fattovich G, Pontisso P, et al. (1998) Retrospective analysis of the effect of interferon therapy on the clinical outcome of patients with viral cirrhosis. Cancer 83: 901–909.
21. Benvegnù L, Gios M, Boccato S, Alberti A (2004) Natural history of compensated viral cirrhosis: a prospective study on the incidence and hierarchy of major complications. Gut 53: 744–749.
22. Borzio M, Bruno S, Roncalli M, Colloredo Mels G, Ramella G, et al. (1995) Liver cell dysplasia is a major risk factor for hepatocellular carcinoma in cirrhosis: A prospective study. Gastroenterology 108: 812–817.
23. Brunetto MR, Oliveri F, Coco B, Leandro G, Colombatto P, et al. (2002) Outcome of anti-HBe positive chronic hepatitis B in alpha-interferon treated and untreated patients: a long term cohort study. Journal of Hepatology 36: 263–270.
24. Chen YC, Chu CM, Yeh CT, Liaw YF (2007) Natural course following the onset of cirrhosis in patients with chronic hepatitis B: a long-term follow-up study. Hepatol Int 1: 267–273.
25. Colombo M, de Franchis R, Del Ninno E, Sangiovanni A, De Fazio C, et al. (1991) Hepatocellular Carcinoma in Italian Patients with Cirrhosis. New England Journal of Medicine 325: 675–680.
26. Cottone M, Turri M, Caltagirone M, Parisi P, Orlando A, et al. (1994) Screening for hepatocellular carcinoma in patients with Child's A cirrhosis: an 8-year prospective study by ultrasound and alphafetoprotein. Journal of Hepatology 21: 1029–1034.
27. de Franchis R, Meucci G, Vecchi M, Tatarella M, Colombo M, et al. (1993) The Natural History of Asymptomatic Hepatitis B Surface Antigen Carriers. Annals of Internal Medicine 118: 191.
28. Di Marco V, Iacono OL, Cammà C, Vaccaro A, Giunta M, et al. (1999) The long-term course of chronic hepatitis B. Hepatology 30: 257–264.
29. Dragosics B, Ferenci P, Hitchman E, Denk H (1987) Long-term follow-up study of asymptomatic HBsAg-positive voluntary blood donors in Austria: a clinical and histologic evaluation of 242 cases. Hepatology 7: 302–306.
30. Guptan RC, Thakur V, Sarin SK, Banerjee K, Khandekar P (1996) Frequency and clinical profile of precore and surface hepatitis B mutants in Asian-Indian patients with chronic liver disease. Am J Gastroenterol 91: 1312–1317.
31. Kim JH, Lee JH, Park SJ, Bae MH, Kim JH, et al. (2008) Factors associated with natural seroclearance of hepatitis B surface antigen and prognosis after seroclearance: a prospective follow-up study. Hepatogastroenterology 55: 578–581.
32. Liaw YF, Lin DY, Chen TJ, Chu CM (1989) Natural course after the development of cirrhosis in patients with chronic type B hepatitis: a prospective study. Liver 9: 235–241.
33. Lo KJ, Tong MJ, Chien MC, Tsai YT, Liaw YF, et al. (1982) The natural course of hepatitis B surface antigen-positive chronic active hepatitis in Taiwan. J Infect Dis 146: 205–210.

34. Lok AS, Lai CL (1989) alpha-Fetoprotein monitoring in Chinese patients with chronic hepatitis B virus infection: role in the early detection of hepatocellular carcinoma. Hepatology 9: 110–115.

35. Ma H, Wei L, Guo F, Zhu S, Sun Y, et al. (2008) Clinical features and survival in Chinese patients with hepatitis B e antigen-negative hepatitis B virus-related cirrhosis. Journal of Gastroenterology and Hepatology 23: 1250–1258.

36. Manzillo G, Piccinino F, Sagnelli E, Izzo CM, Pasquale G, et al. (1983) Treatment of HBsAg-positive chronic active hepatitis with corticosteroids and/ or azathioprine. A prospective study. Ric Clin Lab 13: 261–268.

37. Mazzella G, Accogli E, Sottili S, Festi D, Orsini M, et al. (1996) Alpha interferon treatment may prevent hepatocellular carcinoma in HCV-related liver cirrhosis. J Hepatol 24: 141–147.

38. Nakazawa T, Shibuya A, Takeuchi A, Shibata Y, Hidaka H, et al. (2011) Viral level is an indicator of long-term outcome of hepatitis B virus e antigen-negative carriers with persistently normal serum alanine aminotransferase levels. J Viral Hepat 18: e191–e199.

39. Oka H, Kurioka N, Kim K, Kanno T, Kuroki T, et al. (1990) Prospective study of early detection of hepatocellular carcinoma in patients with cirrhosis. Hepatology 12: 680–687.

40. Papatheodoridis GV, Manesis E, Hadziyannis SJ (2001) The long-term outcome of interferon-alpha treated and untreated patients with HBeAg-negative chronic hepatitis B. J Hepatol 34: 306–313.

41. Paul SB, Sreenivas V, Gulati MS, Madan K, Gupta AK, et al. (2007) Incidence of hepatocellular carcinoma among Indian patients with cirrhosis of liver: an experience from a tertiary care center in northern India. Indian J Gastroenterol 26: 274–278.

42. Sherman M, Peltekian KM, Lee C (1995) Screening for hepatocellular carcinoma in chronic carriers of hepatitis B virus: Incidence and prevalence of hepatocellular carcinoma in a North American urban population. Hepatology 22: 432–438.

43. Solmi L, Primerano AM, Gandolfi L (1996) Ultrasound follow-up of patients at risk for hepatocellular carcinoma: results of a prospective study on 360 cases. Am J Gastroenterol 91: 1189–1194.

44. Sulaiman HA (1989) The development of hepatocellular carcinoma from liver cirrhosis during a follow-up study. Gastroenterol Jpn 24: 567–572.

45. Tong MJ, Blatt LM, Kao VWC (2001) Surveillance for hepatocellular carcinoma in patients with chronic viral hepatitis in the United States of America. J Gastroenterol Hepatol 16: 553–559.

46. Tong MJ, Blatt LM, Tyson KB, Kao VWC (2006) Death from liver disease and development of hepatocellular carcinoma in patients with chronic hepatitis B virus infection: a prospective study. Gastroenterol Hepatol 2: 41–47.

47. Tsubota A, Arase Y, Ren F, Tanaka H, Ikeda K, et al. (2001) Genotype may correlate with liver carcinogenesis and tumor characteristics in cirrhotic patients infected with hepatitis B virus subtype adw. J Med Virol 65: 257–265.

48. Yu MW, Hsu FC, Sheen IS, Chu CM, Lin DY, et al. (1997) Prospective Study of Hepatocellular Carcinoma and Liver Cirrhosis in Asymptomatic Chronic Hepatitis B Virus Carriers. Am J Epidemiol 145: 1039–1047.

49. Yu MW, Shih WL, Lin CL, Liu CJ, Jian JW, et al. (2008) Body-mass index and progression of hepatitis B: a population-based cohort study in men. J Clin Oncol 26: 5576–5582.

50. Zacharakis GH, Koskinas J, Kotsiou S, Papoutselis M, Tzara F, et al. (2005) Natural history of chronic HBV infection: A cohort study with up to 12 years follow-up in North Greece (part of the Interreg I-II/EC-project). J Med Virol 77: 173–179.

51. Loomba R, Yang HI, Su J, Brenner D, Barrett-Connor E, et al. (2013) Synergism between obesity and alcohol in increasing the risk of hepatocellular carcinoma: a prospective cohort study. American Journal of Epidemiology 177: 333–342.

52. Chen CH, Hung CH, Lee CM, Hu TH, Wang JH, et al. (2007) Pre-S Deletion and Complex Mutations of Hepatitis B Virus Related to Advanced Liver Disease in HBeAg-Negative Patients. Gastroenterology 133: 1466–1474.

53. Chiaramonte M, Stroffolini T, Vian A, Stazi MA, Floreani A, et al. (1999) Rate of incidence of hepatocellular carcinoma in patients with compensated viral cirrhosis. Cancer 85: 2132–2137.

54. Chu CM, Liaw YF (2007) HBsAg seroclearance in asymptomatic carriers of high endemic areas: Appreciably high rates during a long-term follow-up. Hepatology 45: 1187–1192.

55. Fattovich G, Giustina G, Realdi G, Corrocher R, Schalm SW (1997) Long-term outcome of hepatitis B e antigen–positive patients with compensated cirrhosis treated with interferon alfa. Hepatology 26: 1338–1342.

56. Gheorghe L, Iacob S, Simionov I, Vadan R, Gheorghe C, et al. (2005) Natural history of compensated viral B and D cirrhosis. Rom J Gastroenterol 14: 329–335.

57. Ikeda K, Arase Y, Kobayashi M, Someya T, Saitoh S, et al. (2003) Consistently Low Hepatitis B Virus DNA Saves Patients from Hepatocellular Carcinogenesis in HBV-Related Cirrhosis. Intervirology 46: 96–104.

58. Ikeda K, Saitoh S, Suzuki Y, Kobayashi M, Tsubota A, et al. (1998) Interferon decreases hepatocellular carcinogenesis in patients with cirrhosis caused by the hepatitis B virus. Cancer 82: 827–835.

59. Ishikawa T, Ichida T, Yamagiwa S, Sugahara S, Uehara K, et al. (2001) High viral loads, serum alanine aminotransferase and gender are predictive factors for the development of hepatocellular carcinoma from viral compensated liver cirrhosis. Journal of Gastroenterology and Hepatology 16: 1274–1281.

60. Macias Rodriguez MA, Rendon Unceta P, Tejada Cabrera M, Infante Hernandez JM, Correro Aguilar F, et al. (2000) Risk factors for hepatocellular carcinoma in patients with liver cirrhosis. Rev Esp Enferm Dig 92: 458–469.

61. Maeshiro T, Arakaki S, Watanabe T, Aoyama H, Shiroma J, et al. (2007) Different natural courses of chronic hepatitis B with genotypes B and C after the fourth decade of life. World J Gastroenterol 13: 4560–4565.

62. Romeo R, Del Ninno E, Rumi M, Russo A, Sangiovanni A, et al. (2009) A 28-Year Study of the Course of Hepatitis Δ Infection: A Risk Factor for Cirrhosis and Hepatocellular Carcinoma. Gastroenterology 136: 1629–1638.

63. Sato A, Kato Y, Nakata K, Nakao K, Daikoku M, et al. (1996) Relationship between sustained elevation of serum alanine aminotransferase and progression from cirrhosis to hepatocellular carcinoma: comparison in patients with hepatitis B virus- and hepatitis C virus-associated cirrhosis. J Gastroenterol Hepatol 11: 944–948.

64. Tai DI, Lin SM, Sheen IS, Chu CM, Lin DY, et al. (2009) Long-term outcome of hepatitis B e antigen-negative hepatitis B surface antigen carriers in relation to changes of alanine aminotransferase levels over time. Hepatology 49: 1859–1867.

65. Tong MJ, Hsien C, Song JJ, Kao JH, Sun HE, et al. (2009) Factors associated with progression to hepatocellular carcinoma and to death from liver complications in patients with HBsAg-positive cirrhosis. Dig Dis Sci 54: 1337–1346.

66. Trerè D, Borzio M, Morabito A, Borzio F, Roncalli M, et al. (2003) Nucleolar hypertrophy correlates with hepatocellular carcinoma development in cirrhosis due to HBV infection. Hepatology 37: 72–78.

67. Yuen MF, Wong DKH, Sablon E, Tse E, Ng IOL, et al. (2004) HBsAg seroclearance in chronic hepatitis B in the Chinese: Virological, histological, and clinical aspects. Hepatology 39: 1694–1701.

68. Yuen MF, Yuan HJ, Wong DK, Yuen JC, Wong WM, et al. (2005) Prognostic determinants for chronic hepatitis B in Asians: therapeutic implications. Gut 54: 1610–1614.

69. Bolukbas C, Bolukbas FF, Kendir T, Akbayir N, Ince AT, et al. (2006) The effectiveness of lamivudine treatment in cirrhotic patients with HBV precore mutations: a prospective, open-label study. Dig Dis Sci 51: 1196–1202.

70. Das K, Das K, Datta S, Pal S, Hembram JR, et al. (2010) Course of disease and survival after onset of decompensation in hepatitis B virus-related cirrhosis. Liver International 30: 1033–1042.

71. IIHCSG (1998) Effect of interferon-α on progression of cirrhosis to hepatocellular carcinoma: a retrospective cohort study. The Lancet 351: 1535–1539.

72. Lin CC, Wu JC, Chang TT, Huang YH, Wang YJ, et al. (2001) Long-term evaluation of recombinant interferon α2b in the treatment of patients with hepatitis B e antigen-negative chronic hepatitis B in Taiwan. J Viral Hepat 8: 438–446.

73. Lin SM, Yu ML, Lee CM, Chien RN, Sheen IS, et al. (2007) Interferon therapy in HBeAg positive chronic hepatitis reduces progression to cirrhosis and hepatocellular carcinoma. J Hepatol 46: 45–52.

74. Manolakopoulos S, Karatapanis S, Elefsiniotis J, Mathou N, Vlachogiannakos J, et al. (2004) Clinical course of lamivudine monotherapy in patients with decompensated cirrhosis due to HBeAg negative chronic HBV infection. Am J Gastroenterol 99: 57–63.

75. Matsumoto A, Tanaka E, Rokuhara A, Kiyosawa K, Kumada H, et al. (2005) Efficacy of lamivudine for preventing hepatocellular carcinoma in chronic hepatitis B: A multicenter retrospective study of 2795 patients. Hepatology Research 32: 173–184.

76. Niederau C, Heintges T, Lange S, Goldmann G, Niederau CM, et al. (1996) Long-Term Follow-up of HBeAg-Positive Patients Treated with Interferon Alfa for Chronic Hepatitis B. New England Journal of Medicine 334: 1422–1427.

77. Sinn DH, Choi MS, Gwak GY, Paik YH, Lee JH, et al. (2013) Pre-s mutation is a significant risk factor for hepatocellular carcinoma development: a long-term retrospective cohort study. Digestive Diseases & Sciences 58: 751–758.

78. Tangkijvanich P, Thong-ngam D, Mahachai V, Kladchareon N, Suwangool P, et al. (2001) Long-term effect of interferon therapy on incidence of cirrhosis and hepatocellular carcinoma in Thai patients with chronic hepatitis B. Southeast Asian J Trop Med Public Health 32: 452–458.

79. Tseng TC, Liu CJ, Yang HC, Su TH, Wang CC, et al. (2012) High levels of hepatitis B surface antigen increase risk of hepatocellular carcinoma in patients with low HBV load. Gastroenterology 142: 1140–1149.e1143; quiz e1113–1144.

80. Yuen MF, Seto WK, Chow DH, Tsui K, Wong DK, et al. (2007) Long-term lamivudine therapy reduces the risk of long-term complications of chronic hepatitis B infection even in patients without advanced disease. Antivir Ther 12: 1295–1303.

81. Heleno B, Thomsen MF, Rodrigues DS, Jørgensen KJ, Brodersen J (2013) Quantification of harms in cancer screening trials: literature review. BMJ 347.

82. Aggestrup LM, Hestbech MS, Siersma V, Pedersen JH, Brodersen J (2012) Psychosocial consequences of allocation to lung cancer screening: a randomised controlled trial. BMJ Open 2.

83. Iloeje UH, Yang HI, Jen CL, Su J, Wang LY, et al. (2007) Risk and predictors of mortality associated with chronic hepatitis B infection. Clin Gastroenterol Hepatol 5: 921–931.

84. Ioannou GN, Splan MF, Weiss NS, McDonald GB, Beretta L, et al. (2007) Incidence and predictors of hepatocellular carcinoma in patients with cirrhosis. Clin Gastroenterol Hepatol 5: 938–945, 945 e931–934.

85. Bedogni G, Miglioli L, Masutti F, Ferri S, Castiglione A, et al. (2008) Natural Course of Chronic HCV and HBV Infection and Role of Alcohol in the General Population: The Dionysos Study. Am J Gastroenterol 103: 2248–2253.

86. Chao LT, Wu CF, Sung FY, Lin CL, Liu CJ, et al. (2011) Insulin, glucose and hepatocellular carcinoma risk in male hepatitis B carriers: results from 17-year follow-up of a population-based cohort. Carcinogenesis 32: 876–881.

14

MALDI Imaging Mass Spectrometry Profiling of N-Glycans in Formalin-Fixed Paraffin Embedded Clinical Tissue Blocks and Tissue Microarrays

Thomas W. Powers[1], Benjamin A. Neely[1], Yuan Shao[2], Huiyuan Tang[5], Dean A. Troyer[3], Anand S. Mehta[4], Brian B. Haab[5], Richard R. Drake[1,2]*

1 Department of Cell and Molecular Pharmacology and Experimental Therapeutics and MUSC Proteomics Center, Medical University of South Carolina, Charleston, South Carolina, United States of America, 2 Hollings Cancer Center Biorepository and Tissue Analysis Resource, Medical University of South Carolina, Charleston, South Carolina, United States of America, 3 Departments of Pathology and Microbiology and Molecular Cell Biology, Eastern Virginia Medical School, Norfolk, Virginia, United States of America, 4 Drexel University College of Medicine, Department of Microbiology and Immunology and Drexel Institute for Biotechnology and Virology, Doylestown, Pennsylvania, United States of America, 5 Laboratory of Cancer Immunodiagnostics, Van Andel Research Institute, Grand Rapids, Michigan, United States of America

Abstract

A recently developed matrix-assisted laser desorption/ionization imaging mass spectrometry (MALDI-IMS) method to spatially profile the location and distribution of multiple N-linked glycan species in frozen tissues has been extended and improved for the direct analysis of glycans in clinically derived formalin-fixed paraffin-embedded (FFPE) tissues. Formalin-fixed tissues from normal mouse kidney, human pancreatic and prostate cancers, and a human hepatocellular carcinoma tissue microarray were processed by antigen retrieval followed by on-tissue digestion with peptide N-glycosidase F. The released N-glycans were detected by MALDI-IMS analysis, and the structural composition of a subset of glycans could be verified directly by on-tissue collision-induced fragmentation. Other structural assignments were confirmed by off-tissue permethylation analysis combined with multiple database comparisons. Imaging of mouse kidney tissue sections demonstrates specific tissue distributions of major cellular N-linked glycoforms in the cortex and medulla. Differential tissue distribution of N-linked glycoforms was also observed in the other tissue types. The efficacy of using MALDI-IMS glycan profiling to distinguish tumor from non-tumor tissues in a tumor microarray format is also demonstrated. This MALDI-IMS workflow has the potential to be applied to any FFPE tissue block or tissue microarray to enable higher throughput analysis of the global changes in N-glycosylation associated with cancers.

Editor: Surinder K. Batra, University of Nebraska Medical Center, United States of America

Funding: This work was supported by grants from the National Institutes of Health/National Cancer Institute grants R21CA137704 and R01CA135087, and the state of South Carolina SmartState Endowed Research program to R.R.D. Additional resources and support were from the Biorepository & Tissue Analysis Shared Resource, Hollings Cancer Center (P30 CA138313), and by the South Carolina Clinical & Translational Research (SCTR) Institute (UL1 RR029882 & UL1 TR000062) for R.R.D. This work was supported by grants R01 CA120206 and U01 CA168856 from the National Cancer Institute (NCI), the Hepatitis B Foundation, and an appropriation from The Commonwealth of Pennsylvania to A.M. This work was supported by a grant from the National Institutes of Health/National Cancer Institute, U01CA168896, to B.B.H. The funders had no role in study design, data collection and analysis, decision to publish or preparation of the manuscript.

Competing Interests: The authors confirm that Anand S. Mehta is a current member of the Editorial Board. This does not alter the authors' adherence to PLOS ONE Editorial policies and criteria.

* Email: draker@musc.edu

Introduction

Tissues obtained from surgeries or diagnostic procedures are most commonly preserved in formalin-fixed paraffin-embedded (FFPE) tissue blocks. These tissues are fixed in formalin and processed as paraffin-embedded tissue blocks. The embedding process preserves the cellular morphology and allows tissues to be stored at room temperature, causing FFPE fixation to be used by many tissue banks and biorepositories [1,2]. For cancer biomarker discovery, FFPE tissues are particularly attractive because they are archived for years and are much more widely available than cryopreserved tissue. When combined with clinical outcomes, FFPE tissues are a rich source of samples for biomarker discovery and validation in retrospective studies. While the fixation method has many benefits, the formalin treatment results in the formation of methylene bridges between the amino acids of the proteins, complicating further analysis by mass spectrometry. There has been continued progress in improving extraction methods of trypsin digested peptides from FFPE tissues in recent years, in parallel with improved high resolution sequencing analysis of peptides by mass spectrometry [3,4]. Incorporation of multiple FFPE tumor tissue cores in a tissue microarray (TMA) format also has proven to be effective for immunohistochemistry analysis of potential biomarker candidates [5], and TMAs are increasingly being used for validation of alterations in protein expression associated with emerging genetic mutation phenotypes and transcriptional profiling studies [6,7]. The main advantages of experiments performed with TMAs are the ability to include multiple cores from the same subject tumors, improved sample throughput, statistical relevance and multiplexed analysis of diverse molecular targets [5,8]. Thus, it is possible to place up to 100 samples with duplicates and controls on a single slide. When correlated with associated clinical outcomes, this provides a powerful method for biomarker discovery and validation while minimizing reagent use and assuring that each core in the TMA is treated under identical conditions.

It is well documented that malignant transformation and cancer progression result in fundamental changes in the glycosylation patterns of cell surface and secreted glycoproteins [9–11]. Glycosylation of proteins are post-translational modifications most commonly involving either N-linked addition to asparagine residues or O-linked additions to serine or threonine residues. Current approaches to evaluate glycosylation changes generally involve bulk extraction of glycans and glycoproteins from tumor tissues for analysis by mass spectrometry or antibody array platforms, however, this disrupts tissue architecture and distribution of the analytes. Broad affinity carbohydrate binding lectins and a small number of glycan antigen antibodies can be used to target glycan structural classes in tissues, but not individual glycan species. Additionally, these detection methods for global alterations in glycosylation requires staining on many adjacent tissue sections, making large scale assessments on many samples difficult, expensive and time consuming. There are only a few reported studies examining glycosylation related changes of proteins or glycolipids in FFPE cancer tissues [12–14], and these focus primarily on determining the levels of the protein carriers or glycosyltransferases through immunostaining.

One potential approach to assess glycan changes in tissues is matrix-assisted laser desorption/ionization imaging mass spectrometry (MALDI-IMS). This technique has been used to directly profile multiple protein [15,16], lipid [17,18] and drug metabolite [19–21] in tissue, generating molecular maps of the relative abundance and spatial distribution of individual analytes linked to tissue histopathology. MALDI-IMS analysis of peptides following trypsin digestion of FFPE TMAs have also been reported [22–24]. Recently, our group reported a MALDI-IMS method workflow to directly profile N-linked glycan species in fresh/frozen tissues [25]. Adapting this method for the analysis of N-glycans in FFPE tissues would serve to extend the application of the technique to larger retrospective sample sets and TMAs.

In this report, we describe the application of MALDI-IMS glycan imaging to various formalin-fixed tissues. Formalin-fixed mouse kidney tissues were used to optimize antigen retrieval, PNGaseF digestion and glycan detection conditions for MALDI-IMS. This was followed by N-glycan analysis of clinical FFPE tissue blocks from prostate and pancreatic cancers, as well as a commercial tissue microarray of hepatocellular carcinoma (HCC). Glycan identity was confirmed by on-tissue collision-induced dissociation (CID) and off-tissue permethylation analysis. An optimized MALDI-IMS workflow is presented that allows routine simultaneous analysis of 30 or more glycans per FFPE tissue, including TMA formats. The approach is amenable to any FFPE tissue, and represents an additional molecular correlate assay for use with the TMA format. Furthermore, depending on the construction of the TMA and targeted tumor type, the approach has the potential to identify novel glycan biomarker panels for cancer detection and prognosis. To our knowledge, this represents the first instance of using MALDI-IMS to profile N-glycans in FFPE tissue blocks or TMAs.

Materials and Methods

Materials

The glycan standard NA2 was obtained from ProZyme (Hayward, CA). Trifluoroacetic acid, sodium hydroxide, dimethyl sulfoxide, iodomethane and α-cyano-4-hydroxycinnamic acid (CHCA) were obtained from Sigma-Aldrich (St. Louis, MO). HPLC grade methanol, ethanol, acetonitrile, xylene and water were obtained from Fisher Scientific (Pittsburgh, PA). ITO slides were purchased from Bruker Daltonics (Billerica, MA) and Tissue Tack microscope slides were purchased from Polysciences, Inc (Warrington, PA). Citraconic anhydride for antigen retrieval was from Thermo Scientific (Bellefonte, PA). Recombinant Peptide N-Glycosidase F (PNGaseF) from *Flavobacterium meningosepticum* was expressed and purified as previously described [25].

FFPE Tissues and TMA

All human tissues used were de-identified and determined to be not human research classifications by the respective Institutional Review Boards at MUSC and Van Andel. Mouse kidneys were excised from euthanized C57BL/6 mice and immediately placed in 10% formalin prior to processing for routine histology and paraffin embedding. Mice were housed in an Institutional Animal Care and Use Committee-approved small animal facility at MUSC, and tissues obtained were harvested as part of approved projects unrelated to glycan tissue imaging. A liver TMA was purchased from BioChain consisting of 16 cases of liver cancer in duplicates, and one adjacent non-tumor tissue for each case. Tissues were from 14 male and two female patients with an average age of 47.5 with a range of 33 to 68 years old, with additional information provided in Table S1. A de-identified prostate tumor FFPE block, stored for 10 years representing a Gleason grade 6 (3+3)/stage T2c adenocarcinoma from a 62 year old Caucasian male, was obtained from the Hollings Cancer Center Biorepository at the Medical University of South Carolina. A pathologist confirmed the presence of approximately 10% prostate cancer gland content in the sample. A de-identified large-cell undifferentiated pancreatic carcinoma FFPE tissue section with low CA19-9 staining was obtained from the Van Andel Institute Biospecimen Repository. For each section analyzed, histological analysis and staining with hematoxylin and eosin (H & E) were performed.

Washes for Deparaffinization and Rehydration

Tissue and TMA blocks were sectioned at 5 μm and mounted on positively charged glass slides measuring 25×75 mm, compatible with the Bruker slide adaptor plate. The slides were heated at 60°C for 1 hr. After cooling, tissue sections were deparaffinized by washing twice in xylene (3 minutes each). Tissue sections were then rehydrated by submerging the slide twice in 100% ethanol (1 minute each), once in 95% ethanol (one minute), once in 70% ethanol (one minute), and twice in water (3 minutes each). Following the wash, the slide was transferred to a coplin jar containing the citraconic anhydride buffer for antigen retrieval and the jar was placed in a vegetable steamer for 25 minutes. Citraconic anhydride (Thermo) buffer was prepared by adding 25 μL citraconic anhydride in 50 mL water, and adjusted to pH 3 with HCl. After allowing the buffer to cool, the buffer was exchanged with water five times by pouring out ½ of the buffer and replacing with water, prior to replacing completely with water on the last time. The slide was then desiccated prior to enzymatic digestion. Tris buffer pH 9–10 was also effective, but citraconic anhydride buffer was used for all experiments in this study.

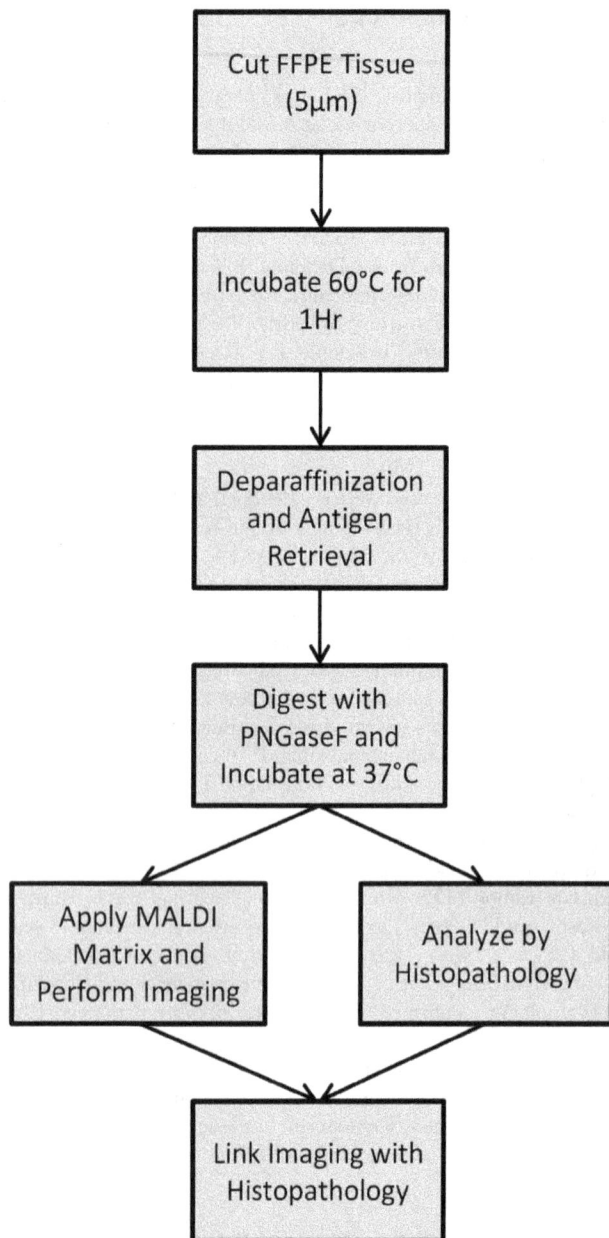

Figure 1. Schematic of the methodology for imaging N-glycans from FFPE tissues. Prior to enzyme application, FFPE blocks are cut at 5 µm, incubated, deparaffinized and undergo antigen retrieval. PNGaseF is then applied and the slide is incubated before MALDI-IMS. The data is then linked with histopathology either on the same tissue slice or a serial tissue slice.

N-glycan MALDI-IMS

An ImagePrep spray station (Bruker Daltonics) was used to coat the slide with a 0.2 ml aqueous solution of PNGaseF (20 µg total/slide) as previously described [25]. Adjacent control tissue slices lacking PNGaseF were generated by covering them with a glass slide during the spraying process. Following application of PNGaseF, slides were incubated at 37°C for 2 hr in a humidified chamber, then dried in a desiccator prior to matrix application. α-Cyano-4-hydroxycinnamic acid matrix (0.021 g CHCA in 3 ml 50% acetonitrile/50% water and 12 µL 25% TFA) was applied using the ImagePrep sprayer. Released glycan ions were detected

using a Solarix dual source 7T FTICR mass spectrometer (Bruker Daltonics) (m/z = 690–5000 m/z) with a SmartBeam II laser operating at 1000 Hz, a laser spot size of 25 µm. Images of differentially expressed glycans were generated to view the expression pattern of each analyte of interest using FlexImaging 4.0 software (Bruker Daltonics). Following MS analysis, data was loaded into FlexImaging Software focusing on the range m/z = 1000–4000 and reduced to 0.95 ICR Reduction Noise Threshold. Observed glycans were searched against the glycan database provided by the Consortium for Functional Glycomics (www.functionalglycomics.org). Glycan structures were generated by Glycoworkbench [26] and represent putative structures determined by combinations of accurate m/z, CID fragmentation patterns and glycan database structures.

Permethylation of Tissue Extracted N-glycans

PNGaseF sprayed mouse kidney tissue slides were incubated for 2 hr at 37°C; 50 µL water was applied on top of the tissue and incubated for 20 minutes to extract the released native N-glycans. The water was removed from the tissue, and then concentrated under vacuum by centrifugation. Permethylation was performed as described [25], and glycans analyzed by MALDI. Masses detected in the permethylation experiments were searched against the permethylated glycan database provided by the Consortium for Functional Glycomics (www.functionalglycomics.org).

Collision-Induced Dissociation of N-linked Glycans

Glycan standards were spotted on a stainless steel MALDI plate using CHCA matrix and desiccated to yield a homogenous layer. Tissues were prepared as previously described for MALDI imaging of FFPE tissues. 10 spectra of 1000 laser shots with a laser frequency of 1000 Hz were averaged for each spectra provided. The collision energy varied between 60–70V.

TMA Statistics

Mass spectra from TMA tissue Regions of Interest (ROIs) representing each tissue core were exported directly from FlexImaging and analyzed using an in-house workflow. The peak lists were first deconvoluted followed by calculating the mean peak intensity of points in each ROI, resulting in a monoisotopic peak list corresponding to signal intensity in each region. Comparison of tumor versus non-tumor was accomplished with a Wilcoxon rank sum test. Individual peaks were also evaluated to discriminate between tumor and non-tumor using receiver operator characteristic curves.

Results

Analysis of Formalin-Fixed Mouse Kidneys and Human Cancer Tissues

Mouse kidney tissues were fixed in formalin and used as an initial model system to develop MALDI-IMS glycan imaging workflows for FFPE tissues. These tissues were chosen due to the availability of reference glycan structures and spectra (Consortium for Functional Glycomics; www.functionalglycomics.org), and previous MALDI-IMS glycan imaging data from our laboratory for fresh/frozen tissue analysis [21]. A summary workflow schematic is provided (Figure 1). Tissues were cut at 5 microns, deparaffinized and rehydrated in sequential xylene/ethanol/water rinses, followed by antigen retrieval in citraconic anhydride pH 3. The rehydrated tissues were sprayed with PNGaseF, incubated for glycan release, sprayed with CHCA matrix, and then analyzed by MALDI-IMS. While all data shown herein uses CHCA, 2,5-dihydroxybenzoic acid (DHB) matrix could also be used success-

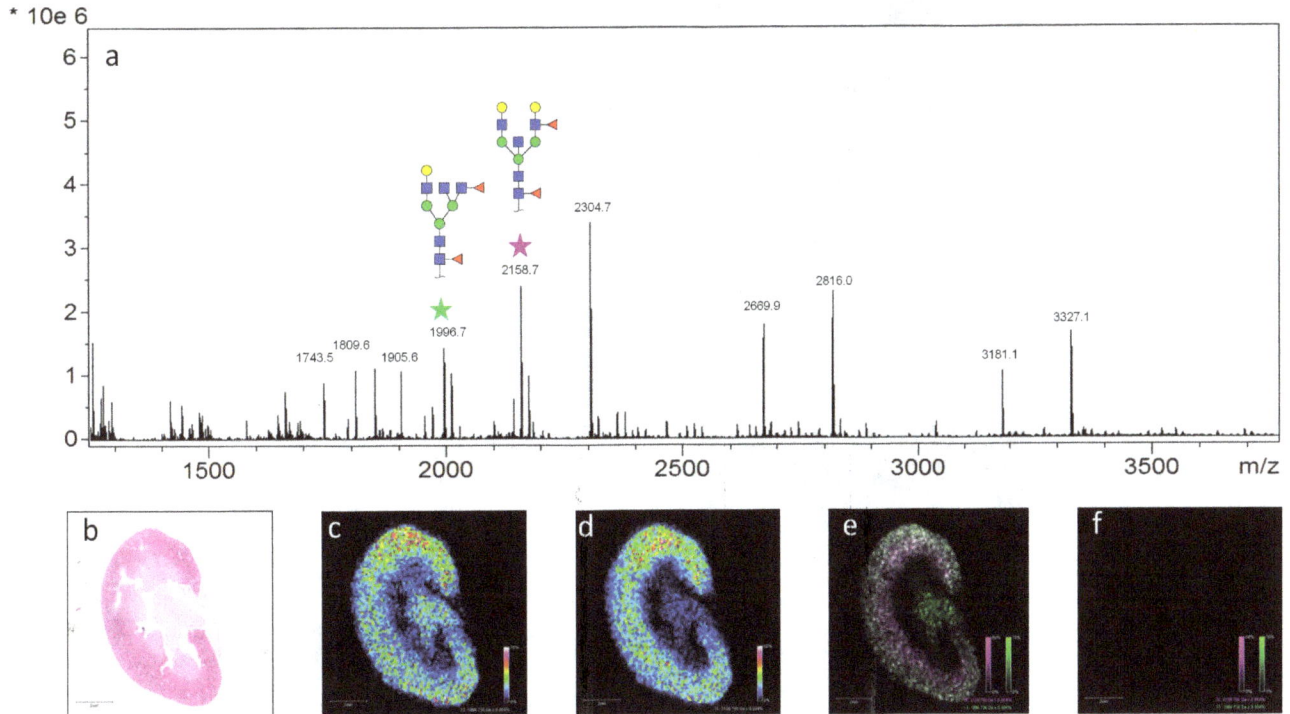

Figure 2. MALDI-IMS of N-Glycans on Mouse Kidney Tissue. Two mouse kidneys were sliced at 5 um prior to proceeding with the MALDI-IMS workflow. One tissue was covered with a glass slide during PNGaseF application to serve as an undigested control tissue. An average annotated spectra from the tissue that received PNGaseF application is provided (a). Tissue regions were assessed by H&E stain (b). The labeled peaks correspond to native N-glycans that have been reported for the mouse kidney on the Consortium for Functional Glycomics mouse kidney database. Two of these ions were selected and their tissue localization was assessed. Hex4dHex2HexNAc5 at m/z = 1996.7 (c) is located in the cortex and medulla while Hex5dHex2HexNAc5 m/z = 2158.7 (d) is more abundant in the cortex of the mouse kidney. An overlay image of these two masses is also shown (e), as well as the corresponding image from untreated PNGaseF control tissues (f).

fully for N-glycan imaging of FFPE tissues. As shown in Figure 2, there were multiple ions detectable only in the tissue incubated with PNGaseF that were not present in the control tissue with no PNGaseF application. Different glycans were distributed across the cortex or medulla regions. For example, a Hex4dHex2Hex-NAc5 ion (m/z = 1996.74) is present in the cortex and medulla (Figure 2c), while a Hex5dHex2HexNAc5 glycan (m/z = 2158.76) is more specific to the cortex (Figure 2d). An overlay of the MALDI-IMS images for these two ions from the PNGaseF treated sections (Figure 2e) and the control tissue (Figure 2f) demonstrates that these two ions are released by PNGaseF. In control kidney tissues that were only sprayed with aqueous PNGaseF solution lacking enzyme, or tissue slices that were not processed by antigen retrieval plus and minus PNGaseF digestion, only matrix ions or paraffin/formalin polymer were detected (data not shown). A summary glycan image panel of 28 glycan ions detected in these kidneys, sodium adducts and observed/expected m/z values is provided in Figure S1. Additionally, N-glycans were extracted from the tissue following on-tissue PNGaseF digestion, permethylated and analyzed by MALDI. A representative spectra from this analysis is provided in Figure S2. These permethylated values were also compared with MALDI reference spectra for mouse kidney glycans from the Consortium for Functional Glycomics. The imaged glycan ions were correlated to the reference spectra glycans, illustrated in Figure S3, and could be matched to all 28 glycan species highlighted in the reference spectra.

We next assessed whether the method was compatible with two representative archived pathology FFPE tissue blocks, one for

pancreatic cancer and one for prostate cancer. A section of human pancreatic cancer tissue of complex histology was processed, incubated with PNGaseF and glycans detected by MALDI-IMS (Figure 3). Different N-glycans were detected that could distinguish between non-tumor, tumor, tumor necrotic and fibroconnective tissue regions. A representative glycan image overlay of four m/z values that correspond to the sodium adducts of potential N-glycan species is shown in Figure 3a, each representing a specific region of the tissue (Figure 3b). A glycan of m/z = 1891.80 (red)/Hex3dHex1HexNAc6 was detected primarily in the non-tumor region of the pancreas, while a glycan of m/z = 1743.64 (blue)/Hex8HexNAc2 was predominant in the tumor region of the tissue. A region of desmoplasia surrounding the tumor region, an area of increased extracellular matrix proteins and myofibroblast-like cells resulting in a dense fibrous connective tissue [27], is represented by a glycan of m/z = 1809.69 (green)/Hex5dHex1-HexNAc4. A region of tumor necrosis is represented by a different glycan of m/z = 1663.64 (orange)/Hex5HexNAc4. Additional examples of tissue distributions of other individual glycan species are shown in Figure 3c.

A human prostate tissue block containing both tumor and non-tumor gland regions was also analyzed by MALDI-IMS. A heterogeneous N-glycan distribution reflective of the tissue histology was observed, and as an example of stroma and gland distributions, two glycan ions and two sub-regions within the tissue are highlighted in Figure 4. Distribution of glycans of m/z = 1663.56 (Hex5HexNAc4) and m/z = 1850.65 (Hex4dHex1-HexNAc5) are shown in Figure 4b and 4c. A higher resolution

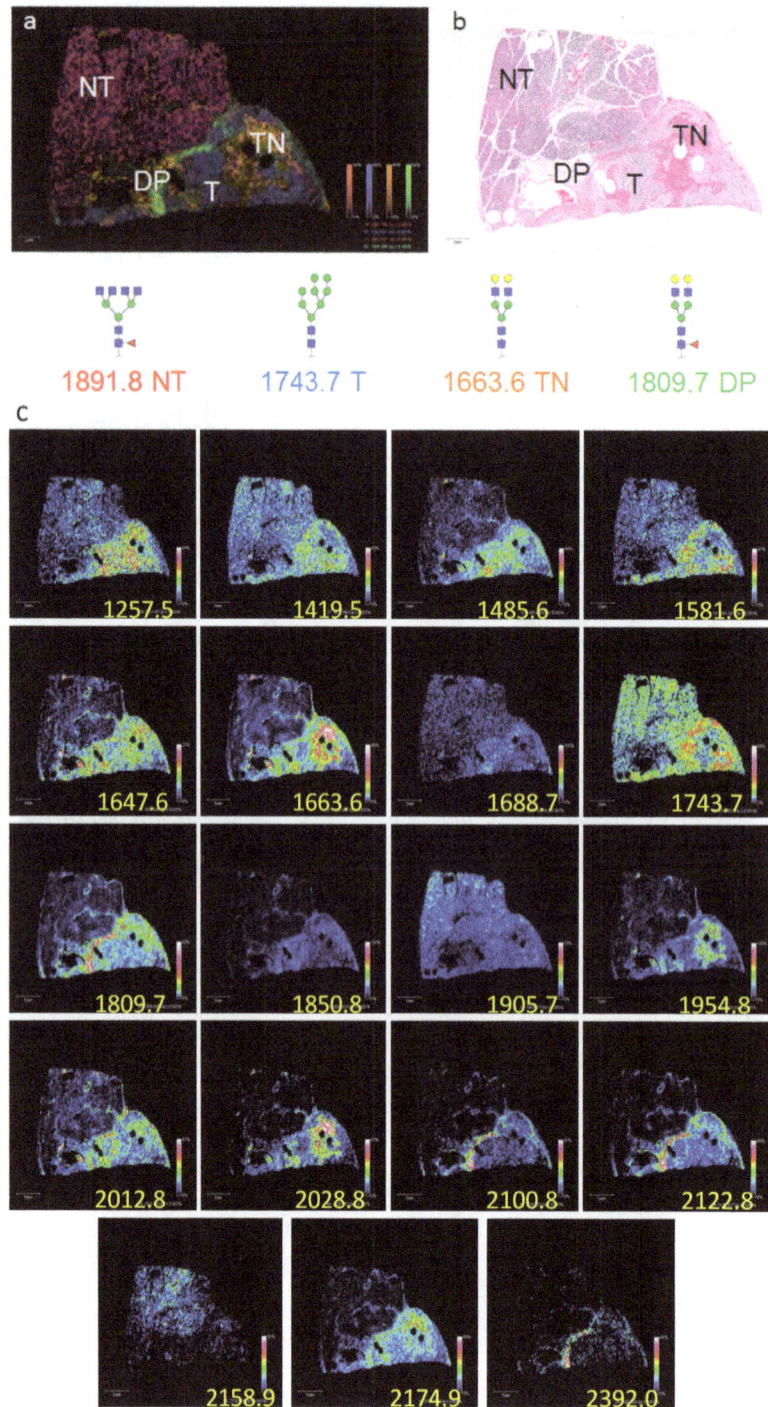

Figure 3. MALDI-IMS of a Human Pancreas FFPE Tissue Block. An FFPE block of pancreatic tissue from a human patient was cut at 5 um prior to and selected for MALDI-IMS. Histopathology found four unique regions in the H&E of this tissue block. The tissue block contained tumor tissue, non-tumor tissue, fibroconnective tissue representing desmoplasia surrounding the tumor tissue, and necrotic tissue (b). MALDI-IMS was able to distinguish these four regions based off of specific ions after MALDI-IMS. M/z = 1891.80 (red) is found in the non-tumor (NT) region of the pancreas and corresponds to Hex3dHex1HexNAc6, while m/z = 1743.64 (blue) represents Hex8HexNAc2 and is predominant in the tumor region (T) of the tissue. Desmoplasia (DP) is represented by m/z = 1809.69 (green) corresponding to Hex5dHex1HexNAc4. In the region where necrosis was identified (TN), m/z = 1663.64 (orange) was elevated corresponding to Hex5HexNAc4. Image spectra were acquired at 200 μm raster. (c). Representative individual glycan images for the pancreatic FFPE tissue slice.

tissue imaging analysis was done for selected regions as marked in the panel, with the H&E images (Figure 4d–4f) highlighting stroma and gland substructures. In both instances, m/z = 1850.65 is present in both the stroma and glands, while m/z = 1663.56 is predominantly located in the stroma. An overlay of these two ions depicts the stroma as an orange color, demonstrating the presence

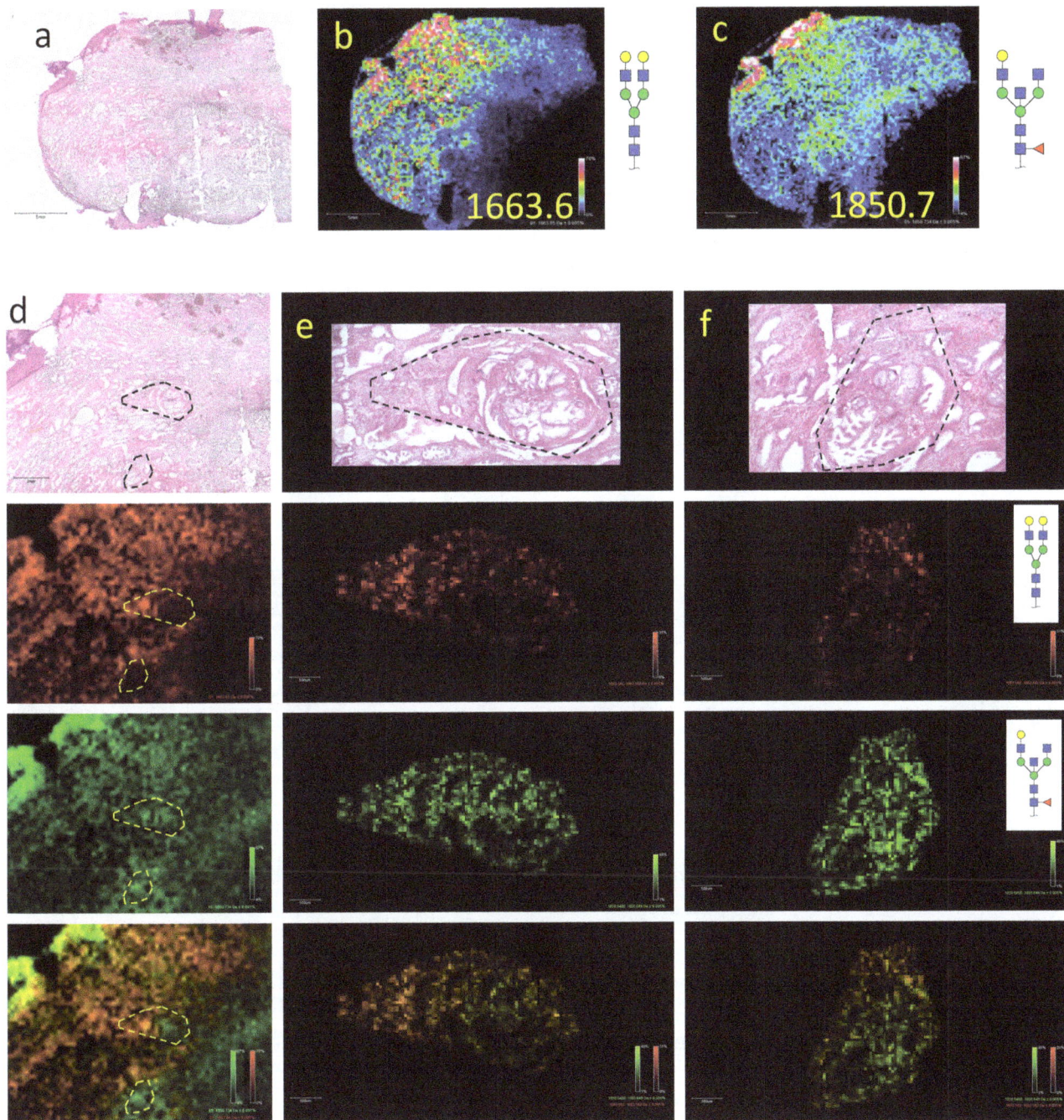

Figure 4. MALDI-IMS of a Human Prostate FFPE Tissue Block. An archived FFPE block of prostate tissue from a human patient was cut at 5 μm and prepared for MALDI-IMS glycan analysis, (a). H&E image. A global glycan imaging experiment performed with a raster of 225 μm demonstrated a heterogeneous expression of two glycan ions (b). at m/z = 1663.56 and (c). m/z = 1850.65. Stromal versus gland distribution were further assessed in a high resolution experiment at 50 μm raster (d–f). Column (d) indicates a 2× amplification of the H&E, and distribution of the same two glycans are shown at this magnification for m/z = 1663.56 (red) and m/z = 1850.65 (green), and an overlay image. Column (e) (enlargement of upper region shown in d). and (f) (enlargement of lower region shown in d), show two highlighted regions of stroma and glands enhanced at 10× resolution, with the same colors and glycans shown for column (d).

of both red and green, while the glands are predominantly green. The distribution of other representative individual glycan ions is provided in Figure S4, including the distribution of high-mannose glycan species (Man5–Man9) associated with the heterogeneous tumor region in this tissue.

On-tissue Glycan Fragmentation and Structural Composition

The glycan structures identified by imaging of the FFPE tissue blocks were assigned based on the comparison to permethylated species, glycan reference databases and previous studies [24]. An on-tissue approach to further verify N-glycan structures was done

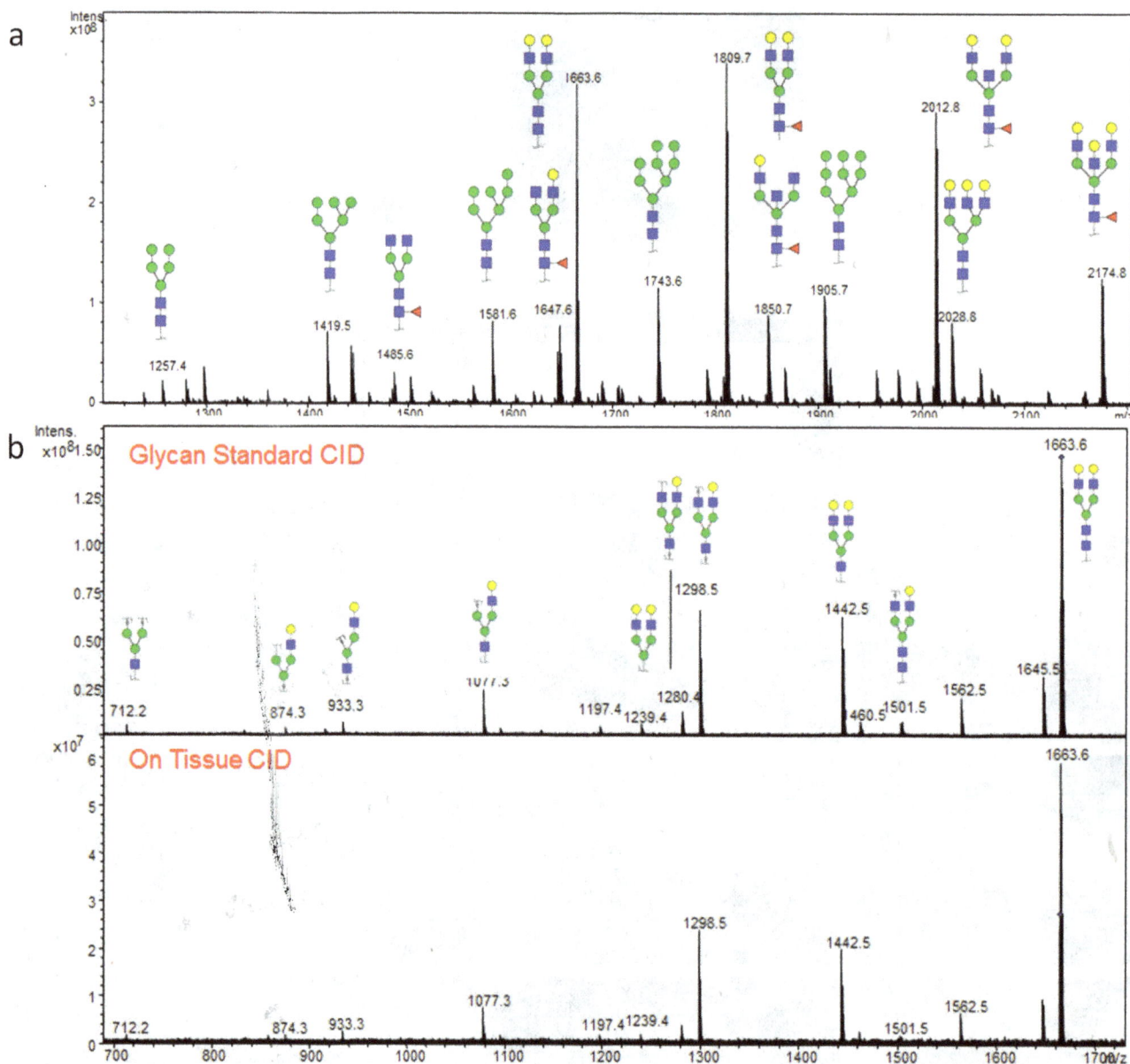

Figure 5. Comparison of the Fragmentation Pattern of a Glycan Standard with the same Ion on Tissue. (a). A representative MALDI spectra for native N-linked glycans from pancreatic cancer FFPE tissue. (b). NA2 glycan standard (m/z = 1663.6) was fragmented using CID, revealing a variety of cleavages across glycosidic bonds as demonstrated in the spectrum (a). When the same ion was fragmented on the pancreatic tissue, the fragmentation pattern was the same, verifying that we were detecting Hex5HexNAc4 in the human pancreas.

using collision-induced dissociation (CID) directly on the human pancreatic tissue. Released native glycans from pancreatic cancer FFPE tissues were used as a source for on-tissue CID analysis, and a representative MALDI spectra of these glycans is shown in Figure 5a. For comparison, a Hex5HexNAc4 (m/z = 1663.6) purified standard (also termed NA2) was spotted on a stainless steel MALDI target plate and fragmented by CID, generating a robust fragmentation pattern of glycans for this ion as previously reported by Harvey et al [28]. The same glycan ion was abundant in pancreatic tissue after PNGaseF release of N-glycans (Figure 3) and was selected for CID. As shown in Figure 5b, the CID fragmentation pattern of m/z 1663.6 in pancreatic tissue was the same as the N-glycan standard, confirming detection of NA2 directly in pancreatic tissue (Figure 3). Mass shifts due to loss of

individual sugar ions were detected, such as Hex (resulting in m/z = 1502.5), HexNAc (resulting in m/z = 1460.5), and Hex + HexNAc (resulting in m/z = 1298.5) (Figure 5b). An ion at m/z = 712.2, which has been previously characterized [28] as the sodium adduct of Hex3HexNAc1, was also detected. The structures of 13 other glycan ions were confirmed using this CID approach, and additional fragmentation data and spectra are provided in Figures S5 & S6.

Glycan MALDI-IMS of a Hepatocellular Carcinoma Tissue Microarray

The ability to perform N-glycan analysis on FFPE tissues potentially enables the analysis of multiple FFPE tissue cores in a TMA format. Initial experiments were performed using a

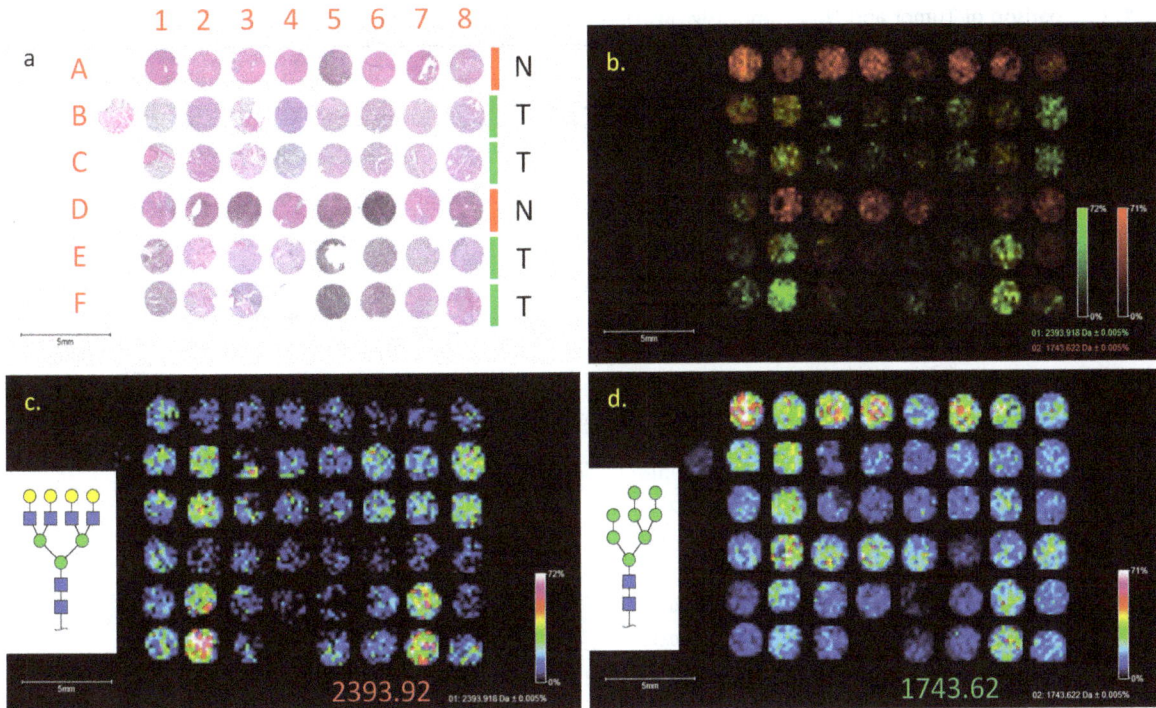

Figure 6. N-Glycan Imaging of a Liver TMA. A liver TMA purchased by BioChain consisting of 2 tumor tissue cores and one normal tissue core from 16 patients was imaged (200 μm raster). The H&E (a) provides the TMA location (red letters and numbers) and classifies whether the row is tumor (green bar) or non-tumor (red bar). M/z = 2393.95 (c) and m/z 1743.64 (d) were able to distinguish between hepatocellular carcinoma and uninvolved liver tissue. An overlay of these ion demonstrates that m/z = 2393.95 is elevated in tumor tissue and m/z = 1743.64 is elevated in normal tissue (b). Statistical data for these two ions is provided in Table 1.

commercially available hepatocellular carcinoma (HCC) TMA (BioChain) consisting of samples from 16 individual patients, with two tumor tissue cores and one non-tumor tissue core per patient (Figure 6). Additional patient data are provided in Table S1. Glycan MALDI-IMS was done as described for the other FFPE tissues, and imaging data for two representative glycan ions at m/z = 2393.92 (Hex7HexNAc6) and m/z = 1743.62 (Hex8HexNAc2) are shown in Figure 6. Analysis of the cumulative MALDI spectra and detected ions for each tissue core were processed and compared using an in-house bioinformatic workflow followed by statistical analysis. Of the 176 identified ions from the HCC TMA, 132 were increased in tumor cores, and 83 ions had a p-value< 0.05. Interestingly 78 (94%) of the significantly different ions were elevated in tumor cores. After cross-referencing this list of 176 ions with glycans presented in this paper and our previous study [21], 26 N-glycans of high-confidence structure determinations were selected, listed in Table 1. Of these 26 known glycans, ion intensities of 13 species were significantly different in tumor and normal tissue (p<0.05), and 21 were increased in tumor relative to normal. FlexImaging was then used to demonstrate the distribution and relative ion intensities of each glycan across the TMA (images provided in Figure S7). Additionally, ROC curves were used to evaluate how well each of the glycan ion intensities discriminates tumor versus non-tumor. Of the 176 identified ions, 61 had area under the ROC curve (AuROC)>0.80, indicating they are strong classifiers. For two glycans at m/z = 2393.95 (Hex7HexNAc6) and m/z = 1743.64 (Hex8HexNAc2), both had an AuROC>0.80 and a p-value<0.05, with m/z 2393.95 being elevated in tumor tissue and m/z 1743.64 being elevated in non-tumor tissue, as demonstrated by the log2-fold change value (tumor/non-tumor) (Figure 6). In the overlay (Figure 6b) tumor

tissue is predominantly green and non-tumor tissue is predominantly red, confirming results from our statistical analysis. This data, although from limited numbers of samples, demonstrates the potential ability of a panel of glycans to be used to accurately discriminate cell types or outcomes on a TMA by MALDI-IMS.

Discussion

Multiple N-linked glycans can be directly profiled from FFPE tissue blocks and TMAs while maintaining intact architecture. The basic methodology, which mirrors that of MALDI-IMS analysis of peptides in FFPE tissues and TMAs [18–20], requires deparaffinization and antigen retrieval prior to PNGaseF application. The ability to adapt the N-glycan imaging method originally designed for fresh/frozen tissues [25] to encompass FFPE tissue and TMA blocks increases the scope and speed of glycan-based studies that can be performed in tissues. In initial studies of formalin-fixed mouse kidney slices, the MALDI-IMS workflow successfully identified all 28 of the glycans in the mouse kidney database provided by the Consortium for Functional Glycomics. Many of the structures of these glycans were verified by permethylation (Figure S2) and CID experiments (Figures S5 & S6). As observed with the mouse brain [25], these glycans were not homogenously present across the entire mouse kidney slice, but were either predominantly located in the cortex, or distributed across the cortex and medulla (Figure S1). This unique distribution of N-glycans associated with tissue sub-structure or disease status was also observed in human pancreas and prostate tissue slices. In the pancreas, an overlay of four different glycans was able to map the normal pancreas tissue, tumor pancreas tissue, a region of desmoplasia, and a necrotic region (Figure 3a). Similarly, an

Table 1. Comparison of Tumor and Non-Tumor Glycans Detected in Hepatocellular Carcinoma Tissue Microarrays.

m/z	AuROC	log2-fold change	p-val
1866.76	0.895	3.045	<.001
2393.95	0.879	1.819	<.001
2378.01	0.869	3.495	<.001
1743.64	0.831	−0.967	<.001
1850.78	0.827	1.953	<.001
1257.42	0.821	0.780	<.001
1501.60	0.813	2.223	0.001
2686.02	0.764	4.316	0.003
1905.71	0.742	−0.572	0.007
1298.44	0.742	0.910	0.007
2012.82	0.734	1.165	0.010
2320.89	0.707	2.146	0.022
2540.03	0.707	1.493	0.022
3271.15	0.657	2.004	0.082
2028.74	0.657	0.360	0.082
1647.62	0.649	0.683	0.099
1581.57	0.635	−0.190	0.135
2174.89	0.633	0.598	0.141
1976.71	0.617	0.398	0.197
2100.77	0.597	0.295	0.266
1954.79	0.593	−0.114	0.307
1419.48	0.577	−0.076	0.400
1809.67	0.548	0.973	0.598
1485.54	0.488	0.149	0.902
1663.66	0.490	0.255	0.920
1282.46	0.494	0.703	0.991

A list of 26 monoisotopic ions that were identified in the HCC TMA were cross-referenced against a library of known glycan m/z values listed in this paper or our previous paper (21). The ability of individual glycan ions to distinguish tumor tissue from non-tumor tissue were assessed using AuROC, log2-fold changes (tumor/non-tumor), and p-values. Localization of m/z = 2393.95 and m/z = 1743.62 (highlighted in yellow) are depicted in Figure 6.

overlay of two glycans could distinguish between prostate stroma and glands (Figure 4).

In general, the peak intensities of PNGaseF-released glycans in the FFPE tissues seems to be more intense than that obtained with fresh/frozen tissue sections. This may be a result of the more extensive heating and washing steps required in the deparaffinization and rehydration steps. It is this increased detection sensitivity that facilitated CID fragmentation of N-glycans directly from the tissue (Figure 5b, Figures S5 & S6). Under the conditions used, CID generated mainly fragments across the glycosidic bonds, which were useful in characterizing that the structure was an intact hexose or HexNAc. This did not provide any information regarding anomeric linkages between sugar residues. The amount of fragmentation observed was directly related to the relative intensity of each parent N-glycan ion, and inversely related to the mass of the parent ion observed. This is typified by the extensive fragmentation of two glycans of m/z = 1663.50 and m/z = 1809.64 (Figure 5b, Figures S5 & S6).

One drawback to using FFPE tissues is residual polymer from the paraffin block adjacent to the tissue. Detection of this polymer is more predominant in the lower mass range of the imaging runs, and can overlap with potential glycan masses, complicating detection and further statistical analysis. This polymer can be observed in the average spectra of the mouse kidney tissue after PNGase application (Figure 2a) from m/z = 1250–1300, 1450–1500, and 1650–1700. An additional key to distinguishing polymer peaks is the analysis of spectra from the non-PNGaseF treated control tissues. Particularly for the TMA format, the ion selection program that we report can detect and account for polymer peaks relative to glycan ions. These polymer peaks seem to vary in terms of intensity compared to N-glycan ions depending on what tissue is being used. It is possible that this variation is a function of different formalin formulations, variations is tissue processing (i.e. amount of time in formalin), storage time or variations in the tissue itself [1,2]. These considerations will be further monitored and evaluated as more glycans from FFPE tissues are analyzed.

In relation to potential cancer diagnostic applications, the most significant aspect to developing a method to image N-glycans on FFPE tissue blocks could be the ability to use TMAs for high-throughput glycan-based experiments. Not only does the method increase the number of tumor samples that can be analyzed in one experiment, but it could also be used to compare the glycans detected in a TMA core versus the larger source FFPE tissue. N-glycan MALDI-IMS of the HCC TMA (Figure 6) is provided as an example, but we have already obtained initial glycan profiling data from TMAs representing prostate, kidney, lung, breast, colon and pancreatic cancers. In the HCC TMA, a statistically significant increase in tetra-antennary N-glycan (m/z = 2393.95) and decrease in Man-8 glycan (m/z = 1743.64) was detected in HCC cores compared to adjacent non-tumor tissue (Figure 6 and Table 1). The tetra-antennary N-glycan has been previously demonstrated to be elevated in HCC compared to matched adjacent non-tumor tissue by Mehta et al. [29]. Continued investigations will be performed on whether these two ions can distinguish between matched HCC and non-tumor tissues in other HCC TMAs. Our data analysis identified a total of 176 ions in the tissue, with the majority of significantly different ions being increased in HCC relative to non-tumor tissue, including 21 known or previously identified glycans. It is unclear how this trend of increased glycan levels relates specifically to tumor related biochemical changes, though the role of glycosylation in tumor development is well documented. Future work will also focus on determining the identity of the remaining ions to distinguish other glycan species from the aforementioned polymer peak contaminants.

Currently, MALDI-IMS provides a new approach to effectively visualize and evaluate N-glycan localization in tissue sections. It does not solve the known limitations of MALDI analysis of underivatized glycans like loss of sialic acids, nor does it provide anomeric linkage information for N-glycan structure. Established tandem mass spectrometry methods of glycan extraction, modification and fragmentation are more capable of providing this structural information. Combining the glycan tissue maps generated by MALDI-IMS to target regions of interest for further tandem mass spectrometry analysis of glycans could be a new synergistic approach to more effectively identify tumor-associated glycans and glycoproteins in situ. Use of other glycosidases like sialidase, as we have previously reported [25], or fucosidases, could further extend the utility of the combined methods. Overall, the ability to effectively profile N-glycans on FFPE tissue blocks and TMAs provides new opportunities to evaluate glycan profiles associated with disease status.

Supporting Information

Figure S1 Panel of Mouse Kidney N-Glycans. Ions detected in the kidney with enzyme application were compared to the control tissue. Ions that were only observed in the tissue following PNGaseF application were compared to the glycans found in the mouse kidney database on the Consortium for

Functional Glycomics. The panel provides the glycan species, the projected mass for the sodium adduct, and our observed mass for the sodium adduct.

Figure S2 Permethylation of Mouse Kidney N-Glycans. Mouse kidney N-glycans were extracted from the imaging slide after PNGaseF application and digestion. Glycans were dried down and underwent permethylation as previously described. The permethylated m/z values were then compared to the permethylation data from the Consortium for Functional Glycomics mouse kidney database (www.functionalglycomics.org).

Figure S3 Panel of Mouse Kidney N-Glycans Linked to Known Glycan Database.

Figure S4 Individual N-Glycans from Prostate Cancer FFPE Tissue. The orange ovals highlight the areas of heterogeneous tumor for high mannose glycans.

Figure S5 CID of N-Glycans from Human Pancreas Tissue I.

Figure S6 CID of N-Glycans from Human Pancreas Tissue II.

Figure S7 Images From Ions Corresponding to N-Glycans. The Ions identified in Table 1 were viewed in FlexImaging Software.

Table S1 Patient Data Summary for Hepatocellular Carcinoma TMA from Biochain.

Author Contributions

Conceived and designed the experiments: TWP BAN DAT ASM BBH RRD. Performed the experiments: TWP BAN YS HYT. Analyzed the data: TWP BAN DAT ASM BBH RRD. Contributed reagents/materials/analysis tools: YS ASM BAH RRD. Contributed to the writing of the manuscript: TWP BAN DAT ASM BBH RRD.

References

1. Thompson SM, Craven RA, Nirmalan NJ, Harnden P, Selby PJ, et al. (2013) Impact of pre-analytical factors on the proteomic analysis of formalin-fixed paraffin-embedded tissue. Proteomics Clin Appl 7; 241–251.

2. Craven RA, Cairns DA, Zougman A, Harnden P, Selby PJ, et al. (2013) Proteomic analysis of formalin-fixed paraffin-embedded renal tissue samples by label-free MS: assessment of overall technical variability and the impact of block age. Proteomics Clin Appl 7; 273–282.

3. Magdeldin S, Yamamoto T (2012) Toward deciphering proteomes of formalin-fixed paraffin-embedded (FFPE) tissues. Proteomics 12: 1045–1058.

4. Wiśniewski JR, Duś K, Mann M (2013) Proteomic workflow for analysis of archival formalin-fixed and paraffin-embedded clinical samples to a depth of 10 000 proteins. Proteomics Clin Appl 7; 225–233.

5. Takikita M, Chung JY, Hewitt SM (2007) Tissue microarrays enabling high-throughput molecular pathology. Curr Opin Biotechnol 18: 318–325.

6. Franco R, Caraglia M, Facchini G, Abbruzzese A, Botti G (2011) The role of tissue microarray in the era of target-based agents. Expert Rev Anticancer Ther 11; 859–869.

7. Hewitt SM (2006) The application of tissue microarrays in the validation of microarray results. Methods Enzymol 410: 400–415.

8. Camp RL, Neumeister V, Rimm DL (2008) A decade of tissue microarrays: progress in the discovery and validation of cancer biomarkers. J Clin Oncol 26; 5630–5637.

9. Ludwig JA, Weinstein JN (2005) Biomarkers in cancer staging, prognosis and treatment selection. Nat Rev Cancer 5; 845–856.

10. Schultz MJ, Swindall AF, Bellis SL (2012) Regulation of the metastatic cell phenotype by sialylated glycans. Cancer Metastasis Rev 31; 501–518.

11. Miwa HE, Song Y, Alvarez R, Cummings RD, Stanley P (2012) The bisecting GlcNAc in cell growth control and tumor progression. Glycoconjugate J 8–9; 609–618.

12. van Cruijsen H, Ruiz MG, van der Valk P, de Gruijl TD, Giaccone G (2009) Tissue micro array analysis of ganglioside N-glycolyl GM3 expression and signal transducer and activator of transcription (STAT)-3 activation in relation to dendritic cell infiltration and microvessel density in non-small cell lung cancer. BMC Cancer 9:180.

13. Chen CY, Jan YH, Juan YH, Yang CJ, Huang MS, et al. (2013) Fucosyltransferase 8 as a functional regulator of nonsmall cell lung cancer. Proc Natl Acad Sci U S A 110; 630–635.

14. Kobayashi M, Nakayama J (2010) Immunohistochemical analysis of carbohydrate antigens in chronic inflammatory gastrointestinal diseases. Methods Enzymol 479; 271–289.

15. Chaurand P, Norris JL, Cornett DS, Mobley JA, Caprioli RM (2006) New developments in profiling and imaging of proteins from tissue sections by MALDI mass spectrometry. J Proteome Res 5; 2889–2900.

16. Cazares LH, Troyer D, Mendrinos S, Lance RA, Nyalwidhe JO, et al. (2009) Imaging mass spectrometry of a specific fragment of mitogen-activated protein

kinase/extracellular signal-regulated kinase kinase kinase 2 discriminates cancer from uninvolved prostate tissue. Clin Cancer Res 15; 5541–5551.

17. Berry KA, Hankin JA, Barkley RM, Spraggins JM, Caprioli RM, et al. (2011) MALDI imaging of lipid biochemistry in tissues by mass spectrometry. Chem Rev 111; 6491–6512.

18. Chaurand P, Cornett DS, Angel PM, Caprioli RM (2011) From whole-body sections down to cellular level, multiscale imaging of phospholipids by MALDI mass spectrometry. Mol Cell Proteomics 10: O110.004259.

19. Castellino S, Groseclose MR, Wagner D (2011) MALDI imaging mass spectrometry: bridging biology and chemistry in drug development. Bioanalysis 3; 2427–2441.

20. Cornett DS, Frappier SL, Caprioli RM (2008) MALDI-FTICR imaging mass spectrometry of drugs and metabolites in tissue. Anal Chem 80; 5648–5653.

21. Nilsson A, Fehniger TE, Gustavsson L, Andersson M, Kenne K, et al. (2010) Fine mapping the spatial distribution and concentration of unlabeled drugs within tissue micro-compartments using imaging mass spectrometry. PLoS One; e11411.

22. Groseclose MR, Massion PP, Chaurand P, Caprioli RM (2008) High-throughput proteomic analysis of formalin-fixed paraffin-embedded tissue microarrays using MALDI imaging mass spectrometry. Proteomics 8 3715–3724.

23. Quaas A, Bahar AS, von Loga K, Seddiqi AS, Singer JM, et al. (2013) MALDI imaging on large-scale tissue microarrays identifies molecular features associated with tumour phenotype in oesophageal cancer. Histopathology 63; 455–462.

24. Casadonte R, Caprioli RM (2011) Proteomic analysis of formalin-fixed paraffin-embedded tissue by MALDI imaging mass spectrometry. Nat Protoc 6; 1695–1709.

25. Powers TW, Jones EE, Betesh LR, Romano PR, Gao P, et al. (2013) Matrix assisted laser desorption ionization imaging mass spectrometry workflow for spatial profiling analysis of N-linked glycan expression in tissues. Anal Chem 85; 9799–9806.

26. Ceroni A, Maass K, Geyer H, Geyer R, Dell A, et al. (2008) GlycoWorkbench: A Tool for the Computer-Assisted Annotation of Mass Spectra of Glycans, J Proteome Res 7; 1650–1659.

27. Shi C, Washington MK, Chaturvedi R, Drosos Y, Revetta FL, et al. (2014) Fibrogenesis in pancreatic cancer is a dynamic process regulated by macrophage-stellate cell interaction. Lab Invest 94; 409–421.

28. Harvey DJ (2005) Structural determination of N-linked glycans by matrix-assisted laser desorption/ionization and electrospray ionization mass spectrometry. Proteomics 5; 1774–1786.

29. Mehta A, Norton P, Liang H, Comunale MA, Wang M, et al. (2012) Increased levels of tetraantennary N-linked glycan but not core fucosylation are associated with hepatocellular carcinoma tissue. Cancer Epidemiol Biomarkers Prev 21; 925–933.

15

The Transcriptional Profiling of Glycogenes Associated with Hepatocellular Carcinoma Metastasis

Tianhua Liu[1,2], Shu Zhang[1], Jie Chen[1], Kai Jiang[1,2], Qinle Zhang[1,2], Kun Guo[1], Yinkun Liu[1,2]*

1 Liver Cancer Institute, Zhongshan Hospital, Fudan University, Shanghai, People's Republic of China, **2** Cancer Research Center, Institute of Biomedical Science, Fudan University, Shanghai, People's Republic of China

Abstract

Background and objective: Metastasis is one of the important reasons for the poor prognosis of hepatocellular carcinoma (HCC), abnormal glycosylation plays a pivotal role in HCC metastasis. The goal of this study was to screen and validate the transcriptional profiling of glycogenes associated with HCC metastasis.

Methodology: The differentially transcribed glycogenes were screened out by the Human Glycosylation RT^2 Profiler PCR Array, and were identified by qRT-PCR in human HCC cell lines and their orthotopic xenograft tumors. Further analyses were performed with *K-mean* clustering, Gene Ontology (GO) and ingenuity pathways analysis (IPA). Four differentially transcribed glycogenes were validated in clinical cancer specimens by qRT-PCR.

Results: A total of thirty-three differentially transcribed glycogenes were obtained by comparison the transcription in the metastatic human HCC cell lines (MHCC97L, MHCC97H and HCCLM3) with the transcription in the non-metastatic HCC cell line Hep3B. Seven differentially transcribed glycogenes were selected to further identification in human HCC cell lines and their orthotopic xenograft tumors. According to their trends by *K-mean* clustering, all of the differentially transcribed glycogenes were classified in six clusters. GO analysis of the differentially transcribed glycogenes described them in biological process, subcellular location and molecular function. Furthermore, the partial regulatory network of the differentially transcribed glycogenes was acquired through the IPA. The transcription levels of *galnt3*, *gcnt3*, *man1a1*, *mgat5b* in non-metastatic and metastatic HCC clinical cancer specimens showed the same changing trends with the results in human HCC cell lines and their orthotopic xenograft tumors, and the divergent transcription levels of *gcnt3* and *mgat5b* were statistically significant.

Conclusions: The transcriptional profiling of glycogenes associated with HCC metastasis was obtained and validated in this study and it might provide novel drug targets and potential biological markers for HCC metastasis.

Editor: Xin-Yuan Guan, The University of Hong Kong, China

Funding: This work was supported by National Basic Research Program of China (973 Program: 2011CB910 604), China National Key Projects for Infectious Diseases (2008ZX 10002-021 and 2008ZX10002-017). The funders had no role in study design, data collection and analysis, decision to publish, or preparation of the manuscript.

Competing Interests: The authors have declared that no competing interests exist.

* Email: liu.yinkun@zs-hospital.sh.cn

Introduction

Hepatocellular carcinoma (HCC), which is the sixth common neoplasm, ranks the third in cancer mortality in the world [1]. 80% of the HCC are mainly found in eastern Asia and sub-Saharan Africa [2]. HCC is a complex process mediated by multiple genes. The risk factors for the development of HCC, which interact and cooperate with each other, could increase the probability of HCC tumorigenesis. Most people suffering from HCC will die within one year after its detection [3]. One reason for the high mortality can in part be attributed to extrahepatic metastasis [4] and the bottleneck in treatment of HCC is to prevent extrahepatic metastasis. The understanding of the gene transcription profiling underlying HCC metastasis will provide us new theoretical basis for HCC diagnosis and treatment.

Glycosylation, which can be found in a variety of physiological and pathological events, is one of the most important kinds of posttranslational modifications. More than 50% of proteins in nature are presumed to have undergone glycosylation [5]. These glycans not only alter the structures and functions of glycoproteins, but also are crucial for cell adhesion and cellular signal transduction. Other than that, aberrant glycosylation also plays a key role in the underlying mechanism of a variety of diseases [6]. Glycans are formed by the catalytic activity of enzymes such as glycosyltransferases and glycosidases. The alterations in transcription and translation levels of enzymes are related to corresponding changes in the glycan branched structures. Currently, studies of the aberrant glycosylation in HCC have been paid much attention and certain achievements have been made. *mgat3* and *mgat5* were proved to be over-expressed in human HCC cell lines, knockdown of *mgat3* could promote cells invasion and increase the resistance to 5-fluorouracil in vitro [7]. However, the silence of *mgat5* in cells could inhibit invasion and increase sensitivity to 5-fluorouracil in vitro. *mgat4a* was vital to tumor migration and metastasis through altering the glycosylation of CD147 [8]. It was also reported that transcription levels of *mgat4b*, and *mgat5* were increased in mice with HCC [9]. Recently, further analysis revealed that *mgat5* could partially decrease cell adhesion and promote cell proliferation through RPTPκ [10].

In this study, we obtained and identified the transcriptional profiling of glycogenes in human HCC cell lines with or without metastasis potential and orthotopic xenograft tumors by PCR Array and qRT-PCR. The differentially transcribed glycogenes were classified and described by *K*-mean clustering and GO analysis, respectively. The possible regulatory network of them was built by the IPA. Furthermore, the differently transcribed glycogenges were validated in clinical cancer specimens by PCR Array. This work might provide the novel potential drug targets and the potential biological markers of HCC.

Materials and Methods

Ethics Statement

Access to human tissues complied with both Chinese laws and the guidelines of the Ethics Committee and this study was approved by the Research Ethics Committee of Zhongshan Hospital and First Affiliated Hospital of Guangxi Medical University. All participants have given written informed consent.

Cell Culture

The Human HCC cell lines with different metastatic potentials (MHCC97L, MHCC97H and HCCLM3) have the same genetic background and were established in our Liver Cancer Institute [11–14]. All of them were cultured in Dulbecco's modified Eagle's (DMEM) medium (Gibco, USA) supplemented with 10% fetal bovine serum (FBS, Gibco, USA). Hep3B, the non-metastatic HCC cell line (ATCC number HB-8065), was generously provided by Cornell University and was cultured in minimum essential medium (MEM) medium (Gibco, USA) supplemented with 10% FBS (Gibco, USA). All of these cells were incubated at 37°C with a 5% CO_2 in air atmosphere.

HCC orthotopic xenograft tumor model in nude mice

The male BALB/C nude mice (5 to 6-week-old) we obtained were from Shanghai Institute of Materia Medica (Chinese Academy of Sciences, Shanghai, China). The orthotopic xenograft tumor models were established as described previously [15–17]. Simply, 1×10^7 Hep3B, MHCC97L, MHCC97H or HCCLM3 cell lines were injected subcutaneously into the upper left flank region of nude mice, respectively. After tumor formation, the tumors were cut into 2 mm×2 mm×2 mm sized pieces. Nude mice that were anaesthetized with pentobarbital 45 mg/kg by intraperitoneal injection after regular disinfection were dissected and then the tumor tissue lumps were implanted into livers of nude mice. The mice were slaughtered at the 35th day after tumor implantation and the orthotopic xenograft tumors were immediately placed in liquid nitrogen. All of the in vivo experiments carried out were strictly complied with the protocol which was approved by the Shanghai Medical Experimental Animal Care Committee (Permit Number: 2009-0082).

Clinical cancer specimens

Fifteen HCC patients under-going resection in 2012 in Zhongshan Hospital, Fudan University (Shanghai, China) and First Affiliated Hospital of Guangxi Medical University (Nanning, China) were enrolled in this study, including ten patients with non-metastatic HCC and five patients with metastatic HCC. All the tissue samples collected from the patients were performed to qRT-PCR analysis. The detailed information of these fifteen patients was described in Table S1.

Table 1. Sequences of qRT-PCR primers.

Glycogene	Primer Sequence
c1galt1	F: 5′-ATGAGTGGAGGAGCAGGATA-3′
	R: 5′-TCTGGCACAAAGGGATGAA-3′
galnt3	F: 5′-CTGCCTCTCCAGGCAACG-3′
	R: 5′-GTAGTACCTGGCGGGTGGG-3′
gcnt3	F: 5′-AGATGTTGAATGGGAGGAATAG-3′
	R: 5′-TGTTGGTTAGGTGTAATGTGTCTC-3′
man1a1	F: 5′-CTCTCAGCCTACTATCTGTCTGG-3′
	R: 5′-CAGTTCCTTCCAATACCACTTT-3′
mgat4a	F: 5′-GCAACGGAAGAACAGGAGTTTC-3′
	R: 5′-AGGTTGGCTACAACACCATGT-3′
mgat5	F: 5′-GCTGCCCCTGTAGGAGAC-3′
	R: 5′-GAATCAAGGACTCGGAGCAT-3′
mgat5b	F: 5′-ATGAGTGGAGGAGCAGGATA-3′
	R: 5′-TCTGGCACAAAGGGATGAA-3′
st3gal1	F: 5′-CACGAATGGCGTTGGTCTAC-3′
	R: 5′-CTCAATCAAAAGGGATGGCA-3′
β-Actin	F: 5′-CATGTACGTTGCTATCCAGGC-3′
	R: 5′-CTCCTTAATGTCACGCACGAT-3′

Table 2. Up-regulated glycogenes in HCC cell lines with different metastatic potentials.

	Gene Symbol	UniGene ID	GeneBank ID	Functional Gene Grouping	Fold Change (MHCC 97L/Hep3B)	Fold Change (MHCC 97H/Hep3B)	Fold Change (HCC LM3/Hep3B)
1	b3gnt3	Hs.657825	NM_014256	N-acetylglucosaminyltransferases	14.32	10.34	10.13
2	b4galt5	Hs.370487	NM_004776	Galactosyltransferases	2.07	2.25	2.99
3	edem1	Hs.224616	NM_014674	Mannosidases	14.12	3.05	2.31
4	edem2	Hs.356273	NM_018217	Mannosidases	2.68	2.48	2.71
5	galnt11	Hs.647109	NM_022087	N-acetylgalactosaminyltransferases	1.80*	2.14	2.39
6	galnt4	Hs.25130	NM_003774	N-acetylgalactosaminyltransferases	3.25	2.03	2.16
7	galnt7	Hs.548088	NM_017423	N-acetylgalactosaminyltransferases	2.38	3.48	5.24
8	gcnt3	Hs.194710	NM_004751	N-acetylglucosaminyltransferases	47.18	41.36	28.84
9	hexa	Hs.604479	NM_000520	Galactosides & Glucosidases & Hexosaminidases	2.50	2.36	2.41
10	man1b1	Hs.279881	NM_016219	Mannosidases	2.27	1.73*	2.33
11	man1c1	Hs.197043	NM_020379	Mannosidases	30.06	11.55	11.47
12	mgat5	Hs.651869	NM_002410	N-acetylglucosaminyltransferases	7.94	4.69	9.85
13	mgat5b	Hs.144531	NM_144677	N-acetylglucosaminyltransferases	240.52	71.51	292.04
14	ogt	Hs.405410	NM_181673	N-acetylglucosaminyltransferases	3.97	2.51	4.00
15	pomgnt1	Hs.525134	NM_017739	N-acetylglucosaminyltransferases	2.25	1.92**	2.30
16	st3gal1	Hs.374257	NM_173344	Sialyltransferases	117.78	91.77	166.57
17	st6galnac1	Hs.105352	NM_018414	Sialyltransferases	280.14	404.50	119.43
18	st8sia4	Hs.308628	NM_175052	Sialyltransferases	288.02	42.52	81.01

Note: Fold Change>2, P≤0.5; *: Fold Change<2, P≤0.5; **: Fold Change<2, P≥0.5.

Table 3. Down-regulated glycogenes in HCC cell lines with different metastatic potentials.

Gene Symbol	UniGene ID	GeneBank ID	Functional Gene Grouping	Fold Change (MHCC 97L/Hep3B)	Fold Change (MHCC 97H/Hep3B)	Fold Change (HCC LM3/Hep3B)
1 a4gnt	Hs.278960	NM_016161	N-acetylglucosaminyltransferases	0.20	0.09	0.17
2 c1galt1	Hs.592180	NM_020156	Galactosyltransferases	0.33	0.45	0.48
3 galnt1	Hs.514806	NM_020474	N-acetylgalactosaminyltransferases	0.38	0.36	0.39
4 galnt12	Hs.47099	NM_024642	N-acetylgalactosaminyltransferases	0.01	0.00	0.01
5 galnt13	Hs.470277	NM_052917	N-acetylgalactosaminyltransferases	0.00	0.00	0.01
6 galnt3	Hs.170986	NM_004482	N-acetylgalactosaminyltransferases	0.01	0.01	0.00
7 galntl1	Hs.21035	NM_020692	N-acetylgalactosaminyltransferases	0.22	0.03	0.04
8 gant4	Hs.272404	NM_016591	N-acetylglucosaminyltransferases	0.06	0.15	0.18
9 man1a1	Hs.102788	NM_005907	Mannosidases	0.14	0.09	0.12
10 man2a2	Hs.116459	NM_006122	Mannosidases	0.63*	0.45	0.27
11 man2b1	Hs.356769	NM_000528	Mannosidases	0.19	0.15	0.11
12 mgat1	Hs.519818	NM_002406	N-acetylglucosaminyltransferases	0.85*	0.49	0.50
13 mgat4a	Hs.177576	NM_012214	N-acetylglucosaminyltransferases	0.01	0.01	0.00
14 st8sia3	Hs.23172	NM_015879	Sialyltransferases	0.01	0.01	0.01
15 uggt2	Hs.193226	NM_020121	Glucosyltransferases	0.34	0.33	0.36

Note: Fold Change<0.5, P≤0.5; *Fold Change>0.5, P≤0.5.

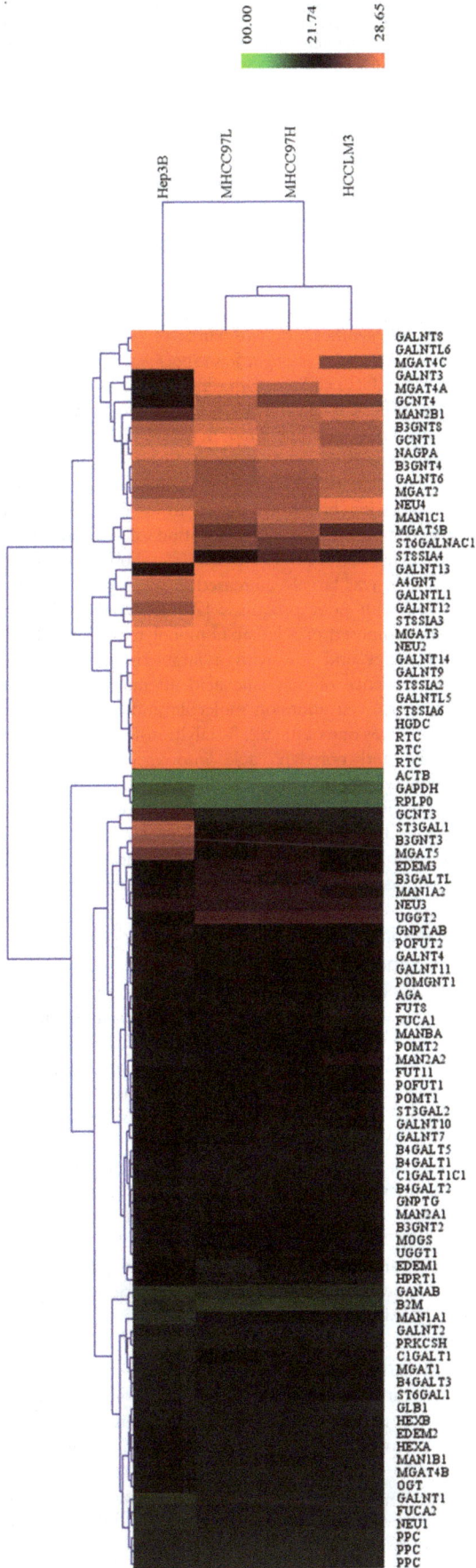

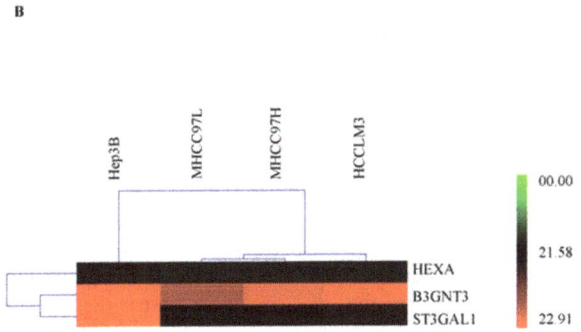

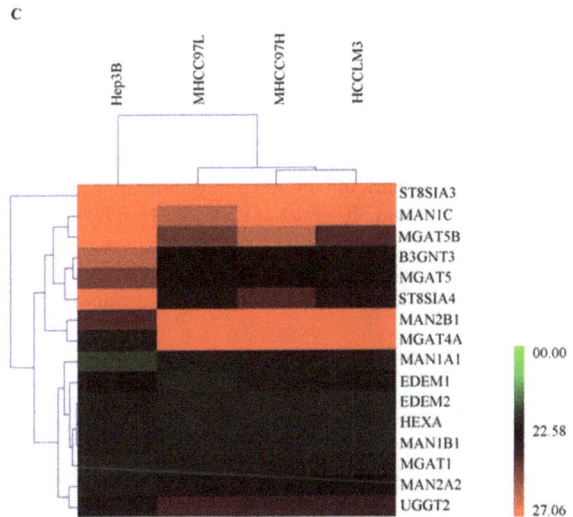

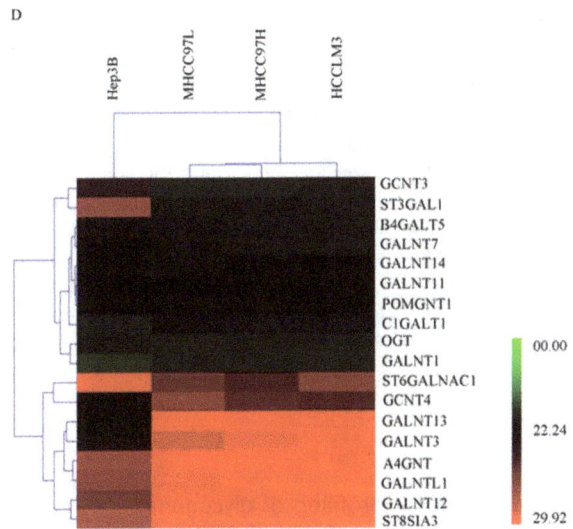

Figure 1. Hierarchical clustering. (A) Hierarchical clustering of 84 glycogenes. Each row represented a single gene; each column represented a cell line. The expression levels of glycogenes, which were the average value of three test results, were shown by the color scale: red represents a target gene with high Ct value while green represents a target gene with low Ct value. (B) Hierarchical clustering of 3 glycogenes acted on glycosphingolipids. (C) Hierarchical clustering of 16 glycogenes generated and altered mature N-linked glycans. (D) Hierarchical clustering of 18 glycogenes generated and altered mature O-linked glycans.

Human Glycosylation PCR Array and qRT-PCR

Total RNA was harvested from cultured cells, orthotopic xenograft tumors and clinical cancer specimens with TRIzol (Invitrogen) and purified with the RNeasy MinElute Cleanup Kit (Qiagen) according to the manufacturer's instruction. After quantification using a Nanodrop spectrophotometer, 10 µg total RNA was reversed transcribed into cDNA using the Revert Aid First Strand cDNA Synthesis Kits (Fermentas), respectively. Besides, cDNA prepared respectively with Super Array PCR master mix (Cat. No. PA-112) was needed in order to perform PCR Array.

The Human Glycosylation RT^2 Profiler PCR Array, including 84 key genes encoding glycan processing enzymes i.e. glycosyl-transferase and glycosidase for several important sugars: galactose, glucose, mannose, N-acetylgalactosamine, N-acetylglucosamine, fucose and sialic acid, was designed and produced by the Qiagen company (German).

The PCR Array and qRT-PCR were performed on IQ5 machine (Bio-Rad) and the PCR cycling condition was set as follows: 95°C for 5 min, 40 cycles of 95°C for 15 s, 60°C for 15 s and 72°C for 20 s. Each test was run three times and the mean was taken to eradicate any discrepancies.

The used primer sequences in qRT-PCR were summarized in Table 1.

Statistical analysis and database searching

Take advantage of the Ct obtained from PCR-Array, the MeV 4.8.1 was used to map the hierarchical clustering of all the glycogenes in the PCR Array, the differentially transcribed glycogenes generated and altered N-linked glycans, O-linked glycans and glycosphingolipids, respectively.

The fold change was normalized to the expression of the housekeeping gene, *β-Actin*, and was calculated respectively for each cell using $2^{-\Delta\Delta Ct}$, where $\Delta\Delta Ct = $ (Ct target gene-*β-Actin*) MHCC97L/MHCC97H/HCCLM3-(Ct target gene-*β-Actin*) Hep3B. Glycogene with differences greater than 2-fold (P≤0.05) was considered as the differentially transcribed glycogenes and they were divided into six clusters by a *K*-means approach, which is a kind of clustering algorithm for grouping genes or proteins with a similar expression pattern [17,18] and the GO was used to describe. IPA (Ingenuity System Inc, USA) is a proof of knowledge based comprehensive software of data analysis that can help researchers model, analyze, and understand the complex biological and chemical systems in life science research [19,20]. The differentially transcribed glycogenes were uploaded to the database to explore regulatory network. In the analysis of validation in clinical cancer specimens, the housekeeping gene *β-Actin* was as the reference and the relative expressions value were expressed by $\Delta Ct = $ Ct target gene-*β-Actin*, which means that the higher value of ΔCt of the glycogene, the lower its transcription level.

Results

The transcriptional profiling of glycogenes

The transcriptional profiling of the 84 glycogenes was obtained by the Human Glycosylation RT^2 Profiler PCR Array and was used to produce a hierarchical clustering scheme (Figure. 1A). A total of thirty-three glycogenes were differentially transcribed. Among them, sixteen glycogenes generated and altered mature N-linked glycans, eighteen glycogenes were concerned in the synthesis and processing of O-linked glycans, three glycogenes acted on glycosphingolipids (Figure 1B–D). Double counting did occur among four glycogenes *b3gnt3, hexa, st3gal1, st8sia3*, which took part in the synthesis of two kinds of glycans. A total of eighteen mRNA, such as *mgat5, st3gal1, st8sia4*, were up-regulated in the HCC cell lines with different metastatic potentials (MHCC97L, MHCC97H and HCCLM3) compared with the non-metastatic HCC cell line Hep3B, while fifteen mRNA like *c1galt1, gcent4, man1a1* were down-regulated (Table 2 and 3). *st3gal1* could mediate the sialylation of T antigen and the increase of *st3gal1* expression had been shown to be one of the major mechanisms responsible for the sialylation of T antigen [21]. Sialyl-T antigen was tumor-associated carbohydrate antigen whose expression was largely increased in some types of cancers and associated with poor prognosis [22]. Polysialic acid was a carbohydrate composed of a linear homopolymer of α2, 8-linked sialic acid residues and was with a large amount of negative charge. The presence of polysialic acid attenuates the adhesive property of neural cell adhesion molecule and increases cellular motility. *st8sia4* was one of the α2, 8-sialyltransferases which could add oligosialic and polysialic acid into various sialylated N-acetyllactosaminyl oligosaccharides [23–25]. Amounts of β-1, 6-GlcNAc branched N-Glycan were commonly increased in malignancies and correlated with disease progression. *mgat5* was required in the biosynthesis of β-1, 6-GlcNAc-branched N-linked glycans attaching to cell surface and secreted glycoproteins.

Identification in human HCC cell lines and their orthotopic xenograft tumors by qRT-PCR

Seven glycogenes: *c1galt1, galnt3, gcnt3, man1a1, mgat4a, mgat5, mgat5b*, were selected to identify the results of the PCR Array by qRT-PCR in human HCC cell lines (Hep3B, MHCC97L, MHCC97H, HCCLM3) and their orthotopic xenograft tumors. The housekeeping gene *β-Actin* was as the reference and normalized the obtained fold changes of differential glycogenes. The results of the human HCC cell lines were shown in Figure 2A, C, E, G, I, K, M, meanwhile the results from the orthotopic xenograft tumors were in Figure 2B, D, F, H, J, L, N. *c1ganlt1, man1a1, mgat4a, galnt3* were all down-regulated whereas *gcnt3, mgat5, mgat5b* were all obviously up-regulated, almost all the transcription levels of the glycogenes had significant difference. These results supported the transcriptional profiling from the PCR Array.

K-mean clustering and GO analysis

The thirty-three differentially transcribed glycogenes were classified in six clusters according to their trends by *K*-means clustering (Figure 3, Table S2). Among these, only *b4galt5, galnt7, galnt11* were up-regulated gradually while *man2a2, mgat1* were down-regulated step by step, which implied that changes of diverse glycogenes transcription had little related with the level of metastatic potentials. GO teams were used to describe three attributes of the differentially transcribed glycogenes

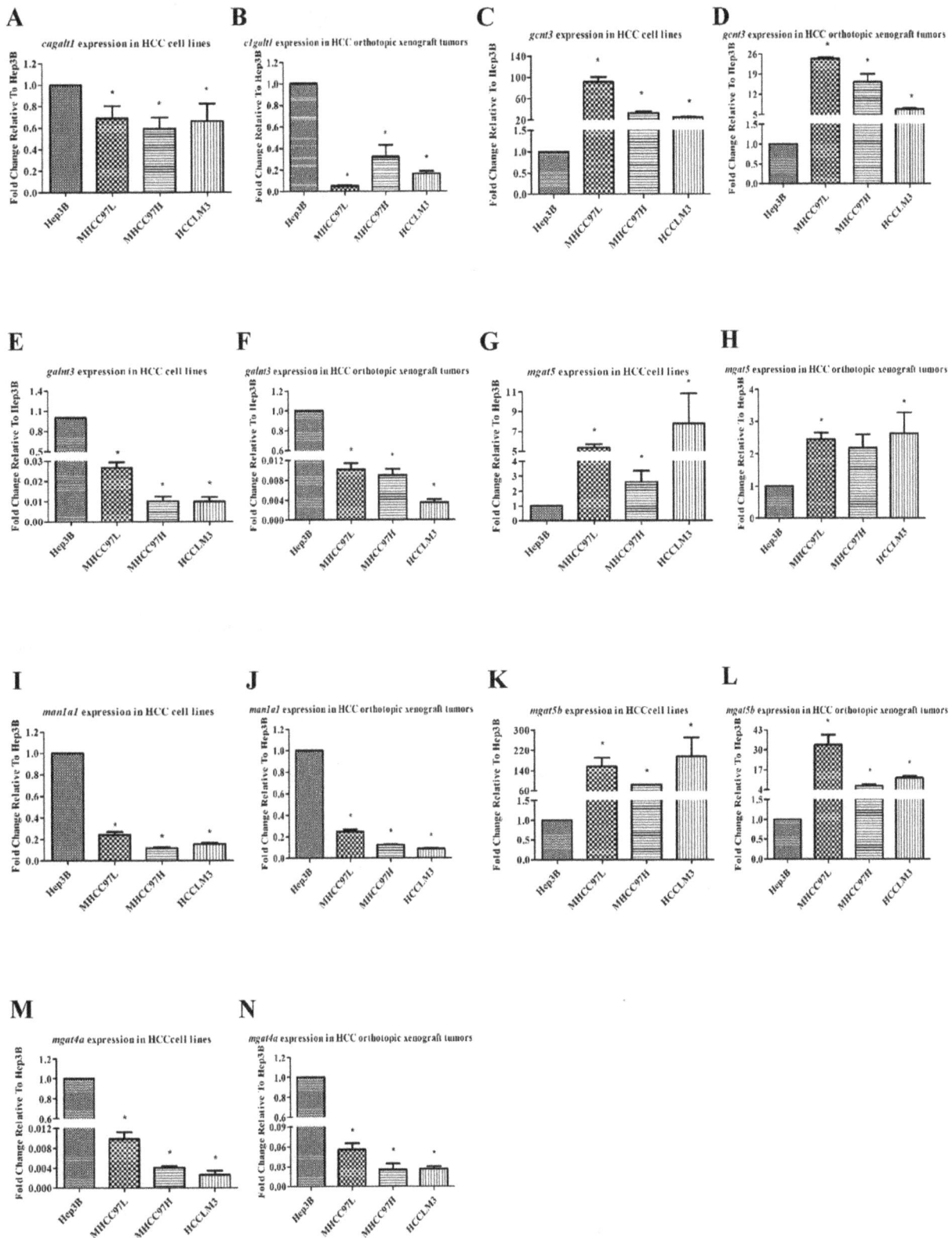

Figure 2. Identification of the differentially transcribed glycogenes in human HCC cell lines and their orthotopic xenograft tumors by qRT-PCR. A, C, E, G, I, K and M were the HCC cell lines with different metastatic potentials (MHCC97L, MHCC97H, HCCLM3) with the comparison to the no-metastatic Hep3B cell line, respectively. B, D, F, H, J, L and N were the orthotopic xenograft tumors of the HCC cell lines MHCC97L, MHCC97H, HCCLM3 comparison to the orthotopic xenograft tumor of the Hep3B cell line. The expression of these glycogenes were normalized against endogenous mRNA of the housekeeping gene, β-Actin.

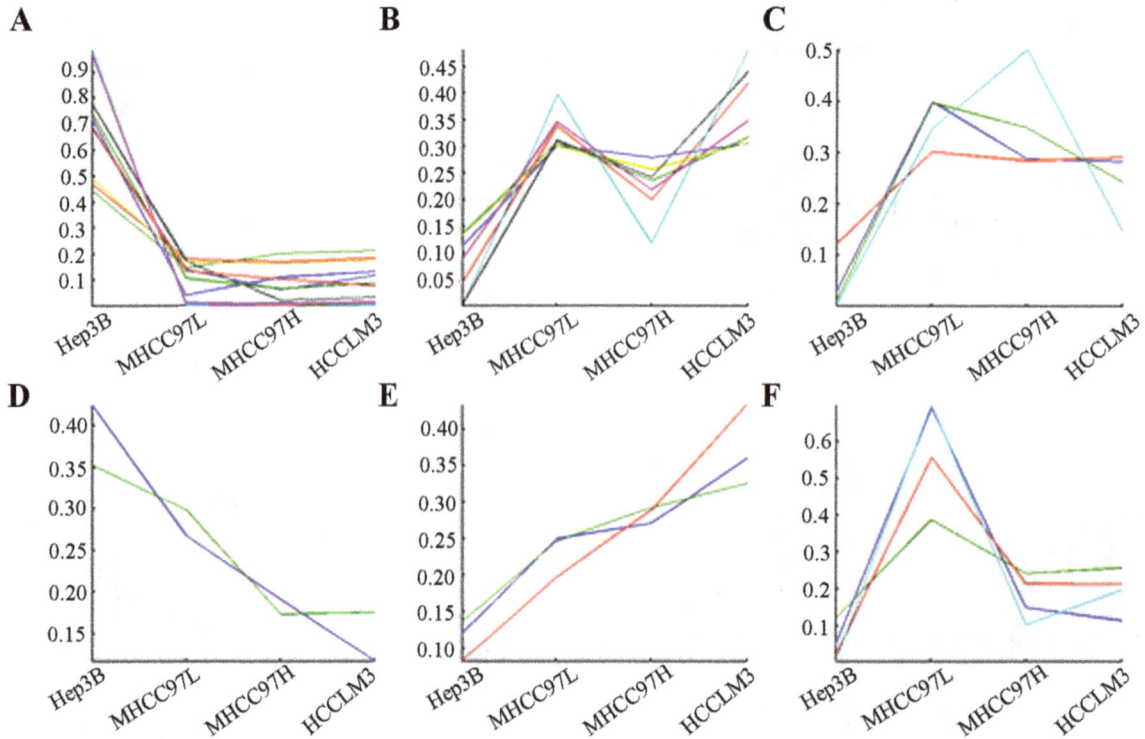

Figure 3. K-means clustering of differentially transcribed glycogenes. Each line represented one differentially transcribed glycogene, the shape of lines displayed the expression trend of the differentially transcribed glycogenes in the no-metastatic HCC cell line Hep3B and the HCC cell lines with different metastatic potentials (MHCC97L, MHCC97H and HCCLM3).

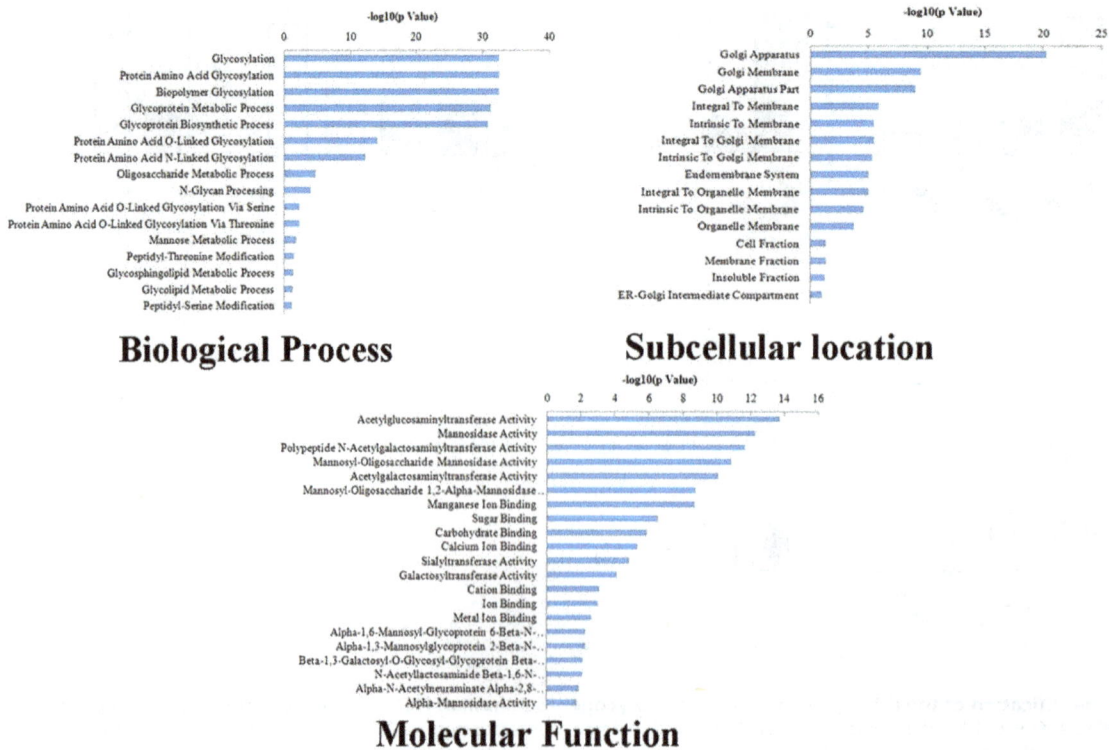

Figure 4. GO analysis of differentially transcribed glycogenes. The differentially transcribed glycogenes were described in 3 categories: biological process, subcellular location, molecular function. GO teams were used to describe three as their attributes of the differentially transcribed glycogenes.

Table 4. Upstream regulators and target molecules in the regulatory network.

Upstream Regulator	EntrezID	Molecule Type	p-value of overlap	Target molecules in dataset
ACSL5	51703	enzyme	0.0246	galnt13
ADCYAP1	116	other	0.0467	galnt7, man1a1
AIRE	326	transcription regulator	0.0023	mgat1, mgat5
BAK1	578	other	0.0416	edem1
CCND1	595	other	0.0418	galnt11, st6galnac1
CLOCK	9575	transcription regulator	0.0186	galnt11, pomgnt1
ETS1	2113	transcription regulator	0.0352	b4galt5, mgat5
ETV4	2118	transcription regulator	0.0416	b4galt5
HIST1H1A	3024	other	0.0003	b4galt5, man2b1, ogt
HIST1H1T	3010	other	0.0003	b4galt5, man2b1, ogt
IDH1	3417	enzyme	0.0416	edem1
KCNIP3	30818	transcription regulator	0.0232	edem1
NCF4	4689	enzyme	0.0146	st3gal1
SDC1	6382	enzyme	0.0117	galnt3
SIRT1	23411	transcription regulator	0.0125	edem1, mgat1
STAT5B	6777	transcription regulator	0.0229	hexa, st8sia4
TFEB	7942	transcription regulator	0.0445	hexa
TMBIM6	7009	other	0.0189	edem1
XBP1	7494	transcription regulator	0.0340	edem1, edem2

(Figure 4). The differentially transcribed glycogenes were closely related with some types of biological process, such as protein amino acid glycosylation, glycoprotein metabolic process, glycoprotein biosynthetic process. The subcellular distributions of these glycogenes were enriched in golgi apparatus, golgi membrane, and so on. They were associated with molecular functions, like acetylglucosaminyltransferase activity, mannosidase activity, polypeptide N-acetylgalactosaminyltransferase activity.

Regulatory network by IPA

All of the thirty-three differentially transcribed glycogenes were uploaded to the database to analyze upstream regulatory events and build the possible regulatory network by the IPA (Figure 5). The molecule type, p-value of overlap and target molecules of the transcription regulators in the regulatory network were described and listed in Table 4. We found that a transcription regulator may control more than one glycogene, such as SIRT1 which can act on edem1 and mgat1. At the same time, it was not difficult to detect that a glycogene may be simultaneously affected by two or more transcription regulators. Instances were described as following: galnt11 was direct regulated by CLOCK, meanwhile it was indirectly regulated by CCND1. Moreover, edem1 was directly influenced by XBP1, KCNIP3 and SIRT1, in the meantime, it was indirectly influenced by TMBIM6, IDH1, BAK1. As expected, results showed that the different transcription regulators tended to have different degree of regulation on glycogene expressions and these influences could be measured by the p-value of overlap. The smaller p-value of overlap there was, the greater influence of the regulation there was. For a given glycogene, which of the transcription regulator(s) had more influence could be discriminated by the p-value of overlap. Like edem1 as a glycogene was influenced by XBP1, SIRT1, TMBIM6, IDH1, BAK1, KCNIP3, nevertheless, KCNIP3 and TMBIM6 play much more important roles. For the seventeen glycogenes in

the regulatory network, NCF4, SDC1, SIRT1, CLOCK, TMBIM6 had smaller p-values and it suggested that they may play more important roles in the transcriptional regulation of the differentially transcribed glycogenes.

Validation in clinical cancer specimens by qRT-PCR

Four differentially transcribed glycogenes, including galnt3, gcnt3, man1a1, mgat5b were selected to detect the expressions in clinical cancer specimens and their results were shown in Figure 6. Although the transcription levels of galnt3 and man1a1 in metastatic HCC clinical cancer specimens were lower than in the non-metastatic ones, there were no significant differences (P = 0.246, P = 0.108, respectively). While the divergent trends of gcnt3 and mgat5b between non-metastatic and metastatic HCC clinical cancer specimens were statistically significant (P = 0.002, P = 0.04, respectively) and they were all up-regulated in metastatic HCC clinical cancer specimens, which trends were as same as in human HCC cell lines and their orthotopic xenograft tumors. gcnt3 (glucosaminyl (N-acetyl) transferase 3, mucin type) is required to form GlcNAcβ1→6Gal/GalNAc (Figure 6E) [26] and mgat5b (mannosyl (α-1,6-)-glycoprotein β-1,6-N-acetyl-glucosaminyltransferase, isozyme B) acts on the GlcNAc β1,2-Manα1-Ser/Thr moiety, forms a 2,6-branched structure in brain O-mannosyl glycan (Figure 6F) [27].

Discussion

A growing number of researches indicated that the structural modifications of cell membrane glycans had correlation with disease progression, metastasis, and poor prognosis [28,29]. Essentially, cancer could be regarded as a molecular disease of cell membrane glycans because cancer cells were characterized by aberrant glycosylation of the surface membrane [30]. Abnormal glycosylation was also highly associated with HCC progression.

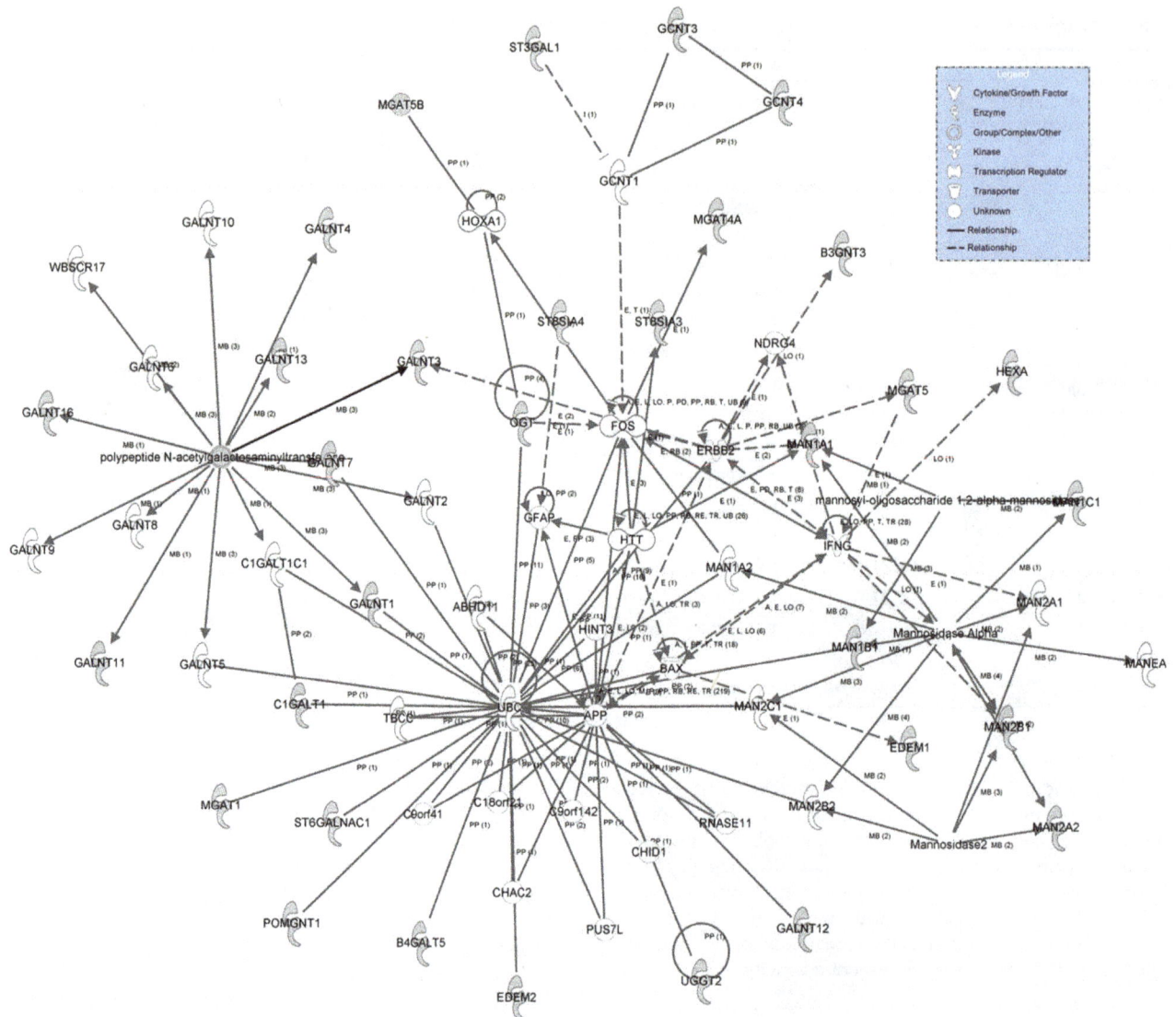

Figure 5. Regulatory network of glycogenes by IPA. The network of glycogenes was derived from the thirty-three differentially transcribed glycogenes. The grey ones represented they were included in the differentially transcribed glycogenes whereas the white ones represented they were not. There were six types of relationship in the network, A: activation, E: expression, M: modification, PD: protein-DNA interaction, PP: protein-protein interaction, T: transcription. Full lines meant a direct action between two nodes, while the dotted lines meant an indirect relationship between two nodes.

The alterations of glycan branched structures of glycoproteins, such as GlcNAc-branched N–glycans, sialic acid and core fucosylation, were demonstrated to be highly expressed in HCC and these changes were closely related to the transcriptional and translational levels of the glycogenes [31–34]. It was generally known that AFP-L3, which was the LCA-bound fraction of AFP, as a new generation of tumor marker for HCC had been widely used in clinic. It had been reported that malignant liver cells produce AFP-L3, even when HCC was at its early stage [34]. In the meantime, *fut8* was known to be a key enzyme of fucosylation and it had been implicated in the production of AFP-L3 [35,36]. This example suggested that some abnormal glycosylation and the differentially transcribed glycogenes might be potential markers of biologic malignancy of HCC and maybe they could be used for identifying subtypes of HCC and elevating the possibility of individual treatment, hence the further research was needed.

In current study, we obtained and validated the transcriptional profiling of glycogenes. This was the first study to select the transcriptional profiling of glycogenes associated with HCC metastasis by PCR Array and it was a comprehensive analysis of glycogenes with relevant N-linked glycosylation, O-Linked glycosylation, glycosphingolipids in human HCC cell lines, orthotopic xenograft tumors and clinical cancer specimens.

The metastatic potential of HCC cell lines in our experiments were strengthening step by step. Hep3B, the non-metastatic cell line from ATCC, was established from a patient of 8-year-old black boy. Nevertheless, MHCC97L, MHCC97H and HCCLM3, all of them can metastasize, whose metastatic potential were increasing in general [35]. The original source of these cell lines was MHCC97 which derived from the LCI20 tumor line (male HCC) and their lung metastatic rate were 40%, 100% and 100%, respectively. The node rate of HCCLM3 was 60% [36]. We found thirty-three differentially transcribed glycogenes by the Human

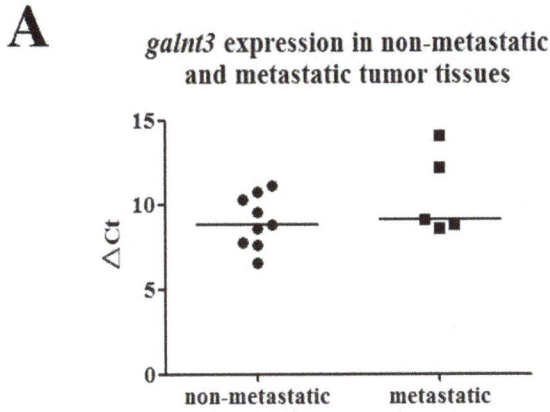

A *galnt3* expression in non-metastatic and metastatic tumor tissues

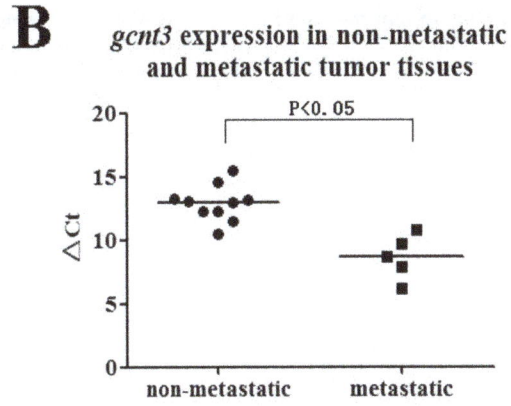

B *gcnt3* expression in non-metastatic and metastatic tumor tissues

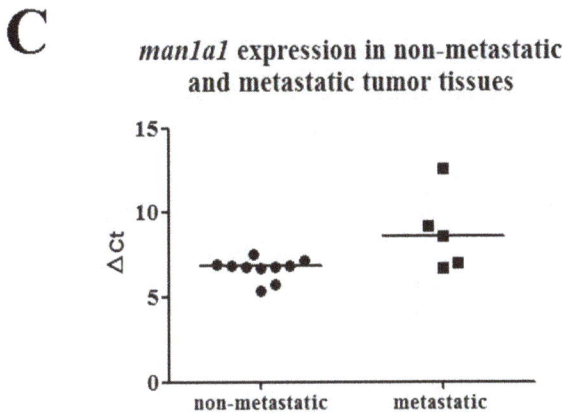

C *man1a1* expression in non-metastatic and metastatic tumor tissues

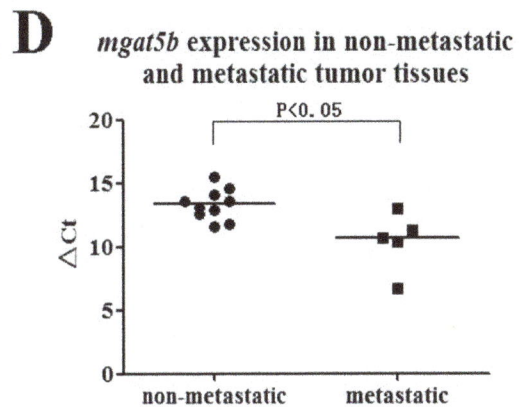

D *mgat5b* expression in non-metastatic and metastatic tumor tissues

E

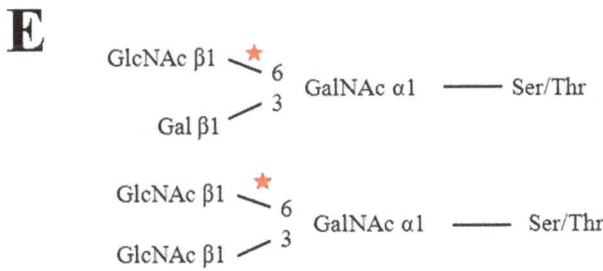

F

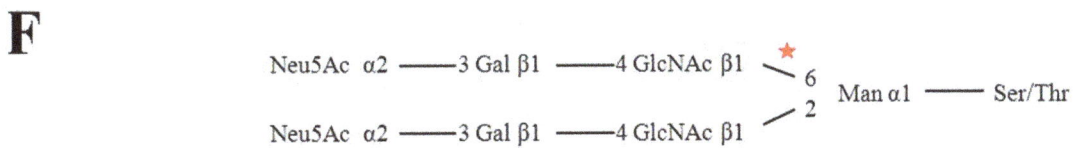

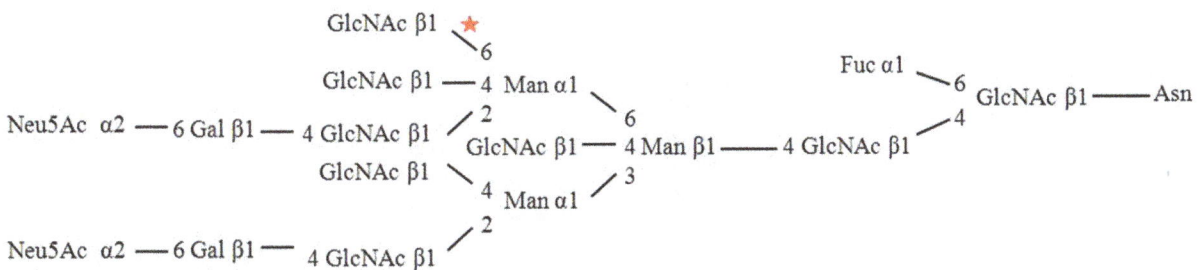

Figure 6. Validation in non-metastatic and metastatic tissue samples by qRT-PCR. A, B, C, D were the transcription levels of *galnt3*, *gcnt3*, *man1a1*, *mgat5b*, respectively. The housekeeping gene, *β-Actin* was used to normalize the expression levels in the subsequent quantitative analyses, and the higher value of ΔCt of the glycogene, the lower its transcription level. E, *gcnt3* involved in the glycan biosynthetic pathways. F, *mgat5b was* correlated with the pathway of glycan biosynthetic.

Glycosylation RT^2 Profiler PCR Array with differences greater than 2-fold (P≤0.05) as a criteria. A glycomics study using glycogene microarray which contained 115 genes by Kang et.al reported eighteen glycogenes were up-regulated in high metastatic potential HCCLM3 cell lines in comparison to Hep3B cell lines, while eleven glycogenes were down-regulated [4]. Guo et.al's study using qRT-PCR for quantification found that six glycogenes *b3galt1, fut8, gal3st2, mgat5, st3gal5 and st6gal1* were overexpressed in MHCC97H cell lines compared with those in MHCC97L cell lines; conversely, five glycogenes, *b3gnt6, b3gnt7, galnt6, mgat3 and st8sia2* were down-regulated [7]. However, Kang et.al only compared the high metastatic potential HCC cell lines HCCLM3 to non-metastasis cell lines Hep3B and Guo et.al only compared two metastasis cell lines (MHCC97L and MHCC97H). Comparisons both of them carried out were between two cell lines, while our results were more confident than theirs with four cell lines to be compared, and all of the differently transcribed glycogenes had been identificated in orthotopic xenograft tumors and validated in clinical cancer specimens. Kang et.al used glycogene microarray, by contrast, we used the PCR-Array. It was cheaper than by gene microarrays and its experimental conditions could be easily controlled [37]. In contrast with Guo et.al's result by qRT-PCR, our findings obtained more differentially transcribed genes. Additionally, apart from the glycogenes which have been reported previously like *mgat1, mgat5 and st3gal1*, some glycogenes such as "UDP-N-acetyl-α-D-galactosamine: polypeptide N-acetylgalactosaminyl-transferase" family members: *galnt3, galnt4, galnt11, galnt13,* and "mannosidase, α class" family members, for instance, *man1b1, man1c1, man2a2*, their different expressions were associated with HCC metastasis are the first reported. This research revealed that glycogenes which could generate and alter sialylated glycan structures or β-1, 6-GlcNAc branched N-Glycan were significantly up-regulated in the metastatic HCC cell lines and their orthotopic xenograft tumors. Sialic acids could prevent cell-cell interactions through charge repulsion effects [38]. Tumor cell lines with more invasive ability expressed more heavily sialylated glycan structures. *mgat5* could advance tumor growth and metastasis by destructing the extracellular matrix or boost the production of angiogenic factors by a metal ion-dependent serine protease. *mgat5* could also promote tumor metastasis by catalyzing sugar chain which can change the function of angiogenic factors or by directly increasing the gene transcription of angiogenic factors [39].

The qRT-PCR analysis of the transcribed glycogenes in the human HCC cell lines and their orthotopic xenograft tumors provided evidences of the same changing trends in statistics (P< 0.05) to support the analysis of PCR-array results. Nevertheless, we found that the respective fold-change value of comparison results within metastatic HCC cell lines and their orthotopic xenograft tumors had no obvious gradually change trend. It revealed that the transcriptional of glycogenes was highly related with metastasis no matter whether their metastatic potentials were high or low. Therefore, we suggested that our future studies about glycosyltransferases should more focus on comparison of whether these cells or orthotopic xenograft tumors were able to metastatic or not rather than the difference of their metastatic potentials.

The regulatory network of part of the differentially transcribed glycogenes was obtained by the IPA, and it included six types of relationship and nineteen upstream regulators. Aside from regulators, current data suggests that miRNA is related with the expressions of glycogenes. Human and rodents HCC cell lines were transfected with miR-122 and miR-34a and the result demonstrated that forced expression of these miRNAs was able to induce a decrease of *fut8* levels and also to affect core fucosylation of secreted proteins [40]. The passenger strand miR-17-3p repressed expression of *galnt7*, which regulates metabolism of liver toxin galactosamine [41]. Further analysis including glycogenes regulation may elucidate the changes of the expressions of glycogenes.

The validation in clinical cancer specimens showed some differences of the transcription levels of glycogenes in clinical tissue samples were not significant. It might be caused by the part of the differences among cell lines, orthotopic xenograft tumors and clinical tissue samples themselves. But it was important to note there were still a substantial part of glycogenes which were differentially transcribed between non-metastatic and metastatic tissues. This evidence suggested there might be some potential novel drug targets and biological markers to predict metastasis of HCC in the differentially transcribed genes. To validate the transcription levels of the remaining differentially transcribed glycogenes, further investigation is needed and this part of the work is undergoing. Moreover, it could not be neglected that our study is the first time to provide evidences in human HCC cell lines, orthotopic xenograft tumors and clinical tissue samples that the up-regulated of *gcnt3* and *mgat5b* were associated with HCC metastasis.

In summary, this study identified thirty-three differentially transcribed glycogenes by the Human Glycosylation RT^2 Profiler PCR Array. A total of seven glycogenes, including *c1galt1, galnt3, gcnt3, man1a1, mgat4b, mgat5, mgat5b*, were further identified by qRT-PCR in HCC cell lines and their orthotopic xenograft tumors. All of these differentially transcribed glycogenes were analyzed by *K*-means and GO analysis, and were uploaded to the IPA database for regulatory network analysis. What was more, *galnt3, gcnt3, man1a1* and *mgat5b* were selected to further validation in clinical cancer specimens and this is the first report that the up-regulated of *gcnt3* and *mgat5b* were associated with HCC metastasis. The differentially transcribed glycogenes could be the potential targets for the novel drugs and might act as the potential biological markers to predict metastasis of HCC.

Supporting Information

Table S1 General information of non-metastatic and metastatic HCC patients.

Table S2 The K-means class of the differentially expression glycogenes.

Author Contributions

Conceived and designed the experiments: YKL. Performed the experiments: THL. Analyzed the data: KG THL. Contributed reagents/

materials/analysis tools: SZ JC QLZ KJ. Contributed to the writing of the manuscript: THL.

References

1. Ferlay J, Shin HR, Bray F, Forman D, Mathers C, et al. (2010) Estimates of worldwide burden of cancer in 2008: GLOBOCAN 2008. Int J Cancer 127: 2893–2917.
2. El-Serag HB (2011) Hepatocellular carcinoma. N Engl J Med 365: 1118–1127.
3. Zhang JY (2007) Mini-array of multiple tumor-associated antigens to enhance autoantibody detection for immunodiagnosis of hepatocellular carcinoma. Autoimmun Rev 6: 143–148.
4. Kang X, Wang N, Pei C, Sun L, Sun R, et al. (2012) Glycan-related gene expression signatures in human metastatic hepatocellular carcinoma cells. Exp Ther Med 3: 415–422.
5. Apweiler R, Hermjakob H, Sharon N (1999) On the frequency of protein glycosylation, as deduced from analysis of the SWISS-PROT database. Biochim Biophys Acta 1473: 4–8.
6. Taniguchi N, Korekane H (2011) Branched N-glycans and their implications for cell adhesion, signaling and clinical applications for cancer biomarkers and in therapeutics. BMB Rep 44: 772–781.
7. Guo R, Cheng L, Zhao Y, Zhang J, Liu C, et al. (2013) Glycogenes mediate the invasive properties and chemosensitivity of human hepatocarcinoma cells. Int J Biochem Cell Biol 45: 347–358.
8. Fan J, Wang S, Yu S, He J, Zheng W, et al. (2012) N-acetylglucosaminyltransferase IVa regulates metastatic potential of mouse hepatocarcinoma cells through glycosylation of CD147. Glycoconj J 29: 323–334.
9. Blomme B, Heindryckx F, Stassen JM, Geerts A, Colle I, et al. (2013) Serum protein N-glycan alterations of diethylnitrosamine-induced hepatocellular carcinoma mice and their evolution after inhibition of the placental growth factor. Mol Cell Biochem 372: 199–210.
10. Wang C, Li Z, Yang Z, Zhao H, Yang Y, et al. (2010) The effect of receptor protein tyrosine phosphatase kappa on the change of cell adhesion and proliferation induced by N-acetylglucosaminyltransferase V. J Cell Biochem 109: 113–123.
11. Li Y, Tang ZY, Ye SL, Liu YK, Chen J, et al. (2001) Establishment of cell clones with different metastatic potential from the metastatic hepatocellular carcinoma cell line MHCC97. World J Gastroenterol 7: 630–636.
12. Li Y, Tang Y, Ye L, Liu B, Liu K, et al. (2003) Establishment of a hepatocellular carcinoma cell line with unique metastatic characteristics through in vivo selection and screening for metastasis-related genes through cDNA microarray. J Cancer Res Clin Oncol 129: 43–51.
13. Zhou Z, Deng H, Yan W, Luo M, Tu W, et al. (2014) AEG-1 promotes anoikis resistance and orientation chemotaxis in hepatocellular carcinoma cells. PLoS One 9: e100372.
14. Li X, Jiang J, Zhao X, Wang J, Han H, et al. (2013) N-glycoproteome analysis of the secretome of human metastatic hepatocellular carcinoma cell lines combining hydrazide chemistry, HILIC enrichment and mass spectrometry. PLoS One 8: e81921.
15. Sun FX, Tang ZY, Lui KD, Ye SL, Xue Q, et al. (1996) Establishment of a metastatic model of human hepatocellular carcinoma in nude mice via orthotopic implantation of histologically intact tissues. Int J Cancer 66: 239–243.
16. Sun C, Sun L, Jiang K, Gao DM, Kang XN, et al. (2013) NANOG promotes liver cancer cell invasion by inducing epithelial-mesenchymal transition through NODAL/SMAD3 signaling pathway. Int J Biochem Cell Biol 45: 1099–1108.
17. Wang C, Guo K, Gao D, Kang X, Jiang K, et al. (2011) Identification of transaldolase as a novel serum biomarker for hepatocellular carcinoma metastasis using xenografted mouse model and clinic samples. Cancer Lett 313: 154–166.
18. Yu Y, Shen H, Yu H, Zhong F, Zhang Y, et al. (2011) Systematic proteomic analysis of human hepotacellular carcinoma cells reveals molecular pathways and networks involved in metastasis. Mol Biosyst 7: 1908–1916.
19. Nehme A, Lobenhofer EK, Stamer WD, Edelman JL (2009) Glucocorticoids with different chemical structures but similar glucocorticoid receptor potency regulate subsets of common and unique genes in human trabecular meshwork cells. BMC Med Genomics 2: 58.
20. Lv H, Liu L, Zhang Y, Song T, Lu J, et al. (2010) Ingenuity pathways analysis of urine metabonomics phenotypes toxicity of gentamicin in multiple organs. Mol Biosyst 6: 2056–2067.
21. Brockhausen I (1999) Pathways of O-glycan biosynthesis in cancer cells. Biochim Biophys Acta 1473: 67–95.
22. Videira PA, Correia M, Malagolini N, Crespo HJ, Ligeiro D, et al. (2009) ST3Gal.I sialyltransferase relevance in bladder cancer tissues and cell lines. BMC Cancer 9: 357.
23. Tanaka F, Otake Y, Nakagawa T, Kawano Y, Miyahara R, et al. (2001) Prognostic significance of polysialic acid expression in resected non-small cell lung cancer. Cancer Res 61: 1666–1670.
24. Rutishauser U, Landmesser L (1996) Polysialic acid in the vertebrate nervous system: a promoter of plasticity in cell-cell interactions. Trends Neurosci 19: 422–427.
25. Angata K, Suzuki M, McAuliffe J, Ding Y, Hindsgaul O, et al. (2000) Differential biosynthesis of polysialic acid on neural cell adhesion molecule (NCAM) and oligosaccharide acceptors by three distinct alpha 2,8-sialyltransferases, ST8Sia IV (PST), ST8Sia II (STX), and ST8Sia III. J Biol Chem 275: 18594–18601.
26. Gonzalez-Vallinas M, Molina S, Vicente G, Zarza V, Martin-Hernandez R, et al. (2014) Expression of microRNA-15b and the glycosyltransferase GCNT3 correlates with antitumor efficacy of Rosemary diterpenes in colon and pancreatic cancer. PLoS One 9: e98556.
27. Inamori K, Endo T, Gu J, Matsuo I, Ito Y, et al. (2004) N-Acetylglucosaminyltransferase IX acts on the GlcNAc beta 1,2-Man alpha 1-Ser/Thr moiety, forming a 2,6-branched structure in brain O-mannosyl glycan. J Biol Chem 279: 2337–2340.
28. Yamamoto E, Ino K, Miyoshi E, Shibata K, Takahashi N, et al. (2007) Expression of N-acetylglucosaminyltransferase V in endometrial cancer correlates with poor prognosis. Br J Cancer 97: 1538–1544.
29. Handerson T, Camp R, Harigopal M, Rimm D, Pawelek J (2005) Beta1,6-branched oligosaccharides are increased in lymph node metastases and predict poor outcome in breast carcinoma. Clin Cancer Res 11: 2969–2973.
30. Hakomori S (1989) Aberrant glycosylation in tumors and tumor-associated carbohydrate antigens. Adv Cancer Res 52: 257–331.
31. Ang IL, Poon TC, Lai PB, Chan AT, Ngai SM, et al. (2006) Study of serum haptoglobin and its glycoforms in the diagnosis of hepatocellular carcinoma: a glycoproteomic approach. J Proteome Res 5: 2691–2700.
32. Yamashita K, Koide N, Endo T, Iwaki Y, Kobata A (1989) Altered glycosylation of serum transferrin of patients with hepatocellular carcinoma. J Biol Chem 264: 2415–2423.
33. Chen GQ, Zhang Q, Xu YF, Zhang WZ, Guan M, et al. (2003) Changes of alkaline phosphatase sugar chains in hepatocellular carcinoma tissue. Zhonghua Gan Zang Bing Za Zhi 11: 739–741.
34. Pettersen I, Andersen JH, Bjornland K, Mathisen O, Bremnes R, et al. (2003) Heterogeneity in gamma-glutamyltransferase mRNA expression and glycan structures. Search for tumor-specific variants in human liver metastases and colon carcinoma cells. Biochim Biophys Acta 1648: 210–218.
35. Li Y, Tian B, Yang J, Zhao L, Wu X, et al. (2004) Stepwise metastatic human hepatocellular carcinoma cell model system with multiple metastatic potentials established through consecutive in vivo selection and studies on metastatic characteristics. J Cancer Res Clin Oncol 130: 460–468.
36. Tian J, Tang ZY, Ye SL, Liu YK, Lin ZY, et al. (1999) New human hepatocellular carcinoma (HCC) cell line with highly metastatic potential (MHCC97) and its expressions of the factors associated with metastasis. Br J Cancer 81: 814–821.
37. Kurokawa Y, Matoba R, Nakamori S, Takemasa I, Nagano H, et al. (2004) PCR-array gene expression profiling of hepatocellular carcinoma. J Exp Clin Cancer Res 23: 135–141.
38. Dall'Olio F, Chiricolo M (2001) Sialyltransferases in cancer. Glycoconj J 18: 841–850.
39. Qi JJ, Wang LY, ZHA XL (2011) Functional mechanisms of N-acetylglucosaminyltransferase V. in oncogenesis and tumor metastasis. CHEMISTRY OF LIFE 625–629.
40. Bernardi C, Soffientini U, Piacente F, Tonetti MG (2013) Effects of microRNAs on fucosyltransferase 8 (FUT8) expression in hepatocarcinoma cells. PLoS One 8: e76540.
41. Shan SW, Fang L, Shatseva T, Rutnam ZJ, Yang X, et al. (2013) Mature miR-17-5p and passenger miR-17-3p induce hepatocellular carcinoma by targeting PTEN, GalNT7 and vimentin in different signal pathways. J Cell Sci 126: 1517–1530.

16

CAV1 Promotes HCC Cell Progression and Metastasis through Wnt/β-Catenin Pathway

Hongxiu Yu[1], Huali Shen[1], Yang Zhang[1], Fan Zhong[1], Yinkun Liu[1,2], Lunxiu Qin[1,2], Pengyuan Yang[1,3]*

1 Institutes of Biomedical Sciences of Shanghai Medical School, Fudan University, Shanghai, P. R. China, **2** Zhongshan Hospital, Fudan University, Shanghai, P. R. China, **3** Department of Chemistry, Fudan University, Shanghai, P. R. China

Abstract

Caveolin-1 (CAV1) has significant roles in many primary tumors and metastasis, despite the fact that malignant cells from different cancer types have different profiles of CAV1 expression. There is little information concerning CAV1 expression and role in hepatocellular carcinoma (HCC) progresion and metastasis. The role of CAV1 in HCC progression was explored in this study. We reported that CAV1 was overexpressed in highly invasive HCC cell lines compared with poorly invasive ones. The immunohistochemical staining was obviously stronger in metastatic HCC samples than in the non-metastatic specimens via tissue microarrays. Furthermore, CAV1 overexpression enhanced HCC cell invasiveness *in vitro*, and promoted tumorigenicity and lung metastasis *in vivo*. By contrast, CAV1 stable knockdown markedly reduced these malignant behaviors. Importantly, we found that CAV1 could induce EMT process through Wnt/β-catenin pathway to promote HCC metastasis. We also identify MMP-7 as a novel downstream target of CAV1. We have determined that CAV1 acts as a mediator between hyperactive ERK1/2 signaling and regulation of MMP-7 transcription. Together, these studies mechanistically show a previously unrecognized interplay between CAV1, EMT, ERK1/2 and MMP-7 that is likely significant in the progression of HCC toward metastasis.

Editor: Yick-Pang Ching, The University of Hong Kong, Hong Kong

Funding: This work was supported in part by Natural Science Foundation of Shanghai (11ZR1403800), National Key Basic Research Program of China (2013CB910502), National Natural Science Foundation of China (81201534), National Science and Technology Major Project (2012ZX10002012-006) and Shanghai Pujiang Program. The funders had no role in study design, data collection and analysis, decision to publish, or preparation of the manuscript.

Competing Interests: The authors have declared that no competing interests exist.

* Email: pyyang@fudan.edu.cn

Introduction

Hepatocellular carcinoma (HCC) is one of the most common and aggressive human malignancies, and like other tumors, how HCC invade and spread remains a mysterious [1]. There are a number of genes found to play important roles in HCC malignance and metastasis, including Caveolin-1 (CAV1). CAV1 is the main component of caveolae membrane structures, and has been implicated in diverse human cancers. The function of CAV1 in cancer is reported to be cancer type- and stage-dependent [2,3]. In HCC, stepwise increase in CAV1 expression during hepatocellular carcinogenesis has been reported [4]. Increased expression of CAV1 was associated with metastasis and with a worse prognosis of HCC [5,6]. CAV1 expression correlates positively with vascular endothelial growth factor (VEGF), microvessel density (MVD) and unpaired artery (UA) [6,7]. These results suggest that CAV1 may play an important role in the progression of HCC.

However, few reports gave some evidences that CAV1 could be considered as an tumor suppressor and anti-metastatic effector in HCC, for example, Yan et al reported that CAV1 expression is significantly decreased in hepatitis B virus (HBV)-infected HCC tissues and reversely correlates with HCC tumor progression [8]. Yang et al also reported that CAV1 may play a tumour-suppressive role in HCC [9]. CAV1's function as a tumor suppressor or promoter in HCC is still debated. CAV1 inhibits metastatic potential in melanomas through suppression of the integrin/Src/FAK signaling pathway in melanoma has been reported [10]. These observations do not provide clear evidence about the role of CAV1 in HCC progression.

In present study, we aimed to identify the expression status of CAV1 in HCC cell lines and tumor samples, in order to investigate the changes of CAV1 expression in HCC progression. CAV1 expression was examined in a panel of human HCC cell lines using western blotting analysis and quantitative RT-PCR and human tissues by immunohistochemistry. To investigate the functions of CAV1 in HCC metastasis, CAV1 overexpressing and knockdown stable clones were established in HCC cells. It's *in vitro* cellular effects and tumourigenicity and metastatic potential *in vivo* were examined. We complemented these descriptive analyses by studying its molecular mechanisms behind the increase in the motility and invasion.

Materials and Methods

Cell Culture

Cell-lines were cultured at 37°C in 5% CO_2 in Dulbeccos modified Eagle medium (DMEM)(Gibco, U.S.A) supplemented with 10% fetal bovine serum (FBS, Life Technologies) in a 5% CO_2-humidified chamber.

Extraction of RNA and Quantitative Real-time RT-PCR

Total RNA was extracted using Trizol solution (Invitrogen) according to the protocols recommended by the manufacturer.

RNAase-free DNase I was used to remove DNA contamination. The total RNA concentration and quantity were assessed by absorbance at 260 nm, using a DNA/Protein Analyzer (Nano-DROP2000C; Thermo). Reverse transcription was performed on 5 μg of total RNA with an ologo(dT) primer.

To perform quantitative analysis of the expression of the CAV1 gene in cell lines, the relative mRNA level of CAV1 was measured by quantitative real-time RT-PCR, using the ABI 7500 Detection System and SYBR green dye (TaKaRa), according to the protocols recommended by the manufacturer. The following primers were used to amplify a 144-bp PCR product for CAV1: forward, 5′- GCAACATCTACAAGCCCA -3′; reverse, 5′-CTTCAAAGTCAA TCTTGACCAC-3′. The following primers were used to amplify E-cadherin: forward, 5′- GACCGGTG-CAATCTTCAAA -3′; reverse, 5′-TTGACGCCGAGAGCTA-CAC-3′. The following primers were used to amplify Vimetin: forward, 5′-ATTCCAC TTTGCGTTCAAGG-3′; reverse, 5′-CTTCAGAGAGAGGAAGCCGA-3′. The following primers were used to amplify TWIST: forward, 5′- TCCATTTTCTC CTTCTCTGGAA -3′; reverse, 5′-GTCCGCGTCCCACTAGC -3′. A housekeeping gene, 18S RNA, was used as an endogenous control. The following primers were used to amplify 18S RNA: forward, 5′-CAGCCACCCGAGATTGAGCA-3′; reverse: 5′-TAGTAGCGACGGGCG GTGTG-3′. Measurements were repeated at least 3 times to ensure the reproducibility of the results.

Preparation of stable CAV1-expressing cells

To construct CAV1 recombinant adenovirus vector, full length CAV1 cDNA was amplified by PCR from HCCLM3 cells cDNA. The primers were as follows: forward, 5′-GAATTCATGTCT-GGGGGGC-3′; reverse, 5′- GTCGACTTATATTTC TTTCT-GC-3′. After digestion with *ECORI* and *Sal I*, the PCR product was inserted into the pBABE-Puro vector. After verified by sequencing, lentivirus production and transduction Virus was produced by triple transfection of pBABE-CAV1, VSVG and GAG into 293T cells using Lipofectamine 2000 (Invitrogen). Five hours after transfection, the medium was changed to DMEM containing 10% FBS. The medium was harvested 48 hours after transfection. HepG2 was infected by overnight incubation with medium containing the pBABE-CAV1 retrovirus and 8 ug/ml of Polybrene (Sigma). Stable pools were selected with 2 ug/ml puromycin (Sigma) for 7 days. Cells were stably transfected with pBABE-GFP as control.

Construction and Transfection of Lentivial Vectors with Specific shRNAs for CAV1

For the construction of the RNAi plasmid, the oligonucleotides for the double-stranded shRNA were inserted into the expression plasmid pLKO.1 (Sigma). The oligonucleotides for shRNA were synthesized as follows: shRNA-1, forward, CCGGGACCCAC-TCTTTGAAGCTGTTCTCGAGAACAGCTTCAAAGAGTG-GGTCTTTTTG; shRNA-1, reverse, AATTCAAAAAGACC-CACTCTTTGAAGCTGTT CTCGAGAACAGCTTCAAA-GAGTGGGTC, shRNA-2, forward, CCGGGACCCTAAA-CACCTCAACGATCTCGAGATCGTTGAGGTGTTTAGGG-TCTTTTTG, shRNA-2, reverse, AATTCAAAAAGACCC-TAAACACCTCAACGAT CTCGAGATCGTTGAGGTGTT-TAGGGT for pLKO.1 CAV1; The negative control oligos served as the nonspecific control. To generate lentiviral particles, the desired plasmid and lentiviral packaging plasmids psPAX2 and pMD2. G (Sigma) were transfected into 293 T cells using FuGENE 6 (Roche, Germany). Medium was changed 24 hours after transfection and viral particles were harvested twice over the next 72 hours. Cells were infected with the lentiviral supernatant

for 24 hours in the presence of 8 μg/ml of Polybrene (Sigma). Infected MHCC97-H and HCCLM3 cells were selected by addition of 5 μg/ml puromycin (Sigma).

Tissue Microarray (TMA) Construction

TMA was constructed from 96 human HCCs to test CAV1 expression. The TMA contains 48 patients with metastatic HCC whose primary HCC lesions were accompanied by intrahepatic spreading, which had been regarded as the most frequently metastatic site of HCC, in portal vein, hepatic vein, or bile duct, and 48 patients who had only solitary HCC without metastases. Both staining intensity and percentage of positive cells were scored by two experienced pathologists. This TMA was constructed by a standard method from patients who underwent curative resection at the Liver Cancer Institute and Zhongshan Hospital (Fudan University, Shanghai, China). Ethical approval from Fudan University (Shanghai, PR China) Research Ethics Committee was obtained. The original tissues had been fixed in 4% buffered formalin and paraffin embedded according to routine procedures. New hematoxylin and eosin-stained slides from each case were performed for review and selection of the most representative areas. Briefly, for each sample, two 1 mm diameter cylinders of tissue were obtained from representative areas of each archived paraffin block and arrayed into a new recipient paraffin block with a custom-built precision instrument (Beecher Instruments, Silver Spring, MD, USA). After construction, initial sections of the TMA were stained for hematoxylin and eosin and reviewed by clinical pathologists to verify the histopathological findings.

Immunohistochemistry Staining (IHC)

Immunohistochemical staining for CAV1 was carried out on sections of the formalin-fixed samples on the TMA. Briefly, the sections were deparaffinized in xylene and rehydrated by transfer through graded concentrations of ethanol to distilled water, and endogenous peroxidase activity was blocked by incubation with 30 mL/L H_2O_2 in methanol for 10 minutes at room temperature. Then, sections were submitted to antigen retrieval in a pressure cooker containing 0.01 mmol/L sodium citrate buffer for 10 minutes. Slides were subsequently incubated in 100 mL/L normal goat serum for 20 minutes at room temperature. Antibodies to CAV1 (SC-894, Santa Cruze) were incubated at 37°C for 2 hours and placed at 4°Covernight. Then, the slides were incubated with a horseradish peroxidase–conjugated mouse anti-rabbit secondary antibody (Genscript, P.R.China) at 37°C for 1 hour. Finally, the sections were reacted with 0.02% 3,3′-diaminoberzidine and 0.005% H_2O_2 in 0.05 mmol/L Tris-HCl buffer, and counter-staining was performed with hematoxylin. Negative control slides were treated by incubation with PBS instead of the primary mouse antibody. Stained slides were observed under light microscopy. All slides were reviewed independently by 2 pathologists who were blinded to each other's readings. CAV1 immunostaining were semi-quantitatively estimated based on proportion (percentage of positive cells). The proportion of caveolin-1 staining was classified into two categories: −(0~25%), +(26~100%) for statistical analysis. Antibodies to E-cadherin(610181) and Vimentin (ab92547) are purchased from BD Transduction Laboratories and Abcam respectively.

In vivo metastasis assay via orthotopic implantation

We employed the orthotopic implantation assay to assess the effect of CAV1 on tumor metastasis. Mice were anesthetized with 2.5% sodium pentobarbital (40 mg/kg; Sigma), the right side of the abdomen was sterilely prepped. The abdomen was entered through a small opening in the muscle and peritoneum. Small

A

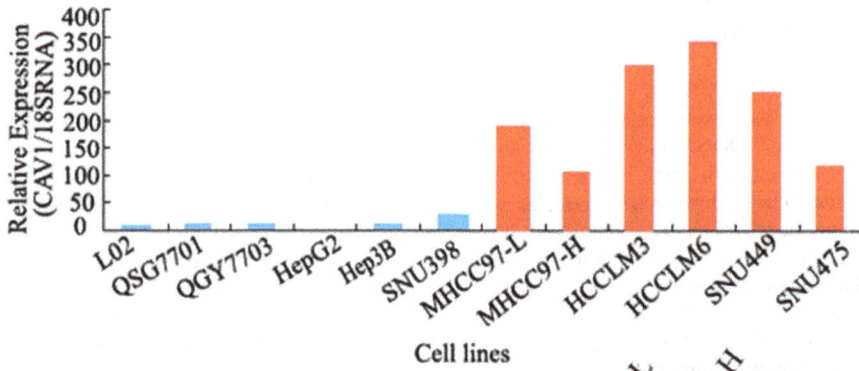

C

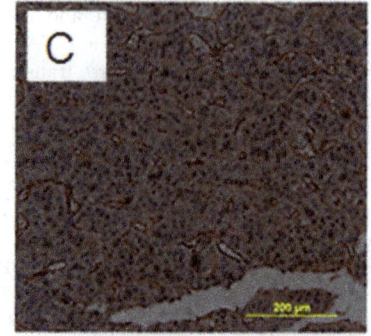

B

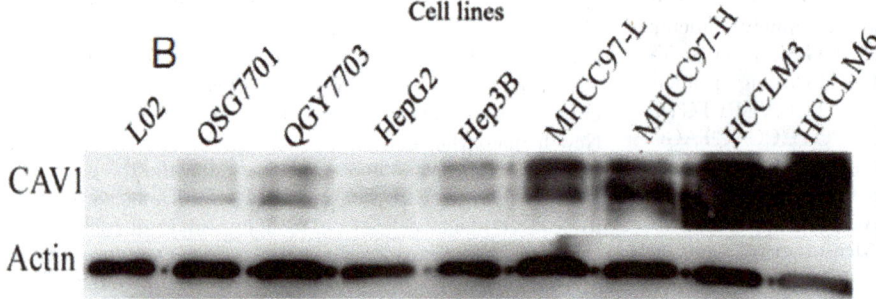

D

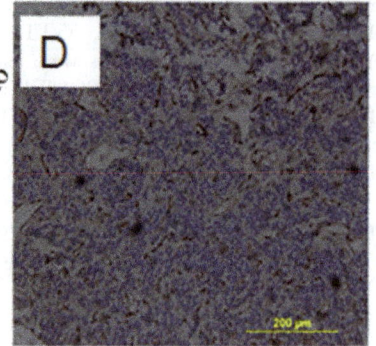

E

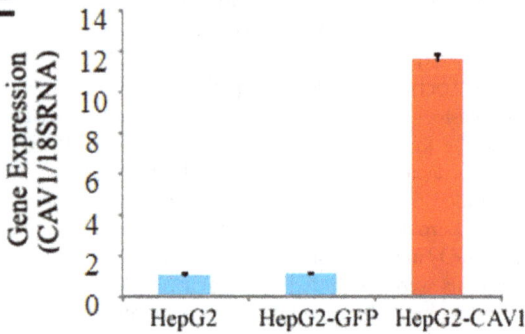

F

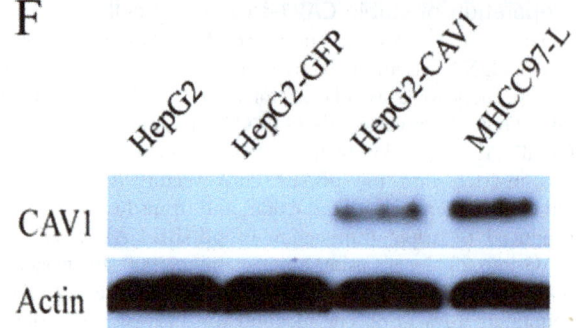

G

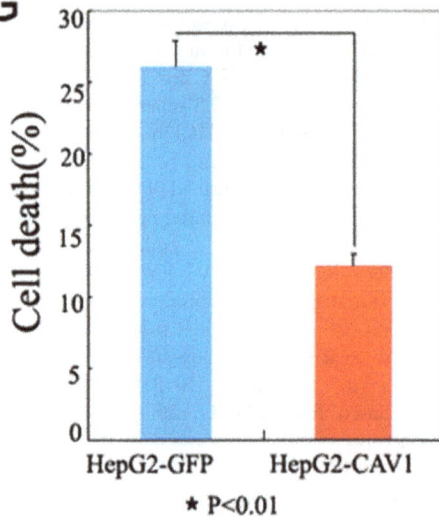

★ P<0.01

H

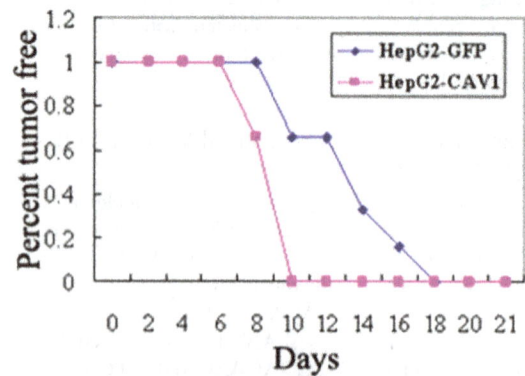

I

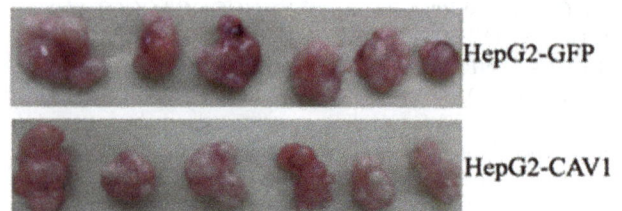

Figure 1. Expression levels of CAV1 in various HCC samples. 1A, 1B: CAV1 mRNA and protein levels of HCC cell lines detected by Q-PCR and Western Blotting. 1C, Membranous and strong cytoplasmic CAV1 expression in a metastatic HCC; 1D, Weak CAV1 expression in hepatocytes of a non-metastatic HCC and strong CAV1 expression in the endothelium of the blood vessels. Original magnification, ×200; 1E and 1F, Q-PCR and Western blot analysis indicated the expressed CAV1 in HepG2 cell lines. The CAV1 expression levels upon CAV1 adenovirus expression are comparable to the endogenous CAV1 level in MHCC97-L cell lines; 1G, Cell anoikis assays using poly-HEMA. Data are presented as mean values (n = 3); error bars represent ± SD; 4H, Stable CAV1 overexpression pools from HepG2 cells were injected subcutaneously into mice; each group contained 6 mice. A Kaplan-Meier survival plot 4 weeks after injection indicates that the mice injected with the CAV1 cells survived for a significantly longer period of time than the controls (P<0.01); 4I, all xenograft tumors were removed from the experimental mice.

piece of subcutaneous tumor was removed, minced to produce fresh tumor pieces about $1 \times 1 \times 1$ mm^3, and implanted into the liver of each of six nude mice. Then, the skin was closed. After 6 weeks, the mice were killed and autopsied.

The abdominal organs, including the liver, the lungs were sampled for standard histopathological studies as detailed above. Liver tumor wet weights were compared using the t test in SPSS (version 11.5; SPSS). Consecutive sections were made for every tissue block of the lung. Take first one of the every five consecutive sections for hematoxylin-eosin staining and examination for the lung metastasis. Based on the number of HCC cells in the maximal section of the metastatic lesion, the lung metastases were classified into four grades: grade I, ~20 cells; grade II, 20–50 cells; grade III, 50–100 cells; and grade IV, ~100 cells. This study was approved by the The Animal Care and Use Committee of Fudan University, China. All surgery was performed under sodium pentobarbital anesthesia, and all efforts were made to minimize suffering.

Experimental procedure for cell migration, wound-healing, anoikis, WB, reporter gene, and tumorigenicity are mentioned in Supplemental Experimental Procedures (File S1).

Results

CAV1 overexpression was necessary for HCC malignance and metastasis but has minor effect for HCC growth

To investigate the function of CAV1 in HCC progression, we first determined the CAV1 levels in metastatic HCC cell lines and tissues compared with non-metastatic ones. By using Q-PCR (Fig. 1A) and western blotting (Fig. 1B), the expression levels of CAV1 in12 HCC cell lines were determined. Metastatic HCC cell lines such as MHCC97-L, MHCC97-H, HCCLM3, HCCLM6,

SNU449 and SNU475 express much higher CAV1 expression than that in L02, QGY7701, QGY7703, HepG2, Hep3B and SNU398, while the lowest level of CAV1 among the 12 HCC cells tested was in HepG2 cells. These results provide evidence that CAV1 is associated with the metastatic phenotype of HCC cells. Therefore, HepG2 was selected late on for constructing stable overexpression cells, while MHCC97-H and HCCLM3 were selected and used in RNAi experiments.

In order to determine the expression level of CAV1 in HCC tissues, we performed TMA analysis then. The TMA was constructed from a total of 96 HCC cases (Table 1), consisting of 48 liver cancer tissues each from patients with and without metastasis. TMA analysis showed that HCC tissues with metastasis had higher CAV1 expression levels than those without metastasis (p<0.05, Fig. 1C and 1D, Table 1). This tendency in HCC tissues confirms likely the expression pattern observed in the cell lines.

Based on the CAV1 expression pattern in HCC-derived cell lines, we stably transfected adenoviral vectors containing CAV1 into HepG2 cells. Stable pools were established (Fig. 1E, F) and used for measuring cell characteristics. For localization of CAV-1 before and after the transfection procedures, we carried out immunofluorescence staining experiments and found that CAV1 is highly enriched in the cytoplasm (Figure S1 in File S1). CAV1 overexpression suppressed the poly-HEMA induced apoptosis of these cells relative to cells transfected with empty pBABE vector (P<0.01; Fig.1G), where it has no effect on cell proliferation and cell cycle (data not shown). Furthermore, we subcutaneously injected HepG2-CAV1 cells into nude mice in order to assess their tumorigenicity. The results showed that CAV1 overexpression can promote the occurrence of visible tumors. Indeed, in our experiments the tumors formed in cells of overexpressing CAV1 were significantly earlier than those of tumors formed from control

Table 1. Relationship between CAV1 expression and clinicopathological variables in the 96 HCC patients

Parameters	Variable	No. of patients	CAV-1 (+)	%	p
Gender	Male	88	28	32	>0.05
	Female	8	4	50	
Age	<65 year	85	45	53	>0.05
	>65 year	11	9	82	
Tumor size	<5 cm	43	23	53	>0.05
	>5 cm	53	30	57	
TNM stage	I-II	66	32	48	>0.05
	III-IV	30	15	50	
Metastasis	No	48	25	52	<0.05*
	Yes	48	38	79	

* Statistically significant.

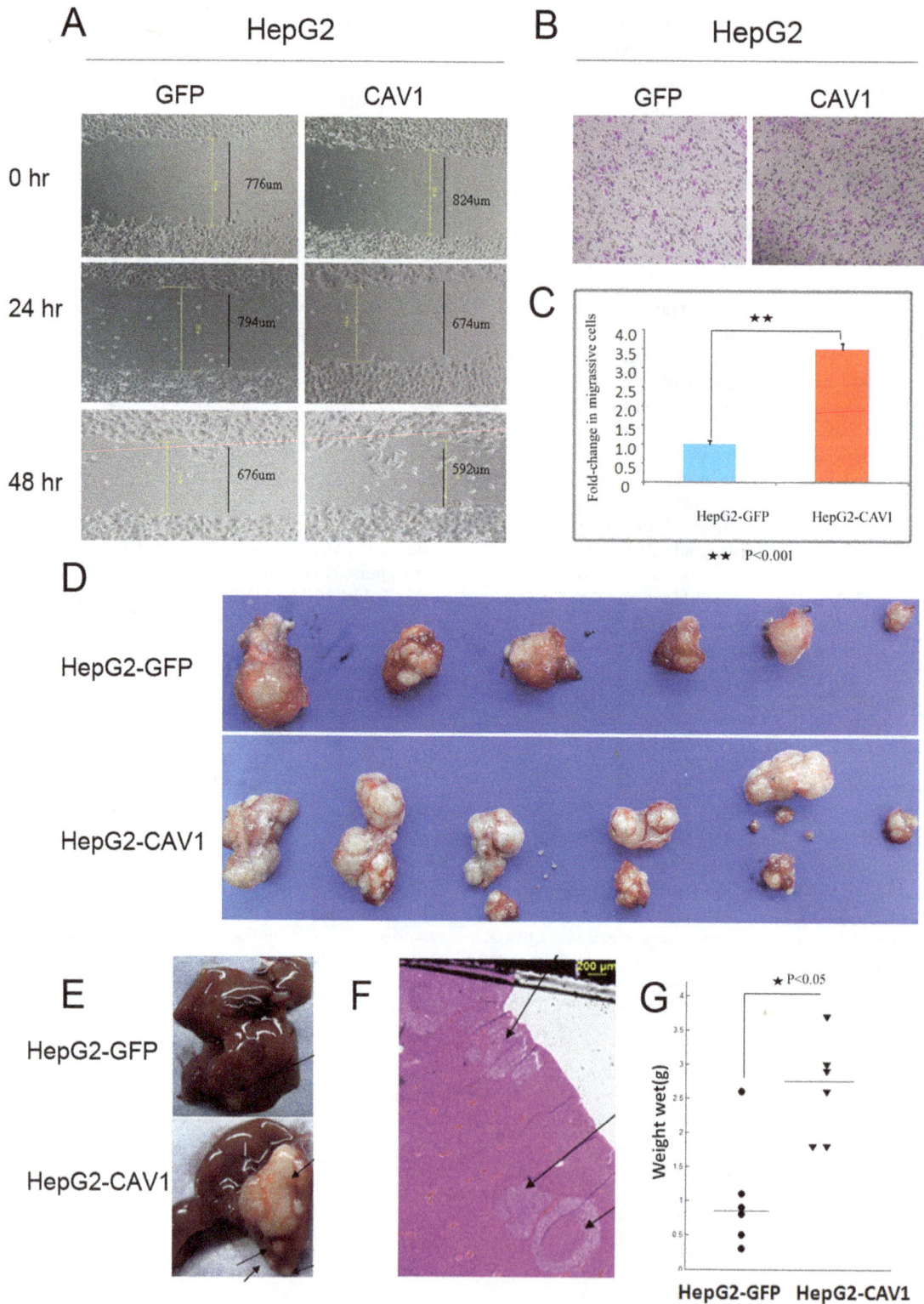

Figure 2. CAV1 modulates HCC cell migration, growth, and metastasis. A, CAV1 overexpression promotes cell migration in HepG2 cells that express GFP and CAV1 using a wound-healing assay. B, Transwell migration assay of HepG2 cell, viewed at ×200 and stained with purple for three independent experiments. C, Comparison analysis with data as *mean ± SD*, and the statistically significant differences with Student's t-test. D and E, Effect of CAV1 overexpression on the HepG2 cell metastasis using letivirus–CAV1 via orthotopic implantation. Locoregional metastases, classified as abdominal wall metastases and intrahepatic metastases (black arrow) were observed by day 40. F, representative images show intrahepatic metastases (black arrow) and H&E-stained sections. G, The quantification of average weight of xenograft tumors at 6 weeks is shown. * P<0.05.

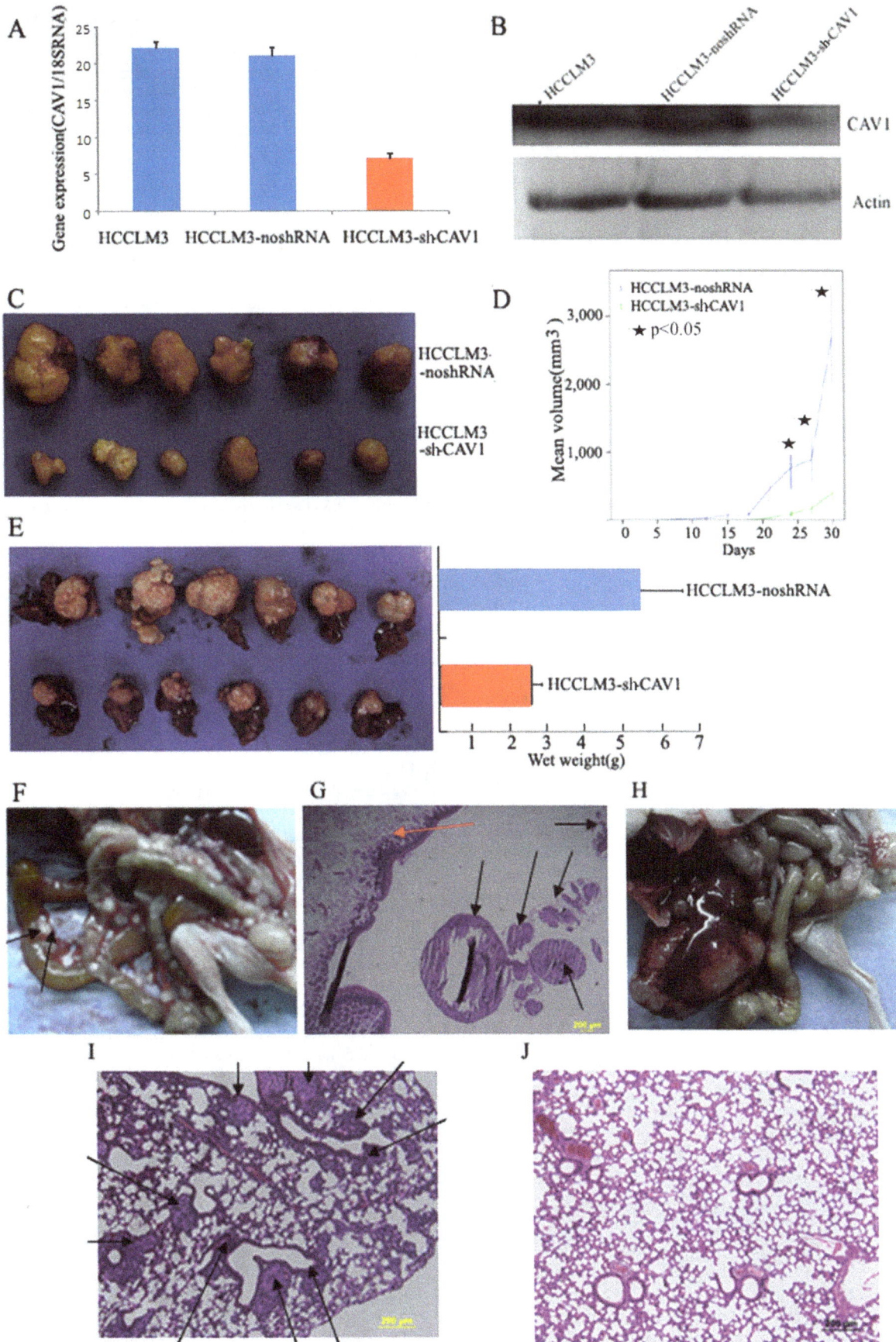

Figure 3. CAV1 knockdown inhibited HCC tumor growth and metastasis. A and B, CAV1 knockdown in MHCCLM3 cells by shRNA-CAV1-1, as demonstrated by qPCR and western blot analysis, with noshRNA as the control. C and D, The growth of subcutaneous tumors was recorded for 30 days, monitored in terms of tumor diameter after 3 days (*mean ± SD*), and photographed as mice killed. Cells (5×10^6) in 0.2 mL of PBS were injected s.c. into right upper flank region of each of the six nude mice. E, After orthotopic implantation, tumor growth was assayed using small piece of subcutaneous tumor. The mice were killed after 6 weeks, and autopsied for photo (left panel) and weight (right panel, *mean ± SD*). F, Abdominal metastases to mesenteric lymph nodes (black arrow) in noshRNA tumors. G, Representative images of liver cancer metastasis (black arrow) on the mesenteric fold (red arrow, intestine) (H&E-stain, original magnification, ×40). H, No abdominal metastasis was observed in shRNA-CAV1-1 tumors. I and J, Representative images of metastases formed in lungs of each nude mouse ($n = 6$) at 6 weeks after orthotopic implantation with MHCCLM3 no-shRNA or shRNA-CAV1-1 tumors (black arrow, metastatic tumors).

cells transfected with empty vector. As shown in Fig. 1H, mice injected with CAV1 cells survived for longer than control. The average tumor size and weight were similar between the two group mice (Fig. 1I).

CAV1 overexpression in non-metastatic cells enables invasion *in vivo*, whereas CAV1 knockdown in metastatic cells inhibits metastasis *in vivo*

Above observations that CAV1 was overexpressed in metastatic live cell lines and tissues suggested the promoting role of CAV1 in HCC metastasis. The wound-healing assay (Fig. 2A) and the Transwell experiments (Fig. 2B and 2C) revealed that CAV1 overexpression can enhance non-metastatic HepG2 cell migration. CAV1 overexpression HepG2 stable clones were then injected subcutaneously into six athymic mice to assess tumorigenicity. By the end of four weeks, no difference in the proliferation could be observed (data not shown). Then, two envelope intact HCC tumors from control or CAV1 overexpression HepG2 stable clones were implanted respectively into the liver of six athymic recipient mice in vivo. Widespread loco regional effects were observed by day 40 (Fig. 2D and 2E), with three mice exhibiting abdominal wall metastases and the other three intrahepatic metastases. The presence of intrahepatic metastatic tumors in mice was confirmed by histologic analysis (Fig. 2F). Distant lung metastasis was not observed. Furthermore, the tumors in the mice injected with CAV1-expressing cells were significantly larger than those injected with control cells ($P < 0.001$; Fig. 2D and 2G).

Results also show that the CAV1 shRNA can efficiently knock down the endogenous CAV1 expression in highly-metastatic MHCCLM3 cells, as indicated by the qPCR and western blot analysis (Fig. 3A and 3B). MHCCLM3 cells (5×10^6 cells) from each of the stable subclones were injected subcutaneously into six athymic mice to assess tumorigenicity. By the end of four weeks, the shRNA-free tumors grew to an average size of $2,747.7$ mm^3 whereas the shRNA-CAV1-1 403.6 mm^3, being an approximately 65% inhibition in tumor growth statistically (Fig. 3C and 3D). Furthermore, when small s.c. CAV1-1 shRNA tumor tissues were implanted into the liver of new recipient mice, the tumors were significantly smaller than the tumors in the control mice after 6 weeks ($p < 0.01$; Fig. 3E).

We have checked the effects of CAV1 knockdown in MHCCLM3 on long-distance tumor metastasis *in vivo*. Widespread locoregional and distant metastases were observed in the six mice that were orthotopically implanted with MHCCLM3-noshRNA tumors (Fig. 3F). Locoregional metastasis to the abdominal wall occurred in 100% of the cases, 67% metastasized intrahepatically, and 19% metastasized to the abdominal cavity and involved the mesenteric lymph nodes (Fig. 3F and 3G). Lung metastases were observed, and the hematoxylin and eosin (H&E)-stained tissue block sections showed numerous massive metastases in the lung parenchyma (Fig. 3I). However, bare- or tiny-visible locoregional metastasis or metastatic tumors were found in mice

lungs that were orthotopically implanted with the MHCCLM3 cells of CAV1 knockdown tumor (Fig. 3H and 3J).

Furthermore, we also verified that CAV1 knockdown not only can inhibit xenograft tumor growth and metastasis in HCCLM3 cells (Fig. 3), but it had the same effect in the other HCC lines, such as MHCC97-H (Figure S2 in File S1). These data suggest that CAV1 downregulation plays a crucial role in the malignant aggression and metastasis of aggressive HCC cells.

CAV1 overexpression can activate Wnt/β-catenin pathway and induce EMT process

We have proved that the expression of Epithelial-Mesenchymal Transition (EMT)-markers can be regulated by CAV1 likely through Wnt/β-catenin pathway. The CAV1-overexpression HepG2 cells exhibited downregulation of E-cadherin, a epithelial-marker, whereas the CAV1-knockdown clones showed an upregulation of E-cadherin (Fig. 4A). Vimetin, the mesenchymal marker in EMT, can be upregulated in CAV1-overexpression HepG2 cells, but was downregulated in CAV1-knockdown MHCC97-H cells (Fig. 4A). The corresponding mRNA levels of E-cadherin and Vimetin, were examined respectively by qPCR and showed the same results (Fig. 4B). In addition, the CAV1-overexpression HepG2 cells has high mRNA level of Twist, a transcription factor highly expressed and crucial in promotion of EMT and consequently tumor cell invasion as well [11], while the CAV1-knockdown MHCC97-H cells resulted in a decrease in Twist mRNA level (Fig. 4B).

E-cadherin is a main binding partner of β-catenin and plays an important role in regulating its nuclear localization. The translocation of β-catenin can be investigated by measuring the protein level in the nuclear and cytosolic fractions. We have verified that the CAV1-overexpressed HepG2 cells displayed nuclear accumulation of β-catenin (Fig. 4C). In contrast, markedly increased cytosolic β-catenin and decreased nuclear β-catenin are induced by CAV1 depletion in MHCC97-H (Fig. 4C). The subcellular relocalization of β-catenin can subsequently regulate the transcriptional activities of the Tcf/Lef DNA-binding factors [12,13]. We have found that reduced nuclear localization of β-catenin in the CAV1-depletion clones is associated with decreased β-catenin transcriptional activity, as detected with the responsive reporter plasmid of β-catenin-Tcf/Lef transfected into cells (Fig. 4D).

Metastasis is an in vivo process and in vitro data showing differential expression of EMT markers is not sufficient. Then we investigated the CAV1-dependent expression of E-cadherin and Vimentin by immunohistochemical staining in the tumors in vivo. The immunohistochemistry results showed that the tumors from CAV1-overexpression HepG2 cells exhibited downregulation of E-cadherin, an epithelial-marker, whereas Vimetin, the mesenchymal marker in EMT, can be upregulated in CAV1-overexpression HepG2 cells. The data have been presented in Fig 4E. We have tried to study the mechanism of how the signal is transduced to the nucleus. It was shown that membrane-type-1

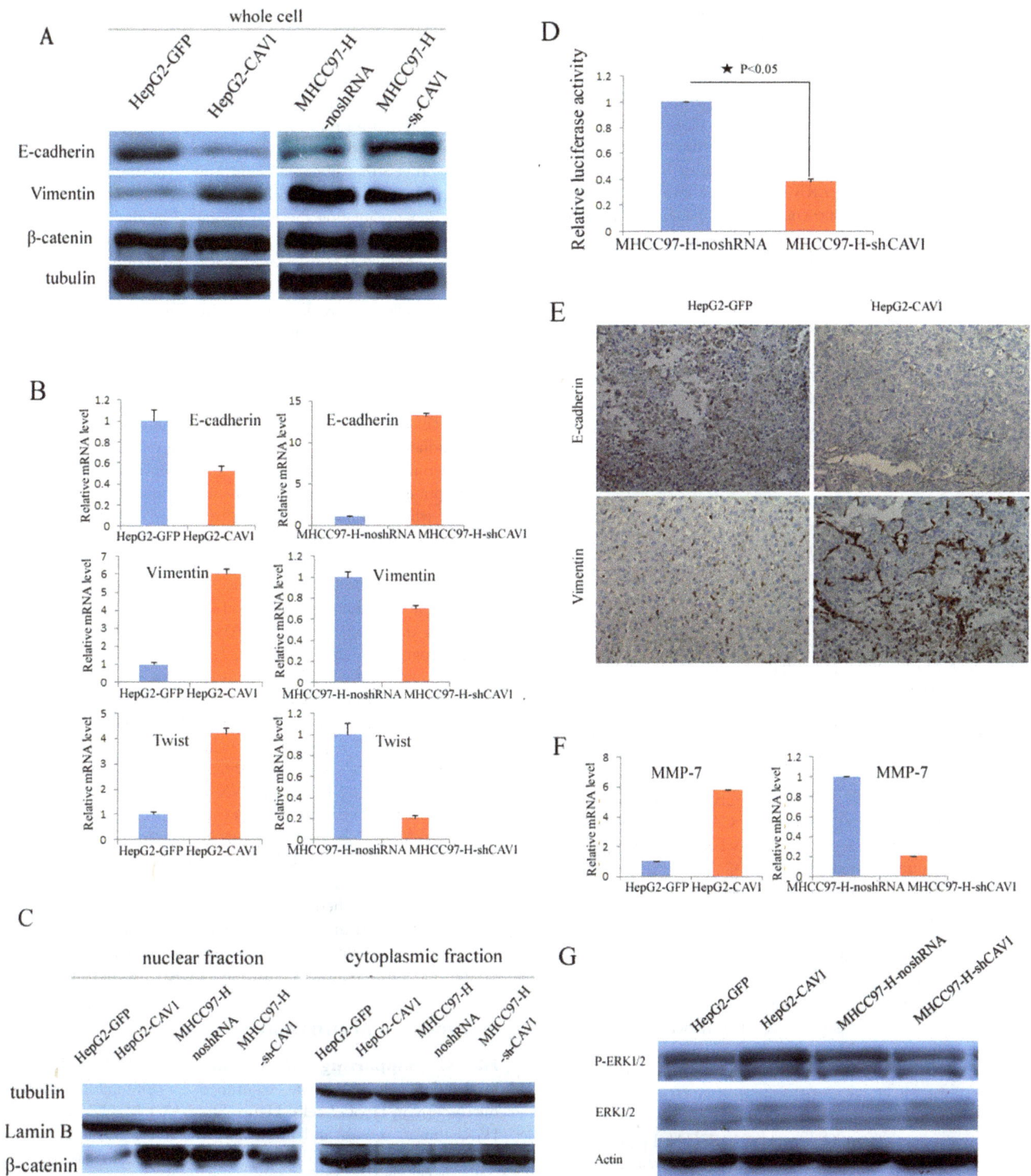

Figure 4. CAV1 changes the subcellular distribution and signaling of β-catenin in EMT. A, CAV1 induce EMT in HCC cells. Whole cell lysates from the control, CAV1-expressing, and sh-CAV1 HCC cells were separated and probed with antibodies for epithelial and mesenchymal markers as indicated. B, CAV1 decreases E-cadherin mRNA level, increases Vimentin and Twist mRNA level. C, The β-catenin distribution in CAV1-expressing and sh-CAV1 HCC cells was determined. The purity of nuclear and cytoplasmic fractions was confirmed by immunoblotting. D, The control and CAV1-RNAi MHCC97-H cells were transiently transfected with TOP-tk to determine the transcriptional activity of β-catenin–mediated signaling. The activity levels are represented as fold activation compared with the control in triplicate wells. E, Immunohistochemistry staining of E-cadherin and Vimentin in the tumors from control and CAV1-overexpression HepG2 cells. F, mRNA level of MMP-7 was determined by Q-PCR. G, Protein levels of phospho-ERK 1/2, and total ERK1/2 were analyzed by western blot. Actin is a loading control.

matrix metalloproteinase (MT1-MMP) co-localizes with CAV1 at the perinuclear region and it may be translocated to the nucleus via caveolae mediated endocytosis in HCC [14]. Data has also shown that CAV1 is needed in epidermal growth factor (EGF)-induced mouse embryonic stem cell migration, extracellular signal-regulated protein kinase (ERK) phosphorylation and MMP-2 expression [15]. However, CAV1 has been reported as a negative regulator of MMP-1 gene expression in human dermal fibroblasts via inhibition of ERK signaling pathway [16]. Han et al has shown that CAV1 gene could inhibit pancreatic carcinoma cell invasion, at least in part, probably through ERK-MMP signal pathway [17]. Since EMT is always dependent on the activation of ERK signaling pathways [18], so we investigated the effect of CAV1 in ERK phosphorylation level and MMPs mRNA expression in HCC metastatic process.

We found MMP-7 was increased in CAV1 expressing HepG2 cells (Fig 4F), while MMP-1 and MMP-2 mRNA level have no significant change (data not shown). For activity of ERK examined by Western blot, we observed that overexpression of CAV1 induced activation of ERK in CAV1 overexpressing HepG2 cells compared with those of control cells (Fig 4G).

Discussion

CAV1 has been implicated in the tumorogenesis. It was shown that CAV1 expression difference is tumor cells type-dependent. For instance, while CAV1 downregulation is typical for ovarian, lung, and mammary carcinomas, it is upregulated in bladder, thyroid and prostate carcinomas [2]. Furthermore, CAV1 contributes to metastatic phenotype in different types of carcinomas [19,20]. De-regulation of CAV1 expression in HCC tissues has been documented [3]. Yokomori et al. reported that CAV1 expression elevated in cirrhotic liver and HCC, while it was almost undetectable in normal liver [21]. On the other hand, it was shown that CAV1 expression was inactivated in HCC cell lines by aberrant methylation [22]. These observations do not provide clear evidence about the role of CAV1 in hepatocellular carcinogenesis, yet the function of CAV1 in HCC metastasis still remain poorly understood.

Our observation in human HCC samples was in accordance with previous reports. CAV1 was absent in non-metastatic liver cell lines but was exclusively expressed in metastatic cell lines. Together with the significant overexpression in metastatic liver tissues, it is conceivable that CAV1 positively regulates HCC progression and metastasis. Cell migration and invasion are critical events in metastasis which involve the relocation of signaling molecules that establish the polarity and induce dynamic cytoskeletal changes of the cell. CAV1 overexpressing and knockdown stable clones were established in HCC cells and their *in vitro* cellular effects and *in vivo* tumourigenicity and metastatic potential were examined. Overexpression of CAV1 promoted liver cancer cell motility and invasiveness *in vitro*, as well as metastasis *in vivo*. Conversely, knockdown of CAV1 in metastatic HCC cells markedly inhibited the tumour metastatic potential *in vivo*. In summary, our results have shown the exclusive expression of CAV1 in metastatic HCC cell lines and clinical samples. The definitive role of CAV1 promoting HCC metastasis was demonstrated.

EMT and related pathways have been studied in metastatic HCCs, to investigate whether EMT is a crucial step in the conversion of early stage tumors into invasive malignancies [13,23]. Sun reported that Twist1 (an EMT trigger marker) was frequently overexpressed in the nuclear relocation occurring in VM (vasculogenic mimicry)-positive HCCs, and Twist1 nuclear expression in EMT was likewise associated with VM formation, and with the tumor invasion and metastasis of HCC [24]. Yang discovered that a comprehensive profile of EMT markers in HCC, and the independent and collaborative effects of Snail (the other trigger marker) and Twist on HCC metastasis were confirmed through different assays [25].

β-catenin signaling pathways is important in metastatic HCC. Liu has proven that hypoxia could induce β-catenin overexpression and/or intracellular accumulation in four HCC cell lines through downregulating the endogenous degradation machinery, and hypoxia can also promote an invasion *in vitro* and metastasis *in vivo* for MHCC97 and Hep3B cells [26]. Hypoxic MHCC97 and Hep3B cells exhibited molecular alterations consistent with EMT, characterized by the loss of epithelial cell markers and up-regulation of mesenchymal markers, as well as the increase of MMP2. However, silencing of β-catenin in these hypoxic cells reversed EMT and repressed metastatic potential.

Preventing caveolae assembly through CAV1 reducing results in E-cadherin accumulation at cell borders and the formation of tightly adherent cells [27]. Accordingly, the nuclear translocation of β-catenin occurred after E-cadherin down-regulation, and Lef transcription was activated after β-catenin translocated into the nucleus, where the Tcf/Lef transcript can be activated [28]. We also prove evidence that the CAV1 up-regulation induced E-cadherin downregulation. Consequently, CAV1 stimulation can induce an activation of the Wnt/β-catenin-Tcf/Lef pathway, especially at the transcriptional level.

Due to the crucial roles of CAV1 and MMPs in regulating tumor progression and metastasis, a growing number of studies have investigated a possible relationship between these molecules. Published data suggests that CAV1 can be an important regulator of the expression and activity of MMPs, including CAV1 unregulated MMP-2 and 9 in melanoma cells [29]. Various signaling pathways have been shown to induce MMPs gene expression, including ERK1/2, JNK and p38 MAPK et al [30–31]. In this study, we have investigated the specific contribution of CAV1 to MMPs gene expression in human HCC cell lines. Additionally we show that CAV1 increases MMP-7 expression via activation of ERK1/2 signaling pathways.

Taken together, these results suggest that CAV1 induces the HCC cell invasion and metastasis partial by enhancing MMP-7 expression, associated with decreased E-cadherin expression, resulting in EMT and acting through ERK activation.

Supporting Information

File S1 Supporting information. Figure S1. Subcellular localization of CAV1 was examined by immunofluorescence microscopy in HepG2 cells. Figure S2. CAV1 knockdown inhibit HCC tumor growth and metastasis in MHCC97H cells. A, B, shRNA-CAV1-1was used to knockdown CAV1 in MHCC97H cells, as demonstrated by real time RT-PCR and western blotting, where noshRNA was used as control. C, D, Cells (5×10^6) in 0.2 mL PBS were injected s.c. into the right upper flank region of each of 6 nude mice. The growth of subcutaneous tumor was recorded for 30 days, tumor growth was monitored for 3 days by measuring the tumor diameters (*mean $\pm$ SD*) then the mice were killed and tumors were removed. E, orthotopic implantation was assayed using small piece of subcutaneous tumor. The mice were observed for 6 weeks, killed, and autopsied. Tumors were weighed at 6 weeks; the weight is indicated (*mean $\pm$ SD*). F, G, Representative images of metastases that formed in lungs of each nude mouse ($n = 6$) at 6 weeks after orthotopicly implanted with

MHCC97H no-shRNA or shRNA-CAV1-1 tumors. Black arrows indicate metastatic tumors in lung. Original magnification, ×100.

Acknowledgments

We thank Yinkun Liu for high density tissue microarray construction, Huali Shen for manuscript preparation. Many technical assistance and helpful discussions with Yinkun Liu and Yang Zhang are also gratefully acknowledged.

Author Contributions

Conceived and designed the experiments: PYY LXQ YKL. Performed the experiments: HXY HLS. Analyzed the data: YZ FZ. Contributed reagents/materials/analysis tools: YKL. Wrote the paper: HXY.

References

1. Gupta GP, Massague J (2006) Cancer metastasis: building a framework. Cell 127: 679–695.
2. Williams TM, Lisanti MP (2005) Caveolin-1 in oncogenic transformation, cancer, and metastasis. Am J Physiol Cell Physiol 288: C494–506.
3. Liu P, Rudick M, Anderson RG (2002) Multiple functions of caveolin-1. J Biol Chem 277: 41295–41298.
4. Cokakli M, Erdal E, Nart D, Yilmaz F, Sagol O, et al. (2009) Differential expression of Caveolin-1 in hepatocellular carcinoma: correlation with differentiation state, motility and invasion. BMC Cancer 9: 65.
5. Tang Y, Zeng X, He F, Liao Y, Qian N, et al. (2012) Caveolin-1 is related to invasion, survival, and poor prognosis in hepatocellular cancer. Med Oncol 29: 977–984.
6. Zhang ZB, Cai L, Zheng SG, Xiong Y, Dong JH (2009) Overexpression of caveolin-1 in hepatocellular carcinoma with metastasis and worse prognosis: correlation with vascular endothelial growth factor, microvessel density and unpaired artery. Pathol Oncol Res 15: 495–502.
7. Choi HN, Kim KR, Park HS, Jang KY, Kang MJ, et al. (2007) Expression of caveolin in hepatocellular carcinoma: association with unpaired artery formation and radiologic findings. Korean J Hepatol 13: 396–408.
8. Yan J, Lu Q, Dong J, Li X, Ma K, et al. (2012) Hepatitis B virus X protein suppresses caveolin-1 expression in hepatocellular carcinoma by regulating DNA methylation. BMC Cancer 12: 353.
9. Yang SF, Yang JY, Huang CH, Wang SN, Lu CP, et al. (2010) Increased caveolin-1 expression associated with prolonged overall survival rate in hepatocellular carcinoma. Pathology 42: 438–445.
10. Trimmer C, Whitaker-Menezes D, Bonuccelli G, Milliman JN, Daumer KM, et al. (2010) CAV1 inhibits metastatic potential in melanomas through suppression of the integrin/Src/FAK signaling pathway. Cancer Res 70: 7489–7499.
11. Kang Y, Massague J (2004) Epithelial-mesenchymal transitions: twist in development and metastasis. Cell 118: 277–279.
12. Stockinger A, Eger A, Wolf J, Beug H, Foisner R (2001) E-cadherin regulates cell growth by modulating proliferation-dependent beta-catenin transcriptional activity. J Cell Biol 154: 1185–1196.
13. Conacci-Sorrell M, Simcha I, Ben-Yedidia T, Blechman J, Savagner P, et al. (2003) Autoregulation of E-cadherin expression by cadherin-cadherin interactions: the roles of beta-catenin signaling, Slug, and MAPK. J Cell Biol 163: 847–857.
14. Ip YC, Cheung ST, Fan ST (2007). Atypical localization of Membrane Type 1-Matrix Metalloproteinase in the nucleus is associated with aggressive features of hepatocellular carcinoma. Mol Carinog 46: 225–230
15. Park JH and Han HJ (2009) Caveolin-1 plays important role in EGF-induced migration and proliferation of mouse embryonic stem cells: involvement of PI3K/Akt and ERK. Am J Physiol Cell Physiol 297: C935–C944.
16. Haines P, Samuel GH, Cohen H, Trojanowska M, Bujor AM (2011) Caveolin-1 is a negative regulator of MMP-1 gene expression in human dermal fibroblasts via inhibition of Erk1/2/Ets1 signaling pathway. J Dermatol Sci 64: 210–6
17. Han FI, Zhu HG (2010) Caveolin-1 regulating the invasion and expression of matrix metalloproteinase (MMPs) in pancreatic carcinomacells. J Surg Res 159: 443–50.
18. Lin ZH, Wang L, Zhang JB, Liu Y, Li XQ, Guo L, Zhang B, Zhu WW, Ye QH (2014) MST4 promotes hepatocellular carcinoma epithelial-mesenchymal transition and metastasis via activation of the p-ERK pathway. Int J Oncol 45: 629–640
19. Ho CC, Huang PH, Huang HY, Chen YH, Yang PC, et al. (2002) Up-regulated caveolin-1 accentuates the metastasis capability of lung adenocarcinoma by inducing filopodia formation. Am J Pathol 161: 1647–1656.
20. Lu Z, Ghosh S, Wang Z, Hunter T (2003) Downregulation of caveolin-1 function by EGF leads to the loss of E-cadherin, increased transcriptional activity of beta-catenin, and enhanced tumor cell invasion. Cancer Cell 4: 499–515.
21. Yokomori H, Oda M, Yoshimura K, Nomura M, Wakabayashi G, et al. (2003) Elevated expression of caveolin-1 at protein and mRNA level in human cirrhotic liver: relation with nitric oxide. J Gastroenterol 38: 854–860.
22. Hirasawa Y, Arai M, Imazeki F, Tada M, Mikata R, et al. (2006) Methylation status of genes upregulated by demethylating agent 5-aza-2'-deoxycytidine in hepatocellular carcinoma. Oncology 71: 77–85.
23. Garber K (2008) Epithelial-to-mesenchymal transition is important to metastasis, but questions remain. J Natl Cancer Inst 100: 232–233, 239.
24. Sun T, Zhao N, Zhao XL, Gu Q, Zhang SW, et al. (2010) Expression and functional significance of Twist1 in hepatocellular carcinoma: its role in vasculogenic mimicry. Hepatology 51: 545–556.
25. Yang MH, Chen CL, Chau GY, Chiou SH, Su CW, et al. (2009) Comprehensive analysis of the independent effect of twist and snail in promoting metastasis of hepatocellular carcinoma. Hepatology 50: 1464–1474.
26. Liu L, Zhu XD, Wang WQ, Shen Y, Qin Y, et al. (2010) Activation of beta-catenin by hypoxia in hepatocellular carcinoma contributes to enhanced metastatic potential and poor prognosis. Clin Cancer Res 16: 2740–2750.
27. Orlichenko L, Weller SG, Cao H, Krueger EW, Awoniyi M, et al. (2009) Caveolae mediate growth factor-induced disassembly of adherens junctions to support tumor cell dissociation. Mol Biol Cell 20: 4140–4152.
28. Vincan E, Barker N (2008) The upstream components of the Wnt signalling pathway in the dynamic EMT and MET associated with colorectal cancer progression. Clin Exp Metastasis 25: 657–663.
29. Felicetti F, Parolini I, Bottero L, Fecchi K, Errico MC, Raggi C, et al (2009) Caveolin-1 Tumor - promoting role in human melanoma. Int J Cancer 125: 1514–1522.
30. Sternlicht MD, Werb Z (2001) How matrix metalloproteinases regulate cell behavior. Annu Rev Cell Dev Biol 17: 463–516.
31. Vincenti MP, Brinckerhoff CE (2002) Transcriptional regulation of collagenase (MMP-1, MMP-13) genes in arthritis: integration of complex signaling pathways for the recruitment of gene-specific transcription factors. Arthritis Res 4: 157–164.

17

Role of *IL-4* Gene Polymorphisms in HBV-Related Hepatocellular Carcinoma in a Chinese Population

Yu Lu[1]⊘, Zhitong Wu[2]⊘, Qiliu Peng[1], Liping Ma[1], Xiaolian Zhang[1], Jiangyang Zhao[1], Xue Qin[1]*, Shan Li[1]*

1 Department of Clinical Laboratory, First Affiliated Hospital of Guangxi Medical University, Nanning, Guangxi, China, **2** Department of Clinical Laboratory, Guigang People's Hospital, Guigang, Guangxi, China

Abstract

Background: Interleukin-4 (IL-4) is best known as an important mediator and modulator of immune and inflammatory responses. Hepatocellular carcinoma (HCC) is a typical inflammation-related cancer, and genetic variations in the *IL-4* gene may be associated with the risk of hepatitis B virus (HBV)-related HCC. However, few studies have been conducted on their association.

Objectives: To clarify the effects of *IL-4* gene polymorphisms on the risk of HBV-related HCC, two common variants, −590C/T (rs2243250) and −33C/T (rs2070874), and their relationship with HBV-related disease risk were investigated in a Chinese population.

Methods: IL-4 −590C/T and −33C/T polymorphisms were examined in 154 patients with HBV-related HCC, 62 patients with HBV-induced liver cirrhosis (LC), 129 patients with chronic hepatitis B (CHB), and 94 healthy controls, using the polymerase chain reaction-restriction fragment length polymorphism method and DNA sequencing.

Results: Overall, no significant differences were observed regarding the *IL-4* −590C/T and −33C/T polymorphism genotypes, alleles, or haplotypes between the patient groups and the healthy controls. However, the CC genotypes of *IL-4* −590C/T and −33C/T polymorphisms were observed to be significantly associated with CHB in subgroup analysis in males [CC versus TT (OR: 4.193, 95% CI: 1.094−16.071, $P = 0.037$; and OR: 3.438, 95% CI: 1.032−11.458, $P = 0.044$) and CC versus TT+ CT (OR: 4.09, 95% CI: 1.08−15.49, $P = 0.038$; and OR: 3.43, 95% CI: 1.04−11.28, $P = 0.042$)].

Conclusions: These findings suggest that genetic variants in *IL-4* −590C/T and −33C/T polymorphisms may be a risk factor for CHB in Chinese males but not for HBV-related LC or HCC.

Editor: William B. Coleman, University of North Carolina School of Medicine, United States of America

Funding: This research was supported by National Natural Science Foundation of China (No. 81260302) and Youth Science Foundation of Guangxi Medical University (GXMUYSF201334). The funders had no role in study design, data collection and analysis, decision to publish, or preparation of the manuscript.

Competing Interests: The authors have declared that no competing interests exist.

* Email: qinxue919@126.com (XQ); lis8858@126.com (SL)

⊘ These authors contributed equally to this work.

Introduction

Hepatitis B virus (HBV) infection is one of the leading causes of liver disease, with more than 2 billion people infected worldwide [1,2]. Among them, approximately 350 million individuals persistently infected with HBV develop chronic hepatitis, which results in liver cirrhosis (LC) in one third of all cases, more than three quarters of which progress to hepatocellular carcinoma (HCC) [3]. It is widely accepted that chronic hepatitis B (CHB), LC, and HCC are progressive stages of chronic HBV infection [4]. Nevertheless, the mechanisms underlying such progression are not yet well understood, although immune system-mediated chronic inflammation is believed to play a pivotal role in HCC development. HBV clearance depends on an effective host immune response [5] and, thus, ineffective host immunity may create a hepatocarcinogenic microenvironment in the presence of HBV infection [6–8].

Interleukin-4 (IL-4), a multifunctional pleiotropic cytokine mainly produced by activated T helper 2 (Th2) cells, plays important roles as a mediator and modulator of immune and inflammatory responses [9]; it is not only involved in humoral and cell-mediated immunity, but also an essential regulator in the immune response of B cells, T cells, and macrophages to fight against infections and malignant cells [10]; Th2 diseases are, in their majority, driven by IL-4 [11]. In addition, IL-4 and IL-13 are the archetypal inducers of M2 [12]- an alternatively activated macrophage [13] that has been proved to promote HCC development [14]. Any alterations that influence the expression and function of IL-4 can lead to weakened immune responses, and thus increase the susceptibility to infections and inflammation-related diseases [15]. Due to their highly polymorphic nature, genetic mutations in this gene might be the major contributor.

The human *IL-4* gene is located on chromosome 5q31 and consists of 25 kbps [16]. So far, more than 50 allelic variant polymorphisms have been found (http://www.ncbi.nlm.nih.gov/ SNP/), including −590C/T (rs2243250), −33C/T (rs2070874), + 3437C/G (rs2227282), and 2979G/T (rs2227284) [17]. The impact of *IL-4* gene polymorphisms in the pathogenesis of HBV infection has been investigated, and numerous studies have suggested that *IL-4* variants play pivotal roles in hepatitis B vaccine response and HBV infection risk [18–21]. However, to date, few studies have been conducted to investigate the role of these polymorphisms in HCC development [22]. In the present study, the two most common promoter polymorphisms of *IL-4*, − 590C/T (rs2243250) and −33C/T (rs2070874), were evaluated in four Chinese patient groups – patients with CHB, LC, and HBV-related HCC, and a healthy control group – to determine whether these *IL-4* gene polymorphisms contribute to the susceptibility of HBV-related HCC.

Materials and Methods

Study population

A hospital-based series of 345 unrelated patients were recruited from the First Affiliated Hospital of Guangxi Medical University (Guangxi, China) between June and November 2013, including 154 patients with HBV-related HCC, 62 patients with HBV-induced LC, and 129 patients with CHB. To confirm that all patients had a chronic HBV infection for a period of at least 6 months, hepatitis B surface antigen (HBsAg), hepatitis B virus core antibody, and hepatitis Be antigen or hepatitis Be antibody were confirmed as seropositive. CHB was further diagnosed with serum HBV-DNA levels >1,000 copies/mL, as well as elevated alanine aminotransferase or aspartate aminotransferase (>2 times the upper limit of normal) [23]. LC was diagnosed by histologic analysis of liver biopsy specimens or typical morphologic findings from computed tomography or ultrasonography, together with laboratory features. For the HCC group, the patients enrolled fulfilled the following criteria: i) positive cytologic or pathologic findings or ii) elevated α-fetoprotein levels (≥400 ng/mL) combined with a positive image on computed tomography or ultrasonography; iii) were newly diagnosed HCC patients without a prior medical history of HCC; and iv) not diagnosed with other

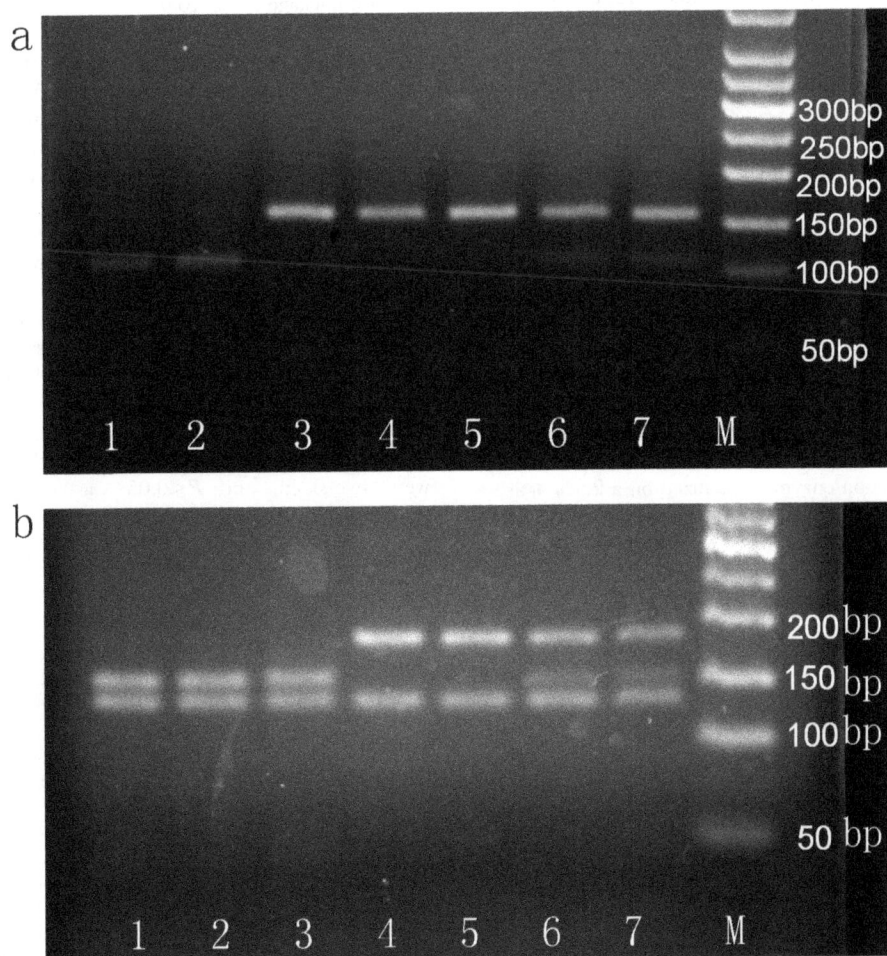

Figure 1. PCR-RFLP assay for analyzing the IL-4 −589C/T and −33C/T polymorphisms of the IL-4 gene. PCR product was digested by restriction enzyme and visualized on a 2.5% agarose gel. a −589C/T polymorphism. Lanes 1 and 2 show CC genotype; lanes 3, 4 and 5 show TT genotype; lanes 6 and 7 show CT genotype. b −33C/T polymorphism. Lanes 1, 2 and 3 show TT genotype; lanes 4 and 5 show CC genotype; lanes 6 and 7 show CT genotype. M, marker.

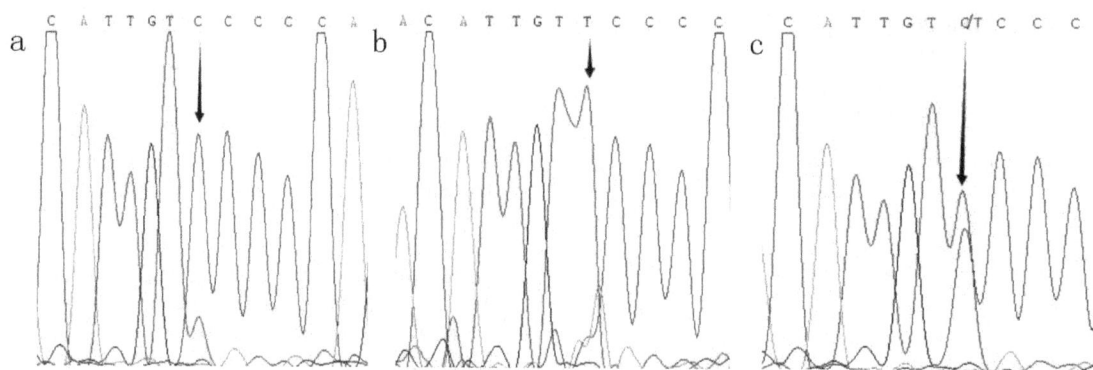

Figure 2. Sequencing map of the genotype for the IL-4 −589C/T polymorphism. Arrow in parts a−c indicates CC, TT and C/T genotypes, respectively.

cancers [24]. For comparison, 170 HBV free healthy controls were randomly selected from the Health Examination Center of the First Affiliated Hospital of Guangxi Medical University during the same period. The selection criteria for controls were absence of any malignancy or other serious illness, as well as other inflammatory status such as autoimmune hepatitis which may generate possible bais. All subjects were Chinese from the Guangxi District. Written informed consent was obtained from each participant, and the study was approved by the ethics committee of the First Affiliated Hospital of Guangxi Medical University, Nanning, Guangxi, China.

DNA extraction and single nucleotide polymorphism (SNP) genotyping

By using the standard phenol-chloroform method, genomic DNA was extracted from 2 mL peripheral white blood cells. The −589C/T and −33C/T SNPs in *IL-4* were detected by polymerase chain reaction-restriction fragment length polymorphism (PCR-RFLP). Primers and probes were designed by Sangon Biotech Company (Shanghai, China). The primer sequences, annealing temperature, length of the PCR products, and corresponding restriction enzyme used for genotyping are presented in Table S1. After amplification, the PCR product was digested by restriction enzyme, visualized on a 2.5% agarose gel, and stained with ethidium bromide (Promega Corporation, Madison, WI, USA) for genotyping (Figure 1). The genotyping was performed for all participants under blinded conditions. For quality control, 50% of samples were repeated and direct

sequencing was also performed by Sangon Biotech Company using 10% randomly selected samples (Figures 2 and 3); a 100% concordance rate was achieved.

Statistical analysis

The statistical analyses were performed using the statistical software package SPSS 16.0 (SPSS Inc., Chicago, IL, USA). The Hardy-Weinberg equilibrium (HWE) was firstly tested with a goodness-of-fit χ^2 test. General characteristics among the four groups were determined via Analysis of Variance (ANOVA) and the allele frequency and genotype distribution of *IL-4* gene polymorphisms were compared using the χ^2 test and Fisher's exact test, when appropriate. Binary logistic regression was used to calculate the odds ratios (ORs) and 95% confidence intervals (CIs) after age and gender status adjustments. Globally, HCC rates are more than twice as high in males as in females [25] and, therefore, gender may be a possible confounder. Thus, a stratification of the study population into males and females was further performed to evaluate the association within each stratum. Considering the possible linkage disequilibrium between the polymorphisms, Shi's standardized coefficient D' was used for quantification [26]; using the Phase program [27,28], haplotypes and their frequencies were also estimated based on a Bayesian algorithm. All significance tests were two-sided, and $P<0.05$ was considered a statistically significant difference.

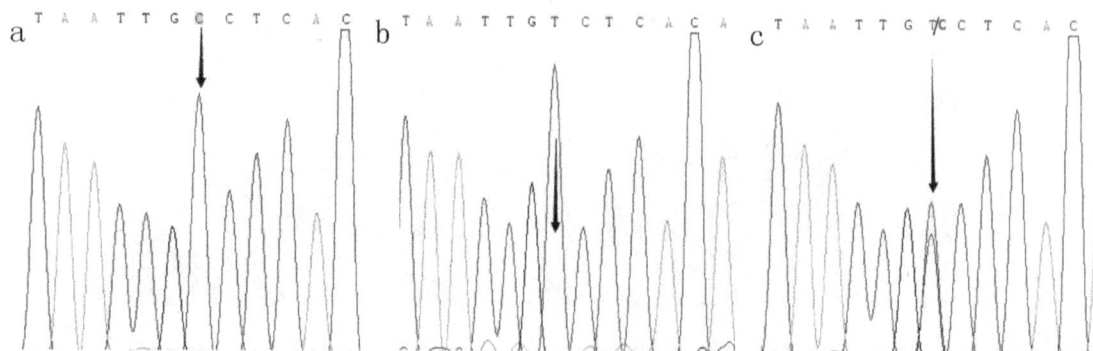

Figure 3. Sequencing map of the genotype for the IL-4 −33C/T polymorphisms. Arrow in parts a−c indicates CC, TT and C/T genotypes, respectively.

Table 1. Basic characteristic of the study population.

Variable	Healthy Controls (n = 170)	CHB patients (n = 129)	P-value	LC patients (n = 62)	P-value	HCC patients (n = 154)	P-value
Age(year, mean±SD)	37.68±11.76	37.67±7.78	0.994	47.38±9.64	<0.001	49.19±11.33	<0.001
Gender, N(%)							
Male	147(86.5)	115(89.1)	0.488	52(83.9)	0.618	135(87.7)	0.751
Female	23(13.5)	14(10.2)		10(16.1)		19(12.3)	

Results

Characteristics of the study participants

Table 1 summarizes the basic characteristics of the 170 healthy controls and the 129 CHB, 62 LC, and 154 HCC patients. Briefly, the LC and HCC patients were, on average, 10 years older than CHB patients and healthy controls, with the difference being statistically significant (both $P<0.001$). As for gender distribution, there were no significant differences between the case and control groups ($P = 0.488$, $P = 0.618$, and $P = 0.751$, respectively).

Genotype polymorphisms and the risk of HBV-related diseases

The genotype and allele frequencies of the −589C/T and −33C/T $IL-4$ gene polymorphisms for patients with HBV-related diseases and healthy controls are shown in Table 2. According to the HWE test, the genotype distribution of the two SNPs in the patient groups and healthy controls were all agreed with HWE ($P>0.05$ for all). However, no significant differences between the genotype and allele frequencies of the −589C/T and −33C/T $IL-4$ gene polymorphisms and CHB risk were observed. Binary logistic regression analyses adjusted for age and gender also failed to reveal any significant difference between them. Further, when considering LC and HCC patients, similar non-significant results were also found.

Nevertheless, when subgroup analyses between males and females were conducted, significant differences were found in males in the CC genotype in co-dominant genetic model CC versus TT and recessive genetic model CC versus TT+CT. Both 589C/T CC and −33C/T CC genotypes in males were associated with a significantly increased risk of CHB compared with the TT genotype (OR: 4.193, 95% CI: 1.094–16.071, and $P = 0.037$; and OR: 3.438, 95% CI: 1.032–11.458, and $P = 0.044$); similar situation was also found in the recessive model (OR: 4.09, 95% CI: 1.08–15.49, and $P = 0.038$; and OR: 3.43, 95% CI: 1.04–11.28, and $P = 0.042$) (Table 3). On the other hand, significant differences between case and control groups were not observed for any genotype in females (Table S2).

Considering that the $IL-4$ genetic background may be distinct between different populations, the genotype and allele frequencies of the two SNPs in our control group were further compared with those in different races from the Haplotype Map (HapMap) project (http://www.ncbi.nlm.nih. gov/snp/) as well as in previous reports [29]. The data shown in Table 4 suggests that the distribution of the two SNPs in the present study is significantly different from that in JPT (Japanese in Tokyo) and CEU (Utah residents with northern and western European ancestry) populations. For the 589C/T polymorphism, the frequencies of genotype TT and allele T in JPT and CEU populations are significantly lower, and the rate of CC genotype and C allele are significantly higher. With respect to the −33C/T polymorphism, significant genotype differences between the present study and YRI (Yoruba in Ibadan) were also found. Further, there were significantly lower detection rates of the TT genotype and T allele and higher detection rates of the CC genotype and C allele in the JPT, CEU, and YRI populations when compared with our data.

Estimated haplotype frequencies and the risk of HBV-related diseases

Haplotype analyses were performed for all patient groups and healthy controls using the SHEsis software, and the four possible haplotype frequencies of the two SNPs are shown in Table 5. According to the results, the $T^{-589} T^{-33}$ haplotype is the most common haplotype and represents >50% in all groups, whereas

Table 2. Genotype and allele frequencies of −589C/T and −33C/T polymorphisms between HBV-related patients and healthy controls.

Polymorphisms	Healthy controls, N=170(%)	CHB patients N=129(%)	LC patients, N=62(%)	HCC patients, N=154(%)	CHB patients vs. Healthy controls	LC patients vs. Healthy controls	HCC patients vs. Healthy controls
					OR (95%CI)[a]		
−589C/T							
TT	115(67.6)	77(59.7)	37(59.7)	111(72.1)	1.00	1.00	1.00
CT	51(30.0)	43(33.3)	22(35.5)	39(25.3)	1.28(0.78–2.12)	1.58(0.80–3.10)	0.90(0.52–1.56)
CC	4(2.4)	9(7.0)	3(4.8)	4(2.6)	3.35(0.99–11.28)	2.10(0.39–11.34)	1.13(0.26–5.06)
Dominant model[b]	55(32.4)	52(40.3)	25(40.3)	43(27.9)	1.44(0.89–2.33)	1.56(0.81–2.99)	0.921(0.54–1.56)
Recessive model[c]	166(97.6)	120(93.0)	59(95.2)	150(97.4)	3.08(0.93–10.25)	1.92(0.87–7.36)	1.17(0.27–5.13)
T allele	281(82.6)	197(76.4)	96(77.4)	261(84.7)	1.00	1.00	1.00
C allele	59(17.4)	61(23.6)	28(22.6)	47(15.3)	1.49(0.99–2.23)	1.51(0.87–2.61)	0.95(0.60–1.51)
P_{HWE}	0.550	0.383	0.907	0.796			
−33C/T							
TT	113(66.5)	77(59.7)	36(58.1)	97(63.0)	1.00	1.00	1.00
CT	52(30.6)	42(32.6)	22(35.4)	49(31.9)	1.21(0.73–2.00)	1.59(0.81–3.13)	1.29(0.76–2.20)
CC	5(2.9)	10(7.8)	4(6.5)	8(5.2)	2.92(0.96–8.92)	2.33(0.52–10.56)	2.24(0.65–7.74)
Dominant model[b]	57(33.5)	52(40.3)	26(41.9)	57(47.1)	1.36(0.84–2.20)	1.67(0.87–3.19)	1.38(0.83–2.30)
Recessive model[c]	165(97.1)	119(92.2)	58(93.5)	146(94.8)	2.74(0.91–8.25)	1.98(0.25–8.74)	2.06(0.60–7.01)
T allele	278(81.8)	196(76.0)	94(75.8)	263(78.9)	1.00	1.00	1.00
C allele	62(18.2)	62(24.0)	30(24.2)	65(21.1)	1.43(0.96–2.13)	1.56(0.91–2.66)	1.38(0.90–2.12)
P_{HWE}	0.737	0.219	0.797	0.581			

[a]Adjusted by age and gender;
[b]Dominant model: CT+CC versus TT;
[c]Recessive model: CC versus TT+CT.

Table 3. Genotype and allele frequencies of −589C/T and −33C/T polymorphisms between HBV-related patients and healthy controls in males.

Polymorphisms	Healthy controls, N = 147(%)	CHB patients N = 115(%)	LC patients, N = 52(%)	HCC patients, N = 135(%)	CHB patients vs. Healthy controls, OR(95%CI)[a]	LC patients vs. Healthy controls, OR (95%CI)[a]	HCC patients vs. Healthy controls, OR (95%CI)[a]
−589C/T							
Genotypes							
TT	100(68.0)	72(62.6)	31(59.6)	95(70.4)	1.00	1.00	1.00
CT	44(30.0)	34(29.6)	19(36.5)	36(26.6)	1.08(0.63–1.86)	1.92(0.92–4.01)	1.01(0.57–1.81)
CC	3(2.0)	9(7.8)	2(3.9)	4(3.0)	4.19(1.09–16.07)*	2.83(0.42–18.88)	1.59(0.32–7.98)
Dominant model[b]	47(32.0)	43(37.4)	21(40.4)	40(29.6)	1.28(0.76–2.15)	1.98(0.99–4.08)	1.05(0.60–1.85)
Recessive model[c]	144(98.0)	106(92.2)	50(96.1)	131(97.0)	4.09(1.08–15.49)*	2.23(0.35–14.43)	1.58(0.32–7.88)
T allele	244(83.0)	178(77.4)	81(77.9)	226(83.7)	1.00	1.00	1.00
C allele	50(17.0)	52(22.6)	23(22.1)	44(16.3)	1.43(0.93–2.06)	1.76(0.97–3.18)	1.085(0.67–1.77)
−33C/T							
Genotypes							
TT	98(66.7)	72(62.6)	30(57.7)	84(62.2)	1.00	1.00	1.00
CT	45(30.6)	33(28.7)	19(36.5)	43(31.9)	1.01(0.58–1.74)	1.84(0.89–3.82)	1.37(0.78–2.43)
CC	4(2.7)	10(8.7)	3(5.7)	8(5.9)	3.44(1.03–11.46)*	2.76(0.51–14.96)	2.96(0.78–11.22)
Dominant model[b]	49(33.3)	43(37.4)	22(42.3)	51(37.8)	1.20(0.72–2.01)	1.92(0.95–3.89)	1.51(0.87–2.61)
Recessive model[c]	143(97.3)	105(91.3)	49(94.2)	127(94.1)	3.43(1.04–11.28)*	2.22(0.43–11.54)	2.65(0.71–9.90)
T allele	241(82.0)	177(77.0)	79(76.0)	211(78.1)	1.00	1.00	1.00
C allele	53(18.0)	53(23.0)	24(24.0)	59(21.9)	1.37(0.89–2.10)	1.73(0.97–3.07)	1.52(0.96–2.41)

[a]Adjusted by age and gender;
[b]Dominant model: CT+CC versus TT;
[c]Recessive model: CC versus TT+CT;
*p<0.05.

Table 4. Comparison of genotype and allele frequencies in the healthy control subjects of our study and that from the HapMap project.

Polymorphisms	Samples, N	Genotype frequency, n(%)				Alleles frequency, n(%)		
		TT	CT	CC	P values	T	C	P values
−589C/T								
Present study	170	115(67.6)	51(30.0)	4(2.4)		281(82.6)	59(17.4)	
HCB*	86	50(58.1)	34(39.5)	2(2.3)	0.307	134(77.9)	38(22.1)	0.196
JPT*	170	90(52.9)	66(38.8)	14(8.2)	0.005	246(72.4)	94(27.6)	0.001
CEU*	226	4(1.8)	54(23.9)	168(74.3)	0.000	62(13.7)	390(86.3)	0.000
YRI*	226	140(61.9)	76(33.6)	10(4.4)	0.356	356(78.8)	96(21.2)	0.172
Chinese†	151	92(60.9)	50(33.1)	9(6.0)	0.185	234(77.5)	68(22.5)	0.101
−33C/T								
Present study	170	113(66.5)	52(30.6)	5(2.9)		278(81.8)	62(18.2)	
HCB*	86	50(58.1)	34(39.5)	2(2.3)	0.357	134(77.9)	38(22.1)	0.298
JPT*	172	90(52.3)	68(39.5)	14(8.1)	0.011	248(72.1)	96(27.9)	0.003
CEU*	226	4(1.8)	54(23.9)	168(74.3)	0.000	62(13.7)	390(86.3)	0.000
YRI*	226	44(19.5)	126(55.8)	56(24.8)	0.000	214(47.3)	238(52.7)	0.000
HCH†	159	104(65.4)	51(32.1)	4(2.5)	0.939	259(81.4)	59(18.6)	0.916

*Data from HapMap Project;
†Data from previous reports; HCB, Han Chinese in Beijing, China; JPT, Japanese in Tokyo, Japan; CEU, Utah residents with northern and western European ancestry; YRI, Yoruba in Ibadan, Nigeria; HCH, Han Chinese in Hunan province, China.

Table 5. Frequencies of the haplotypes formed by −589C/T and −33C/T polymorphisms in HBV-related patients and healthy controls.

Haplotype	Healthy control (%)	CHB Patients (%)	OR (95%CI)	p	LC Patients (%)	OR (95%CI)	p	HCC Patients (%)	OR (95%CI)	p
CC	17.1	23.3	1.47(0.98–2.20)	0.061	16.5	0.96(0.55–1.66)	0.878	14.9	0.85(0.56–1.30)	0.459
CT	0.3	0.4	-	-	6.1	-	-	0.3	-	-
TC	1.2	0.8	-	-	7.7	-	-	6.2	-	-
TT	81.5	75.6	0.68(0.45–1.02)	0.061	69.7	0.52(0.33–0.84)	0.064	78.6	0.83(0.57–1.23)	0.356

the C^{-589} C^{-33} haplotype accounts for 14.9% to 23.3% among the four groups and represents the second highest haplotype. After haplotype analyses, however, no significant differences in these haplotype frequencies were found in any group. Finally, C^{-589} T^{-33} and T^{-589} C^{-33} are rare haplotypes that account for less than 2% in the control subjects and therefore further analyses were not conducted for these.

Discussion

China, a region with 94 million HBsAg carriers, accounts for 50% of the total HCC cases worldwide [30,31]. The predominant mode of HBV transmission in this hyperendemic region is vertical transmission from infected mothers during or shortly after birth [32]. However, only 5% to 10% of perinatally-infected infants become persistent carriers as adults, despite the approximately 90% risk; further, from these persistent infectors, 10% to 30% will progress to LC and HCC [33]. Such highly variable disease outcomes cannot be fully explained by differences in immunological, viral, or environmental factors. Thus, differences in host genetic factors may play essential roles in these processes.

IL-4, a typical pleiotropic Th2 cytokine [9], is best known for defining the Th2 phenotype of lymphocytes, as well as being involved in regulating cell proliferation, apoptosis, and expression of numerous genes in lymphocytes, macrophages, and fibroblasts, among others [34–39]. Functional variations in this gene may contribute to viral clearance as well as HBV-associated HCC in high-risk Chinese patients. However, in the present study, we did not observe any association of *IL-4* genotypes, alleles, and haplotypes with the overall CHB, LC, and HCC patients. Nevertheless, in subgroup analysis, CC genotypes of the *IL-4* −589C/T and −33C/T polymorphisms were observed to be significantly associated with CHB in males as compared with the TT genotypes and TT+CT genotypes. In females, a similar trend towards an increased risk effect of CC genotypes in CHB was also observed, but the difference was not significant. These results indicate that *IL-4* gene polymorphisms may be a risk factor for CHB in the Chinese male population only.

Data from previous epidemiological studies was consistent with our results. In a meta-analysis conducted by Zheng et al. [20] exploring the *IL-4* 590C/T polymorphism and its susceptibility to liver disease (including HBV infection, HCV infection, liver cirrhosis, etc.), significant associations between the *IL-4* 590T polymorphism and increased risk of liver diseases was found in Caucasian populations, but not in Asian populations. Another meta-analysis investigating the association of *IL-4* polymorphisms with response to HBV vaccine and susceptibility to HBV infection, also found no evidence indicating a correlation between *IL-4* polymorphisms (rs2243250 C>T) and susceptibility to HBV infection [21]. It is noted that all "Asian population" studies included in the two meta-analyses mentioned above were conducted in China [40–45].

It is noteworthy that, in the present study, the significant association between CHB in males was found in the CC genotypes of −589C/T and −33C/T polymorphisms, as opposed to the T allele in the Caucasian populations studied in the meta-analysis of Zheng et al. [20]. The fact that the same polymorphism site has distinct genotype frequencies which play different roles in the same disease may be principally explained by differences in the *IL-4* genetic background among ethnicities; results from the comparison of genotype and allele frequencies in the healthy control subjects in the present study and those from the HapMap project provide evidence to this effect. In the current study, the *IL-4* −590T and −33T allele frequencies among healthy controls were

82.6% and 81.8%, respectively, which were significantly higher than those observed in healthy Caucasians (both were 13.7%), while the C allele frequencies accounted for 17.4% in −590C/T mutations and 18.2% in −33C/T mutations, which were significantly lower than in Caucasians (both were 86.3%). Thus, the T allele may be the major allele in −589C/T and −33C/T SNPs in the Chinese population, and the C allele is the variant responsible for various diseases, while the opposite is true for Caucasians.

With respect to HCC, only two studies were found regarding the *IL-4* −590 C/T polymorphism and HCC risk in a high-risk Chinese population [46] and in low-risk non-Asians in the USA [22], both conducted by Ognjanovic et al. [22,46]. Contrary to our results, the authors noted a substantial decrease in HCC risk associated with the *IL-4* −590 CC genotype in Guangxi, China, and a non-significant result in Los Angeles non-Asians. However, in the present study, no association was found for either *IL-4* − 590C/T or −33C/T polymorphisms and HCC risk in the Chinese population. Drinking status may be a possible factor in the disparate associations between our study and theirs. According to their results [46], the *IL-4* −590 CC genotype was not associated with a lower risk of HCC when initially adjusted for age, gender, and ethnicity (CC vs. CT/TT, OR: 0.46, 95% CI: 0.16–1.31); however, after further adjustment for HBsAg seropositivity and the number of alcoholic drinks per day (0, <3, or >3), the CC genotype was found to be negatively associated with HCC risk (CC vs. CT/TT, OR: 0.05, 95% CI: 0.01–0.40); in contrast, individuals included in our study were all HBsAg seropositive. In addition, the difference in study design and sample size may also be possible confounders.

For *IL-4* polymorphism haplotypes, previous experimental data has demonstrated some to be associated with respiratory syncytial virus [47], multiple sclerosis [48], oral cancer [49], and systemic lupus erythematosus [50], suggesting that certain important

polymorphisms could affect the regulation of this cytokine. In addition, the T allele of the *IL-4* −590C/T polymorphism has been reported to be in linkage disequilibrium with −33T [51], and was associated with an increased expression of IL-4 [52]. However, we did not find an association between any of the estimated haplotype frequencies and the risk of HBV-related diseases, indicating that the *IL-4* gene haplotypes may not play any facilitative role in the development of HCC.

In conclusion, we could not detect an effect of genetic variants between *IL-4* and HBV-related HCC in a Chinese population. Interestingly, in subgroup analysis, the CC genotype of *IL-4* − 589C/T and −33C/T polymorphisms were observed to be significantly correlated with the risk of CHB in the Chinese male population. However, considering the relatively small sample size of this study, more studies with a larger sample size are warranted in an attempt to confirm the observed association.

Supporting Information

Table S1 **The sequences of forward and backward primers and restriction enzymes for genotyping IL-4 polymorphisms.**

Table S2 **Genotype and allele frequencies of −589C/T and −33C/T polymorphisms between HBV-related patients and healthy controls in females.**

Author Contributions

Conceived and designed the experiments: XQ SL. Performed the experiments: YL ZTW. Analyzed the data: QLP LPM. Contributed reagents/materials/analysis tools: XLZ JYZ. Contributed to the writing of the manuscript: YL.

References

1. Liaw YF, Chu CM (2009) Hepatitis B virus infection. Lancet 373: 582–592.
2. Lavanchy D (2005) Worldwide epidemiology of HBV infection, disease burden, and vaccine prevention. J Clin Virol 34 Suppl 1: S1–3.
3. Perz JF, Armstrong GL, Farrington LA, Hutin YJ, Bell BP (2006) The contributions of hepatitis B virus and hepatitis C virus infections to cirrhosis and primary liver cancer worldwide. J Hepatol 45: 529–538.
4. Yin J, Xie J, Liu S, Zhang H, Han L, et al. (2011) Association between the various mutations in viral core promoter region to different stages of hepatitis B, ranging of asymptomatic carrier state to hepatocellular carcinoma. Am J Gastroenterol 106: 81–92.
5. Chisari FV, Ferrari C (1995) Hepatitis B virus immunopathogenesis. Annu Rev Immunol 13: 29–60.
6. Chen L, Zhang Q, Chang W, Du Y, Zhang H, et al. (2012) Viral and host inflammation-related factors that can predict the prognosis of hepatocellular carcinoma. Eur J Cancer 48: 1977–1987.
7. Chemin I, Zoulim F (2009) Hepatitis B virus induced hepatocellular carcinoma. Cancer Lett 286: 52–59.
8. Han YF, Zhao J, Ma LY, Yin JH, Chang WJ, et al. (2011) Factors predicting occurrence and prognosis of hepatitis-B-virus-related hepatocellular carcinoma. World J Gastroenterol 17: 4258–4270.
9. Durie FH, Foy TM, Masters SR, Laman JD, Noelle RJ (1994) The role of CD40 in the regulation of humoral and cell-mediated immunity. Immunol Today 15: 406–411.
10. Landi S, Bottari F, Gemignani F, Gioia-Patricola L, Guino E, et al. (2007) Interleukin-4 and interleukin-4 receptor polymorphisms and colorectal cancer risk. Eur J Cancer 43: 762–768.
11. Luzina IG, Keegan AD, Heller NM, Rook GA, Shea-Donohue T, et al. (2012) Regulation of inflammation by interleukin-4: a review of "alternatives". J Leukoc Biol 92: 753–764.
12. Gordon S (2003) Alternative activation of macrophages. Nat Rev Immunol 3: 23–35.
13. Stein M, Keshav S, Harris N, Gordon S (1992) Interleukin 4 potently enhances murine macrophage mannose receptor activity: a marker of alternative immunologic macrophage activation. J Exp Med 176: 287–292.
14. Capece D, Fischietti M, Verzella D, Gaggiano A, Cicciarelli G, et al. (2013) The

inflammatory microenvironment in hepatocellular carcinoma: a pivotal role for tumor-associated macrophages. Biomed Res Int 2013: 187204.
15. Jiang H, Harris MB, Rothman P (2000) IL-4/IL-13 signaling beyond JAK/STAT. J Allergy Clin Immunol 105: 1063–1070.
16. Marsh DG, Neely JD, Breazeale DR, Ghosh B, Freidhoff LR, et al. (1994) Linkage analysis of IL4 and other chromosome 5q31.1 markers and total serum immunoglobulin E concentrations. Science 264: 1152–1156.
17. Naslednikova IO, Konenkov VI, Ryazantseva NV, Novitskii VV, Tkachenko SB, et al. (2007) Role of genetically determined production of immunoregulatory cytokines in immunopathogenesis of chronic viral hepatitides. Bull Exp Biol Med 143: 706–712.
18. Aithal GP, Ramsay L, Daly AK, Sonchit N, Leathart JB, et al. (2004) Hepatic adducts, circulating antibodies, and cytokine polymorphisms in patients with diclofenac hepatotoxicity. Hepatology 39: 1430–1440.
19. Zhu QR, Ge YL, Gu SQ, Yu H, Wang JS, et al. (2005) Relationship between cytokines gene polymorphism and susceptibility to hepatitis B virus intrauterine infection. Chin Med J (Engl) 118: 1604–1609.
20. Zheng Z, Li X, Li Z, Ma XC (2013) IL-4 -590C/T polymorphism and susceptibility to liver disease: a meta-analysis and meta-regression. DNA Cell Biol 32: 443–450.
21. Cui W, Sun CM, Deng BC, Liu P (2013) Association of polymorphisms in the interleukin-4 gene with response to hepatitis B vaccine and susceptibility to hepatitis B virus infection: a meta-analysis. Gene 525: 35–40.
22. Ognjanovic S, Yuan JM, Chaptman AK, Fan Y, Yu MC (2009) Genetic polymorphisms in the cytokine genes and risk of hepatocellular carcinoma in low-risk non-Asians of USA. Carcinogenesis 30: 758–762.
23. Lok AS, McMahon BJ (2007) Chronic hepatitis B. Hepatology 45: 507–539.
24. Peng Q, Qin X, He Y, Chen Z, Deng Y, et al. (2013) Association of IL27 gene polymorphisms and HBV-related hepatocellular carcinoma risk in a Chinese population. Infect Genet Evol 16: 1–4.
25. Jemal A, Bray F, Center MM, Ferlay J, Ward E, et al. (2011) Global cancer statistics. CA Cancer J Clin 61: 69–90.
26. Shi YY, He L (2005) SHEsis, a powerful software platform for analyses of linkage disequilibrium, haplotype construction, and genetic association at polymorphism loci. Cell Res 15: 97–98.

27. Li Z, Zhang Z, He Z, Tang W, Li T, et al. (2009) A partition-ligation-combination-subdivision EM algorithm for haplotype inference with multiallelic markers: update of the SHEsis (http://analysis.bio-x.cn). Cell Res 19: 519–523.

28. Stephens M, Smith NJ, Donnelly P (2001) A new statistical method for haplotype reconstruction from population data. Am J Hum Genet 68: 978–989.

29. Tang ZY YQ, Feng XL, Zhou L, Zhang YL, Chen B (2009) Association between IL-4 C+33T and serum levels of IL-4 and atherothrombotic cerebral infarction in Chinese Han. Stroke and nevous diseases 16: 11–14.

30. Yin J, Zhang H, He Y, Xie J, Liu S, et al. (2010) Distribution and hepatocellular carcinoma-related viral properties of hepatitis B virus genotypes in Mainland China: a community-based study. Cancer Epidemiol Biomarkers Prev 19: 777–786.

31. Siegel R, Naishadham D, Jemal A (2012) Cancer statistics, 2012. CA Cancer J Clin 62: 10–29.

32. Yu MC, Yuan JM (2004) Environmental factors and risk for hepatocellular carcinoma. Gastroenterology 127: S72–78.

33. Zeng Z (2014) Human genes involved in hepatitis B virus infection. World J Gastroenterol 20: 7696–7706.

34. Nelms K, Keegan AD, Zamorano J, Ryan JJ, Paul WE (1999) The IL-4 receptor: signaling mechanisms and biologic functions. Annu Rev Immunol 17: 701–738.

35. Kelly-Welch A, Hanson EM, Keegan AD (2005) Interleukin-13 (IL-13) pathway. Sci STKE 2005: cm8.

36. Chomarat P, Banchereau J (1998) Interleukin-4 and interleukin-13: their similarities and discrepancies. Int Rev Immunol 17: 1–52.

37. Kelly-Welch AE, Hanson EM, Boothby MR, Keegan AD (2003) Interleukin-4 and interleukin-13 signaling connections maps. Science 300: 1527–1528.

38. LaPorte SL, Juo ZS, Vaclavikova J, Colf LA, Qi X, et al. (2008) Molecular and structural basis of cytokine receptor pleiotropy in the interleukin-4/13 system. Cell 132: 259–272.

39. Iseki M, Omori-Miyake M, Xu W, Sun X, Takaki S, et al. (2012) Thymic stromal lymphopoietin (TSLP)-induced polyclonal B-cell activation and autoimmunity are mediated by CD4+ T cells and IL-4. Int Immunol 24: 183–195.

40. Chen TY, Hsieh YS, Wu TT, Yang SF, Wu CJ, et al. (2007) Impact of serum levels and gene polymorphism of cytokines on chronic hepatitis C infection. Transl Res 150: 116–121.

41. Gao QJ, Liu DW, Zhang SY, Jia M, Wang LM, et al. (2009) Polymorphisms of some cytokines and chronic hepatitis B and C virus infection. World J Gastroenterol 15: 5610–5619.

42. Liu Q, Long H., Wang J.G., Du J.H. (2007) Relationship between genetic polymorphisms of interleukin-4 (IL-4), interleukin-4 receptor a chain with susceptibility to HBVinduced liver cirrhosis. Chin J Integr Tradit West Med Liver Dis 17: 211–213.

43. Zhu QR, Ge YL, Gu SQ, Yu H, Wang JS, et al. (2005) Relationship between cytokines gene polymorphism and susceptibility to hepatitis B virus intrauterine infection. Chin Med J 26: 1604–1069.

44. Wang K, Shi CW, Gao Y, Yu ZH, Ning T, et al. (2006) The association of IL-2 and IL-4 polymorphisms and hepatitis B in population of north China. Chin J Curr Adv Gen Surg 9: 171–176.

45. Gao QJ, Sun DX, Zhang YH, Chen SP, Wang XH, et al. (2012) Association of IL-4-589 polymorphisms with chronic hepatitis B and hepatitis C virus infection. Med Pharm J Chin People's Liberation Army 24: 8–10.

46. Nieters A, Yuan JM, Sun CL, Zhang ZQ, Stoehlmacher J, et al. (2005) Effect of cytokine genotypes on the hepatitis B virus-hepatocellular carcinoma association. Cancer 103: 740–748.

47. Puthothu B, Krueger M, Forster J, Heinzmann A (2006) Association between severe respiratory syncytial virus infection and IL13/IL4 haplotypes. J Infect Dis 193: 438–441.

48. Suppiah V, Goris A, Alloza I, Heggarty S, Dubois B, et al. (2005) Polymorphisms in the interleukin-4 and IL-4 receptor genes and multiple sclerosis: a study in Spanish-Basque, Northern Irish and Belgian populations. Int J Immunogenet 32: 383–388.

49. Tsai MH, Chen WC, Tsai CH, Hang LW, Tsai FJ (2005) Interleukin-4 gene, but not the interleukin-1 beta gene polymorphism, is associated with oral cancer. J Clin Lab Anal 19: 93–98.

50. Wu MC, Huang CM, Tsai JJ, Chen HY, Tsai FJ (2003) Polymorphisms of the interleukin-4 gene in chinese patients with systemic lupus erythematosus in Taiwan. Lupus 12: 21–25.

51. Takabayashi A, Ihara K, Sasaki Y, Kusuhara K, Nishima S, et al. (1999) Novel polymorphism in the 5′-untranslated region of the interleukin-4 gene. J Hum Genet 44: 352–353.

52. Wierenga EA, Messer G (2000) Regulation of interleukin 4 gene transcription: alterations in atopic disease? Am J Respir Crit Care Med 162: S81–85.

18

Is 3-Tesla Gd-EOB-DTPA-Enhanced MRI with Diffusion-Weighted Imaging Superior to 64-Slice Contrast-Enhanced CT for the Diagnosis of Hepatocellular Carcinoma?

Bettina Maiwald*, Donald Lobsien, Thomas Kahn, Patrick Stumpp

Department of Diagnostic and Interventional Radiology, University of Leipzig, Leipzig, Germany

Abstract

Objectives: To compare 64-slice contrast-enhanced computed tomography (CT) with 3-Tesla magnetic resonance imaging (MRI) using Gd-EOB-DTPA for the diagnosis of hepatocellular carcinoma (HCC) and evaluate the utility of diffusion-weighted imaging (DWI) in this setting.

Methods: 3-phase-liver-CT was performed in fifty patients (42 male, 8 female) with suspected or proven HCC. The patients were subjected to a 3-Tesla-MRI-examination with Gd-EOB-DTPA and diffusion weighted imaging (DWI) at b-values of 0, 50 and 400 s/mm^2. The apparent diffusion coefficient (ADC)-value was determined for each lesion detected in DWI. The histopathological report after resection or biopsy of a lesion served as the gold standard, and a surrogate of follow-up or complementary imaging techniques in combination with clinical and paraclinical parameters was used in unresected lesions. Diagnostic accuracy, sensitivity, specificity, and positive and negative predictive values were evaluated for each technique.

Results: MRI detected slightly more lesions that were considered suspicious for HCC per patient compared to CT (2.7 versus 2.3, respectively). ADC-measurements in HCC showed notably heterogeneous values with a median of $1.2\pm0.5\times10^{-3}$ mm^2/s (range from 0.07 ± 0.1 to $3.0\pm0.1\times10^{-3}$ mm^2/s). MRI showed similar diagnostic accuracy, sensitivity, and positive and negative predictive values compared to CT (AUC 0.837, sensitivity 92%, PPV 80% and NPV 90% for MRI vs. AUC 0.798, sensitivity 85%, PPV 79% and NPV 82% for CT; not significant). Specificity was 75% for both techniques.

Conclusions: Our study did not show a statistically significant difference in detection in detection of HCC between MRI and CT. Gd-EOB-DTPA-enhanced MRI tended to detect more lesions per patient compared to contrast-enhanced CT; therefore, we would recommend this modality as the first-choice imaging method for the detection of HCC and therapeutic decisions. However, contrast-enhanced CT was not inferior in our study, so that it can be a useful image modality for follow-up examinations.

Editor: Andreas-Claudius Hoffmann, West German Cancer Center, Germany

Funding: This work was supported by a research grant from Bayer Vital, Leverkusen, Germany. This was used to buy contrast media for the MRI-examination. The funders had no role in study design, data collection and analysis, decision to publish, or preparation of the manuscript. None of the author received specific funding for this work. www.bayerpharma.com.

Competing Interests: The study was supported by a research grant from Bayer Vital, Leverkusen, Germany but this did not modify the authors' results and conclusion in any way. It was used to buy contrast media (Gd-EOB-DTPA (Primovist®)) for the MRI-examination of the patients. This contrast medium is a specific tool in imaging liver lesions since it is metabolized by the hepatocytes. It is officially approved by the European Medicines Agency (EMA) as well as by the Food and Drug Administration (FDA) in the USA and the authors currently use it daily in clinical routine. The funders had no role in study design, data collection and analysis, decision to publish or preparation of the manuscript. The authors' employments were not paid by the research grant. None of the authors received personal funding for this work and therefore no personal competing interests exist. This funding does not alter the authors' adherence to PLOS ONE policies on sharing data and materials.

* Email: bettina.maiwald@medizin.uni-leipzig.de

Introduction

Hepatocellular carcinoma (HCC) is one of the most common malignancies worldwide. Liver cirrhosis is a precancerous condition associated with the development of HCC. Other important risk factors include chronic hepatitis B and C, as well as alcohol abuse. The sequential carcinogenesis from regenerative nodules to overt HCC has been described previously, and the *de novo* development of HCC without prior liver cirrhosis has also been delineated [1–5].

HCC can be diagnosed by various imaging modalities, including ultrasound, multidetector computed tomography (CT) and magnetic resonance imaging (MRI). Despite these versatile imaging modalities, correct characterization of HCC versus other liver lesions remains a challenging task, and a definite diagnosis often cannot be made based on imaging alone [6]. However, in cancer patients, a precise diagnosis is important for optimal treatment planning [2,7].

Concerning advanced magnetic resonance techniques, diffusion weighted imaging (DWI) has the ability to differentiate between malignant and benign liver lesions [8–12]. A recently developed liver-specific contrast medium, Gd-EOB-DTPA (Gadolinium-ethoxybenzyl-diethylene-triamine-pentaacetic-acid), is a paramagnetic contrast agent with properties of extracellular and hepatobiliary contrast media for use in MR imaging of the liver. This reagent allows for dynamic perfusion imaging and the evaluation of liver function. Gd-EOB-DTPA is taken up in hepatocytes to approximately 50% via OATP-1 (organic anion transporter protein-1), increasing the signal intensity of the liver parenchyma approximately 20 min after injection [13–16]. Several studies have demonstrated that this reagent improved the detection and characterization of focal liver lesions [17–19].

High field-strength MRI at 3.0 Tesla provides better tissue contrast compared to 1.5 Tesla due to a greater signal-to-noise ratio, improved image quality, higher resolution imaging and faster scanning times [20].

The aim of this study was to compare the diagnostic power of CT with 3 Tesla MRI using Gd-EOB-DTPA for the diagnosis of HCC and to evaluate the diagnostic impact of DWI with apparent diffusion coefficient (ADC) quantification in this setting.

Material and Methods

Patient Selection

Fifty patients (mean age 60.6 years, range 29–84 years, mean body weight 79,8 kg, range 45–120 kg, 42 male, 8 female, Table 1) with suspected or proven HCC were included in this prospective single-centre study to evaluate the diagnostic performance of contrast-enhanced CT and Gd-EOB-DTPA-enhanced MRI in terms of lesion detection. Inclusion criteria were suspicious findings in the US or/and increased laboratory parameters (e.g., alpha-fetoprotein). Exclusion criteria were renal failure, allergy to contrast agents, hyperthyreoidism, pregnancy and, especially for the MRI-examination, pacemaker or other non-compatible implants and claustrophobia. The aetiology of liver cirrhosis in the patient cohort was as follows: 26 patients with alcohol induced liver cirrhosis, 2 with Hepatitis B- and 3 with Hepatitis C-related chronic liver disease, 3 patients with hemochromatosis, one with Budd-Chiari-Syndrome and one with non-alcoholic steatohepatitis. 14 patients had cryptogenic liver cirrhosis. Based on the Child-Pugh-Classification, the severity of liver cirrhosis was classified as class A in 27 patients, class B in 16 patients and class C in 7 patients [Table 1].

The histopathological report after resection or biopsy of a lesion served as the gold standard for diagnosis, whereas a surrogate of follow-up (after 6 months) or complementary imaging technique (ultrasound, digital subtraction angiography) in combination with clinical (loss of weight, general state) and paraclinical parameters (especially alpha-fetoprotein) was used in unresected lesions.

This study was approved by the ethics committee of the medical faculty of the University of Leipzig, and all patients provided written informed consent.

Imaging technique

Multiphase-CT was performed using two different scanners (Brilliance 64/iCT; Philips Healthcare, Eindhoven, Netherlands) with identical parameters to prevent bias within the CT: collimation of 0.625 mm, rotation time of 0.75 s, tube voltage of 120 kV, tube current 200 mAs and adjusted with automatic dose modulation, reconstructed slice thickness of 3 mm, matrix 512*512). The contrast agent (Iopromide Ultravist 370, Bayer Vital GmbH, Leverkusen, Germany) was applied at a constant volume of 100 ml at a rate of 3 ml/s (Power injector mississippi, Ulrich Medical, Ulm, Germany). The unenhanced phase, early arterial phase 10 s after bolustracking (positioning the respective region of interest in the abdominal aorta just above the coeliac trunk, threshold 150 HU) and portal venous phase 60 s after reaching the threshold were acquired.

Subsequent MRI (median time: 2.2 days, range 0–30d) was performed in all subjects using a 3.0 Tesla scanner (TrioTim, Siemens Medical Solutions, Erlangen, Germany). The study protocol consisted of the following sequences:

(1) T2w-HASTE (half-fourier acquisition single-shot turbo spin echo) coronal and axial

(2) T1w-VIBE (volume-interpolated breath-hold examination) coronal unenhanced, axial unenhanced and dynamic after contrast medium was applied (Gd-EOB-DTPA (Primovist), Bayer Vital GmbH, Leverkusen, Germany) at 0.1 ml/kg bodyweight at a rate of 2 ml/s using a power injector (Spectris solaris EP, Medrad, Dusseldorf, Germany), followed by a 30 ml saline flush. Scanning times were as follows: arterial phase, 2 s; portalvenous phase, 30–40, equilibrium phase, 2–3 min; and hepatobiliary phase, 20 min after the contrast bolus reached the abdominal aorta.

(3) Diffusion-weighted sequence coronal and axial (b-value 0, 50 and 400 s/mm^2)

(4) T2w TSE (turbo spin echo) with fat saturation coronal

(5) T1w in phase and opposed phase axial

See Table 2 for more details concerning the sequences.

Imaging analysis

Image analysis focused on the number, size and detectability of liver lesions, as well as image quality. A radiologist with 10 years of experience in abdominal imaging performed the analysis using a picture archiving and communication system workstation (Magic-View 1000, Siemens Medical Solutions, Erlangen, Germany). The observer was aware of the patients being at risk of HCC, but otherwise blinded to all patient data. Diagnosis of HCC was based on hypervascularization in the arterial phase and washout in the portal venous phase or delayed phase, as suggested by the European Association for the Study of the Liver and the American Association for the Study of Liver Disease for MRI and CT [1]. In addition, focal areas with a suspicious hypointense signal in the hepatobiliary phase were used to detect HCC [21] (Figure 1). The radiologist recorded the presence and anatomical location of lesions, as well as diagnostic confidence using the following 5-point scale: 1 = definitely not HCC, 2 = probably not HCC, 3 = equivocal, 4 = probably HCC, 5 = definitely HCC.

Lesion detectability and image quality were evaluated using a 5-point rating-scale (1 = excellent, 2 = good, 3 = fair, 4 = poor, 5 = unacceptable). The average largest tumour diameter was determined using a measuring tool integrated in the workstation software.

ADC-values were measured for each clearly demarcated lesion in ADC-map by drawing a circular region of interest into the tumour that encompassed as much of the lesion as possible while excluding vascular structures and necrotic tissue.

Imaging analysis was accomplished according to the following settings:

Table 1. Demographics, aetiology of liver cirrhosis and patients clinical condition.

Gender	
Male	42
Female	8
Mean age (years)	60.6 (range 29–84)
Mean weight (kg)	79.8 (range 45–120)
Aetiology of liver cirrhosis	
Alcoholic disease	26
Hepatitis B	2
Hepatitis C	3
Haemochromatosis	3
Budd-Chiari-Syndrome	1
Non-alcoholic steatohepatosis	1
Cryptogenic	14
Child Pugh Status	
A (5–6)	27
B (7–9)	16
C (10–15)	7

1) In general, CT-scans were compared with

2) complete MRI-examinations (including conventional dynamic MRI with hepatobiliary phase and DWI).

To estimate the impact of the hepatobiliary phase and diffusion-weighted imaging, MRI-data were subdivided into three sets:

3) conventional dynamic MRI without the hepatobiliary phase and DWI

4) dynamic MRI including the hepatobiliary phase

5) MRI including diffusion-weighted sequences.

In addition, the observer evaluated the reading time.

Statistical analysis

Statistical analysis was performed using SPSS 20.0 for Windows (statistical package for social sciences 20.0, Chicago, IL, USA) and Microsoft Excel (Microsoft, Redmond, WA, USA). The diagnostic performance of each technique was assessed by measuring the area under the curve (AUC) of the free-response receiver operating characteristic analysis (ROC-curve) on a lesion-per-patient-basis.

Sensitivity, specificity, and positive and negative predictive values were calculated for patients assigned a diagnostic confidence level of 4 and 5 (probably and definitely HCC). In addition, we included patients with a confidence level of 3, because in clinical routine, a suspicious lesion must be clarified (e.g., by further imaging or biopsy). The differences in the ROC-curves, sensitivities, specificities, positive predictive value (PPV) and negative predictive value (NPV) were statistically analysed using a binomial test. Student's t-test was used to calculate significant differences for image quality, detectability and reading time between the image modalities, P-values <0.05 were considered significantly different.

Table 2. MR Imaging Parameters.

Parameter	T2-weighted (HASTE)	T1-weighted (VIBE)	DWI	T2-weighted TSE	T1-weighted in and out of phase
Imaging plane	Coronal and axial	Coronal and axial unenhanced, axial enhanced	Coronal and axial	Coronal	Axial
Fat saturation	No	Yes	Yes	Yes	No
Respiratory triggering	Breath-hold (12 s)	Breath-hold (16 s)	Respiratory-triggered	Respiratory-triggered	Breath-hold (18 s)
Repetition time (TR)	800 ms	2.92 ms	2000 ms	2000 ms	212 ms
Echo time (TE)	83 s	0.86 ms	60 ms	81 ms	2.32 ms
Flip angle	160°	10°	-	120°	65°
Bandwidth	781 Hz/Px	540 Hz/Px	1736 Hz/Px	260 Hz/Px	930 Hz/Px
Field of view (FOV)	450 mm	400 mm	380 mm	400 mm	380 mm
Slice thickness	5 mm	3 mm	5 mm	5 mm	5 mm
Matrix	320*256	256*200	192*154	320*224	256*200

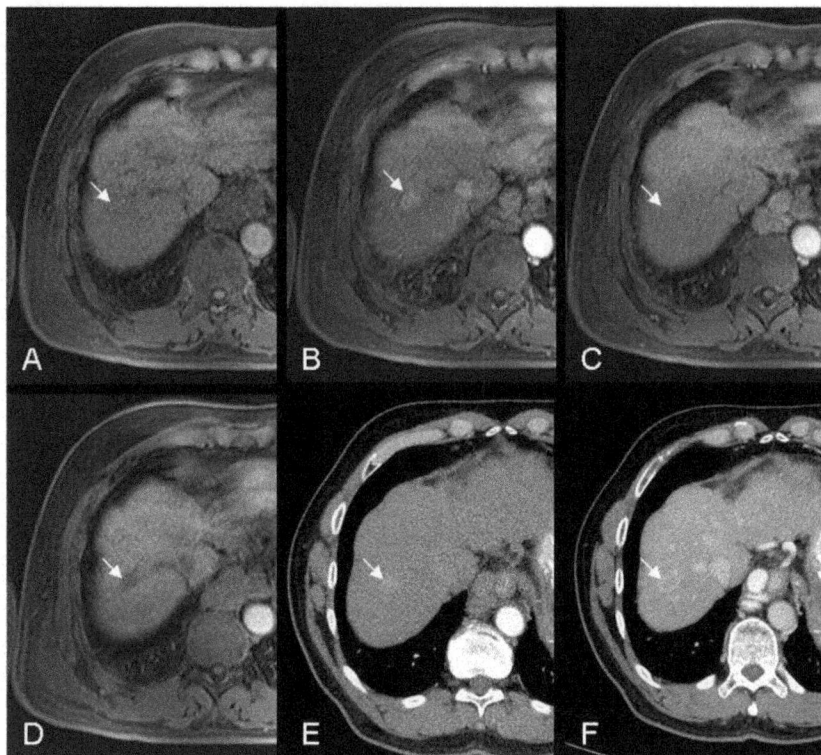

Figure 1. A 59-year-old male patient with liver cirrhosis (Child A) and HCC (arrow) in segment 7. Axial images: A) lesion is barely visible using unenhanced T1w-VIBE, B) marked arterial enhancement in T1w-VIBE following i.v. administration of contrast medium, C) typical washout of the lesion in the equilibrium phase (T1w-VIBE), and D) a clear hypointense lesion in the hepatobiliary phase (20 min after contrast agent injection, T1w-VIBE). Similar behaviour was observed with typical contrast medium enhancement in CT: E) early arterial phase after bolus tracking and F) washout in the portal venous phase with pseudocapsule.

Results

In 35 of 50 patients, the histopathological report after resection or biopsy of a lesion served as the gold standard for diagnosis, and in 24 of these 35 patients, the diagnosis of HCC was proven histopathologically. In 2 additional cases, HCC was diagnosed at follow-up (after 6 months) via clinical and paraclinical parameters.

In our study, 26 of 50 patients were positive for HCC (MRI-related: 9 patients with one lesion, 4 patients with 2 lesions, 3 patients with 3 lesions and 10 patients with 4 or more lesions).

ROC-curves for MRI displayed similar AUCs as observed for CT (0.837 vs. 0.798, p = 0.48). Sensitivity and positive and negative predictive values were measured for both methods (sensitivity 92%, PPV 80% and NPV 90% for MRI vs. sensitivity 85%, PPV 79% and NPV 82% for CT). Specificity was 75% for both techniques (see Table 3 and Figure 2). False positives resulted from numerous metastases of a neuroendocrine carcinoma, one adenoma and regenerative nodules. Because we calculated sensitivity, specificity, and positive and negative predictive values on a per-patient-basis, our subset analyses revealed no differences.

On a *liver-lesion-per-patient basis*, we detected slightly more lesions that were suspicious for HCC using MRI compared to CT, but this value did not reach statistical significance (mean, 2.7 for MRI versus 2.3 for CT, p = 0.256, Figure 3). One additional HCC was identified with aid of the hepatobiliary phase compared to conventional dynamic MRI; this lesion measured 8 mm in diameter (Figure 4). Compared to Gadolinium-EOB-DTPA-enhanced MRI-images evaluated with the hepatobiliary phase, no additional lesions were detected by DWI. However, DWI identified one additional malignant lesion compared to conventional dynamic MRI-scan. This was the same 8 mm diameter lesion that was observed with the hepatobiliary phase, and this finding impacted patient treatment (Figure 4).

Lesion size was similar using both methods, with an average greatest diameter of 33 mm for CT and 32 mm for MRI (measured in the arterial phase T1w VIBE; p = 0.195). Twenty malignant neoplasms were >3 cm, 16 lesions were 2–3 cm and 35 lesions were <2 cm, as determined by MRI-scans.

ADC-measurements in 32 lesions showed extremely heterogeneous values, with a mean of $1.2 \pm 0.5 \times 10^{-3}$ mm^2/s (range, 0.07 ± 0.1 to $3.0 \pm 0.1 \times 10^{-3}$ mm^2/s; Figure 5).

The radiologist reported that the *detectability* of lesions was similar using both methods using a 5-point rating scale (2.6 for CT and 2.7 for MRI, p = 0.807; range from 2.6 to 4.0 between sequences, 1 = excellent, 5 = unacceptable). The ability of MRI to detect lesions was significantly better using the hepatobiliary phase (2.2, range from 1 to 4) compared to conventional dynamic MRI (2.9, p = 0.005), but the difference was not significantly different compared to DWI (2.6, p = 0.125).

Image quality (2.2 for CT vs. 2.3 for MRI, p = 0.249, 2 = good, 3 = fair) was more scattered within MR sequences (1.8 in T1w HASTE and 2.9 in T2w TSE). Image quality was rated better for the hepatobiliary phase and conventional dynamic MRI than for DWI (2.0 for hepatobiliary phase, 2.1 for dynamic MRI without hepatobiliary phase and 2.7 for DWI, p<0.001). No significant disparity was noted between conventional dynamic MRI and the hepatobiliary phase (p = 0.342).

Table 3. Diagnostic accuracy, sensitivity, specificity, PPV and NPV for MRI and CT (binomial test, p<0.05= significant).

	MRI	CT	P-value
Diagnostic accuracy (AUC)	0.837	0.798	0.4795
Sensitivity	0.92	0.85	0.4795
Specificity	0.75	0.75	1.000
PPV	0.80	0.79	0.500
NPV	0.90	0.82	1.000

The average *reading time* for MR-images was16.9 min and significantly longer than the reading time for CT-scans, which averaged 4.5 min. (p<0.001).

Discussion

Accuracy

In our study, MRI showed similar diagnostic accuracy for the detection of HCC compared to CT. Reports by Akai et al. and Lee et al. demonstrated similar results with a tendency to higher diagnostic accuracy for MRI, but also without statistically significant differences [22,23]. One explanation for this discrepancy might be the high number of suspicious lesions with a diameter greater than 3 cm in our study population. Haradome et al. also showed no difference in diagnostic accuracy between conventional dynamic MRI and CT. However, using the hepatobiliary phase, MRI displayed significantly higher accuracy than CT, especially for lesions smaller than 1.5 cm [24]. Kim demonstrated that MRI has better sensitivity for the detection of HCCs due to an increased delineation of hypointensity of HCC at a three-minute late phase and a hepatocyte phase [25], supporting previous reports [26–28]. While these studies report that CT is inferior to MRI, the use of different contrast agents, older scanner technology and different scanning parameters of the CTs must be taken into account. Similar to our study parameters, several groups used an early arterial phase [25,27]. For example, Chan et al. described better conspicuity for hepatocellular carcinomas using a bolus tracking delay of 6s for achieving the arterial phase [29]. Other studies state that the late arterial phase (e.g., approximately 14–30 s from 100 HU-threshold) is the optimal scan window for the detection of HCC [30]. Moreover, differences in histopathological subtypes of HCC might also yield different enhancement patterns [31], making it difficult to clearly specify standard examination protocols.

Detectability and number of lesions

Although the reader rated the subjective detectability of liver lesions similarly for MRI and CT, slightly more liver lesions per patient were detected using 3T MRI. Although this did not reach statistical significance, it is important for therapeutic decisions because liver transplantation can achieve excellent results in patients with HCC according to the benchmark defined by the Milan criteria (solitary HCC of less than 5 cm or with up to three nodules of less than 3 cm) [32–34]. Furthermore, decision to surgically resect tumours or use minimally invasive therapies (i.e., radiofrequency ablation (RFA), laser-induced interstitial thermotherapy (LITT), microwave ablation (MWA), cryoablation and transarterial chemoembolisation (TACE), etc.) depends on number and size of hepatocellular carcinomas, as visualised using CT or MRI [35,36].

In our study, the detectability of lesions using MRI with the hepatobiliary phase 20 min after i.v. injection of Gd-EOB-DTPA was significantly better than conventional dynamic MRI. In one patient a suspicious lesion with a diameter of 8 mm was only observed with the hepatobiliary phase and DWI, but not with conventional dynamic MRI (Figure 4). This lesion changed the therapeutic management of the patient because it was the 4th HCC suspicious lesion in his liver, which excluded him from the liver transplantation list according to the Milan criteria [32]. These data support several studies reporting that Gd-EOB-DTPA enhanced MRI is superior to conventional dynamic MRI [17,21,24].

Gd-EOB-DTPA is a gadolinium-based, liver specific MRI contrast medium that allows diagnosis derived from haemodynamics during the extracellular phase and measures hepatocellular function during the hepatobiliary phase. Information regarding the degree of cellular differentiation might also be possible [18]. Concerning the timing of hepatobiliary phase imaging, Motosugi

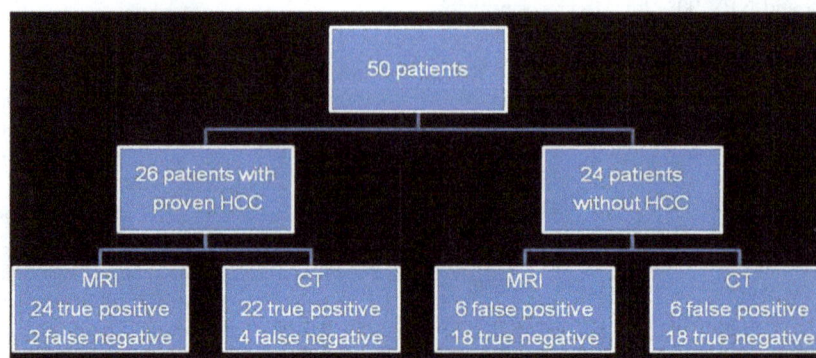

Figure 2. Flow chart for identification of patients with HCC in MRI and CT.

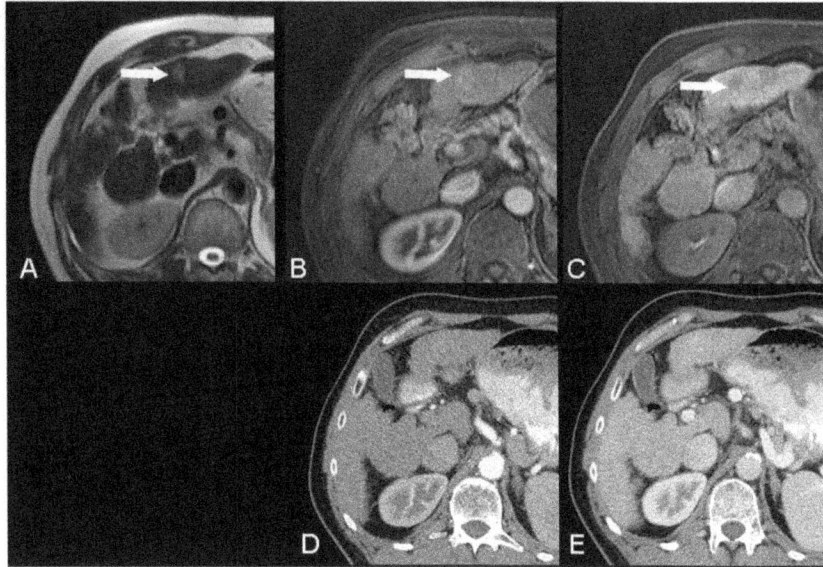

Figure 3. A 59-year-old male patient with liver cirrhosis and HCC (arrow) in S3 was only observed using MRI: *A)* **markedly hyperintense HCC in T2w-HASTE axial,** *B)* **typical arterial enhancement in T1w-VIBE, and** *C)* **hypointense lesion in the hepatobiliary phase.** No lesion was detected using CT: *D)* early arterial phase and *E)* portal venous phase.

et al. described that if the liver parenchyma is sufficiently enhanced 10 min after injection, no further imaging is necessary to detect focal liver lesions. However, the visual liver to spleen contrast scores 20 min after injection were frequently higher than 10 min images in patients with chronic liver diseases. These data indicate that a longer delay of 20 min might be more useful for patients with chronic liver diseases [37]. Because all of our patients

suffered from chronic liver disease, we acquired hepatobiliary phase images 20 min after contrast application.

DWI

DWI is commonly used in liver imaging to assess various focal lesions. In particular, DWI has a higher detection rate and diagnostic performance for small, malignant liver lesions com-

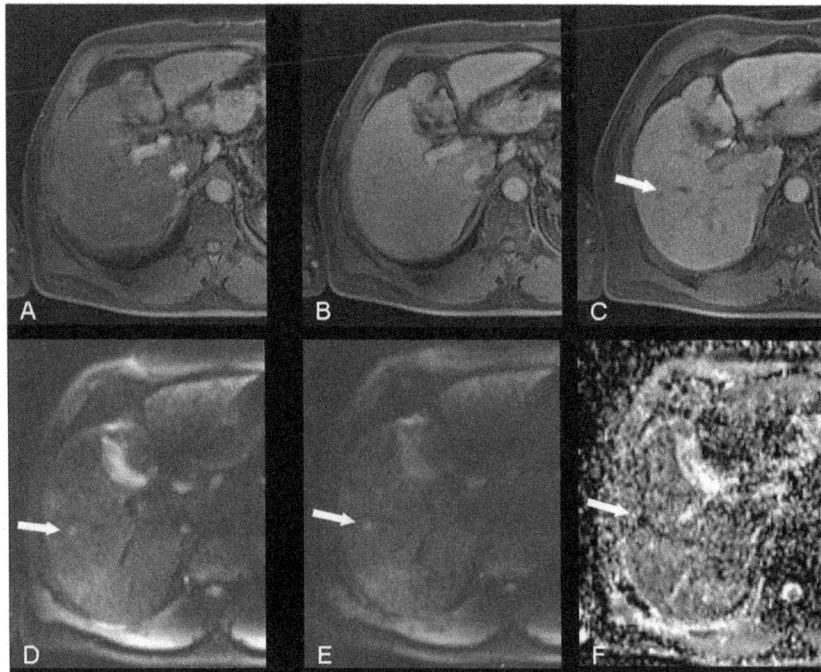

Figure 4. MRI of a 53-years-old male patient with HCC (arrow) in Segment 5: no lesion was identified in the arterial (A) and equilibrium phases (B), a small hypointense lesion was only observed in the hepatobiliary phase (C) and in DWI, where it is seen as a hyperintense lesion in b 50- (D) and b 400-images (E) and hypointense in the ADC-map (F).

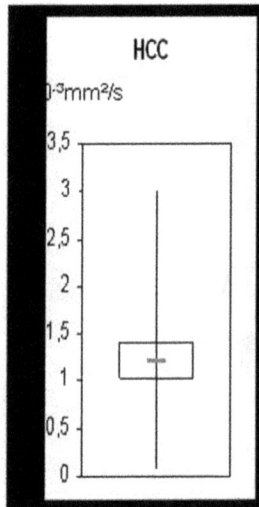

Figure 5. Range of ADC-values (10^{-3} mm²/s) in lesions suspicious for HCC.

pared to conventional dynamic MRI with different contrast agents; however, these results are not always significant [38–40]. A recent study by Holzapfel et al. reported no significant difference in diagnostic accuracy and sensitivity between diffusion weighted imaging, Gd-EOB-DTPA-enhanced imaging and combined imaging for the detection of focal liver lesions. However, for lesions smaller than 10 mm, a combination of DWI and Gd-EOB-DTPA significantly increased the overall detection rate. Similar to our findings regarding HCC-related diagnostic accuracy, Gadolinium-enhanced MRI and the combination of DWI and Gd-EOB-DTPA enhanced MRI demonstrated equal results [41]. In our 50 patients, just one additional HCC suspicious lesion was detected with DWI compared to conventional dynamic MRI, an 8 mm lesion that was also detected with hepatobiliary phase imaging. Therefore, DWI did not improve the detection of HCC compared to imaging with Gd-EOB-DTPA in our study.

Park et al. also demonstrated that DWI was outperformed by contrast enhanced T1-weighted imaging for the detection of HCC, but it represents a reasonable alternative [42]. However, if Gd-EOB-DTPA is used in the hepatic imaging, a time gap occurs between the equilibrium phase and the hepatobiliary phase, and because there is no significant impact of contrast media on achieving diffusion-weighted imaging and ADC-maps [43–45]. This gap can easily be filled with respiratory-triggered, diffusion-weighted imaging, which can provide additional information for the characterization of focal liver lesions. An important advantage of DWI is that no contrast agent is necessary, a property that is especially valuable for patients with poor renal function [39]. In our department, diffusion-weighted MR imaging is part of the routine liver protocol for all patients.

The potential to differentiate between benign and malignant liver lesions using ADC-quantification was previously reported in the literature [8–12]. Several thresholds have been proposed to accomplish this task, but there is still considerable overlap between benign and malignant liver lesions [9]. Vandecavaeye confirmed

that there is no significant difference in ADC between malignant and benign lesions in patients with cirrhotic liver disease [46]. In our study, the mean ADC-value of HCC lesions was $1.2 \pm 0.5 \times 10^{-3}$ mm²/s, which is similar to values reported in the literature. For example, Naoto measured an ADC-value of $1.31 \pm 0.28 \times 10^{-3}$ mm²/s [12], and Holzapfel reported an ADC-value of $1.12 \pm 0.28 \times 10^{-3}$ mm²/s for a small number of HCC samples [9]. These variances are likely due to differential cellularity of the tumours [47]. Another influential factor are the b-values chosen for DWI. In our study, we used relatively low b-values (b = 0, 50 and 400 s/mm²), which have the disadvantage of being influenced by perfusion effects. Measured ADC-values tend to decrease as the b-value increases [48]. However, the use of low (perfusion-sensitive) b-values has several advantages: it provides a higher signal-to-noise ratio and more anatomical information of the liver, it is less sensitive to eddy current-induced distortions and it suppresses signals from the hepatic vasculature, which improves the detectability of perivascular lesions [49–51]. Further investigations are needed to determine the best b-values for liver imaging.

Our study has some limitations. First, there was a bias in patient recruitment because we included patients with proven or suspected HCC. This stipulation might result in an overestimation of specificity. Second, we could not achieve a histological proof for every detected lesion due to ethical reasons, so we had to use follow-up examinations and surrogates of clinical and paraclinical findings to confirm the presence of lesions. For this reason, we calculated sensitivity, specificity, and positive and negative predictive values on a patient basis. Third, our study group was relatively small, and further studies with more patients might yield statistically significant results. Fourth, we used a first generation MR-scanner with 3 Tesla, which can suffer from B0 artefacts within the liver parenchyma. Newer MR-Scanners with different coil and RF impulse designs (i.e., the TrueForm and Multi-Transmit) reduce these artefacts and can increase the diagnostic ability for liver imaging. Finally, we only determined ADC-values for suspicious lesions that were clearly visible in the ADC-map. However, our ADC-values were comparable to the values given in literature.

Conclusions

Our study did not show a statistically significant difference in detection of HCC between 3-Tesla Gd-EOB-DTPA-enhanced MRI with diffusion-weighted imaging and 64-slice contrast-enhanced CT.

As we detected slightly more lesions per patient using MRI, we recommend this imaging modality as the first-choice imaging method for the detection of HCC and individual therapeutic decisions. However, contrast-enhanced CT was not inferior in our study, indicating that it represents a useful image modality when MRI is not available or for follow-up examinations.

Author Contributions

Conceived and designed the experiments: BM PS. Performed the experiments: BM. Analyzed the data: PS DL BM. Contributed reagents/materials/analysis tools: BM PS TK. Wrote the paper: BM DL TK PS.

References

1. Bruix J, Sherman M (2005) Management of hepatocellular carcinoma. Hepatology 42: 1208–36

2. Kudo M (2010) The 2008 Okuda lecture: Management of hepatocellular carcinoma: from surveillance to molecular targeted therapy. J Gastroenterol Hepatol 25: 439–52

3. El-Serag HB (2007) Epidemiology of hepatocellular carcinoma in USA. Hepatol Res 37: S88–94

4. Tannapfel A, Wittekind C (2003) Pathology of hepatocellular carcinoma. Chir Gastroenterol 19: 225–230.

5. Tanimoto A, Lee JM, Murakami T, Huppertz A, Kudo M, et al. (2009) Consensus report of the 2nd International Forum for Liver MRI. Eur Radiol 19: S975–89

6. Zech CJ, Reiser MF, Herrmann KA (2009) Imaging of hepatocellular carcinoma by computed tomography and magnetic resonance imaging: state of art. Dig Dis 27: 114–24

7. Rempp H, Boss A, Helmberger T, Pereira P (2011) The current role of minimally invasive therapies in the management of liver tumors. Abdom Imaging 36: 635–47

8. Bruegel M, Holzapfel K, Gaa J, Woertler K, Waldt S, et al. (2008) Characterization of focal liver lesions by ADC measurements using a respiratory triggered diffusion-weighted single-shot echo-planar MR imaging technique. Eur Radiol 18: 477–85

9. Holzapfel K, Bruegel M, Eiber M, Ganter C, Schuster T, et al. (2010) Characterization of small (≤10 mm) focal liver lesions: value of respiratory-triggered echo-planar diffusion-weighted MR imaging. Eur J Radiol 76: 89–95

10. Moteki T, Ishizaka H, Horikoshi H, Matsumoto M (1995) Differentiation between hemangiomas and hepatocellular carcinomas with the apparent diffusion coefficient calculated from turboFLASH MR images. J Magn Reson Imaging 5: 187–91

11. Kim T, Murakami T, Takahashi S, Hori M, Tsuda K, et al. (1995) Diffusion-weighted single-shot echoplanar MR imaging for liver disease. AJR Am J Roentgenol 173: 393–8

12. Koike N, Cho A, Nasu K, Seto K, Nagaya S, et al. (2009) Role of diffusion-weighted magnetic resonance imaging in the differential diagnosis of focal hepatic lesions. World J Gastroenterol 14; 15: 5805–12

13. Hamm B, Staks T, Mühler A, Bollow M, Taupitz M, et al. (1995) Phase I clinical evaluation of Gd-EOB-DTPA as a hepatobiliary MR contrast agent: safety, pharmacokinetics, and MR imaging. Radiology 195: 785–92

14. Clément O, Mühler A, Vexler V, Berthezène Y, Brasch RC (1992) Gadolinium-ethoxybenzyl-DTPA, a new liver-specific magnetic resonance contrast agent. Kinetic and enhancement patterns in normal and cholestatic rats. Invest Radiol 27: 612–9

15. Schuhmann-Giampieri G, Schmitt-Willich H, Press WR, Negishi C, Weinmann HJ, et al. (1992) Preclinical evaluation of Gd-EOB-DTPA as a contrast agent in MR imaging of the hepatobiliary system. Radiology 183: 59–64

16. Weinmann HJ, Schuhmann-Giampieri G, Schmitt-Willich H, Vogler H, Frenzel T, et al. (1991) A new lipophilic gadolinium chelate as a tissue-specific contrast medium for MRI. Magn Reson Med 22: 233–7

17. Huppertz A, Balzer T, Blakeborough A, Breuer J, Giovagnoni A, et al. (2004) Improved detection of focal liver lesions at MR imaging: multicenter comparison of gadoxetic acid-enhanced MR images with intraoperative findings. Radiology 230: 266–75

18. Huppertz A, Haraida S, Kraus A, Zech CJ, Scheidler J, et al. (2005) Enhancement of focal liver lesions at gadoxetic acid-enhanced MR imaging: correlation with histopathologic findings and spiral CT—initial observations. Radiology 234: 468–78

19. Reimer P, Rummeny EJ, Shamsi K, Balzer T, Daldrup HE, et al. (1996) Phase II clinical evaluation of Gd-EOB-DTPA: dose, safety aspects, and pulse sequence. Radiology 199: 177–83

20. Low RN (2007) Abdominal MRI advances in the detection of liver tumours and characterisation. Lancet Oncol 8: 525–35

21. Ahn SS, Kim MJ, Lim JS, Hong HS, Chung YE, et al. (2010) Added value of gadoxeticacid-enhanced hepatobiliary phase MR imaging in the diagnosis of hepatocellular carcinoma. Radiology 255: 459–66

22. Akai H, Kiryu S, Matsuda I, Satou J, Takao H, et al. (2011) Detection of hepatocellular carcinoma by Gd-EOB-DTPA-enhanced liver MRI: Comparison with triple phase 64 detector row helical CT. Eur J Radiol 80: 310–5

23. Lee CH, Kim KA, Lee J, Park YS, Choi JW, et al. (2012) Using low tube voltage (80kVp) quadruple phase liver CT for the detection of hepatocellular carcinoma: Two-year experience and comparison with Gd-EOB-DTPA enhanced liver MRI. Eur J Radiol 81: e605–11

24. Haradome H, Grazioli L, Tinti R, Morone M, Motosugi U, et al. (2011) Additional value of gadoxetic acid-DTPA-enhanced hepatobiliary phase MR imaging in the diagnosis of early-stage hepatocellular carcinoma: comparison with dynamic triple-phase multidetector CT imaging. J Magn Reson Imaging 34: 69–78

25. Kim YK, Kim CS, Han YM, Kwak HS, Jin GY, et al. (2009) Detection of hepatocellular carcinoma: gadoxetic acid-enhanced 3-dimensional magnetic resonance imaging versus multi-detector row computed tomography. J Comput Assist Tomogr 33: 844–50

26. Di Martino M, Marin D, Guerrisi A, Baski M, Galati F, et al. (2010) Intraindividual comparison of gadoxetate disodium-enhanced MR imaging and 64-section multidetector CT in the Detection of hepatocellular carcinoma in patients with cirrhosis. Radiology 256: 806–16

27. Pitton MB, Kloeckner R, Herber S, Otto G, Kreitner KF, et al. (2009) MRI versus 64-row MDCT for diagnosis of hepatocellular carcinoma. World J Gastroenterol 15: 6044–51

28. Sano K, Ichikawa T, Motosugi U, Sou H, Muhi AM, et al. (2011) Imaging study of early hepatocellular carcinoma: usefulness of gadoxetic acid-enhanced MR imaging. Radiology 261: 834–44

29. Chan R, Kumar G, Abdullah B, Ng Kh, Vijayananthan A, et al. (2011) Optimising the scan delay for arterial phase imaging of the liver using the bolus tracking technique. Biomed Imaging Interv J 7: e12

30. Kim MJ, Choi JY, Lim JS, Kim JY, Kim JH, et al. (2006) Optimal scan window for detection of hypervascular hepatocellular carcinomas during MDCT examination. AJR Am J Roentgenol 187: 198–206

31. Lee JH, Lee JM, Kim SJ, Baek JH, Yun SH, et al. (2012) Enhancement patterns of hepatocellular carcinomas on multiphasicmultidetector row CT: comparison with pathological differentiation. Br J Radiol 85: e573–83

32. Mazzaferro V, Bhoori S, Sposito C, Bongini M, Langer M, et al. (2011) Milan criteria in liver transplantation for hepatocellular carcinoma: an evidence-based analysis of 15 years of experience. Liver Transpl 17: S44–57

33. Cauchy F, Fuks D, Belghiti J (2012) HCC: current surgical treatment concepts. Langenbecks Arch Surg 397: 681–95

34. Mazzaferro V, Regalia E, Doci R, Andreola S, Pulvirenti A, et al. (1996) Liver transplantation for the treatment of small hepatocellular carcinomas in patients with cirrhosis. N Engl J Med 334: 693–709

35. Llovet JM (2005) Updated treatment approach to hepatocellular carcinoma. J Gastroenterol 40: 225–35

36. Kudo M, Okanoue T (2007) Japan Society of Hepatology. Management of hepatocellular carcinoma in Japan: consensus-based clinical practice manual proposed by the Japan Society of Hepatology. Oncology 72: S2–15

37. Motosugi U, Ichikawa T, Tominaga L, Sou H, Sano K, et al. (2009) Delay before the hepatocyte phase of Gd-EOB-DTPA-enhanced MR imaging: is it possible to shorten the examination time? Eur Radiol 19: 2623–9

38. Kim YK, Lee MW, Lee WJ, Kim SH, Rhim H, et al. (2012) Diagnostic accuracy and sensitivity of diffusion-weighted and of gdoxetic acid-enhanced 3-T MR Imaging alone or in combination in the detection of small liver metastasis (≤ 1.5 cm in diameter). Invest Radiol 47: 159–66

39. Yu JS, Chung JJ, Kim JH, Cho ES, Kim DJ, et al. (2011) Detection of small intrahepatic metastases of hepatocellular carcinomas using diffusion-weighted imaging: comparison with conventional dynamic MRI. Magn Reson Imaging 29: 985–92

40. Chung J, Yu JS, Kim DJ, Chung JJ, Kim JH, et al. (2011) Hypervascular hepatocellular carcinoma in the cirrhotic liver: diffusion-weighted imaging versus superparamagnetic iron oxide-enhanced MRI. Magn Reson Imaging 29: 1235–43

41. Holzapfel K, Eiber MJ, Fingerie AA, Bruegel M, Rummeny EJ, et al. (2012) Detection, classification, and characterization of focal liver lesions: value of diffusion-weighted MR imaging, gadoxetic acid-enhanced MR imaging and the combination of both methods. Abdom Imaging 37: 74–82

42. Park MS, Kim S, Patel J, Hajdu CH, Do RK, et al. (2012) Hepatocellular carcinoma: Detection with diffusion-weighted vs. contrast-enhanced MRI in pre-transplant patients. Hepatology 56: 140–8

43. Kinner S, Umutlu L, Blex S, Maderwald S, Antoch G, et al. (2012) Diffusion weighted MR imaging in patients with HCC and liver cirrhosis after administration of different gadolinium contrast agents: Is it still reliable? Eur J Radiol 81: 625–8

44. Choi JS, Kim MJ, Choi JY, Park MS, Lim JS, et al. (2010) Diffusion-weighted MR imaging of liver on 3.0-Tesla system: effect of intravenous administration of gadoxetic acid disodium. Eur Radiol 20: 1052–60

45. Chiu FY, Jao JC, Chen CY, Liu GC, Jaw TS, et al. (2005) Effect of intravenous gadolinium-DTPA on diffusion-weighted magnetic resonance images for evaluation of focal hepatic lesions. J Comput Assist Tomogr 29: 176–80

46. Vandecaveye V, De Keyzer F, Verslype C, Op de Beeck K, Komuta M, et al. (2009) Diffusion-weighted MRI provides additional value to conventional dynamic contrast-enhanced MRI for detection of hepatocellular carcinoma. Eur Radiol 19: 2456–66

47. Koike N, Cho A, Nasu K, Seto K, Nagaya S, et al. (2009) Role of diffusion-weighted magnetic resonance imaging in the differential diagnosis of focal hepatic lesions. World J Gastroenterol 15: 5805–12

48. Hollingsworth KG, Lomas DJ (2006) Influence of perfusion on hepatic MR diffusion measurement. NMR Biomed 19: 231–5

49. Nasu K, Kuroki Y, Nawano S, Kuroki S, Tsukamoto T, et al. (2006) Hepatic metastases: diffusion-weighted sensitivity-encoding versus SPIO-enhanced MR imaging. Radiology 239: 122–30

50. Goshima S, Kanematsu M, Kondo H, Yokoyama R, Kajita K, et al. (2008) Diffusion-weighted imaging of the liver: optimizing b value for the detection and characterization of benign and malignant hepatic lesions. J Magn Reson Imaging 28: 691–7

51. Takahara T, Kwee TC (2012) Low b-value diffusion-weighted imaging: Emerging applications in the body. J Magn Reson Imaging 35: 1266–73

19

MiR-199a Regulates Cell Proliferation and Survival by Targeting FZD7

Jiugang Song[1,2☉], Liucun Gao[2,3☉], Guang Yang[4☉], Shanhong Tang[2,5☉], Huahong Xie[2], Yongji Wang[6], Jingbo Wang[2], Yanping Zhang[7], Jiang Jin[2], Yawen Gou[2], Zhiping Yang[2], Zheng Chen[2], Kaichun Wu[2], Jie Liu[8], Daiming Fan[2]*

1 Department of Gastroenterology, the 309th Hospital of Chinese People's Liberation Army, Beijing, PR China, 2 State Key Laboratory of Cancer Biology, Xijing Hospital of Digestive Diseases, Fourth Military Medical University, Xi'an, PR China, 3 Department of Pharmacology and Toxicology, Beijing Institute of Radiation Medicine, Beijing, PR China, 4 Department of XiShan Outpatient Clinic, the 309th Hospital of Chinese People's Liberation Army, Beijing, PR China, 5 Department of Digestion, General Hospital of Chengdu Military Command, Chengdu, Sichuan Province, PR China, 6 Department of Medical, the 309th Hospital of Chinese People's Liberation Army, Beijing, PR China, 7 Asian Games Village Clinic of Logistics Department, the General Armament Department of PLA, Beijing, PR China, 8 Department of Digestive Diseases, Huashan Hospital, Fudan University, Shanghai, PR China

Abstract

A growing amount of evidence indicates that miRNAs are important regulators of multiple cellular processes and, when expressed aberrantly in different types of cancer such as hepatocellular carcinoma (HCC), play significant roles in tumorigenesis and progression. Aberrant expression of miR-199a-5p (also called miR-199a) was found to contribute to carcinogenesis in different types of cancer, including HCC. However, the precise molecular mechanism is not yet fully understood. The present study showed that miR-199a is frequently down-regulated in HCC tissues and cells. Importantly, lower expression of miR-199a was significantly correlated with the malignant potential and poor prognosis of HCC, and restoration of miR-199a in HCC cells led to inhibition of the cell proliferation and cell cycle *in vitro* and *in vivo*. Furthermore, Frizzled type 7 receptor (FZD7), the most important Wnt receptor involved in cancer development and progression, was identified as a functional target of miR-199a. In addition, these findings were further strengthened by results showing that expression of FZD7 was inversely correlated with miR-199a in both HCC tissues and cells and that over-expression of miR-199a could significantly down-regulate the expression of genes downstream of FZD7, including β-catenin, Jun, Cyclin D1 and Myc. In conclusion, these findings not only help us to better elucidate the molecular mechanisms of hepatocarcinogenesis from a fresh perspective but also provide a new theoretical basis to further investigate miR-199a as a potential biomarker and a promising approach for HCC treatment.

Editor: Xin-Yuan Guan, The University of Hong Kong, China

Funding: This work was supported by grant 81101852 from the National Natural Science Foundation of China (http://www.nsfc.gov.cn/). The funders had no role in the study design, data collection and analysis, decision to publish, or preparation of the manuscript.

Competing Interests: The authors have declared that no competing interests exist.

* Email: fandaim@fmmu.edu.cn

☉ These authors contributed equally to this work.

Introduction

Hepatocellular carcinoma (HCC), the most common primary liver cancer [1], is one of the most prevalent malignant diseases and the second-most frequent cause of cancer deaths worldwide [2]. Half of the new liver cancer cases and liver cancer deaths worldwide were estimated to occur in China [3]. The dismal prognosis of advanced HCC is largely caused by late detection of the tumors and its high rate of recurrence and metastasis [2,4,5]. Etiologically, approximately 90% of HCC cases arise from cirrhosis, and the disease is strongly associated with several risk factors, including viral infections (e.g., hepatitis B and C) and heavy alcohol intake [6].

In the past decades, studies have focused on investigating the deregulation of genes and proteins underlying the development of HCC [7]. MiRNAs are a recently discovered class of small noncoding RNAs that play critical roles in regulating gene expression. MiRNAs have emerged as key factors involved in several biological processes, including development, differentiation, cell proliferation, and tumorigenesis [8,9]. Several studies have shown that alterations in miRNA genes lead to tumor formation, and several miRNAs that regulate either tumor suppression or tumor formation have been identified [10].

Recently, an increasing number of studies have demonstrated that the expression of miRNAs is deregulated in HCC in comparison with normal liver tissue [11,12]. In view of reports from independent studies, consistent deregulation of miR-21, miR-122, miR-199, and miR-221 appears to be particularly important in HCC [13,14,15,16,17,18]. Interestingly, both miR-122 and miR-199a are among the miRNAs that are most highly expressed in normal liver [19].

However, the role and underlying molecular mechanisms of miR-199a in HCC is not completely understood. The present study aimed to analyze the expression of miR-199a in HCC tissues compared with adjacent non-tumor tissues and to analyze its role in the malignant progression of HCC *in vitro* and *in vivo*. In addition, bioinformatics predicted that FZD7, the most important Wnt receptor, might be a target of miR-199a. To further test this hypothesis, we analyzed the influence of miR-199a on FZD7 and on the expression of its downstream genes.

Materials and Methods

Cell Lines and Human Samples

Human HCC cells (SMMC7721 and HepG2) and normal hepatocytes (Chang liver cells) were obtained from the Cell Research Institute of the Chinese Academy of Sciences (Shanghai, China). 293FT cells were obtained from the American Type Culture Collection (ATCC, Manassas, VA). All of the cell lines were cultured in Dulbecco's modified Eagle medium (Gibco BRL, Life Technologies, NY) supplemented with 10% fetal calf serum (FCS), 100 μg/ml penicillin, and 100 μg/ml streptomycin at 37°C in a 5% CO_2 incubator. HCC specimens and paired non-tumor liver tissues were obtained from 40 patients who underwent primary HCC resection between June 2006 and January 2007 at the Department of General Surgery in Xijing Hospital (Xi'an, China). No patient had received radiotherapy or chemotherapy before surgery. Data including sex, age, tumor size, histologic type of neoplasm and tumor-node-metastasis (TNM) stage were obtained from surgical and pathological records, and all samples were thoroughly reviewed by two pathologists. Tissue samples were collected at surgery, immediately snap-frozen in liquid nitrogen and stored at −80°C until RNA extraction. Written informed consent was obtained from all patients and the study was approved by the Ethics Committee of Xijing Hospital, Fourth Military Medical University, China.

RNA Extraction and Real Time-PCR Analysis (qRT-PCR)

In accordance with the manufacturer's instructions, total RNA was extracted from the cell lines and frozen tissue specimens with TRIzol reagent (Invitrogen, Carlsbad, CA, USA), and the concentration of the total RNA was quantitated by measuring the absorbance at 260 nm. Complementary DNA (cDNA) was generated using a miScript Reverse Transcription Kit (QIAGEN), and Real-time PCR was performed using a miScript SYBRGreen PCR Kit from QIAGEN. Primers for miR-199a and the U6 snRNA (internal control) were also purchased from QIAGEN (MS00006741 and MS00033740). The fold-change of the mRNA in HCC tissues (T) relative to the adjacent non-tumor tissues (NT) was calculated using a previously described method [20], where $\Delta\Delta Ct = \Delta Ct(T)-\Delta Ct(NT)$ and $\Delta Ct = Ct(miR-199a)-Ct(U6)$. The relative mRNA levels of genes in HCC cells were also determined using qRT-PCR, and the expression of GAPDH was used as the internal control. Each PCR was performed in triplicate. The primers for the examined genes are presented in Table 1.

Vector Constructs and Lentivirus Production

Lentivirus-expressed miR-199a was constructed as described in a previous study [21]. The precursor sequence of miR-199a was constructed as follows: (Forward) hsa-miR-199a-Xho GGGC-CCGCTCTAGAGACTCGAGATATTTGCATGTCGCTATGTG, (Reverse) hsa-miR-199a- BamH I CGCGGCCGCCTAATG-GATCCAAAAAAGGCACAGTCGAGGCTGATC. The sequence was amplified and cloned into the pGCSIL-GFP Vector (GENECHEM) to generate pGCSIL-GFP-miR-199a. The miR-

199a and the negative-control virus were transfected into HepG2 cells as in a previous study [21]. Cells successfully transfected with GFP were separated by flow cytometry (FACScan; Becton Dickinson, San Jose, CA), and the purified, GFP-positive cell lines were named HepG2-199a and HepG2-NC (NC, negative control).

Cell Proliferation Assays

An MTT assay was used to analyze cellular proliferation according to a previously described protocol [22]. Briefly, log-phase cells were plated in 96-well plates (1×10^3 cells/well at a final volume of 200 μl) in replicates of three. After 1, 2, 3, 4, 5, 6 or 7 days of cell cultivation, 20 μl of 3-(4,5-dimethylthiazol-2-yl)-2,5-diphenyltetrazolium bromide (MTT, 5 mg/ml; Sigma, St. Louis, MO) was added to the cells and incubated for 4 hours at 37°C. The supernatant was then removed, and 150 μl dimethylsulfoxide (DMSO) was added with agitation for 10 minutes at room temperature to dissolve the MTT crystals. The absorbance values were determined by an ELISA reader (Bio-Rad Laboratories, Richmond, CA) at a wavelength of 490 nm. Each experiment was repeated at least thrice.

Soft Agar Assay

The tumorigenicity of the cells *in vitro* was determined by analyzing the formation of colonies in soft agar. Approximately 2×10^3 cells were seeded in 2 ml of 0.3% agar layered onto a 0.5% agar underlay in a six-well plate. Cells were incubated for 3 weeks at 37°C in 5% CO_2 before counting the colonies using a code. Each assay was performed in triplicate.

Flow Cytometry Assay

For cell cycle analysis, cells were harvested and washed twice with ice-cold phosphate-buffered saline (PBS). The cell pellets were fixed in 70% ethanol, treated with RNase A (Boehringer Mannheim, Indianapolis, IN), and stained with propidium iodide (Sigma-Aldrich, St. Louis, MO). Cell cycle analysis was performed with a flow cytometer (FACScan; Becton Dickinson, San Jose, CA). The proliferation index (PI) was calculated as PI = (S+G2)/(S+G2+G1).

Luciferase Reporter Assay

For dual luciferase reporter assays, a luciferase reporter vector (pMir-Report; Ambion) was used to generate luciferase reporter constructs. A fragment of the 3′-UTR of the FZD7 mRNA (region 1974–2508, GenBank accession no. NM_003507), which included the seed sequence of the mature miR-199a-binding site, and a mutated binding site of the 3′-UTR sequence were cloned into the luciferase reporter vector. HepG2-199a or HepG2-NC cells in 24-well plates were co-transfected with 0.2 μg of the firefly luciferase reporter vector and 0.08 μg of the pRL-TK control vector containing Renilla luciferase (Promega) using Lipofectamine 2000 (Invitrogen) according to the manufacturer's protocol. Lysates were prepared after 48 h of transfection. Both firefly luciferase and Renilla luciferase activities were measured using the Dual-Luciferase assay kit (Promega, Madison, WI) according to the manufacturer's instructions. Firefly luciferase activity was normalized to Renilla luciferase activity for each transfected well. Three independent experiments were performed in triplicate. The primers for the 3′-UTR of FZD7 and mutated 3′-UTR of FZD7 sequences are shown in Table 2.

Table 1. Primers for qRT-PCR.

Primers	Sequence
FZD7	F 5′ TTTCGTCCCTGGGCCTCT 3′
	R5′ TGGTCTGGTTGTAGGCGATG3′
GAPDH	F5′ GCACCGTCAAGGCTGAGAAC 3′
	R 5′ TGGTGAAGACGCCAGTGGA 3′

Western Blot Analysis

Western Blot analysis was performed according to our previous study [22]. Total cellular proteins were extracted and separated using sodium dodecyl sulfate–polyacrylamide gel electrophoresis and transferred to nitrocellulose membranes (Immobilin-P; Millipore, Bedford, MA). The membranes were blocked with 5% nonfat milk at room temperature for 2 hours and then incubated overnight with rabbit anti-FZD7 (Santa Cruz, CA, USA), mouse anti-Myc (Santa Cruz, CA, USA), mouse anti-Cyclin D1 (Santa Cruz, CA, USA), mouse anti-β-catenin (Santa Cruz, CA, USA) or mouse anti-β-actin (Sigma, St. Louis, MO, USA) antibodies at 4°C. After incubation with horseradish peroxidase–conjugated anti-rabbit IgG or anti-mouse IgG (Santa Cruz, CA, USA), the specific protein band was visualized by enhanced chemiluminescence (Amersham-Pharmacia Biotech, Beijing, China). β-actin was used as an internal control, and each experiment was repeated at least thrice.

Tumorigenicity Assays in Nude Mice

Female athymic BALB/c nude mice (4–5 weeks old) were purchased from the Animal Center of the Chinese Academy of Science (Shanghai, China), maintained in laminar flow cabinets under specific pathogen-free conditions, and had free access to food and water. All animal studies were undertaken in accordance with the National Institutes of Health Guide for the Care and Use of Laboratory Animals and approved by the Institutional Animal Care and Use Committee (IACUC) of the Fourth Military Medical University (Permit Number: 12020). Twelve mice were assigned to 2 groups and used for *in vivo* tumorigenicity assays. Logarithmically growing cells were trypsinized and resuspended in PBS after washing twice with serum-free medium. HepG2-199a and HepG2-NC cells (2×10^6) were injected subcutaneously into the flanks. Four weeks after inoculation, the tumor-bearing mice were euthanized to recover the tumors for further analysis, and all efforts were made to minimize suffering. Tumor volume was measured using a Vernier caliper, and tumor volumes were calculated following the formula [22]: Tumor volume $(cm^3) = (a/2)(b/2)h\pi$, where a, b, and h are the minor dimension, major dimension, and height of the tumor, respectively ($\pi = 3.1416$).

Statistical Analysis

All data were analyzed using the SPSS software package (SPSS, Chicago, IL), and $P < 0.05$ was considered statistically significant. The significant differences in the expression of miR-199a in the HCC and paired noncancerous tissues were analyzed by the Wilcoxon rank sum test. The Kruskal–Wallis H test or the Mann–Whitney U test was utilized to evaluate the significance of the correlation between the miR-199a expression and the clinical features of HCC. A one-way ANOVA test was adopted to investigate the difference in cell proliferation and soft agar clonogenic assays of three groups, and the least significant difference T test was used to analyze two groups. Overall survival curves were plotted using the Kaplan-Meier method and were evaluated for statistical significance using a log-rank test.

Results

The Expression of miR-199a is Frequently Down-regulated in Human HCC Tissues and Cell Lines

To further determine whether miR-199a is involved in the regulation of tumorigenesis of human HCC, the expression level of miR-199a in HCC and matched nonneoplastic liver tissues from 40 patients was analyzed by qRT-PCR. The results showed that the expression of miR-199a was decreased in 82.5% (33/40) of HCC tissues compared with matched nonneoplastic liver tissues, with an average of 4.79-fold reduction in expression (median = 2.8 vs 5.3; $P < 0.01$; Figure 1A).

The expression of miR-199a in the cell lines displayed a pattern similar to that in the tissues. As shown in Figure 1B, a lower expression of miR-199a was detected in the HCC cell lines HepG2 and SMMC-7721, whereas the expression of miR-199a was higher in the normal Chang liver cell line. MiR-199a expression in HepG2 cells was lower than in SMMC-7721 cells. Therefore, we chose the HepG2 cell lines for further study.

A Lower miR-199a Expression Level in HCC Tissue Correlates with Worse Prognosis of HCC Patients

The correlations between miR-199a expression in HCC tissue and clinical features or prognosis of HCC patients were also

Table 2. Primers for the 3′UTR of FZD7 and Mutant-FZD7.

Primers	Sequence
FZD7	F 5′ CTAG ACTAGT GAAAGCGGTTTGGATGAA 3′
	R 5′ CCC AAGCTT CGTCTCCTTGGCCTTATC 3′
Mutant-FZD7	F 5′ CG ACGCGT GCCAAACTGGAGCCCAGAT 3′
	R 5′ CG ACGCGT AAAAAGAGATTATGGTTTGA 3′

A

B

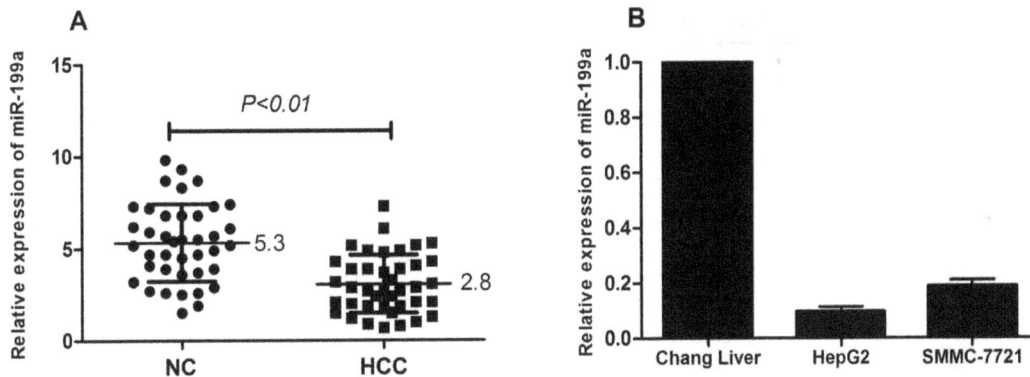

Figure 1. Down-regulation of miR-199a in HCC tissues and cell lines was detected by qRT-PCR. (A) The expression level of miR-199a was lower in 40 HCC tissues than in their pair-matched adjacent normal liver tissues (*P*<0.01). Each sample was analyzed in triplicate and normalized to the U6 snRNA. (B) The relative miR-199a expression in HCC cell lines was much lower compared to the normal Chang liver cell line. The relative expression of miR-199a was normalized to the endogenous control U6 snRNA. Each sample was analyzed in triplicate.

studied. Further analysis of the clinical features of 40 HCC patients revealed that the low expression of miR-199a was positively associated with the patients' TNM stage and tumor metastasis (Table 3). Then, the miR-199a expression levels in HCC samples were used for a survival analysis, and the results revealed that down-regulation of miR-199a expression was significantly associated with poor patient prognosis. The median survival time of these patients was 37 months after operation. A Kaplan-Meier analysis revealed that low miR-199a expression was significantly associated with poor 5-year overall survival time (29.2±3.2 months vs 51.8±3.1 months, P<0.001) (Figure 2). Univariate analysis showed that the patient survival time was also significantly correlated with clinical features such as metastasis (P< 0.001) and T stage (P=0.002), but not with age or gender (Table 4).

Over-expression of MiR-199a Represses the Growth and Tumorigenicity of HCC Cells *In Vitro* and *In Vivo*

To determine whether miR-199a can inhibit the proliferation of HCC cells, lentivirus-mediated miR-199a was transfected into

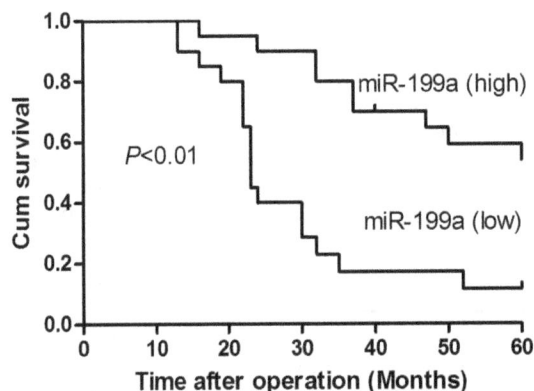

Figure 2. Lower miR-199a expression in HCC tissues is correlated with poorer survival of HCC patients. Five-year cumulative survivals of the HCC patients were analyzed by Kaplan-Meier survival analysis and log-rank tests. The 40 HCC patients were split into high and low miR-199a expression groups based on the median (2.8) for miR-199a. The relative expression of miR-199a in each patient was shown in the supporting information (Table S1).

HepG2 cells (HepG2-199a). As observed in Figure 3A, the expression of miR-199a was markedly up-regulated in HepG2-199a cells compared with those in the controls. MTT assays showed that HepG2 cells with increased miR-199a expression (HepG2-199a) proliferated at a slower rate than did control cells, and statistical analysis showed a significant difference after culture for four days (Figure 3B). The cell cycle of these cells was then measured by flow cytometry. The results indicated that 44.8% of HepG2 cells and 45.1% of HepG2-CN cells were in S-phase, whereas 22.7% of HepG2-199a cells were in S-phase (P<0.01; Figure 3C and Figure 3D), suggesting that miR-199a represses the entry of cells into S-phase. Together, the results show that miR-199a can repress the cell cycle and therefore inhibit the proliferation of HepG2 cells.

Then, colony formation assays of parental and transfected cells were evaluated by determining the plating efficiency in soft agar. As shown in Figure 3E, HepG2 and HepG2-CN cells yielded 34.67±3.51 and 37.33±4.16 colonies, whereas HepG2-199a cells yielded 15.33±2.52 colonies after three weeks (P<0.01). Hence, the results showed that there was a marked reduction in anchorage-independent growth among cells with up-regulated expression of miR-199a compared with the controls.

Furthermore, the repression potential of miR-199a on the growth of HepG2 cells in nude mice was also determined. The result showed that tumor size was dramatically smaller in HepG2-199a cells than in control cells (P<0.05; Figure 3F), suggesting that restoration of miR-199a expression was directly involved in the inhibition of tumor growth in nude mice. In addition, the total RNA and protein of each representative tumor from the mice were used to analyze the expression levels of miR-199a and FZD7 by qRT-PCR and western blotting, respectively. The expression level of miR-199a was much higher in recovered tumors formed in nude mice injected with HepG2-199a cells than in those injected with HepG2-CN cells (Figure 3G). Inversely, the expression of FZD7 was significantly lower in tumors with HepG2-199a cells than those with HepG2-CN cells (Figure 3H). In conclusion, the data suggest that miR-199a plays a suppressive role in inhibiting the tumorigenicity of HCC cells *in vitro* and *in vivo*.

FZD7 is a Novel Direct Target of MiR-199a

To determine the underlying mechanisms by which miR-199a contributes to the progression of HCC, we integrated bioinformatic algorithms, including miRanda, PicTar and TargetScan, to predict the potential target genes of miR-199a. According to the

Table 3. MiR-199a expression is correlated with the clinical features of patients.

| Parameter | Group | MiR-199a | | |
		Low	High	P value
Age	<52	12	10	0.6
	>52	8	10	
Gender	Men	12	9	0.42
	Women	8	11	
Metastasis	With	4	14	0.01*
	Without	16	6	
T stage	I+II	7	15	0.03*
	III+IV	13	5	

*P<0.05 was considered statistically significant.

prediction analysis, FZD7, a HCC tumorigenicity-related gene [23,24], has a putative miR-199a-binding site that maps to the 3'-UTR and is thus of particular interest. To validate the miRNA-target interactions, we constructed luciferase reporters carrying the FZD7 3'-UTR containing the putative miR-199a binding site. As shown in Figure 4A, luciferase assays indicated that the 3'-UTR of FZD7 caused a significant reduction in luciferase activity. However, the variations in the luciferase activity disappeared upon mutation of the key seed region in the 3'UTR of FZD7. The miR-199a binding site in the 3'UTR of FZD7 and the mutated binding site are shown in Figure 4B. The qRT-PCR analysis showed that over-expression of miR-199a significantly repressed the expression of the FZD7 mRNA (Figure 4C). These findings were further verified by the results of the western blot analyses, which revealed that FZD7 expression in HepG2 cells was markedly inhibited by over-expression of miR-199a (Figure 4D). Taken together, these results suggested that miR-199a could significantly suppress the expression of FZD7 through targeting the 3'UTR of its mRNA.

To determine whether miR-199a can inhibit FZD7 expression in clinical HCC tissues. qRT-PCR was performed to measure the expression of FZD7 in HCC samples from 40 patients. As observed in Table 5, Spearman's rank test showed that a significant negative correlation was found between miR-199a and FZD7 expression (r = −0.40, P<0.02). Furthermore, FZD7, as a molecule of the Wnt signaling pathway, and its downstream genes were detected using western blotting. The results indicated that the expression of the FZD7 protein in HCC cell lines was higher compared with that in the normal Chang liver cell line (Figure 4E). In addition, as shown in Figure 4D, over-expression of miR-199a could significantly down-regulate the expression of

FZD7 downstream genes, including β-catenin, Jun, Cyclin D1 and Myc. In conclusion, these results indicated that miR-199a represses the development of HCC partly through inhibiting the FZD7 pathway.

Discussion

A growing number of reports have suggested that miRNAs are important regulators of multiple cellular processes and that miRNAs are expressed aberrantly in different types of cancer, including HCC [25,26]. Studies have revealed that several miRNAs were frequently deregulated in HCC, and some specific miRNAs were found to be associated with the development and progression of HCC [11,18,27,28,29]. However, the roles of miRNAs in the molecular pathogenesis of HCC are still largely unknown because one miRNA may regulate scores of target genes and a single mRNA may be regulated by multiple miRNAs [30], all of which might function alone or in a cooperative manner. Thus, exploring and understanding the more aberrantly expressed miRNAs may help to better reveal the mechanisms underlying HCC carcinogenesis and progression.

MiR-199a is located on chromosome 19 within intron 14 of the dynamin-2 gene. Previous studies showed that miR-199a expression was diversely deregulated in several types of cancer, including HCC. For instance, miR-199a was found to be down-regulated in ovarian cancer [31], renal cancer [32], prostate cancer [33,34], colon cancer, bladder cancer [33] and oral squamous cell carcinoma [35], but it was up-regulated in cervical carcinoma [36], gastric cancer [37,38] and bronchial squamous cell carcinoma [39]. The results of the present study are in line with those of the previous study, which showed that miR-199a

Table 4. Univariate analysis of clinical parameters associated with prognosis.

Parameter	Chi-square	P value
Age	0.21	0.65
Gender	1.78	0.18
Metastasis	13.8	<0.01*
T stage	9. 8	0.002*
miR-199a	15.1	<0.01*

The univariate analysis showed that metastasis, T stage, and miR-199a were statistically significant prognostic factors for HCC patients.

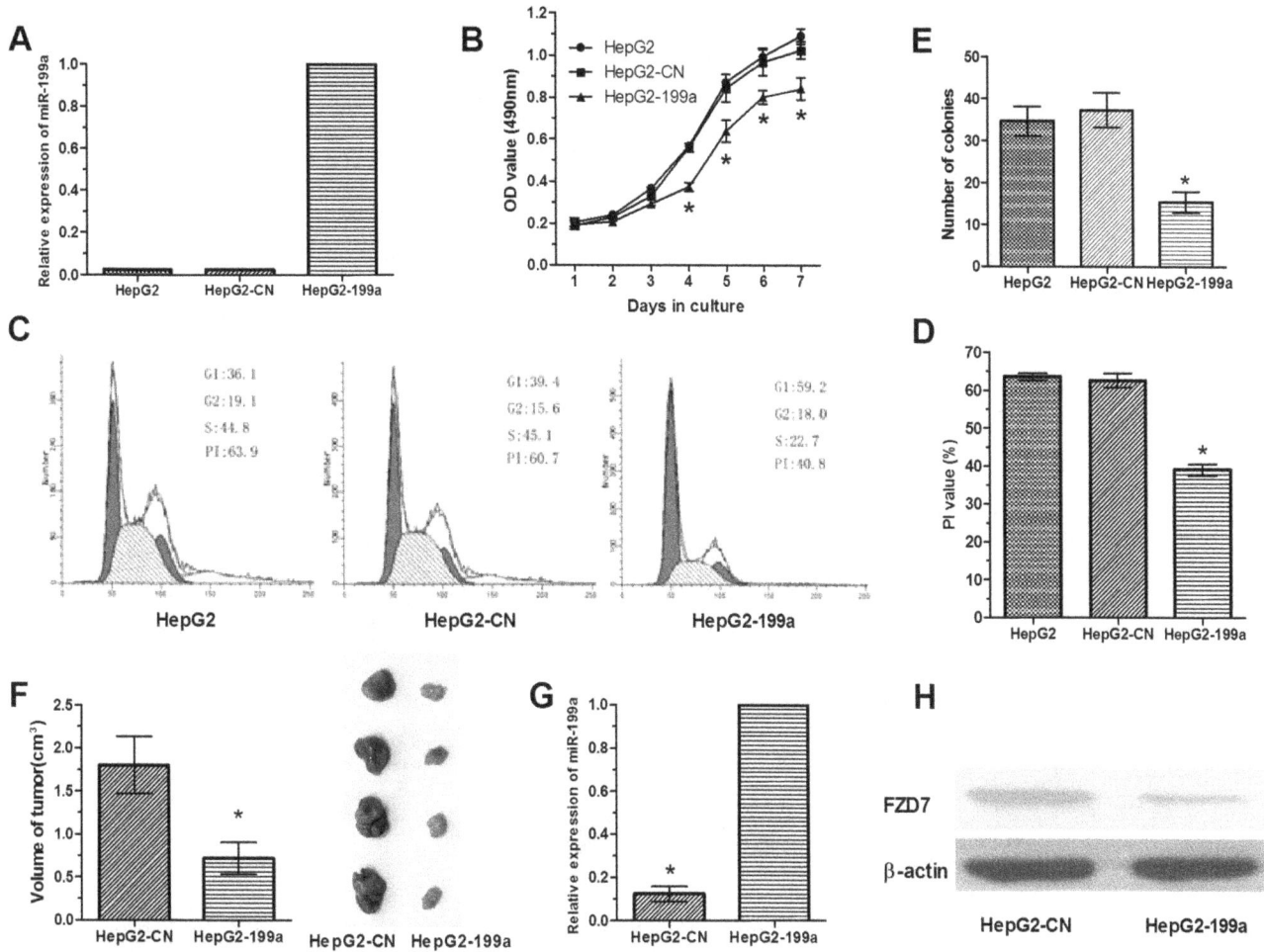

Figure 3. Over-expression of miR-199a represses growth and tumorigenicity *in vitro* and *in vivo*. (A) qRT-PCR analysis confirmed that miR-199a expression was significantly up-regulated in HepG2-199a cells compared with matched controls. U6 snRNA was used as the internal control. (B) The growth curves are plotted based on the MTT assay results. The value shown is the mean of three experiments. *Statistical significance. (C) Cell cycle distribution of HepG2, HepG2-CN, and HepG2-199a cells by flow cytometry. (D) The proliferation index (PI) of HepG2, HepG2-CN, and HepG2-199a cells, as determined by flow cytometry. The PI values that are shown are the mean of three repetitions and are expressed as the mean ± SD. (E) Colony numbers of HepG2-CN and HepG2-199a cells in soft agar. Each soft agar assay was performed in triplicate, and the results are expressed as the mean number of colonies ± SD. (F) Tumor size of HepG2-CN and HepG2-199a cells in nude mice. (G) MiR-199a expression in whole tumor tissue extracts by qRT-PCR analysis. (H) FZD7 expression in whole tumor tissue extracts by Western blot analysis.

expression was frequently down-regulated in HCC tissues compared with matched adjacent nonneoplastic tissues. This finding coincides with our *in vitro* observations that miR-199a is down-regulated in HCC cell lines compared with a normal hepatocyte cell line (Chang liver cells). In addition, lower expression of miR-199a was significantly correlated with the malignant potential and poor prognosis of human HCC. Based on these findings, miR-199a seems to be implicated in HCC development and progression. Lentiviral vectors encoding miR-NAs are useful laboratory tools to study gene function. Lentiviral vectors provide efficient gene delivery *in vitro* and can infect nondividing cells. To explore the functions of miR-199a in HCC, HepG2 cells with lower endogenous expression of miR-199a were transfected using lentiviral vectors, leading to the forced expression of the miRNA. Our findings demonstrated that over-expression of miR-199a could inhibit the proliferation of HepG2 cells and could repress cell cycle progression by inducing G0/G1 cell cycle arrest. In addition, the results showed that enforced expression of miR-199a in HepG2 cells could repress the anchorage-independent

growth of HepG2 cells in soft agar, suggesting that miR-199a might be a tumor suppressor in hepatocarcinogenesis. This finding was further supported by the finding that the over-expression of miR-199a repressed tumor formation and growth in nude mice. In fact, a miRNA is usually down-regulated in a particular human cancer and can have tumor-suppressor-like effects if the main targets for that specific cell type are oncogenes.

It is generally accepted that miRNAs exert their function through regulating the expression of their downstream target genes. We integrated bioinformatic algorithms, including miRan-da, PicTar and TargetScan, to identify the potential target genes of miR-199a. Among the potential mRNAs targeted by miR-199a, FZD7 was particularly interesting. Previous studies indicated that a functional interaction between FZD7 and Wnt3 leads to activation of the Wnt/β-catenin signaling pathway in HCC cells and may play an important role in hepatocarcinogenesis [23]. Among the FZD family, FZD7 appears to be the most important Wnt receptor involved in cancer development and progression, and FZD7 is most commonly up-regulated in a variety of cancers,

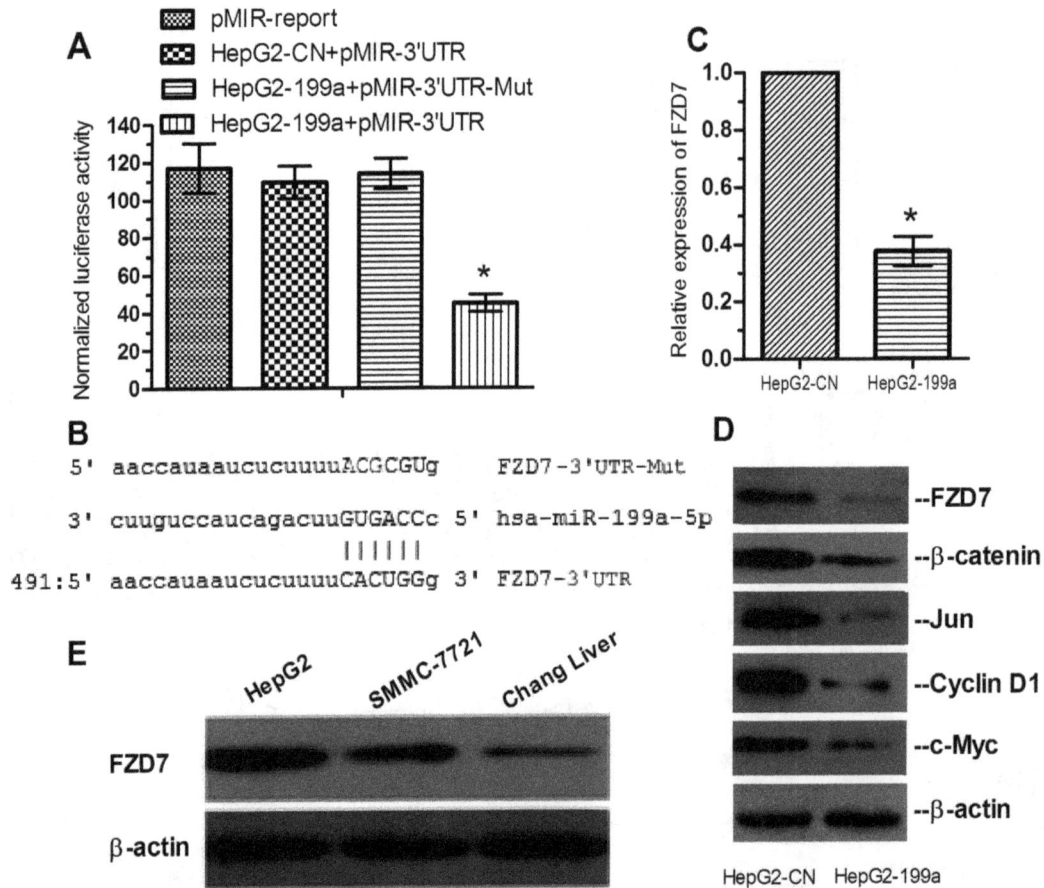

Figure 4. MiR-199a inhibits cell proliferation by directly targeting FZD7. (A) Dual luciferase assays were performed in HepG2-199a and HepG2-NC cells transfected with the firefly luciferase reporter and the control vectors containing Renilla luciferase. The results showed that miR-199a could significantly suppress the luciferase activity of the reporter containing the 3′UTR of FZD7 but had no significant effect on the reporter containing the mutated binding site of FZD7. The data shown are the means ± SD of three independent experiments. (B) The sequences of the miR-199a binding sites within the 3′UTR of FZD7 and the mutated binding site are presented. (C) qRT-PCR analysis showing that the mRNA of FZD7 was significantly decreased in HepG2-199a cells compared with HepG2-NC cells. (D) Western blot analysis confirming that the expression of FZD7 and of its downstream genes was significantly inhibited by miR-199a. β-actin was used as the internal control. (E) The expression of the FZD7 protein in HepG2 and SMMC-7721 cells was higher compared with that in normal Chang liver cells.

including colorectal cancer [40], HCC [24], esophageal cancer [41], breast cancer [42], lung cancer [43], Wilm's tumor [44], gastric cancer [45] and melanoma [43]. The over-activation of Wnt signaling with the up-regulated expression of FZD7 in various types of cancer and the roles of FZD7 in cancer stem cell biology suggest that FZD7 might serve as a therapeutic target for certain cancers [46]. Several research groups have attenuated the action of over-expressed Fzd7 in cancer cells using different methods such as an anti-FZD7 antibody, an extracellular peptide of FZD7

(soluble FZD7 peptide), small interfering peptides or a small molecule inhibitor [40,47,48,49,50,51]. Therefore, targeted inhibition of FZD7 represents a rational and promising new approach for cancer therapy. To experimentally validate this computer prediction, luciferase reporter assays confirmed that FZD7 was a target gene of miR-199a. These data were further strengthened by results from exploring the protein levels of FZD7 in HepG2 cells by western blotting, which showed that the over-expression of miR-199a markedly decreased FZD7 protein expression. Then,

Table 5. The correlations of miR-199a with FZD7 expression in HCC tissues.

		FZD7 expression		R value	P value
		Low	High		
miR-199a	Low	6	14	-0.40	<0.02
expression	High	14	6		

Patients were split into high- and low-expression groups based on the median for miR-199a and FZD7 expression. R: correlation coefficient as evaluated by Spearman's rank correlation coefficient. P<0.05 was considered statistically significant.

the downstream genes of FZD7, including β-catenin, Jun, Cyclin D1 and Myc were investigated using western blot analysis, and the results demonstrated that over-expression of miR-199a could significantly down-regulate the expression of the downstream genes of FZD7. Moreover, the co-expression of miR-199a and its target gene FZD7 were detected in HCC tissues. The results showed that miR-199a was inversely correlated with FZD7 expression in HCC tissues. Taken together, these results strongly suggested that miR-199a might function as a tumor suppressor partly by mediating the repression of FZD7 expression in HCC development.

In conclusion, the data presented here strongly indicate that miR-199a acts as a tumor suppressor in HCC. Our present study showed that miR-199a is frequently down-regulated and inversely correlated with poor prognosis in HCC patients. In addition, restoration of miR-199a expression in HCC cells leads to inhibition of the cell proliferation and of the cell cycle partly through down-regulating FZD7 *in vitro* and *in vivo*. These findings not only help us to better elucidate the molecular mechanisms of hepatocarcinogenesis from a fresh perspective but also provide a new theoretical basis to further investigate miR-199a as a potential biomarker and a promising approach for HCC treatment.

Acknowledgments

We thank Professor Qing Li (Department of Pathology at Xijing Hospital) for pathological analysis and our technician Taidong Qiao for excellent technical assistance.

Author Contributions

Conceived and designed the experiments: JS LG HX JL KW DF. Performed the experiments: JS LG ST JJ YG JW. Analyzed the data: YW JW ZY YZ. Contributed reagents/materials/analysis tools: ZC. Wrote the paper: JS ST LG GY.

References

1. Perz JF, Armstrong GL, Farrington LA, Hutin YJ, Bell BP (2006) The contributions of hepatitis B virus and hepatitis C virus infections to cirrhosis and primary liver cancer worldwide. J Hepatol 45: 529–538.
2. Jemal A, Bray F, Center MM, Ferlay J, Ward E, et al. (2011) Global cancer statistics. CA Cancer J Clin 61: 69–90.
3. Ferlay J, Shin HR, Bray F, Forman D, Mathers C, et al. (2010) Estimates of worldwide burden of cancer in 2008: GLOBOCAN 2008. Int J Cancer 127: 2893–2917.
4. Schwartz M, Roayaie S, Konstadoulakis M (2007) Strategies for the management of hepatocellular carcinoma. Nat Clin Pract Oncol 4: 424–432.
5. Jemal A, Center MM, DeSantis C, Ward EM (2010) Global patterns of cancer incidence and mortality rates and trends. Cancer Epidemiol Biomarkers Prev 19: 1893–1907.
6. Sanyal AJ, Yoon SK, Lencioni R (2010) The etiology of hepatocellular carcinoma and consequences for treatment. Oncologist 15 Suppl 4: 14–22.
7. Aravalli RN, Steer CJ, Cressman EN (2008) Molecular mechanisms of hepatocellular carcinoma. Hepatology 48: 2047–2063.
8. Huang S, He X (2011) The role of microRNAs in liver cancer progression. Br J Cancer 104: 235–240.
9. Bushati N, Cohen SM (2007) microRNA functions. Annu Rev Cell Dev Biol 23: 175–205.
10. Kent OA, Mendell JT (2006) A small piece in the cancer puzzle: microRNAs as tumor suppressors and oncogenes. Oncogene 25: 6188–6196.
11. Negrini M, Gramantieri L, Sabbioni S, Croce CM (2011) microRNA involvement in hepatocellular carcinoma. Anticancer Agents Med Chem 11: 500–521.
12. Braconi C, Henry JC, Kogure T, Schmittgen T, Patel T (2011) The role of microRNAs in human liver cancers. Semin Oncol 38: 752–763.
13. Volinia S, Calin GA, Liu CG, Ambs S, Cimmino A, et al. (2006) A microRNA expression signature of human solid tumors defines cancer gene targets. Proc Natl Acad Sci U S A 103: 2257–2261.
14. Meng F, Henson R, Wehbe-Janek H, Ghoshal K, Jacob ST, et al. (2007) MicroRNA-21 regulates expression of the PTEN tumor suppressor gene in human hepatocellular cancer. Gastroenterology 133: 647–658.
15. Jiang J, Gusev Y, Aderca I, Mettler TA, Nagorney DM, et al. (2008) Association of MicroRNA expression in hepatocellular carcinomas with hepatitis infection, cirrhosis, and patient survival. Clin Cancer Res 14: 419–427.
16. Ladeiro Y, Couchy G, Balabaud C, Bioulac-Sage P, Pelletier L, et al. (2008) MicroRNA profiling in hepatocellular tumors is associated with clinical features and oncogene/tumor suppressor gene mutations. Hepatology 47: 1955–1963.
17. Tsai WC, Hsu PW, Lai TC, Chau GY, Lin CW, et al. (2009) MicroRNA-122, a tumor suppressor microRNA that regulates intrahepatic metastasis of hepatocellular carcinoma. Hepatology 49: 1571–1582.
18. Murakami Y, Yasuda T, Saigo K, Urashima T, Toyoda H, et al. (2006) Comprehensive analysis of microRNA expression patterns in hepatocellular carcinoma and non-tumorous tissues. Oncogene 25: 2537–2545.
19. Hou J, Lin L, Zhou W, Wang Z, Ding G, et al. (2011) Identification of miRNomes in human liver and hepatocellular carcinoma reveals miR-199a/b-3p as therapeutic target for hepatocellular carcinoma. Cancer Cell 19: 232–243.
20. Livak KJ, Schmittgen TD (2001) Analysis of relative gene expression data using real-time quantitative PCR and the 2(-Delta Delta C(T)) Method. Methods 25: 402–408.
21. Gullberg D, Liang S, He L, Zhao X, Miao Y, et al. (2011) MicroRNA Let-7f Inhibits Tumor Invasion and Metastasis by Targeting MYH9 in Human Gastric Cancer. PLoS One 6: e18409.
22. Song J, Xie H, Lian Z, Yang G, Du R, et al. (2006) Enhanced cell survival of gastric cancer cells by a novel gene URG4. Neoplasia 8: 995–1002.
23. Kim M, Lee HC, Tsedensodnom O, Hartley R, Lim YS, et al. (2008) Functional interaction between Wnt3 and Frizzled-7 leads to activation of the Wnt/beta-catenin signaling pathway in hepatocellular carcinoma cells. J Hepatol 48: 780–791.
24. Merle P, Kim M, Herrmann M, Gupte A, Lefrançois L, et al. (2005) Oncogenic role of the frizzled-7/β-catenin pathway in hepatocellular carcinoma. Journal of Hepatology 43: 854–862.
25. Yates LA, Norbury CJ, Gilbert RJ (2013) The long and short of microRNA. Cell 153: 516–519.
26. Nelson KM and Weiss GJ (2008) MicroRNAs and cancer: past, present, and potential future. Mol Cancer Ther 7: 3655–3660.
27. Gramantieri L, Ferracin M, Fornari F, Veronese A, Sabbioni S, et al. (2007) Cyclin G1 is a target of miR-122a, a microRNA frequently down-regulated in human hepatocellular carcinoma. Cancer Res 67: 6092–6099.
28. Budhu A, Jia HL, Forgues M, Liu CG, Goldstein D, et al. (2008) Identification of metastasis-related microRNAs in hepatocellular carcinoma. Hepatology 47: 897–907.
29. Ji J, Shi J, Budhu A, Yu Z, Forgues M, et al. (2009) MicroRNA expression, survival, and response to interferon in liver cancer. N Engl J Med 361: 1437–1447.
30. Miranda KC, Huynh T, Tay Y, Ang YS, Tam WL, et al. (2006) A pattern-based method for the identification of MicroRNA binding sites and their corresponding heteroduplexes. Cell 126: 1203–1217.
31. Nam EJ, Yoon H, Kim SW, Kim H, Kim YT, et al. (2008) MicroRNA expression profiles in serous ovarian carcinoma. Clin Cancer Res 14: 2690–2695.
32. Tsukigi M, Bilim V, Yuuki K, Ugolkov A, Naito S, et al. (2012) Re-expression of miR-199a suppresses renal cancer cell proliferation and survival by targeting GSK-3beta. Cancer Lett 315: 189–197.
33. Su SF, Chang YW, Andreu-Vieyra C, Fang JY, Yang Z, et al. (2013) miR-30d, miR-181a and miR-199a-5p cooperatively suppress the endoplasmic reticulum chaperone and signaling regulator GRP78 in cancer. Oncogene 32: 4694–4701.
34. Porkka KP, Pfeiffer MJ, Waltering KK, Vessella RL, Tammela TL, et al. (2007) MicroRNA expression profiling in prostate cancer. Cancer Res 67: 6130–6135.
35. Yu T, Wang XY, Gong RG, Li A, Yang S, et al. (2009) The expression profile of microRNAs in a model of 7,12-dimethyl-benz[a]anthrance-induced oral carcinogenesis in Syrian hamster. J Exp Clin Cancer Res 28: 64.
36. Lee JW, Choi CH, Choi JJ, Park YA, Kim SJ, et al. (2008) Altered MicroRNA expression in cervical carcinomas. Clin Cancer Res 14: 2535–2542.
37. Ueda T, Volinia S, Okumura H, Shimizu M, Taccioli C, et al. (2010) Relation between microRNA expression and progression and prognosis of gastric cancer: a microRNA expression analysis. Lancet Oncol 11: 136–146.
38. He XJ, Ma YY, Yu S, Jiang XT, Lu YD, et al. (2014) Up-regulated miR-199a-5p in gastric cancer functions as an oncogene and targets klotho. BMC Cancer 14: 218.
39. Mascaux C, Laes JF, Anthoine G, Haller A, Ninane V, et al. (2009) Evolution of microRNA expression during human bronchial squamous carcinogenesis. Eur Respir J 33: 352–359.

40. Ueno K, Hazama S, Mitomori S, Nishioka M, Suehiro Y, et al. (2009) Down-regulation of frizzled-7 expression decreases survival, invasion and metastatic capabilities of colon cancer cells. Br J Cancer 101: 1374–1381.

41. Tanaka S, Akiyoshi T, Mori M, Wands JR, Sugimachi K (1998) A novel frizzled gene identified in human esophageal carcinoma mediates APC/beta-catenin signals. Proc Natl Acad Sci U S A 95: 10164–10169.

42. Yang L, Wu X, Wang Y, Zhang K, Wu J, et al. (2011) FZD7 has a critical role in cell proliferation in triple negative breast cancer. Oncogene 30: 4437–4446.

43. Sagara N, Toda G, Hirai M, Terada M, Katoh M (1998) Molecular cloning, differential expression, and chromosomal localization of human frizzled-1, frizzled-2, and frizzled-7. Biochem Biophys Res Commun 252: 117–122.

44. Li CM, Guo M, Borczuk A, Powell CA, Wei M, et al. (2002) Gene expression in Wilms' tumor mimics the earliest committed stage in the metanephric mesenchymal-epithelial transition. Am J Pathol 160: 2181–2190.

45. Kirikoshi H, Sekihara H, Katoh M (2001) Up-regulation of Frizzled-7 (FZD7) in human gastric cancer. Int J Oncol 19: 111–115.

46. Melchior K, Weiss J, Zaehres H, Kim YM, Lutzko C, et al. (2008) The WNT receptor FZD7 contributes to self-renewal signaling of human embryonic stem cells. Biol Chem 389: 897–903.

47. Ueno K, Hiura M, Suehiro Y, Hazama S, Hirata H, et al. (2008) Frizzled-7 as a potential therapeutic target in colorectal cancer. Neoplasia 10: 697–705.

48. Nambotin SB, Lefrancois L, Sainsily X, Berthillon P, Kim M, et al. (2011) Pharmacological inhibition of Frizzled-7 displays anti-tumor properties in hepatocellular carcinoma. J Hepatol 54: 288–299.

49. Khramtsov AI, Khramtsova GF, Tretiakova M, Huo D, Olopade OI, et al. (2010) Wnt/beta-catenin pathway activation is enriched in basal-like breast cancers and predicts poor outcome. Am J Pathol 176: 2911–2920.

50. Pode-Shakked N, Harari-Steinberg O, Haberman-Ziv Y, Rom-Gross E, Bahar S, et al. (2011) Resistance or sensitivity of Wilms' tumor to anti-FZD7 antibody highlights the Wnt pathway as a possible therapeutic target. Oncogene 30: 1664–1680.

51. Fujii N, You L, Xu Z, Uematsu K, Shan J, et al. (2007) An antagonist of dishevelled protein-protein interaction suppresses beta-catenin-dependent tumor cell growth. Cancer Res 67: 573–579.

20

Multidetector Computed Tomography-Based Microstructural Analysis Reveals Reduced Bone Mineral Content and Trabecular Bone Changes in the Lumbar Spine after Transarterial Chemoembolization Therapy for Hepatocellular Carcinoma

Miyuki Takasu*, Takuji Yamagami, Yuko Nakamura, Daisuke Komoto, Yoko Kaichi, Chihiro Tani, Shuji Date, Masao Kiguchi, Kazuo Awai

Department of Diagnostic Radiology, Graduate School of Biomedical Sciences, Hiroshima University, Hiroshima, Japan

Abstract

Purpose: It is well recognized that therapeutic irradiation can result in bone damage. However, long-term bone toxicity associated with computed tomography (CT) performed during interventional angiography has received little attention. The purpose of this study was to determine the prevalence of osteoporosis and trabecular microstructural changes in patients after transarterial chemoembolization (TACE) for hepatocellular carcinoma therapy using an interventional-CT system.

Materials and Methods: Spinal microarchitecture was examined by 64-detector CT in 81 patients who underwent TACE, 35 patients with chronic hepatitis, and 79 controls. For each patient, the volumetric CT dose index (CTDIv) during TACE (CTDIv (TACE)), the dose-length product (DLP) during TACE (DLP (TACE)), and CTDIv and DLP of routine dynamic CT scans (CTDIv (CT) and DLP (CT), respectively), were calculated as the sum since 2008. Using a three dimensional (3D) image analysis system, the tissue bone mineral density (tBMD) and trabecular parameters of the 12th thoracic vertebra were calculated. Using tBMD at a reported cutoff value of 68 mg/cm^3, the prevalence of osteoporosis was assessed.

Results: The prevalence of osteoporosis was significantly greater in the TACE vs. the control group (39.6% vs. 18.2% for males, $P<0.05$ and 60.6% vs. 34.8% for females, $P<0.01$). Multivariate regression analysis demonstrated that sex, age, and CTDIv (CT) significantly affected the risk of osteoporosis. Of these indices, CTDIv (CT) had the highest area under the curve (AUC) (0.735). Correlation analyses of tBMD with cumulative radiation dose revealed weak correlations between tBMD and CTDIv (CT) ($r^2=0.194$, $P<0.001$).

Conclusion: The prevalence of osteoporosis was significantly higher in post TACE patients than in control subjects. The cumulative radiation dose related to routine dynamic CT studies was a significant contributor to the prevalence of osteoporosis.

Editor: Joseph P. R. O. Orgel, Illinois Institute of Technology, United States of America

Funding: MT was supported by Grant-in-Aid for Scientific Research (KAKENHI) (C) [23591768] in Japan. The funder had no role in study design, data collection and analysis, decision to publish, or preparation of the manuscript.

Competing Interests: The authors have declared that no competing interests exist.

* Email: my-takasu@syd.odn.ne.jp

Introduction

The number of computed tomography (CT)-guided interventional procedures has increased because they are less invasive and more cost-effective than open surgery [1–3]. Transarterial embolization therapies involve the transcatheter delivery of solid particles into an artery feeding a target tumor for the purpose of blocking its blood supply. These therapies include bland embolization, transarterial chemoembolization (TACE), and chemoembolization using drug-eluting beads. TACE is a method in which chemotherapeutic drugs are combined with embolization particles and then injected into the artery that supplies the tumor. TACE

via the hepatic artery has been used as treatment for hepatocellular carcinoma (HCC) in cases where surgical resection is not a viable option or as a means of downstaging HCC to fit within Milan criteria for the possibility of further management with orthotopic liver transplantation. Trials performed by Hong Kong [4] and Barcelona [5] researchers showed a significant increase in survival rates of subjects compared to controls. In some institutions, CT arterial portography and CT during hepatic arteriography are performed to confirm the existence or to evaluate the characteristics of liver tumors during TACE [6]. Additionally, two-dimensional or three-dimensional CT images are acquired to generate a road map of the targets and their positions relative to the interventional instruments. This valuable information provides guidance for the operator to locate the target, plan an interventional path, adjust the interventional instruments, and evaluate the efficacy of the procedure. A priori knowledge of the distribution of contrast material in the tumor from performance of CT arteriography through the selected arterial branch ensures that anticancer drugs and embolic agents are infused effectively.

A concern regarding the use of CT during angiography may be the radiation exposure to the patients, because the number of CT scans performed during TACE with the interventional-CT system is high; around ten times per procedure. It is well recognized that therapeutic irradiation can result in bone damage and may increase fracture risk. The main evidence for the effect of irradiation on fracture risk comes from a long-term follow-up study of two European randomized trials (Stockholm I and II) [7,8] evaluating the effect of short-course irradiation on patients with operable rectal cancer [9]. Pathologically, vascular injury and decrease of osteoblast cells following irradiation have been reported [10–14].

Recently, a case of 12th thoracic vertebral fracture that occurred after multiple TACE procedures to treat multiple hepatocellular carcinomas was seen. Fluorodeoxyglucose (FDG)-positron-emission tomography (FDG-PET)-CT performed to screen for pathologic fractures revealed diffusely decreased FDG uptake within the lower thoracic to lumbar spine (Figure 1). This finding gave us the impression that this area might have corresponded to the radiation field during the TACE procedures because the liver and vessels such as hepatic arteries, their branches, superior mesenteric artery, and portal vein, which are repeatedly imaged during TACE procedures, are all located around the same spinal level. Therefore, we hypothesized that radiation exposure from CT scans during angiographies led to

decreased bone density and bone strength associated with secondary osteoporosis.

Bone strength and fracture susceptibility are governed in large part by the amount of bone, which can be assessed by dual-energy X-ray absorptiometry measurements of areal bone mineral density. However, many other structural and material properties of bone, including microarchitecture, contribute considerably and independently to fragility [15–17]. Recently, high-resolution peripheral quantitative CT [18,19] and multidetector CT (MDCT) [20,21] have been used noninvasively to visualize the details of trabecular microarchitecture.

The long-term bone toxicity associated with CT during interventional angiography has received little attention. The purpose of this study was to determine the prevalence of osteoporosis and trabecular microstructural changes using clinical MDCT-based microstructural analysis in patients after TACE with the interventional-CT system to treat hepatocellular carcinoma.

Materials and Methods

Ethics Statement

This retrospective, single-institution study was approved by the Institutional Review Board of Hiroshima University Hospital, with a waiver of informed consent. Patient records and information were anonymized and de-identified prior to analyses.

Subjects

First, consecutive patients who underwent unenhanced abdominal CT performed with a specific CT unit in our institution from September 2010 to January 2014 were selected. Next, a total of 195 of these patients were enrolled in the study after exclusion of subjects with a history of chemotherapy (n = 4), total or partial gastrectomy (n = 4), esophagectomy (n = 1), radiation therapy to the pelvis (n = 1), vertebral fracture (n = 1), chronic steroid use

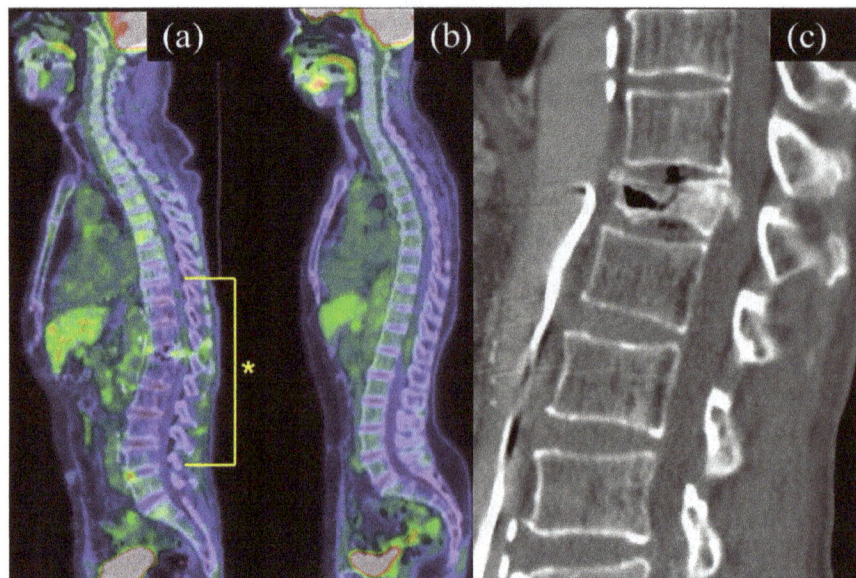

Figure 1. Sagittal reconstructed fluorodeoxyglucose-positron-emission tomography (FDG-PET)-CT image (a) and MDCT image (c) of the spine obtained from a 62-year-old man after eight transarterial chemoembolization procedures for hepatocellular carcinomas. FDG-PET-CT reveals diffusely decreased FDG uptake within the lower thoracic to lumbar spine (*). Sagittal reconstructed FDG-PET-CT image is accompanied by that of a 72-year old woman performed five years after resection of a uterine cervical cancer, in which there is normal spinal FDG uptake, for comparison (b). Sagittal reconstructed CT shows a vertebral fracture of the 12th thoracic vertebra.

(n = 1), and patients with a gait disturbance caused by cerebrovascular disease (n = 4) or myopathy (n = 1). There were no patients with a history of rheumatoid arthritis, inflammatory bowel disease, chronic obstructive pulmonary disease, or organ transplantation. Patients in the TACE group (n = 81) had HCC with a history of TACE and a diagnosis of either type B or type C hepatitis. Patients in the chronic hepatitis (CH) group (n = 35) had a diagnosis of either type B or type C hepatitis and had no history of any angiographic or CT-guided fluoroscopic procedures. The majority of HCC patients had persistent infection from hepatitis B virus or hepatitis C virus. Therefore, we established the CH group to determine whether there were radiation effects from TACE procedures only. Subjects in the control group (n = 79) were randomly selected from our hospital's radiology information system; they had undergone MDCT of the body to screen for tumor recurrences other than liver tumors, to rule out internal malignancy, and to diagnose abdominal or back pain. We did not recruit healthy control subjects from the local community for ethical reason.

Tables 1 and 2 summarize the characteristics of these patients.

TACE Procedure

All patients in the TACE group had adequate hepatic function to undergo TACE. The interventional procedures were performed using an interventional-CT system consisting of a unified CT and angiography unit (Aquilion LB combined with Infinix Celeve-i INFX-8000V, Toshiba Medical Systems, Tokyo, Japan). In addition to angiographic examinations, CT scans were performed

during common or proper hepatic arteriography to evaluate hemodynamics in the HCC, map the arterial anatomy, and assess portal flow. Further selective hepatic arteriograms were also performed using CT scanning to confirm the distribution of contrast material in the HCC from the selected arterial branch just before infusing anti-cancer drugs and embolic agents.

The X-ray tube was equipped with a built-in kerma area product (KAP) meter at the collimator exit with capability to display the cumulative KAP for fluoroscopic and radiographic examinations. The KAP is the integral of air kerma (the energy extracted from an X-ray beam per unit mass of air in a small irradiated air volume; for diagnostic X-rays, the dose delivered to that volume of air) across the entire X-ray beam emitted from the X-ray tube. It is a surrogate measure of the amount of energy delivered to the patient [22]. Entrance skin dose was calculated from KAP, beam area, and the calibration coefficient of the KAP meter at the calibrated distance for the focal-to-skin distance. It is important to estimate entrance skin dose during and after fluoroscopically guided interventions because a skin dose that exceeds 15 Gy is thought to be a sentinel event [23]. The volumetric CT dose index during TACE (CTDIv (TACE)) and dose-length product during TACE (DLP (TACE)) were obtained directly from the scanner console. The computed tomography dose index (CTDI) is a measure of the radiation output of the CT slice comprising the quality of the X-rays produced, the type of filtration and the geometry of the X-ray beam including focus size and collimation [24]. CTDIv, which was introduced for modern CT scanners, is obtained from the average CTDI in an irradiated

Table 1. Comparison of clinical characteristics and cumulative radiation doses.

Men	TACE	CH	Control
Background data	n = 48	n = 17	n = 33
Age (years)	67.1±9.0	66.3±7.6	66.5±7.1
BMI (kg/m^2)	23.2±2.8	21.8±2.4	23.8±3.9
Radiation exposure			
CTDIv (CT) (mGy)	350[††][50, 1950]	200** [50, 950]	50 [0, 700]
CTDIv (TACE) (mGy)	148 [15, 528]		
DLP (CT) (mGy×cm)	14350[††,*][2000, 78000]	7600 [0, 22900]	4500 [0, 22200]
DLP (TACE) (mGy×cm)	2818 [305, 17985]		
Entrance skin dose (mGy)	790.9 [36, 5911]		
Women	**TACE**	**CH**	**Control**
Background data	n = 33	n = 18	n = 46
Age (years)	67.4±7.8	61.7±6.9	62.5±9.3
BMI (kg/m^2)	23.0±3.4	22.9±4.4	22.5±3.4
Radiation exposure			
CTDIv (CT) (mGy)	374[††, **] [100, 1650]	250 [0, 1150]	0 [0, 200]
CTDIv (TACE) (mGy)	101 [26, 1723]		
DLP (CT) (mGy×cm)	9450[†, **] [2800, 33000]	6900 [0, 36000]	1900 [0, 13000]
DLP (TACE) (mGy×cm)	1880 [489, 6599]		
Entrance skin dose (mGy)	817 [76, 4465]		

Note. Values represent the means ± standard deviation or medians [range].
BMI, body mass index; CTDIv (CT): CTDIv of routine dynamic CT scan; CTDIv (TACE): CTDIv during TACE; DLP (CT): DLP of routine dynamic CT scan; DLP (TACE): DLP during TACE.
**P<0.01, control vs. CH group.
[††]P<0.01, [†]P<0.05 control vs. TACE group.
[+]P<0.05, TACE group vs. CH group.

slice divided by a helical pitch. To obtain a dose quantity describing the radiation exposure for a full scan, the DLP was introduced [25,26]. DLP can be obtained by CTDIv divided by the scan length, which means it depends on the patient's height.

For each patient, cumulative radiation doses obtained from each index were calculated as the sum of all TACE procedures performed since 2008.

Imaging by MDCT

All patients were scanned with a 64-section MDCT (LightSpeed VCT; GE Healthcare, Little Chalfont, UK) with spatial resolution equivalent to 16.4 line pair per centimeter at a 2% setting for the modulation transfer function. The collimation was 64×0.625 mm, and table translation speed was 23.4 cm/sec. The tube parameters were 300 mA and 120 kV, with a pitch of 0.586. Unenhanced and three-phase contrast-enhanced helical scans of the entire liver were obtained.

For each patient, the cumulative radiation doses obtained from each of two indices (e.g., CTDIv (CT) and DLP (CT)) were calculated as the sum from all dynamic CT scans since 2008.

Bone mineral density measurement and MDCT-based microstructural analysis

To obtain tissue bone mineral density (tBMD) data by MDCT, the patients were scanned simultaneously with a bone mineral reference phantom (B-MAS2000; Kyotokagaku Co., Kyoto, Japan) containing calibration objects with equivalent densities of 0, 50, 100, 150, and 200 mg/cm^3 calcium hydroxyapatite.

Images of the whole lumbar spine obtained by unenhanced scanning were reconstructed using an acquisition matrix of 512×512 and a field of view of 100 mm, resulting in a voxel size of 0.20×0.20×0.16 mm^3. An edge-enhancing reconstruction kernel (Bone Plus; GE Healthcare, Little Chalfont, UK) was used. The 12th thoracic vertebra (T12) was chosen for the analysis in this study because vertebral fractures typically occur at the thoracolumbar junction (T12 and the first lumbar vertebra) [26,27].

For microstructural analysis, the volume of interest (VOI) was defined manually as a 10-mm thickness of the central part of the T12 vertebral body to avoid the cortex, the basivertebral foramen, and both endplates.

Microstructural parameters were calculated using a computer program for a three dimensional (3D) image analysis system (TRI/3D-BON; RATOC System Engineering, Tokyo, Japan), as described elsewhere [20]. Briefly, using a volumetric bone mineral density value for trabecular bone, >150 mg/cm^3 within the bone marrow was extracted. We used a global threshold method. A standardized method of image threshold levels based on the attenuation histogram of a selected region of interest was used to ensure consistency in the image threshold levels across all subjects studied.

The following trabecular microstructural parameters were obtained: apparent trabecular bone volume fraction (app BV/TV), apparent trabecular number (app Tb.N), apparent trabecular separation (app Tb.S), Euler's number (E), degree of anisotropy (DA), and the structure model index (SMI). Details of these methods are described elsewhere [20,21] but briefly, bone volume (BV) was calculated using tetrahedrons corresponding to the enclosed volume of the triangulated surface. Total tissue volume (TV) analyzed was the entire marrow area volume including trabecular bone. Apparent BV/TV was calculated from these values. App Tb.S was determined by filling maximal spheres into the structure according to the method described by Hildebrand and Rügsegger [28]. App Tb.N was estimated as a trabecular bone

number crossing the line perpendicular to the growing direction of vertebrae based on the plate model [29]. Euler's number was calculated by using the Euler method of Odgaard and Gundersen [30]. Degree of anisotropy was determined from the ratio between the maximal and minimal radii of the mean intercept length ellipsoid [31]. By displaying the surface of the structure to an infinitesimal amount, SMI was calculated according to the method described by Hildebrand and Rügsegger [28]. The SMI quantifies the plate vs. rod characteristics of trabecular bone. An SMI of 0 reflects a purely plate-shaped bone and an SMI of 3 indicates a purely rod-like bone.

A cutoff value of 68 mg/cm^3 was determined from a previous study that evaluated tBMD (bone mineral content/tissue volume (BMC/TV)) in 67 patients with osteoporosis using the 64-section MDCT and the same 3D image analysis system [32].

One author (M.T.) performed microstructural analysis, and precision was confirmed as described elsewhere [20].

Statistical Analysis

The characteristics, cumulative radiation doses, trabecular microstructural parameters, and tBMD of the three groups were compared by the Kruskal-Wallis test followed by the Steel-Dwass test because some indices were non-normally distributed. The Kolmogorov-Smirnov test was used to determine whether values were normally distributed. The prevalence of osteoporosis in the three groups was calculated. For patients in the TACE group, a multivariate general linear model with binomial distribution and logit-link was constructed to identify the predictors of osteoporosis. We calculated the odds ratios for osteoporosis associated with risk factors. To evaluate the diagnostic performance of contributors to osteoporosis, comparisons of the receiver operating characteristic (ROC) curves were performed, and the areas under the curves (AUCs) were calculated. Correlations of tBMD with cumulative radiation dose were determined. The raw datasets of tBMD and CTDIv (CT) showed significant heteroscedasticity and data were transformed to a log scale. Since log-transformed tBMD and CTDIv (CT) were non-normally distributed, the Spearman rank correlation test was used for simple regression analysis. All analyses were performed with a spreadsheet application (Microsoft Office Excel 2010, Redmond, WA, USA) and ROC analysis software (ROCKIT 0.9.1; Charles E. Metz, University of Chicago, Chicago, IL, USA).

Results

Table 1 summarizes the patients' characteristics and cumulative radiation doses. In male subjects, CTDIv (CT) and DLP (CT) were significantly greater in the TACE group than in the control group ($P<0.01$). CTDIv (CT) was significantly greater in the CH group than in the control group ($P<0.01$), and DLP (CT) was significantly greater in the TACE group than in the CH group ($P<0.05$). Patients' age and BMI were similar among the three groups. In female subjects, CTDIv (CT) and DLP (CT) were significantly greater in the TACE group and the CH group than in the control group ($P<0.01$). Patients' age and BMI were similar among the three groups.

The prevalence of osteoporosis in the three groups was calculated (Table 2). The prevalence of osteoporosis was significantly greater in the TACE compared to the control group (39.6% vs. 18.2%, $P<0.05$ for males and 60.6% vs. 34.8%, $P<0.01$ for females, respectively). The prevalence of osteoporosis in the CH group was less than in the TACE group and greater than in the control group, but these results were not statistically significant.

Table 2. Comparison of bone mineral density of the lumbar spine among the three groups.

Male	TACE	CH	Control
tBMD (mg/cm³)	78.6±35.4†	82.0±26.5	91.6±24.9
<68 mg/cm³ (osteoporosis)	19	6	6
≥68 mg/cm³	29	11	27
Prevalence of osteoporosis (%)	39.6	35.3	18.2
Female	**TACE**	**CH**	**Control**
tBMD (mg/cm³)	60.3±31.0††	76.4±30.6	84.6±29.2
<68 mg/cm³ (osteoporosis)	20	9	16
≥68 mg/cm³	13	9	30
Prevalence of osteoporosis (%)	60.6	50.0	34.8

††$P<0.01$, †$P<0.05$, control vs. post TACE.

Results of comparison of microstructural parameters among the three groups are shown in Table 3. Among the microstructural indexes, app Tb.N was significantly lower in the TACE group than in the control group ($P<0.05$). Apparent Tb.S ($P<0.05$ for males, $P<0.01$ for females), structure model index ($P<0.05$ for males, $P<0.01$ for females), and Euler number ($P<0.01$) were significantly higher in the TACE group than in the control group. In female patients, app BV/TV was significantly lower in the TACE group than in the control group ($P<0.01$). These findings indicate that trabecular bones in the patients of the TACE group were fewer, less dense, and more rod-like than in the controls.

Multivariate regression analysis demonstrated that sex, age, and CTDIv (CT) significantly affected the risk of osteoporosis (Table 4). The AUC having the highest discriminatory power to distinguish osteoporotic patients from controls was that for CTDIv (CT) (AUC = 0.735; 95% confidence intervals (CIs), 0.557, 0.732), with an optimal cutoff value of 400 mGy; the sensitivity and specificity were 63.2% (CIs, 0.367, 0.642) and 73.2% (CIs, 0.557, 0.922), respectively. Regarding the same distribution, the AUC for age was 0.692 (CIs, 0.622, 0.771), with an optimal cutoff value of 64 years old; the sensitivity and specificity were 88.6% (CIs, 0.817, 0.972) and 58.8% (CIs, 0.377, 0.811), respectively. Analysis of CTDIv (TACE) revealed no contribution to the risk of osteoporosis.

Correlation analyses of tBMD with cumulative radiation dose showed a weak correlation between tBMD and CTDIv (CT) ($rs = -0.441$, $r^2 = 0.194$, $P<0.001$, Figure 2).

Representative images are shown in Figures 3 and 4.

Discussion

In early 2010, the U.S. Food and Drug Administration introduced the "Initiative to Reduce Unnecessary Radiation Exposure from Medical Imaging" [33]. In this report, CT and associated CT-guided interventions were identified as contributors to increasing the radiation dose to patients, and- the authors pointed out that a lack of awareness of radiation-induced injuries to patients among the users of medical radiation may be contributing to an increase of radiation exposure.

In the current study, weak correlations were found between tBMD and the cumulative radiation dose of patients in the TACE group. Bone loss due to high doses of irradiation therapy has been identified in diagnostic radiographic images [34]. However, to the best of our knowledge, no study has demonstrated an association between bone mass and radiation dose from diagnostic imaging procedures such as CT scans.

The primary effect of irradiation on bone is atrophy. Several pathological findings regarding blood vessels were identified in the radiation-induced changes in bone. They included loss of vasculature [10], sub-intimal fibrosis, and hyaline thickening of the media [12], followed by the later replacement of smooth

Table 3. Comparison of microstructural parameters among the three groups.

	Male			Female		
	TACE	CH	Control	TACE	CH	Control
App BV/TV (%)	27.8±13.5	28.6±8.7	31.9±7.8	21.2±10.5**	27.8±10.8	29.8±9.6
App Tb.N (1/mm³)	0.34±0.08*	0.36±0.06	0.38±0.05	0.30±0.10*	0.35±0.06	0.36±0.07
App Tb.S (μm)	842±281*	775±147	710±109	1003±392**	811±171	770±195
SMI	1.76±0.53*	1.74±0.39	1.61±0.36	2.00±0.44**	1.75±0.48	1.69±0.40
Euler's number	−1426±1149**	−1792±1105	−2185±977	−665±879**	−1074±681	−1402±825
Degree of anisotropy	1.41±0.11	1.43±0.12	1.41±0.09	1.48±0.10	1.52±0.20	1.45±0.11

**$P<0.01$, *$P<0.05$, control vs. post TACE.
app BV/TV, apparent trabecular bone volume fraction; app Tb.N, apparent trabecular number; app Tb.S, apparent trabecular separation; SMI, structure model index.

Table 4. Multivariate regression analysis examining the effects of patients' characteristics and cumulative radiation dose on osteoporosis in the TACE group.

Variable	*β ± Standard error	P Value	Odds ratio (CI)
Sex	0.38±0.62	0.001	1.25 (1.65, 7.43)
Age	0.88±0.02	<0.001	1.11 (1.06, 1.17)
CTDIv (CT)	0.85±0.00	<0.001	1.03 (1.00, 1.01)

*β, Standardized partial regression coefficient.

muscle cells [35]. Other investigators have reported a reduction in the number of osteoblast cells following irradiation, which was associated with decreased collagen production and alkaline phosphatase activity [13]. Since both collagen and alkaline phosphatase play a role in mineralization, it has been proposed that this is a pathway to osteopenia [14].

A radiation dose-effect relationship was also demonstrated by several animal experiments. Bone atrophy was detected after irradiation of the femur of rats with doses of 20–25 Gy, and there was also a significant reduction in the relative amounts of calcium and phosphorus in bone, suggesting that atrophy was associated with bone mineral loss [36]. Although the results from animal studies cannot be applied to patients in clinical settings, they could partly explain the relationship between the cumulative radiation dose and tBMD in this study.

On the basis of the multivariate regression analysis, the greatest contributor to the prevalence of osteoporosis among the indices for radiation exposure was the CTDIv (CT) from routine CT examinations to assess or screen for hepatocellular carcinoma. The cumulative radiation dose from angiographic procedures (e.g., the CTDIv (TACE)) did not significantly contribute to the prevalence of osteoporosis. The cumulative radiation dose from routine CT examinations can be up to four times higher than that of angiographic procedures, as shown in Table 1. Thus, a

reduction in radiation dose for patients who have to undergo repeat TACE treatments will be best achieved by minimizing the dose from routine CT examinations. The most practical methods to achieve this will be to avoid unnecessary CT scans, to use a lower tube current (mA) or peak beam energy (peak kV), and increase the noise settings for tube current modulation [37,38].

Among the microstructural indices in this study, app Tb.N and app BV/TV were significantly lower and app Tb.S and SMI were significantly higher in the TACE group compared to the control group.

There have been several reports of results regarding radiation effects on trabecular morphology that are consistent with those of our study. In 2009, Willey et al. [39] investigated the effect on mice of whole-body irradiation of 2 Gy X-rays. They demonstrated that the trabecular microarchitectural properties of L5 included decreased volumetric BMD, BV/TV, and Tb.N and elevated SMI and Tb.S. In 2014, Xu. et al. [40] reported similar results with X-ray radiation of Wistar rats, which had significantly reduced BMD, BV/TV, and Tb.N, but increased SMI.

We did not include trabecular thickness for microstructural analysis in this study. In 2007, correlation analysis of morphological parameters findings of high-resolution peripheral quantitative CT vs. micro-CT was performed by MacNeil et al. [41]. They showed that, among trabecular parameters, trabecular thickness had the lowest correlation coefficient ($r^2 = 0.59$), whereas other high-resolution peripheral quantitative CT-indices, such as trabecular bone volume fraction, trabecular number and trabecular separation, correlated well with the gold-standards methods results ($r^2 > 0.83$). In addition, regarding changes in trabecular thickness after radiation exposure, several previous studies have had contradictory findings even using micro-CT. For example, Hamilton et al. [42] reported an insignificant increase in trabecular thickness after radiation exposure of 2-Gy to tibiae and femurs of mice. More recently, Chandra et al. [43] demonstrated a slight but significant increase in trabecular thickness after irradiation with a clinically relevant dose of the proximal tibiae of rats. We used clinical MDCT with spatial resolution of 200 μm×200 μm×160 μm to investigate trabecular bones that are known to have about the same size as the imaging spatial resolution. In the previous study [20] performed by using the same CT scanner and 3D image analysis system, the apparent trabecular thickness was around 700 μm, when many studies using micro-CT report an average Tb.Th of 150–200 μm. We speculate that the actual Tb.Th is overestimated by clinical MDCT due to the combined effects of limited spatial resolution and missing thin trabeculae during the thresholding step. Thus, we think that an evaluation of Tb.Th using clinical CT is inappropriate.

There were several limitations to this study. First, there are several other factors that could cause osteoporosis in the CH- and TACE groups. Risk factors for osteoporosis include advanced age, low body mass index, underlying disease (rheumatoid arthritis,

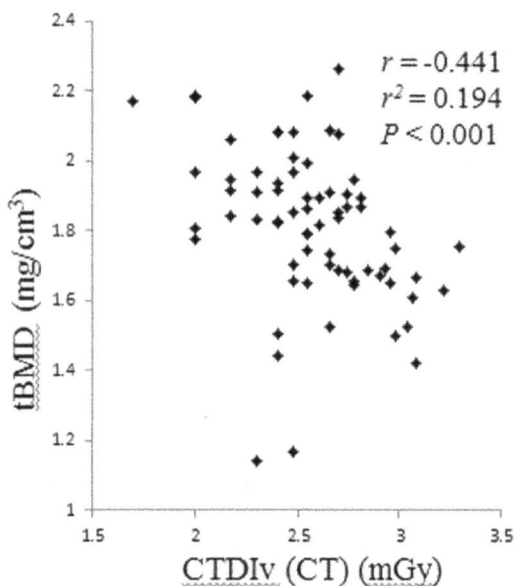

Figure 2. Correlation analysis of tBMD with cumulative radiation dose shows a significant correlation between tBMD and CTDIv (CT).

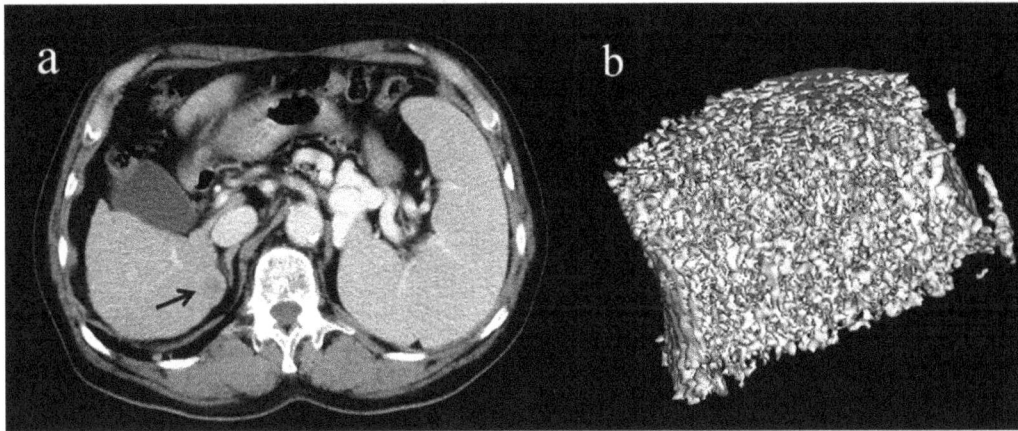

Figure 3. Representative 3D MDCT images of the L3 vertebra obtained from a 71-year-old man after five dynamic CT scans and two transarterial chemoembolization procedures for hepatocellular carcinomas. An axial CT image of the liver shows a recurrence of hepatocellular carcinoma in S7 as a low density area compared to adjacent liver parenchyma(a), (black arrow). The 3D image of the L3 vertebra is shown (b). Tissue bone mineral density (76.8 mg/cm^3) is normal for age. The image is cut in half along the longitudinal midline.

inflammatory bowel disease, chronic obstructive pulmonary disease, history of organ transplantation), smoking, excessive alcohol consumption, and high glucocorticoid dose [44]. Glucocorticoid-induced osteoporosis is the most common and severe form of iatrogenic osteoporosis [44–47]. In patients with glucocorticoid-induced osteoporosis, the loss of bone mineral density occurs at the rate of approximately 3% yearly after the first year [44]. In an animal study [48], peripheral quantitative CT analysis revealed glucocorticoid-induced BMD loss of approximately 7% in wild-type mice. On the other hand, in a rat study [43], radiation from micro-CT scans following the irradiation generated in a clinically relevant range led to more reductions in BMD (26% in BMD and 37% in BV/TV). In fact, we excluded patients with a history of chronic steroid use; in addition, patients' characteristics including age and BMI were similar among the three groups in this study. Thus, we attribute the reduced tBMD in the present study mainly to radiation exposure. Second, there might be some error in the results of this study due to the low

spatial resolution of clinical MDCT, although the results of several previous reports regarding radiation effects on trabecular morphology are consistent with those of our study. Validation of microstructural parameters obtained using clinical MDCT by comparing with results using the gold-standard method, micro-CT, is needed during future studies. Third, the radiation dose per each single CT scan or TACE was not identical, and the intervals between these procedures varied across individuals in this study. One clinical study showed the effects of changes in the dose per fraction on the radiation response of mature bone of post mastectomy patients [49]. Spontaneous rib fracture was significantly higher in the group treated with a larger dose/fraction than in the more standard lower dose/fraction group. The patients who underwent repeat TACE in this study tended to have shorter between-scan intervals than control subjects. Such interindividual variability could have affected our results.

In conclusion, the prevalence of osteoporosis detected with MDCT was significantly higher in post TACE patients than in

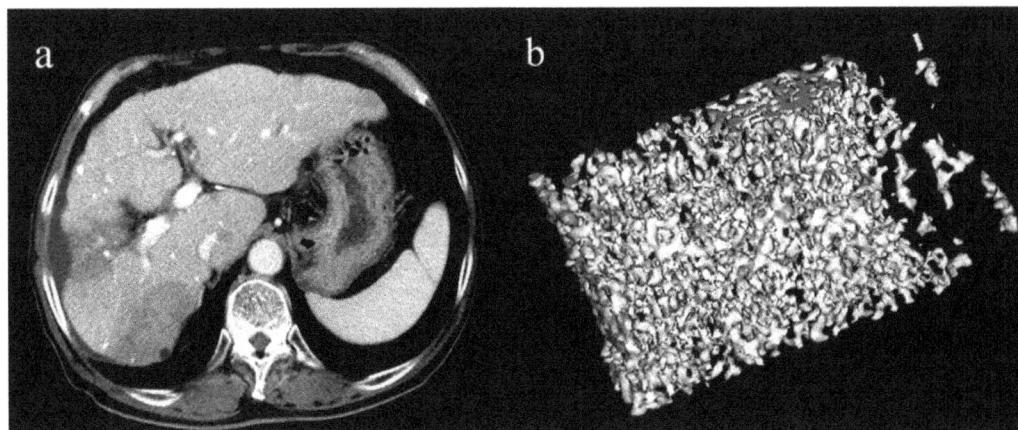

Figure 4. Representative 3D MDCT images of the L3 vertebra obtained from a 71-year-old man after 24 dynamic CT scans and seven transarterial chemoembolization (TACE) procedures for hepatocellular carcinomas. An axial CT image of the liver shows segmental low density areas in the S5 and S7 areas due to previous TACE procedures(a). The 3D image shows sparse trabecular bones (b) compared to those of the patient in Figure 3. Tissue bone mineral density (36.2 mg/cm^3) is lower than the mean value of control subjects. The image is cut in half along the longitudinal midline.

control subjects. The cumulative radiation dose related to routine dynamic CT studies was a significant contributor to the prevalence of osteoporosis. There is a weak relationship between local irradiation to bone and reduced bone density. Based on our study, reduction of the radiation dose for HCC patients might be achieved by minimizing the dose from routine CT examinations; unnecessary CT scans should be avoided.

Author Contributions

Conceived and designed the experiments: MT TY. Performed the experiments: MT YN DK YK CT SD MK. Analyzed the data: MT TY KA. Contributed reagents/materials/analysis tools: MT MK. Wrote the paper: MT.

References

1. Carlson SK, Bender CE, Classic KL, Zink FE, Quam JP, et al. (2001) Benefits and safety of CT fluoroscopy in interventional radiologic procedures. Radiology 219: 515–520.
2. Silverman SG, Deuson TE, Kane N, Adams DF, Seltzer SE, et al. (1998) Percutaneous abdominal biopsy: cost-identification analysis. Radiology 206: 429–435.
3. Fraser-Hill MA, Renfrew DL, Hilsenrath PE (1992) Percutaneous needle biopsy of musculoskeletal lesions. Part 2. Cost-effectiveness. AJR 158: 813–818.
4. Lo CM, Ngan H, Tso WK, Liu CL, Lam CM, et al. (2002) Randomized controlled trial of transarterial lipiodol chemoembolization for unresectable hepatocellular carcinoma. Hepatology 35: 1164–1171.
5. Llovet JM, Real MI, Montaña X, Planas R, Coll S, et al. (2002) Arterial embolisation or chemoembolisation versus symptomatic treatment in patients with unresectable hepatocellular carcinoma: a randomized controlled trial. Lancet 359: 1734–1739.
6. Ishikawa M, Yamagami T, Kakizawa H, Hieda M, Toyota N, et al. (2014) Transarterial therapy of hepatocellular carcinoma fed by the right renal capsular artery. J Vasc Interv Radiol. 25: 389–395.7. Stockholm Colorectal Cancer Study Group. (1995) The Stockholm I trial of preoperative short term radiotherapy in operable rectal carcinoma: a prospective randomized trial. Cancer 75: 2269–2275.
7. Stockholm Colorectal Cancer Study Group (1996) Randomized study on preoperative radiotherapy in rectal carcinoma. Ann Surg Oncol 3: 423–430.
8. Holm T, Singnomklao T, Rutqvist LE, Cedermark B (1996) Adjuvant preoperative radiotherapy in patients with rectal carcinoma: adverse effects during long term follow- up of two randomized trials. Cancer 78: 968–976.
9. Ewing J (1926) Radiation osteitis. Acta Radiol 6: 399–412.
10. Warren S (1994) Histopathology of radiation lesions. Physiol Rev 24: 225–245.
11. Gyorkey Z, Pollock FJ (1940) Radiation necrosis of the ossicles. Arch Otolaryngol 71: 793–799.
12. Sams A (1966) The effects of 2000r of X-rays on the acid and alkaline phosphatase of mouse tibiae. Int J Radiat Biol 10: 123–140.
13. Ergun H, Howland WJ (1980) Post-irradiation atrophy of mature bone. CRC Crit Rev Diagn Imag 12: 225–243.
14. Laib A, Hauselmann HJ, Ruegsegger P (1998) In vivo high resolution 3D-QCT of the human forearm. Technol Health Care 6: 329–337.
15. Laib A, Ruegsegger P (1999) Comparison of structure extraction methods for in vivo trabecular bone measurements. Comput Med Imaging Graph 23: 69–74.
16. Cheung AM, Detsky AS (2008) Osteoporosis and fractures: missing the bridge? JAMA 299: 1468–1470.
17. Stein EM, Liu XS, Nickolas TL, Cohen A, McMahon DJ, et al. (2012) Microarchitectural abnormalities are more severe in postmenopausal women with vertebral compared to nonvertebral fractures. J Clin Endocrinol Metab 97: E1918–E1926.
18. Boutroy S, Bouxsein ML, Munoz F, Delmas PD (2005) In vivo assessment of trabecular bone microarchitecture by high-resolution peripheral quantitative computed tomography. J Clin Endocrinol Metab 90: 6508–6515.
19. Takasu M, Tani C, Ishikawa M, Date S, Horiguchi J, et al. (2011) Multiple myeloma: microstructural analysis of lumbar trabecular bones in patients without visible bone lesions-preliminary results. Radiology 260: 472–479.
20. Ito M, Ikeda K, Nishiguchi M, Shindo H, Uetani M, et al. (2005) Multi-Detector Row CT Imaging of Vertebral Microstructure for Evaluation of Fracture Risk. J Bone Miner Res 20: 1828–1836.
21. Miller DL, Balter S, Cole PE, Lu HT, Schueler BA, et al. (2003) Radiation doses in interventional radiology procedures: the RAD-IR study. I. Overall measures of dose. J Vasc Interv Radiol 14: 711–727.
22. The Joint Commission (2006) Radiation Overdose as a Reviewable Sentinel Event, Update March 7, 2006. Available: http://www.jointcommission.org/assets/1/18/Radiation_Overdose.pdf. Accessed 2014 July 18.
23. Shope TB, Gagne RM, Johnson GC (1981) A method for describing the doses delivered by transmission X-ray computed tomography. Med. Phys 8: 488–495.
24. European commission (1999) European Guidelines on Quality Criteria for Computed Tomography. Report EUR 16262 EN. Luxembourg: Office for Official Publications of the European Communities.
25. Carberry GA, Pooler BD, Binkley N, Lauder TB, Bruce RJ, et al. (2013).
26. Unreported vertebral body compression fractures at abdominal multidetector CT. Radiology 268: 120–126.
27. Cooper C, Atkinson EJ, O'Fallon WM, Melton LJ 3rd (1992) Incidence of clinically diagnosed vertebral fractures: a population-based study in Rochester, Minnesota, 1985–1989. J Bone Miner Res 7: 221–227.
28. Hildebrand T, Ruegsegger P (1997) A new method for the model-independent assessment of thickness in threedimensional images. J Microsc 185: 67–75.
29. Parfitt AM, Drezner MK, Glorieux FH, Kanis JA, Malluche H, et al. (1987) Bone histomorphometry: Standardization of nomenclature, symbols, and units. Report of the ASBMR Histomorphometry Nomenclature Committee. J Bone Miner Res 2: 595–610.
30. Odgaard A, Gundersen HJ (1993) Quantification of connectivity in cancellous bone, with special emphasis on 3-D reconstructions. Bone 14: 173–182.
31. Harrigan TP, Mann RW (1984) Characterization of microstructural anisotropy in orthotropic materials using a second rank tensor. J Mater Sci 19: 761–767.
32. Matsuzaki K, Ito M, Kaneko H, Kato M, Hikata T, et al (2013) Efficacy of osteoporotic agents in trabecular microstructure. Osteoporosis Japan 21: 102–105.
33. U.S. Food and Drug Administration Website, Center for Devices and Radiological Health (2010) Initiative to reduce unnecessary radiation exposure from medical imaging. Available: http://www.fda.gov/Radiation-emittingProducts/RadiationSafety/RadiationDoseReduction/default.htm. Accessed 2014 September 29.
34. Howland WJ, Loeffler RK, Starchman DE, Johnson RG (1975) Postirradiation atrophic changes of bone and related complications. Radiology 117: 677–685.
35. Hopewell JW, Calvo W, Reinhold HS (1989) Radiation effects on blood vessels: Role in normal tissue damage. In: Steel GG, Adams G, Horwich A, editors. Biological basis of radiotherapy. 2nd edition. Amsterdam: Elsevier Scientific; 1989. 101–113.
36. Pitkanen MA, Hopewell JW (1983) Functional changes in the vascularity of the irradiated rat femur: Implications for late effects. Acta Radiol Oncol 22: 253–256.
37. McCollough CH (2008) CT dose: how to measure, how to reduce. Health Phys 95: 508–517.
38. Bankier AA, Tack D (2010) Dose reduction strategies for thoracic multidetector computed tomography: background, current issues, and recommendations. J Thorac Imaging 25: 278–288.
39. Willey JS, Livingston EW, Robbins ME, Bourland JD, Tirado-Lee L, et al. (2010) Risedronate prevents early radiation-induced osteoporosis in mice at multiple skeletal locations. Bone 46: 101–111.
40. Xu D, Zhao X, Li Y, Ji Y, Zhang J, et al. (2014) The combined effects of X-ray radiation and hindlimb suspension on bone loss. J Radiat Res Apr 3. [Epub ahead of print].
41. MacNeil JA, Boyd SK (2007) Accuracy of high-resolution peripheral quantitative computed tomography for measurement of bone quality. Med Eng Phys 29: 1096–1105.
42. Hamilton SA, Pecaut MJ, Gridley DS, Travis ND, Bandstra ER, et al. (2006) A murine model for bone loss from therapeutic and space-relevant sources of radiation. J Appl Physiol (1985) 101: 789–793.
43. Chandra A, Lan S, Zhu J, Lin T, Zhang X, et al. (2013) PTH prevents the adverse effects of focal radiation on bone architecture in young rats. Bone 55: 449–457.
44. Weinstein RS (2011) Clinical practice. Glucocorticoid-induced bone disease. N Engl J Med 365: 62–70.
45. Compston J (2010) Management of glucocorticoid-induced osteoporosis. Nat Rev Rheumatol 6: 82–8.
46. Hofbauer LC, Hamann C, Ebeling PR (2010) Approach to the patient with secondary osteoporosis. Eur J Endocrinol 162: 1009–1020.
47. Maricic M (2011) Update on glucocorticoid-induced osteoporosis. Rheum Dis Clin North Am 37: 415–431.
48. Hofbauer LC, Zeitz U, Schoppet M, Skalicky M, Schüler C, et al. (2009) Prevention of glucocorticoid-induced bone loss in mice by inhibition of RANKL. Arthritis Rheum. 60: 1427–1437.
49. Overgaard M (1998) Spontaneous radiation-induced rib fractures in breast cancer patients treated with post-mastectomy irradiation. Acta Oncol 27: 117–122.

21

Cytoplasmic and/or Nuclear Expression of β-Catenin Correlate with Poor Prognosis and Unfavorable Clinicopathological Factors in Hepatocellular Carcinoma

Jiang Chen[1], Jinghua Liu[1], Renan Jin[1], Jiliang Shen[1], Yuelong Liang[1], Rui Ma[2], Hui Lin[1], Xiao Liang[1], Hong Yu[1], Xiujun Cai[1]*

1 Department of General Surgery, Sir Run Run Shaw Hospital of Zhejiang University, Hangzhou, Zhejiang, China, **2** Department of Surgery, Zhejiang University Hospital, Hangzhou, Zhejiang, China

Abstract

Background: The β-catenin is an important effector in WNT/β-catenin signaling pathway, which exerts a crucial role in the development and progression of hepatocellular carcinoma (HCC). Some researchers have suggested that the overexpression of β-catenin in cytoplasm and/or nucleus was closely correlated to metastasis, poor differentiation and malignant phenotype of HCC while some other researchers hold opposite point. So far, no consensus was obtained on the prognostic and clinicopathological significance of cytoplasmic/nuclear β-catenin overexpression for HCCs.

Methods: Systematic strategies were applied to search eligible studies in all available databases. Subgroup analyses, sensitivity analyses and multivariate analysis were performed. In this meta-analysis, we utilized either fixed- or random-effects model to calculate the pooled odds ratios (OR) and its 95% confidence intervals (CI).

Results: A total of 22 studies containing 2334 cases were enrolled in this meta-analysis. Pooled data suggested that accumulation of β-catenin in cytoplasm and/or nucleus significantly correlated with poor 1-, 3- and 5-year OS and RFS. Moreover, nuclear accumulation combined with cytoplasmic accumulation of β-catenin tended to be associated with dismal metastasis and vascular invasion while cytoplasmic or nuclear expression alone showed no significant effect. Besides, no significant association was observed between cytoplasmic and/or nuclear β-catenin expression and poor differentiation grade, advanced TNM stage, liver cirrhosis, tumor size, tumor encapsulation, AFP and etiologies. Additional subgroup analysis by origin suggested that the prognostic value and clinicopathological significance of cytoplasmic and/or nuclear β-catenin expression was more validated in Asian population. Multivariate analyses of factors showed that cytoplasmic and/or nuclear β-catenin expression, as well as TNM stage, metastasis and tumor size, was an independent risk factors for OS and RFS.

Conclusions: Cytoplasmic and/or nuclear accumulation of β-catenin, as an independent prognostic factor, significantly associated with poor prognosis and deeper invasion of HCC, and could serve as a valuable prognostic predictor for HCC.

Editor: Andreas Krieg, Heinrich-Heine-University and University Hospital Duesseldorf, Germany

Funding: This work was supported by National Natural Science Foundation of China (81201942) and Zhejiang Provincial Natural Science Foundation of China (LZ14H160002). The funders had no role in study design, data collection and analysis, decision to publish, or preparation of the manuscript.

Competing Interests: The authors have declared that no competing interests exist.

* Email: cxjzu@hotmail.com

Introduction

Hepatocellular cancer (HCC) is a global health problem and its incidence has been increasing dramatically since 20 years especially in developed countries [1]. In 2012, it was reported that its annual incidence reached more than half a million worldwide [2]. It ranks No. three on the most frequent cause of cancer-related death list among the global population [3]. Surgery is the main curative treatment, but less than 50% patients survive more than a year following treatment for the poor prognosis of HCC [4]. Until now, few systemic therapies demonstrated a fully positive impact on the prognosis for patients with HCC. Additionally, sorafenib, a multikinase inhibitor, currently used as the targeted anticancer agent, only exhibited comparative efficacy and safety in advanced HCC considering its complicated histologic response and various differentiation of cases [5,6]. Therefore, it is mandatory to have an elemental understanding of the genes and signaling pathways involved in the initiation and progression of

Table 1. Characteristics of studies included in the meta-analysis.

First author & year	Country or region	No. of patients	Mean age	Gender (M/F)	(C+N)/T	Level of evidence	Stage	Clinicopathological features	Method	antibody source	Dilution	Blind evaluation	Definition standard*	Provided-OS data
Jin 2014	Korea	302	54.88(25–77)	254/48	(233+10)/243	5	I–IV	D, T	IHC	NR	NR	Yes	CS	Yes
Lee 2014	USA	89	51 (20–75)	78/11	(21+8)/29	4	I–IV	D	IHC	(BD Biosciences, San Diego, CA)	1:50	Yes	CS	NR
Witjes 2013	Netherlands	47	65 (21–82)	23/24	(0+16)/16	4	NR	D,T	IHC	(DAKO, Japan)	NR	Yes	≥Focal/diffuse	NR
Geng 2012	China	85	NR	77/8	(52+6)/58	4	I–IV	D,T	IHC	(BD Biosciences, USA)	1:400	Yes	CS	Yes
Zhao 2012	China	97	52.86	82/15	(?+?)/66	5	I–IV	D,M	IHC	(Santa Cruz Biotech, USA)	1:100	Yes	CS	Yes
Feng 2011	China	63	45.8±10.6 (24–74)	51/12	(35+0)/35	4	NR	D,M	IHC	(BD Biosciences, San Diego, CA)	NR	Yes	>10%cells	NR
Cheng 2011	Hong Kong	25	47.92(14–72)	23/2	(8+0)/8	3	NR	D	IHC	(DAKO, Japan)	1:100	Yes	CS	NR
Liu 2010	China	200	NR	169/31	(?+?)/87	4	I–IIIa	D,T,M	IHC	(BD Biosciences, San Diego, CA)	NR	Yes	Stronger than non-cancerous	Yes
Zulehner 2010	Austria	133	54.7±9	113/20	(0+78)/78	4	NR	D,M, T	IHC	(Transduction Laboratories, Lexington, UK)	1:100	Yes	> low staining	NR
Du 2009	China	43	49(29–72)	36/7	(17+0)/17	3	NR	D,T,M	IHC	(Abgent Biotechnology, CA)	1:50	Yes	> weak	NR
Yu 2009	China	314	NR	266/48	(?+?)/126	5	I–III	D,T,M	IHC	(Transduction Laboratories, Lexington, KY)	1:200	Yes	>10% cells	Yes
Yang 2009	Taiwan	123	NR	104/19	(?+?)/53	5	I–IV	D,T,M	IHC	(Abcam plc.)	1:1000	Yes	>10% cells	Yes
Korita 2008	Japan	125	63(16–79)	88/37	(0+16)/16	3	NR	D,T	IHC	(Novocastra Laboratories Ltd, Newcastleupon-Tyne, United Kingdom)	1:200	Yes	CS	NR
Zhai 2008	China	97	54(34–72)	67/30	(36+6)/42	3	I–IV	D,T,M	IHC	(Santa Clauze Corporation, USA)	1:200	Yes	CS	Yes
Park 2005	Korea	92	51.6(26–89)	75/17	(?+?)/30	3	I–IV	D	IHC	(Transduction Laboratories, Lexington, KY)	NR	Yes	CS	NR
Tien 2005	Japan	32	64(36–86)	20/8	(7+8)/15	3	NR	D	IHC	(BD Biosciences, San Jose, CA)	1:200	Yes	Stronger than non-cancerous	NR
Schmitt Graff 2003	Germany	196	65.3 (10.7–86.0)	157/39	(84+73)/157	3	I–IV	NR	IHC	(Transduction Laboratories, Lexington, KY, USA)	1:6000	Yes	≥Focal	Yes

Table 1. Cont.

First author & year	Country or region	No. of patients	Mean age	Gender (M/F)	(C+N)/T	Level of evidence	Stage	Clinicopatho-logical features	Method	antibody source	Dilution	Blind evalua-tion	Definition standard*	Provided-OS data
Inagawa 2002	Japan	51	63.5(45–79)	33/18	(0+18)/18	4	NR	D	IHC	(Transduction Laboratories, Lexington, KY)	1:200	Yes	Stronger than non-cancerous	NR
Suzuki 2002	Japan	50	62.4±9.9	38/12	(42+11)/53	3	NR	D,M,T	IHC	(Transduction Laboratories, Lexington, KY)	1:200	Yes	Stronger than non-cancerous	NR
Endo 2000	Japan	107	60(17–80)	87/20	(?+?)/84	4	NR	D	IHC	(Transduction Laboratories, Lexington, KY)	1:100	Yes	CS	Yes
Huang 1999	Japan/Switzerland	22	62.7±6.3 (49–75)	17/5	(0+11)/11	3	NR	D	IHC	(Transduction Laboratories, Lexington, KY)	1:1000–2000	Yes	≥ Focal	NR
Ihara 1996	Japan	41	60.1(42–77)	38/3	(?+?)/58	3	NR	D	IHC	(Transduction Laboratories, Lexington, KY)	10 mg/ml	Yes	CS	NR

CS: complex score combining intensity and percentage; IHC: immunohistochemistry; D: histologic differentiation degree; T: depth of tumor invasion; M: metastasis; OS: overall survival; NR: not reported; *: The definition standard of β-catenin overexpression in cytoplasm or nucleus; (C+N)/T: the number of tissue samples with β-catenin overexpression in cytoplasm(C) (+) nucleus (N); C: cytoplasm; N: nucleus; T: total, T=C+N; ?: no information was provided.

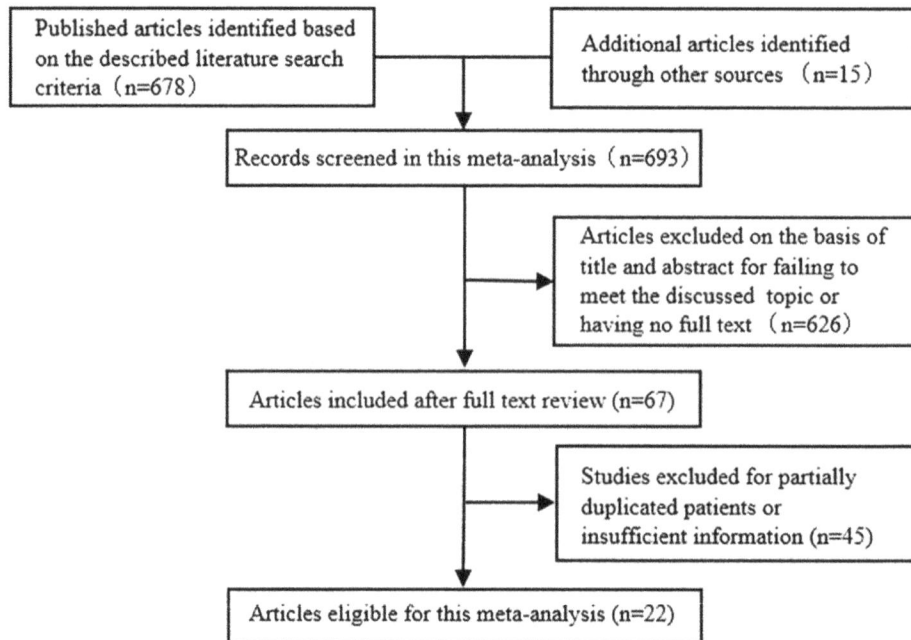

Figure 1. Flow chart of literature search strategies.

this neoplasm and develop more effective therapies to intervene in this process.

Several molecular pathways are implicated in the hepatic oncogenesis such as β-catenin, p53, EGF, HGF, TGF β and others [7]. The WNT/β-catenin mediated signaling pathway has been well studied and exerted an indispensible role in HCC pathogenesis [8]. The aberrantly activated WNT signaling is usually caused by somatic mutations, which contains several hot-spot mutations present in the *CSF1R, CTNNB1, KRAS, BRAF, NRAS, ERBB2, MET, PIK3CA, JAK1,* and *SMO* genes [9]. Among these hot-spot genes, the mutations of *CTNNB1* gene account for the majority of somatic mutations and appear to be the most common cause for activation of WNT signaling pathway. *CTNNB1* is the coding gene for β-catenin, a multifunctional protein that integrates the intercellular E-cadherin–catenin adhesion system with intracellular WNT signaling pathway.

In normal hepatocytes, the great majority of β-catenin is located in cytomembrane where it directly connects the E-catherin to a-catenin, which is in turn bound to the actin-based cytoskeleton, forming an adhesion complex [10,11]. And the unbound cytoplasmic β-catenin is kept at a low level by forming a destruction complex with GSK3β, Axin1, Casein Kinase Iα (CKIα) and APC (Adenomatous Polyposis Coli protein) [12]. The cadherin–catenin adhesion complex can regulate cell-cell adhesion and recognition and hence establish and maintain tissue architecture and function. And the destruction complex can be degraded by undergoing phosphorylation and ubiquitination and hence the unbound β-catenin is removed from cytosol, thereby preventing its translocation to the nucleus [12,13]. When *CTNNB1* mutations occurred, the functional residues of β-catenin may be affected so that the targets usually become invalid of priming phosphorylation by GSK-3β and subsequent catalyzation by proteasome system [14]. Therefore, the unbound β-catenin cannot be removed from the cytosol and accumulates in cytoplasm. The accumulated β-catenin in the cytoplasm could translocate to the nucleus where it serves as a co-factor for the T cell factor (TCF) family of

transcription factors to activate the downstream target genes relevant to cell proliferation, migration, invasion, cell cycle progression and metastasis, including *c-myc, cyclin-D1,* and *survivin* [15]. Finally, the WNT signaling pathway is activated in the context of *CTNNB1* mutations, though the aberrant activation may also occurred in the absence of *CTNNB1* mutations.

The normal hepatocytes are transformed to the malignant ones when the WNT pathway is initiated. Aberrant activation of WNT/β-catenin signaling prevents the formation of the β-catenin destruction complex and further leads to the accumulation of β-catenin in the cytoplasm and/or nucleus [16]. Thus, the cytoplasmic and/or nuclear expression of β-catenin exhibits close relationship with the activated WNT signaling pathway and thereby the hepatic oncogenesis.

Abnormal cytoplasmic and/or nuclear accumulation of β-catenin has been demonstrated in 17–40% of HCCs [17], indicating that β-catenin may be a potential molecular marker for disease development and progression for patients with HCC. In this regard, vast work has been done to investigate the association of cytoplasmic and/or nuclear β-catenin expression with clinicopathological features, etiologies and prognosis for patients with HCC. However, results about their correlation reported by researchers from different institutions or organizations are highly variable and contradictory. Additionally, the number of cases enrolled in each study was not large enough. Therefore, it is necessary to conduct a systematic and comprehensive analysis to achieve a reasonable consensus about the prognostic and clinicopathological significance of β-catenin expression in cytoplasm and/or nucleus.

In this paper, a meta-analysis was performed based on retrospective studies to evaluate the prognostic value and clinicopathological significance of cytoplasmic and/or nuclear β-catenin expression in patients with HCC. In addition, the association between cytoplasmic and/or nuclear β-catenin expression and etiology (HBV and HCV) was also analyzed.

Table 2. Subgroup analysis for prognostic and clinicopathological significance of cytoplasmic and/or nuclear β-catenin expression by its rate (≥50% vs <50%).

Factors	Positive expression rate	Number of studies	OR	95%CI	Z	P	I²
1-year OS	≥50%	5	0.62	0.38–1.00	1.95	0.05	4
	<50%	4	0.58	0.31–1.08	1.72	0.09	6
3-year OS	≥50%	5	0.43	0.21–0.91	2.22	0.03	64
	<50%	4	0.75	0.30–1.84	0.63	0.53	79
5-year OS	≥50%	5	0.36	0.19–0.69	3.11	0.002	54
	<50%	4	0.80	0.22–2.94	0.34	0.73	88
1-year RFS	≥50%	1	0.38	0.14–1.01	1.93	0.05	-
	<50%	3	0.58	0.25–1.35	1.26	0.21	62
3-year RFS	≥50%	1	0.41	0.18–0.93	2.14	0.03	-
	<50%	3	0.35	0.24–0.49	5.86	<0.00001	0
5-year RFS	≥50%	1	0.37	0.16–0.83	2.42	0.02	-
	<50%	3	0.34	0.24–0.49	5.83	<0.00001	-
Metastasis	≥50%	2	0.62	0.30–1.28	1.29	0.2	0
	<50%	6	0.64	0.42–0.97	2.09	0.04	0
Vascular invasion	≥50%	2	0.30	0.14–0.62	3.26	0.001	0
	<50%	5	0.50	0.33–0.78	3.08	0.002	0

Table 3. Subgroup analysis for prognostic and clinicopathological significance of cytoplasmic and/or nuclear β-catenin expression by origin (Asia vs others) and level of evidence (≥4 vs <4).

Factors	subgroup		Number of studies	OR	95%CI	Z	P	I²
1-year OS	Origin							
		Asia	8	0.49	0.30–0.77	3.05	0.002	0
		others	1	1.01	0.50–2.06	0.04	0.97	-
	Level of evidence							
		≥4	7	0.49	0.30–0.77	3.05	0.002	0
		<4	2	1.01	0.50–2.06	0.04	0.97	-
3-year OS	Origin							
		Asia	8	0.5	0.28–0.89	2.35	0.02	70
		others	1	1.24	0.52–2.92	0.49	0.63	-
	Level of evidence							
		≥4	7	0.43	0.32–0.57	5.58	<0.00001	45
		<4	2	1.75	0.92–3.30	1.72	0.09	25
5-year OS	Origin							
		Asia	8	0.41	0.21–0.81	2.57	0.01	77
		others	1	0.99	0.40–2.48	0.02	0.99	-
	Level of evidence							
		≥4	7	0.33	0.19–0.56	4.07	<0.0001	65
		<4	2	6.22	0.07–534.37	0.8	0.42	89
1-year RFS	Origin							
		Asia	4	0.47	0.32–0.70	3.68	0.0002	44
		others	0	-	-	-	-	-
	Level of evidence							
		≥4	4	0.47	0.32–0.70	3.68	0.0002	44
		<4	0	-	-	-	-	-
3-year RFS	Origin							
		Asia	4	0.36	0.26–0.49	6.23	<0.00001	0
		others	0	-	-	-	-	-
	Level of evidence							
		≥4	4	0.36	0.26–0.49	6.23	<0.00001	0
		<4	0	-	-	-	-	-
5-year RFS	Origin							
		Asia	4	0.35	0.25–0.48	6.31	<0.00001	0
		others	0	-	-	-	-	-
	Level of evidence							

Table 3. Cont.

Factors	subgroup		Number of studies	OR	95%CI	Z	P	I²
metastasis		≥4	4	0.35	0.25-0.48	6.31	<0.00001	0
		<4	0	-	-	-	-	-
	Origin	Asia	7	0.65	0.45-0.96	2.19	0.03	0
		others	1	0.44	0.11-1.72	1.18	0.24	-
	Level of evidence	≥4	6	0.58	0.39-0.87	2.63	0.009	0
		<4	2	0.92	0.40-2.12	0.2	0.84	0
Vascular invasion	Origin	Asia	5	0.46	0.30-0.72	3.38	0.0007	4
		others	2	0.38	0.19-0.75	2.8	0.005	0
	Level of evidence	≥4	5	0.35	0.23-0.54	4.68	<0.00001	0
		<4	2	0.86	0.41-1.82	0.39	0.7	0

Methods

Study Selection

The Pubmed, Elsevier, Embase, Cochrane Library and Web of Science databases were searched systematically for identified articles published until June 7th, 2014. The terms used in search was as follows:"β-catenin, Beta-catenin, or CTNNB1", "WNT/β-catenin signal pathway", "prognostic, prognosis, or survival", "HCC", "hepatocellular carcinoma", "hepatic tumor", "hepatic cancer", "liver cancer", "liver tumor" and "liver neoplasms" with all possible combinations. The searched articles were filtered out and the reference lists of eligible ones were taken under scrutiny for additional available studies. The systematic literature search was carried out independently by two reviewers (JC and JL).

Criteria for Inclusion and Exclusion

To make this meta-analysis meet the high standards, studies had to fulfill the following criteria: (1) patients with distinctive hepatocellular carcinoma diagnosis by pathology but without restriction on age or ethnicity; (2) β-catenin expression was measured by immunohistological chemistry (IHC) or other methods in primary HCC tissue; (3) clinical trials or reports were published in English; (4) sufficient information or valid data about β-catenin expression and OS or RFS and the other clinicopathological features were provided directly or could be calculated indirectly; (5) the study with the highest quality assessment was enrolled when several studies reported by one individual author were conducted on the same patients population; (6) the patients were followed-up for at least 3 years.

Abstracts, editorials, letters and expert opinions, conference records, reviews without original data, case reports and studies lack of control groups were excluded. Studies and data were also excluded if: (1) articles about animals or cell lines; (2) the outcomes or parameters of patients were not clearly reported; (3) no related data required for necessary analysis; (4) overlapping articles.

In this process, the title and abstract of studies were first screened to see whether they met the including criteria. Second, the full text was subjected to further examination following the initial screening. Finally, the eligibility of studies was verified by 2 reviewers (JC and JL) after resolving the disagreements by the third reviewer (RJ).

Data Extraction and Literature Quality Assessment

Independently, valid data were retrieved from the set of eligible studies by two reviewers (JC and JL) and relevant characteristics were listed as follows: (1) first author and publication year; (2) number of cases; (3) characteristics of subject population, such as age, gender, origin and clinicopthological features; (4) disease stage; (5) methods of evaluating ORs and 95%CI between β-catenin levels and OS or RFS or other clinicopathological parameters; (6) accumulated percentage of β-catenin expression; (7) the number of cases with accumulated β-catenin expression in specific location (Table 1). Any divergence was ironed out by discussion with the third reviewer (RJ) for final expectation of consensus.

The quality of each included study was assessed by two reviewers (JC and JL) using Newcastle-Ottawa scale (NOS). NOS evaluated various aspects of methodology, which were grouped into the three dimensions of selection, comparability, and outcome. Final scores ranged from 0 (lowest) to 9 (highest); the higher value, the better eligibility of methodology. The study would not be enrolled in the meta-analysis if its value of quality assessment was too low.

A

Study or Subgroup	C(+)/N(+) Events	Total	C(-)&N(-) Events	Total	Weight	Odds Ratio M-H, Fixed, 95% CI
Endo 2000	65	84	20	23	10.4%	0.51 [0.14, 1.91]
Geng 2012	39	58	24	27	15.7%	0.26 [0.07, 0.96]
Jin 2014	8	10	257	292	5.0%	0.54 [0.11, 2.67]
Liu 2010	83	87	113	113	7.4%	0.08 [0.00, 1.54]
Schmitt Graff 2003	69	157	17	39	22.3%	1.01 [0.50, 2.06]
Yang 2009	52	53	49	50	1.4%	1.06 [0.06, 17.44]
Yu 2009	111	126	171	188	23.9%	0.74 [0.35, 1.53]
Zhai 2008	42	42	55	55		Not estimable
Zhao 2012	49	66	27	31	13.9%	0.43 [0.13, 1.40]
Total (95% CI)		683		818	100.0%	0.60 [0.41, 0.89]
Total events	518		733			

Heterogeneity: Chi² = 6.31, df = 7 (P = 0.50); I² = 0%
Test for overall effect: Z = 2.58 (P = 0.010)

Odds Ratio M-H, Fixed, 95% CI
0.01   0.1   1   10   100
Favours [C(-)&N(-)]   Favours [C(+)/N(+)]

B

Study or Subgroup	C(+)/N(+) Events	Total	C(-)&N(-) Events	Total	Weight	Odds Ratio M-H, Random, 95% CI
Endo 2000	40	84	20	23	8.6%	0.14 [0.04, 0.49]
Geng 2012	23	58	16	27	11.2%	0.45 [0.18, 1.15]
Jin 2014	7	10	210	292	8.1%	0.91 [0.23, 3.61]
Liu 2010	61	87	102	113	12.5%	0.25 [0.12, 0.55]
Schmitt Graff 2003	38	157	8	39	11.8%	1.24 [0.52, 2.92]
Yang 2009	41	53	42	50	10.7%	0.65 [0.24, 1.76]
Yu 2009	76	126	133	188	14.8%	0.63 [0.39, 1.01]
Zhai 2008	34	42	34	55	11.1%	2.63 [1.02, 6.74]
Zhao 2012	26	66	23	31	11.1%	0.23 [0.09, 0.58]
Total (95% CI)		683		818	100.0%	0.56 [0.32, 0.96]
Total events	346		588			

Heterogeneity: Tau² = 0.46; Chi² = 26.81, df = 8 (P = 0.0008); I² = 70%
Test for overall effect: Z = 2.12 (P = 0.03)

Odds Ratio M-H, Random, 95% CI
0.01   0.1   1   10   100
Favours [C(-)&N(-)]   Favours [C(+)/N(+)]

C

Study or Subgroup	C(+)/N(+) Events	Total	C(-)&N(-) Events	Total	Weight	Odds Ratio M-H, Random, 95% CI
Endo 2000	33	84	18	23	10.9%	0.18 [0.06, 0.53]
Geng 2012	16	58	16	27	11.7%	0.26 [0.10, 0.68]
Jin 2014	6	10	186	292	9.6%	0.85 [0.24, 3.10]
Liu 2010	34	87	90	113	13.8%	0.16 [0.09, 0.31]
Schmitt Graff 2003	28	157	7	39	12.0%	0.99 [0.40, 2.48]
Yang 2009	28	53	42	50	11.9%	0.21 [0.08, 0.54]
Yu 2009	60	126	112	188	14.8%	0.62 [0.39, 0.97]
Zhai 2008	14	42	0	55	3.7%	56.47 [3.25, 981.34]
Zhao 2012	14	66	10	31	11.7%	0.57 [0.22, 1.47]
Total (95% CI)		683		818	100.0%	0.46 [0.24, 0.85]
Total events	233		481			

Heterogeneity: Tau² = 0.63; Chi² = 34.20, df = 8 (P < 0.0001); I² = 77%
Test for overall effect: Z = 2.45 (P = 0.01)

Odds Ratio M-H, Random, 95% CI
0.01   0.1   1   10   100
Favours [C(-)&N(-)]   Favours [C(+)/N(+)]

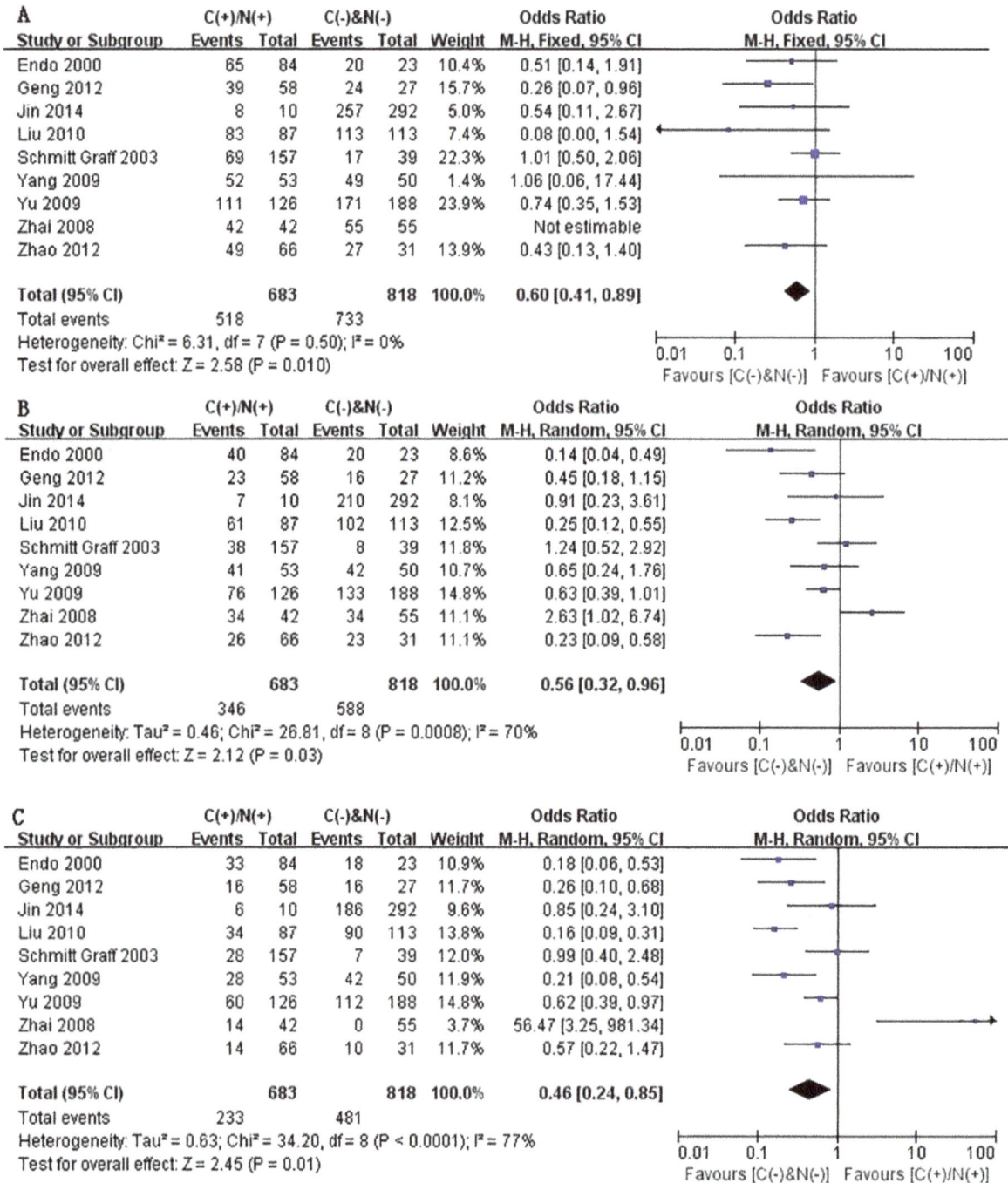

Figure 2. Forest plot of odds ratio for the association of β-catenin expression in cytoplasm and/or nucleus with 1-year (A), 3-year (B) and 5-year (C) overall survival.

Statistical Analysis

This meta-analysis was performed using the Review Manager (RevMan) software (version 5.2; Cochrane collaboration) and STATA (version 12.0, Stata Corp. College Station, Texas) [18]. Odds ratios (OR) combined with 95% confidence intervals (CI) was analyzed to evaluate the association of cytoplasmic and/or nuclear β-catenin accumulation with the prognosis and clinicopathological factors of HCCs. Pooled values of ORs and 95%CIs serve as the recommended summary statistics for meta-analysis of β-catenin expression on prognostic value and clinicopathological features,

such as OS, RFS, differentiation grade, TNM stages, metastasis, vascular invasion and liver cirrhosis. In some studies, these statistical variables were depicted in original studies, and we pooled them directly; otherwise, indirectly, we obtained these variables from the available data or by reading Kaplan-Meier survival curve according to the method described by Parmar MK, which has been widely applied in meta-analysis about prognosis [19]. Heterogeneity among the outcomes of enrolled studies in this meta-analysis was evaluated by using Chi-square based Q statistical test [20]. And I^2 statistic, ranging from 0% to 100%,

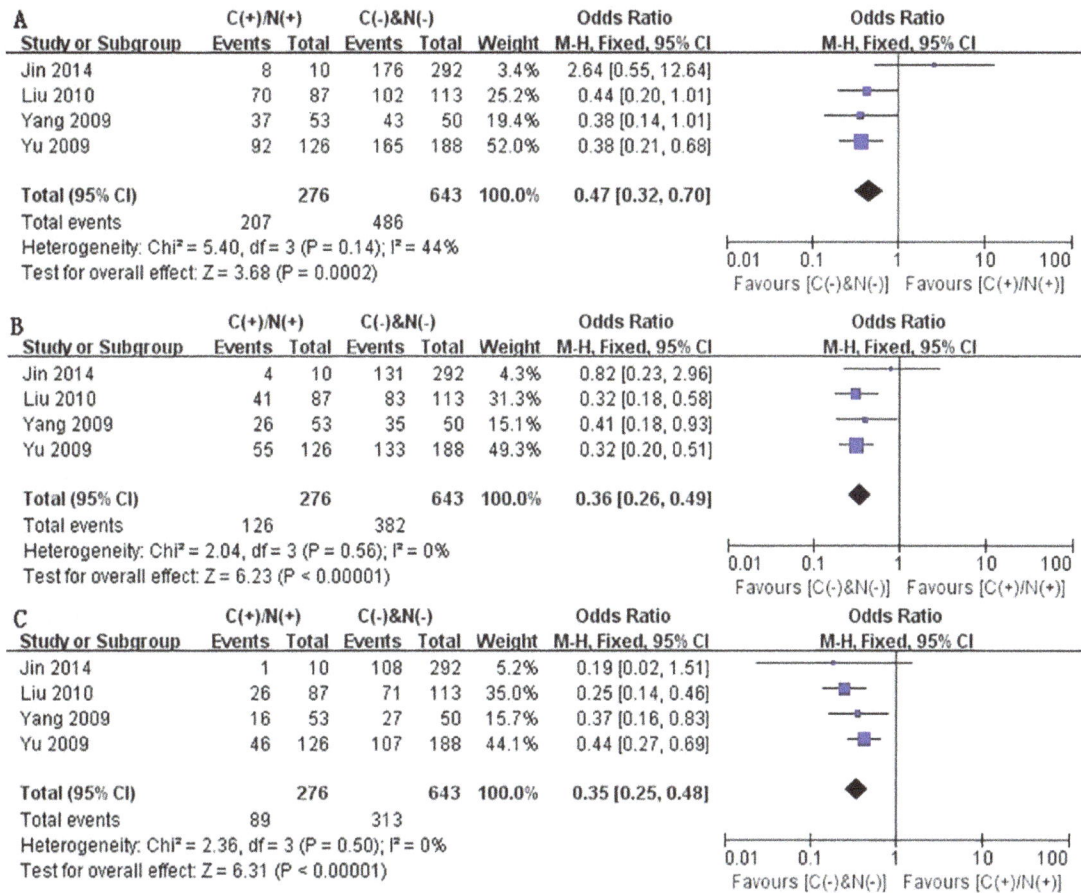

Figure 3. Forest plot of odds ratio for the association of β-catenin expression in cytoplasm and/or nucleus with 1-year (A), 3-year (B) and 5-year (C) recurrence-free survival.

was used to estimate the proportion of total variation caused by inter-study heterogeneity ($I^2 = 0$-50%, no or moderate heterogeneity; $I^2 > 50\%$, significant heterogeneity). By heterogeneity test, according to the result of Q statistical test, a fixed-effects model was selected if $P > 0.05$ and a random-effects model was selected if $P < 0.05$. $P < 0.05$ was considered statistically significant. The funnel plots were made by utilizing Egger's test and Begg's test to examine the risk of potential publication bias. Then, trim and fill analyses were used to evaluate the stability of our meta-analysis results if the plots were asymmetrical.

Results

Selection of Trials

As shown in Figure 1, total 693 potentially eligible studies were screened out in the preliminary search. And then 626 studies were excluded because their titles or abstract failed to meet the discussed topic or these studies had no full text. 67 full papers were captured, among which 45 studies were ultimately excluded due to the lack of adequate data on β-catenin expression level and specific parameters. Thus, 22 studies, with more detailed and sufficient evaluation, met our entry criteria and were retrieved for further analysis. The flow diagram of literature selection procedure was depicted in Figure 1. The major clinical characteristics of these enrolled studies are outlined in Table 1. The total number of cases was 2334. The cases size ranged from 22 to 302 patients. Among these cases, 1853 tissue samples showed cytoplasmic and/or

nuclear accumulation of β-catenin. The data about status of accumulated β-catenin expression, prognostic value, pathological features and etiology had been extracted from these cases. Cytoplasmic and/or nuclear expression rate of β-catenin had a wide range due to the limited number of cases and the circumscribed region of subjects in each study. Subgroup analysis by grouping basing on β-catenin expression rate (≥50% vs <50%) was performed as shown in Table 2. Most of the studies enrolled in this meta-analysis were performed in Asian population. Subgroup analysis by origin (Asia vs others) was conducted in this meta-analysis as shown in Table 3. The ORs and 95%CI between β-catenin expression and overall survival were provided directly or calculated indirectly. Just as shown in Table 1, all studies enrolled in this meta-analysis were performed properly and the expression of β-catenin in specific location (cytomembrane or cytoplasm or nucleus) was determined by using immunohistochemistry without subjective interference.

Quality Assessment

Methodological quality of the 22 studies was assessed according to NOS. The results of quality assessment were shown in the 'level of evidence' column of Table 1. Of the 22 studies, 4 ones [21–24] scored 5 points, 8 [15,25–31] scored 4, 10 [32–41] scored 3. Subgroup analysis by level of evidence (≥4 vs <4) was conducted to investigate if studies with higher or lower level of evidence could make differences in results for prognostic value and clinicopathological significance of cytoplasmic and/or nuclear β-catenin

Table 4. Results of a meta-analysis comparing HCC with C/N β-catenin expression to M β-catenin expression.

Outcome of interest	No. of studies	Number of tissue samples	OR/WMD	95% CI	P value	I^2 (%)
Overall Survival						
1 year	9	C(+)/N(+) = 683, C(-)&N(-) = 818	0.60	0.41–0.89	0.01	0
3 year	9	C(+)/N(+) = 683, C(-)&N(-) = 818	0.56	0.32–0.96	0.03	70
5year	9	C(+)/N(+) = 683, C(-)&N(-) = 818	0.46	0.24–0.85	0.01	77
Recurrence-free Survival						
1 year	4	C(+)/N(+) = 276, C(-)&N(-) = 643	0.47	0.32–0.70	= 0.0002	44
3 year	4	C(+)/N(+) = 276, C(-)&N(-) = 643	0.36	0.26–0.49	<0.00001	0
5 year	4	C(+)/N(+) = 276, C(-)&N(-) = 643	0.35	0.25–0.48	<0.00001	0
Differentiation grade	16	C(+)/N(+) = 627, C(-)&N(-) = 734	1.24	0.71–2.19	0.45	60
Metastasis	8	C(+)/N(+) = 347, C(-)&N(-) = 646	0.63	0.44–0.91	0.01	0
-Subgroup 1	4	N(+) = 117, N(-) = 419	0.66	0.34–1.25	0.20	0
-Subgroup 2	3	C(+) = 310, C(-) = 105	0.93	0.56–1.55	0.79	79
Vascular invasion	7	C(+)/N(+) = 337, C(-)&N(-) = 485	0.44	0.30–0.63	<0.0001	0
- Subgroup 1	4	N(+) = 115, N(-) = 420	0.49	0.28–0.84	0.009	0
- Subgroup 2	2	C(+) = 275, C(-) = 77	0.70	0.42–1.17	0.18	0
TNM stage	7	C(+)/N(+) = 300, C(-)&N(-) = 712	1.18	0.81–1.71	0.39	41
Tumor encapsulation	3	C(+)/N(+) = 179, C(-)&N(-) = 305	1.25	0.64–2.43	0.52	51
Liver cirrhosis	3	C(+)/N(+) = 215, C(-)&N(-) = 307	1.59	0.63–3.97	0.33	51
Tumor size	6	C(+)/N(+) = 260, C(-)&N(-) = 446	1.00	0.49–2.01	0.99	66
HBV	6	C(+)/N(+) = 269, C(-)&N(-) = 349	1.17	0.78–1.76	0.45	0
HCV	4	C(+)/N(+) = 147, C(-)&N(-) = 208	0.52	0.25–1.09	0.08	4
AFP	4	C(+)/N(+) = 214, C(-)&N(-) = 335	0.85	0.59–1.22	0.39	44

C(+)/N(+): β-catenin expression in cytoplasm(C) and/or nucleus (N); C(-)&N(-): none β-catenin expression in cytoplasm(C) and nucleus (N); OR: odds ratio; WMD: weighted mean difference; CI: confidence interval.

expression. Studies with score of 5 or more were regarded as high quality. It indicated that 4 studies obtaining score of 5 in methodological assessment were of high quality.

Impact of Cytoplasmic and/or Nuclear B-Catenin Expression on OS and RFS

Some of the enrolled studies provided the ORs and 95%CI directly or indirectly when they investigated the correlation between cytoplasmic and/or nuclear β-catenin expression and overall survival (OS) or recurrence-free survival (RFS) (Table 4). By pooling these relevant data, we systematically assessed the association of cytoplasmic and/or nuclear expression of β-catenin with OS and RFS of patients with HCC by phasing three periods, one-year, three-year and five-year, respectively. On the basis of 9 retrospective studies [21–24,28,30,31,39,41], it was found that aberrant accumulation of β-catenin in cytoplasm or nucleus significantly correlated with poor 1-, 3- and 5-year OS, just as shown in Fig.2 (A–C). The pooled ORs were 0.60 (n = 9 studies, 95% CI: 0.41–0.89, Z = 2.58, P = 0.010), 0.56 (n = 9 studies, 95% CI: 0.32–0.96, Z = 2.12, P = 0.03) and 0.46 (n = 9 studies, 95% CI: 0.24–0.85, Z = 2.45 P = 0.010) and statistical heterogeneity was 0%, 70% and 77%, respectively for 1-, 3- and 5-year OS. In Fig.3 (A–C), the RFS correlated with cytoplasmic and/or nuclear overexpression of β-catenin was evaluated basing on 4 studies [21,23,24,28], the combined ORs were 0.47 (n = 4 studies, 95% CI: 0.32–0.70, Z = 3.68, P = 0.0002), 0.36 (n = 4 studies, 95% CI: 0.26–0.49, Z = 6.23, P<0.00001) and 0.35 (n = 4 studies, 95% CI: 0.25–0.48, Z = 6.31, P<0.00001), respectively. And no significant heterogeneity was observed (I^2 = 0% for 1-, 3- and 5-year RFS).

Taken together, the above results suggested that β-catenin accumulation in cytoplasm and/or nucleus was significantly correlated with a worse prognosis of HCC. That is to say, patients with HCC showing no β-catenin overexpression in cytoplasm and nuclear were found to have a better prognosis than those patients with HCC showing cytoplasmic and/or nuclear β-catenin overexpression.

Correlation of Cytoplasmic and/or Nuclear B-Catenin Expression with Clinicopathological Parameters

We performed the meta-analysis to evaluate the correlation between β-catenin expression in cytoplasm and/or nucleus with clinicopathological parameters, namely, metastasis, vascular invasion, differentiation grade, TNM stages, liver cirrhosis, tumor size, tumor encapsulation and alpha fetal protein (AFP). Eight studies [21,22,26–29,39,40] investigated the association of cytoplasmic and/or nuclear expression of β-catenin with metastasis of HCC (Fig.4a). The combined OR was 0.63(95%CI: 0.44–0.91, Z = 2.45, P = 0.01) and the statistic heterogeneity is not significant (I^2 = 0%). This result suggested that there was significant correlation between cytoplasmic and/or nuclear accumulation of β-catenin and metastasis of HCC. As depicted in Fig.4b–c, subgroup analysis was also conducted with expectation to further investigate the effect of specific location (cytoplasm or nucleus) of β-catenin accumulation on metastasis. The results showed that nuclear or cytoplasmic overexpression alone was not significantly correlated with metastasis. The pooled ORs were 0.66(n = 4, 95%CI: 0.34–1.25, Z = 1.28, P = 0.20) for the former and 0.93(n = 3, 95%CI: 0.56–1.55, Z = 0.27, P = 0.79) for the latter. Seven studies [23–

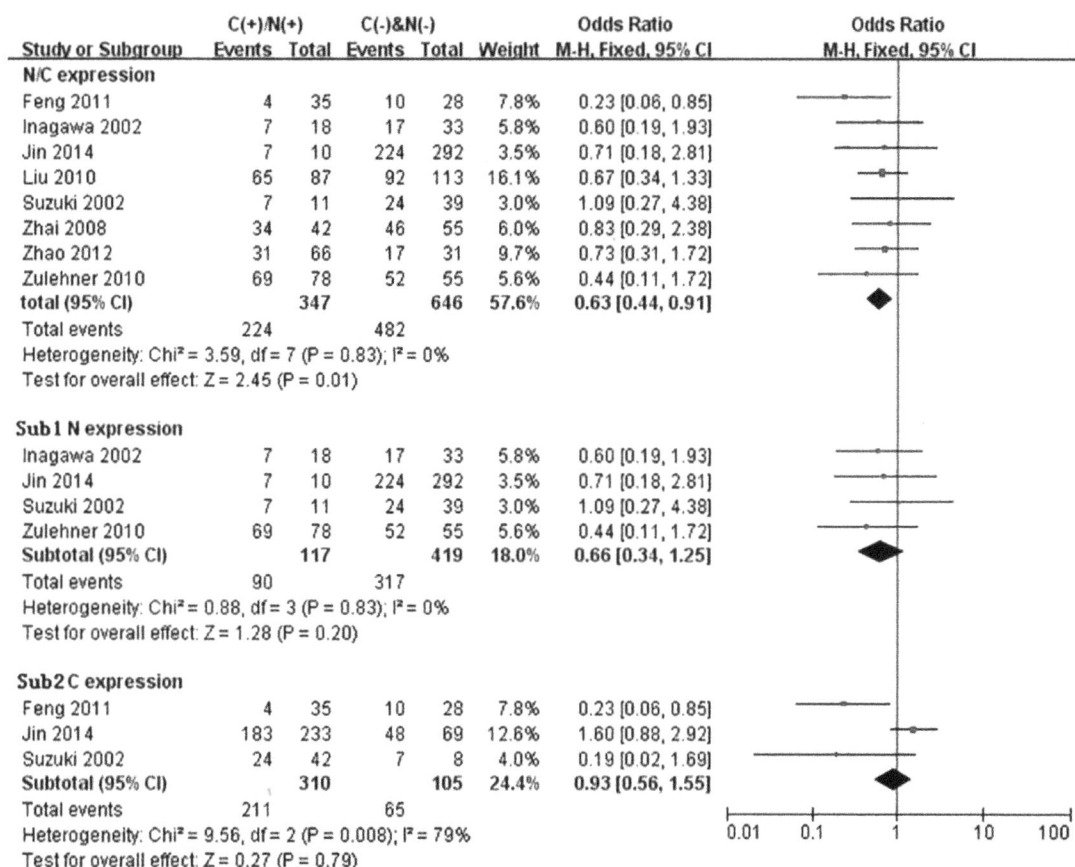

Figure 4. Forest plot of odds ratio for the association of β-catenin expression in cytoplasm and/or nucleus with metastasis by subgroup analysis. Sub1: in cytoplasm alone. Sub2: β-catenin expression in nucleus alone.

25,27,28,39,40] assessed the relationship of aberrant accumulation of β-catenin in cytoplasm and/or nucleus with vascular invasion with no heterogeneity (Fig.5a). The pooled OR was 0.44 (95%CI: 0.30–0.63, Z = 4.37, P<0.0001), indicating that β-catenin accumulation in cytoplasm and/or nucleus was closely correlated with vascular invasion. And then subgroup analysis were also performed just as shown in Fig.5b–c. The results denoted that nuclear overexpression alone had a more close relationship with vascular invasion than cytoplasmic overexpression alone. It indicated that nuclear overexpression alone or combined with cytoplasmic overexpression significantly correlated with vascular invasion. Additionally, we also assessed the relationship of cytoplasmic and/or nuclear β-catenin overexpression with differentiation grade (III/IV versus I/II) and TNM stages (T3/T4 versus T1/T2) on the basis of sixteen studies [15,23–28,30,32–39] and seven studies [15,23,24,28,36,39,42], respectively (Table 4). It was found that β-catenin accumulation in cytoplasm and/or nucleus had no worse effect on the two clinicopathological features. As shown in Fig.6 and Fig.7, the combined ORs were 1.24 (95% CI: 0.71–2.19, Z = 0.75, P = 0.45) and 1.18 (95% CI: 0.81–1.71, Z = 0.86, P = 0.39) and statistic heterogeneity was 60% and 41%. For other clinicopathological parameters, such as liver cirrhosis (Fig.8), tumor size (Fig.9), tumor encapsulation (Fig.10) and AFP level (Fig.11), of HCC showing accumulated expression of β-catenin in cytoplasm and/or nucleus, the pooled ORs were 1.59 (n = 3 studies, 95%CI: 0.63–3.97, Z = 0.98, P = 0.33), 1.00 (n = 6 studies, 95%CI: 0.49–2.01, Z = 0.01, P = 0.99), 1.25 (n = 3 studies, 95%CI: 0.64–2.43, Z = 0.65, P = 0.52) and 0.85 (n = 4

studies, 95%CI: 0.59–1.22, Z = 0.87, P = 0.39) indicating that cytoplasmic and/or nuclear accumulation of β-catenin had no significant correlation with these parameters.

Correlation of Cytoplasmic and/or Nuclear B-Catenin Expression with Etiology

In this meta-analysis, the correlation between cytoplasmic and/or nuclear β-catenin expression and etiology (HBV and HCV) was evaluated basing on the retrospective studies which provided the relevant data. Just as depicted in Fig.12A–B, six studies assessed the association of β-catenin overexpression in cytoplasm and/or nucleus with HBV, and four studies investigated the relationship between β-catenin overexpression in cytoplasm and/or nucleus and HCV. The combined ORs were 1.17 (95%CI: 0.78–1.76, Z = 0.75, P = 0.45) for the former and 0.52(95%CI: 0.25–1.09, Z = 1.74, P = 0.08) for the latter. The statistic heterogeneity was not significant (I^2 = 0%, 4%, respectively). The results suggested that no significant correlation was observed between cytoplasmic and/or nuclear β-catenin expression and etiology (HBV and HCV).

Subgroup Analysis by Grouping Basing on B-Catenin Expression Rate, Origin and Level of Evidence

To critically investigate prognostic and clinicopathological significance of cytoplasmic and/or nuclear β-catenin expression, subgroup analysis by positive β-catenin expression rate was performed and the results showed that in the group of studies

Study or Subgroup	C(+)/N(+) Events	Total	C(-)&N(-) Events	Total	Weight	Odds Ratio M-H, Fixed, 95% CI	Odds Ratio M-H, Fixed, 95% CI
N/C expression							
Liu 2010	60	87	99	113	16.5%	0.31 [0.15, 0.65]	
Suzuki 2002	5	11	19	39	2.8%	0.88 [0.23, 3.36]	
Witjes 2013	5	16	14	34	3.8%	0.65 [0.18, 2.29]	
Yang 2009	46	53	48	50	4.0%	0.27 [0.05, 1.39]	
Yu 2009	4	50	24	139	7.2%	0.42 [0.14, 1.27]	
Zhai 2008	30	42	41	55	6.3%	0.85 [0.35, 2.11]	
Zulehner 2010	45	78	45	55	13.8%	0.30 [0.13, 0.69]	
total (95% CI)		337		485	54.3%	0.44 [0.30, 0.63]	
Total events	195		290				
Heterogeneity: Chi² = 5.42, df = 6 (P = 0.49); I² = 0%							
Test for overall effect: Z = 4.37 (P < 0.0001)							
Sub1 N expression							
Jin 2014	4	10	140	292	3.4%	0.72 [0.20, 2.62]	
Suzuki 2002	5	11	19	39	2.8%	0.88 [0.23, 3.36]	
Witjes 2013	5	16	14	34	3.8%	0.65 [0.18, 2.29]	
Zulehner 2010	45	78	45	55	13.8%	0.30 [0.13, 0.69]	
Subtotal (95% CI)		115		420	23.8%	0.49 [0.28, 0.84]	
Total events	59		218				
Heterogeneity: Chi² = 2.59, df = 3 (P = 0.46); I² = 0%							
Test for overall effect: Z = 2.59 (P = 0.009)							
Sub2 C expression							
Jin 2014	106	233	38	69	19.7%	0.68 [0.40, 1.17]	
Suzuki 2002	20	42	4	8	2.2%	0.91 [0.20, 4.13]	
Subtotal (95% CI)		275		77	21.9%	0.70 [0.42, 1.17]	
Total events	126		42				
Heterogeneity: Chi² = 0.12, df = 1 (P = 0.72); I² = 0%							
Test for overall effect: Z = 1.36 (P = 0.18)							

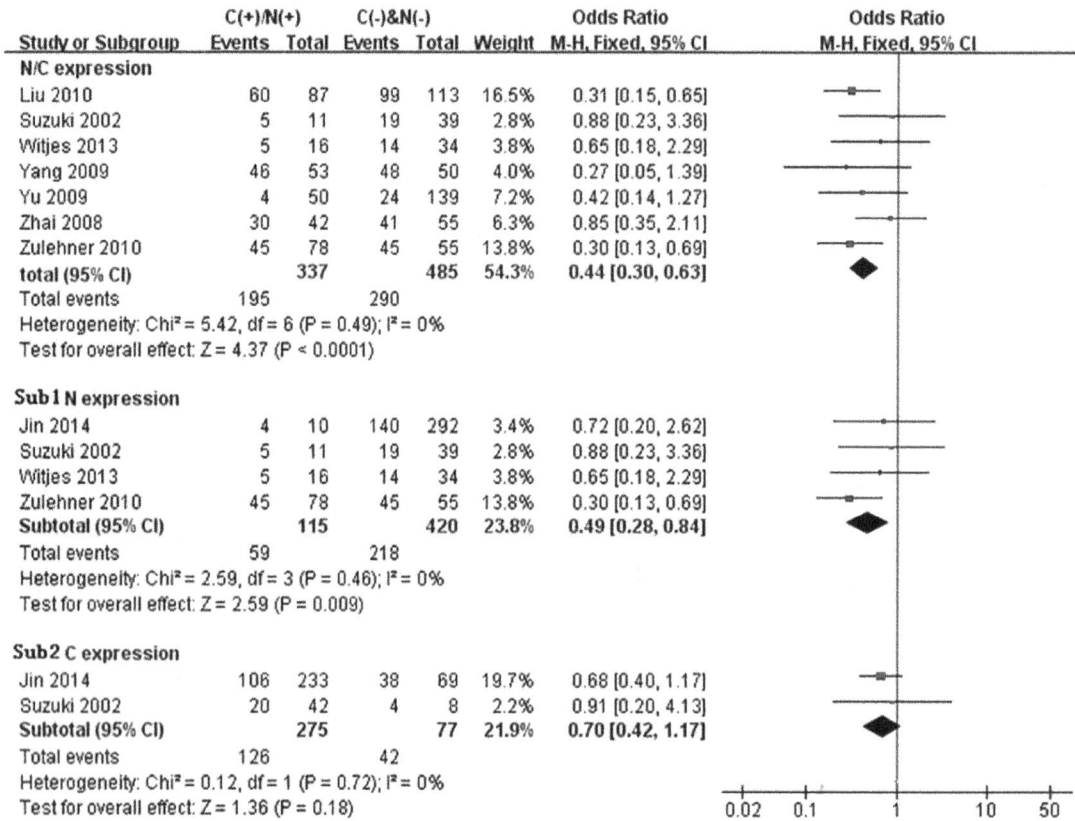

Figure 5. Forest plot of odds ratio for the association of β-catenin expression in cytoplasm and/or nucleus with vascular invasion by subgroup analysis. Sub1: in cytoplasm alone. Sub2: β-catenin expression in nucleus alone.

with higher aberrant β-catenin expression rate, a more significant correlation was observed between cytoplasmic and/or nuclear β-catenin expression and poor prognosis (Table 2). The detailed information was presented in Figure S1, S2, S3, S4, S5, S6, S7, S8 in File S1. However, lower aberrant expression rate of β-catenin (<50%) tended to barely affect the relationship between cytoplas-

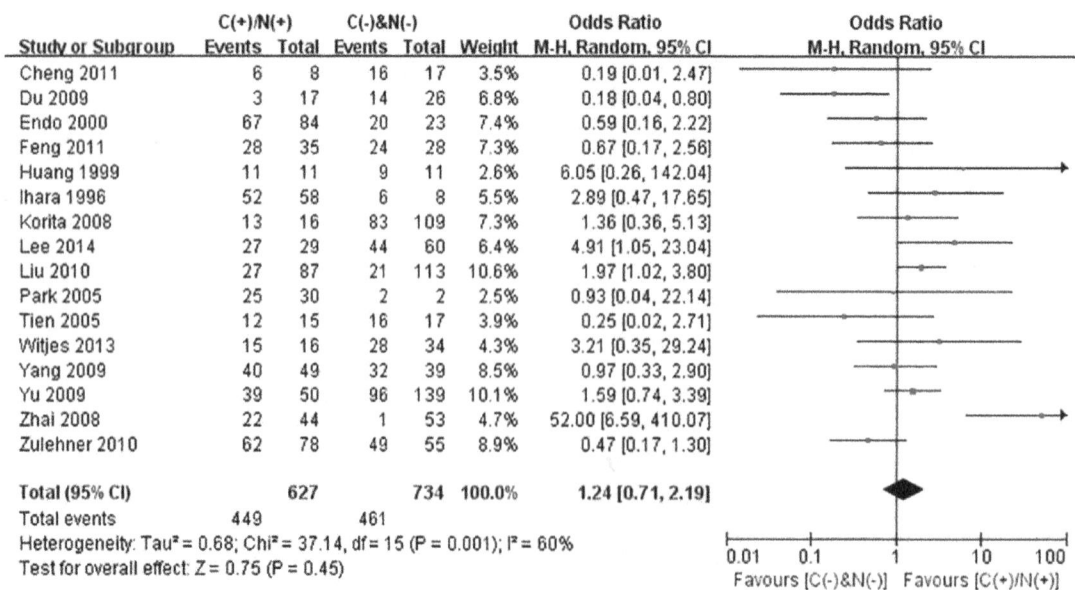

Study or Subgroup	C(+)/N(+) Events	Total	C(-)&N(-) Events	Total	Weight	Odds Ratio M-H, Random, 95% CI	Odds Ratio M-H, Random, 95% CI
Cheng 2011	6	8	16	17	3.5%	0.19 [0.01, 2.47]	
Du 2009	3	17	14	26	6.8%	0.18 [0.04, 0.80]	
Endo 2000	67	84	20	23	7.4%	0.59 [0.16, 2.22]	
Feng 2011	28	35	24	28	7.3%	0.67 [0.17, 2.56]	
Huang 1999	11	11	9	11	2.6%	6.05 [0.26, 142.04]	
Ihara 1996	52	58	6	8	5.5%	2.89 [0.47, 17.65]	
Korita 2008	13	16	83	109	7.3%	1.36 [0.36, 5.13]	
Lee 2014	27	29	44	60	6.4%	4.91 [1.05, 23.04]	
Liu 2010	27	87	21	113	10.6%	1.97 [1.02, 3.80]	
Park 2005	25	30	2	2	2.5%	0.93 [0.04, 22.14]	
Tien 2005	12	15	16	17	3.9%	0.25 [0.02, 2.71]	
Witjes 2013	15	16	28	34	4.3%	3.21 [0.35, 29.24]	
Yang 2009	40	49	32	39	8.5%	0.97 [0.33, 2.90]	
Yu 2009	39	50	96	139	10.1%	1.59 [0.74, 3.39]	
Zhai 2008	22	44	1	53	4.7%	52.00 [6.59, 410.07]	
Zulehner 2010	62	78	49	55	8.9%	0.47 [0.17, 1.30]	
Total (95% CI)		627		734	100.0%	1.24 [0.71, 2.19]	
Total events	449		461				
Heterogeneity: Tau² = 0.68; Chi² = 37.14, df = 15 (P = 0.001); I² = 60%							
Test for overall effect: Z = 0.75 (P = 0.45)							

Favours [C(-)&N(-)]   Favours [C(+)/N(+)]

Figure 6. Forest plot of odds ratio for the association of β-catenin expression in cytoplasm and/or nucleus with differentiation grade.

Cytoplasmic and/or Nuclear Expression of β-Catenin Correlate with Poor Prognosis and Unfavorable...

209

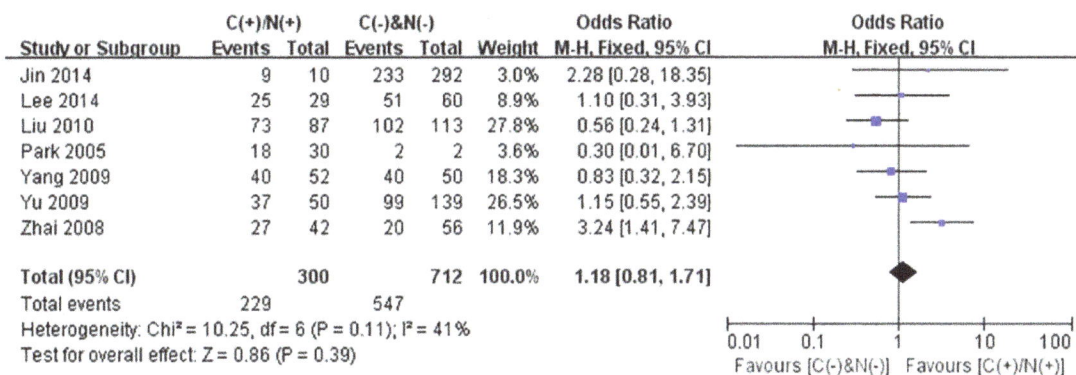

Figure 7. Forest plot of odds ratio for the association of β-catenin expression in cytoplasm and/or nucleus with TNM stage.

mic and/or nuclear β-catenin expression and prognostic value. It indicated that different positive β-catenin expression rate of all tissue samples in each study would make differences in results for the correlation between cytoplasmic and/or nuclear β-catenin expression and prognostic value. Different sample size and wide-scope expression rate involved in each study may induce potential risks of weakening the results of large sample with better quality and strengthening the effect of the small sample with worse quality. In Table 3, the results of subgroup analysis by origin showed that Asian population exhibited a more close association between cytoplasmic and/or nuclear β-catenin expression and poor prognosis and unfavorable clinicopathological factors. In other origins, mainly western population, no significant correlation was observed between cytoplasmic and/or nuclear β-catenin expression and prognostic and clinicopathological value. But the number of studies conducted in western populations was very limited and the limited number may result in no significant changes. Another subgroup analysis was performed by grouping basing on level of evidence (≥4 vs <4), as depicted in Table 3. The results suggested that in the group of studies with higher level of evidence, cytoplasmic and/or nuclear β-catenin expression showed a more robust correlation with poor prognosis and clinicopathological significance. Studies with lower level of evidence usually provided comparatively less adequate data and thus had no advantages during evaluating prognostic value and clinicopathological significance of cytoplasmic and/or nuclear β-catenin expression.

Multivariate Analyses of Factors Associated with Survival and Recurrence

In Table 5, multivariate analyses were performed to determine if cytoplasmic and/or nuclear β-catenin expression has an independent prognostic value compared to other clinical and

pathological features, such as metastasis, vascular invasion, differentiation grade, TNM stage, liver cirrhosis, tumor size, tumor encapsulation and AFP level. The results showed that β-catenin overexpression in cytoplasm and/or nucleus, as well as metastasis, TNM stage and tumor size, was an independent prognostic factor. It implied that β-catenin could serve as a novel independent target of developing clinical therapies for patients with HCC.

Publication Bias

Begg's test indicated that there was no evidence of significant publication bias after assessing the funnel plot (Figure S9, S10, S11, S12, S13, S14, S15, S16, S17, S18, S19 in File S1) for the studies included in our meta-analysis.

Discussion

Hepatocellular carcinoma (HCC) is the third most fatal cancer worldwide and a major health threat [21]. Its high morbidity and mortality makes understanding its cellular and molecular basis and broadening the currently limited treatment options in urgent need [16,21]. The WNT/β-catenin pathway had been well-studied and proven to be involved in progression of several tumors. B-Catenin is a double-functional molecule. In addition to its role in intercellular adhesion, it can also serve as a key downstream effector and a crucial signaling molecule in WNT signaling pathway. In malignant hepatocytes, β-catenin loses its function as a cell-adhesion molecule, accumulates in the cytoplasm, translocates to the nucleus, activates the WNT signaling pathway and switches on transcription of target genes such as c-myc or cyclin D1, resulting in proliferation and metastasis of tumor cells. So far, tremendous work has been done dedicated to investigating the relationship between cytoplasmic and/or nuclear β-catenin

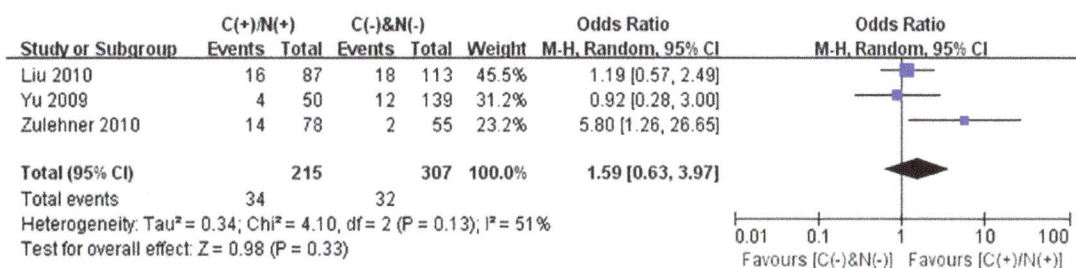

Figure 8. Forest plot of odds ratio for the association of β-catenin expression in cytoplasm and/or nucleus with liver cirrhosis.

Study or Subgroup	C(+)/N(+) Events	Total	C(-)&N(-) Events	Total	Weight	Odds Ratio M-H, Random, 95% CI
Feng 2011	2	35	10	28	11.4%	0.11 [0.02, 0.55]
Korita 2008	8	16	40	109	17.5%	1.73 [0.60, 4.95]
Liu 2010	57	87	76	113	24.0%	0.93 [0.51, 1.67]
Park 2005	15	30	2	2	4.3%	0.20 [0.01, 4.52]
Yu 2009	29	50	77	139	23.1%	1.11 [0.58, 2.14]
Zhai 2008	18	42	11	55	19.6%	3.00 [1.22, 7.38]
Total (95% CI)		260		446	100.0%	1.00 [0.49, 2.01]
Total events	129		216			

Heterogeneity: Tau² = 0.44; Chi² = 14.82, df = 5 (P = 0.01); I² = 66%
Test for overall effect: Z = 0.01 (P = 0.99)

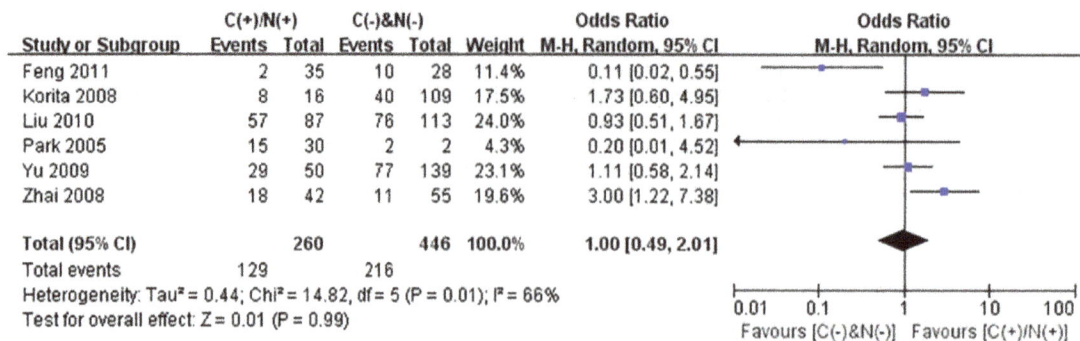

Figure 9. Forest plot of odds ratio for the association of β-catenin expression in cytoplasm and/or nucleus with tumor size.

expression and the prognostic and clinicopathological value of patients with HCC but no conclusive result was achieved. On the other hand, meta-analytical technique, as a useful tool in clinical researches, has been utilized commonly to evaluate the value of prognostic predictors in different clinical trials. Its evaluation was systematically qualitative and quantitative. It can realize the consensus for those subjects still with controversial results by integrating and comparing these results to estimate the outcome of interests. Therefore, we investigated 2334 cases extracted from 22 enrolled studies to conduct a systematic and comprehensive meta-analysis to address the association between cytoplasmic and/or nuclear accumulation of β-catenin and prognosis and clinicopathological factors of patients with HCC. And this effort will also be dedicated to identify β-catenin as a novel independent target of developing clinical therapies for patients with HCC.

Despite new therapies of HCC arising continually, researchers still felt gloomy for its poor prognosis mainly caused by metastasis and recurrence. That's why many researchers have been dedicated to finding out more reliable and exact predicators of prognosis for patients with HCC. The β-catenin protein has been reported to be located at the cell membrane, in the cytoplasm, or in the nucleus [12]. In inactivated cells, the majority of β-catenin is mainly located in the membrane and integrated into adhesion complex responsible for the maintenance of cell junctions and the rest β-catenin, free in cytoplasm, is bound to destruction complex and degraded. Once WNT/β-catenin signaling pathway aberrantly activated, membranous expression of β-catenin is reduced and cytoplasmic degradation of β-catenin is prevented, allowing free β-catenin to accumulate in cytoplasm and translocate to the nucleus, where it interacts with transcription factors of the TCF and LEF family (TCF/LEF) to regulate various target genes [43]. Many researchers have reported that β-catenin overexpression in

cytoplasm and/or nucleus is closely correlated with metastasis and poor prognosis [31]. But other researchers put forward different points suggesting that no significant correlation was found between β-catenin accumulation in cytoplasm and/or nucleus and prognosis [24,39–41]. In this meta-analysis, a systematic and comprehensive analysis was performed and the result denoted that cytoplasmic and/or nuclear accumulation of β-catenin had worse impact on OS and RFS. Additionally, it was found that nuclear combined with cytoplasmic overexpression of β-catenin significantly correlated with metastasis and vascular invasion. However, no significant correlation was observed between cytoplasmic and/or nuclear β-catenin accumulation and other clinicopathological characteristics, such as differentiation grade, TNM stages, liver cirrhosis, tumor size, tumor encapsulation and AFP level. Besides, β-catenin accumulation in cytoplasm and/or nucleus showed no significant association with HBV and HCV. Moreover, multivariate analyses suggested that cytoplasmic and/or nuclear β-catenin expression was a significantly independent prognostic factor. Taken together, all above results suggested that cytoplasmic and/or nuclear expression of β-catenin, as an independent factor, closely correlated with dismal prognosis, disease development and deeper invasion of HCC. The accumulation of β-catenin in cytoplasm and/or nucleus could serve as a biomarker to predict prognostic value and clinicopathological significance of HCC and act as a target of newly developed therapies.

Although we obtained substantial results in this meta-analysis, no more significant conclusions could be reached due to the weakness of the enrolled studies. It was clearly shown from taxonomic studies that different clusters of HCCs with WNT activation can be split depending on CTNNB1 mutation or not. However, the enrolled studies in this meta-analysis failed to provide adequate information about relationship between cyto-

Study or Subgroup	C(+)/N(+) Events	Total	C(-)&N(-) Events	Total	Weight	Odds Ratio M-H, Random, 95% CI
Liu 2010	37	87	34	113	44.4%	1.72 [0.96, 3.09]
Yu 2009	34	50	81	137	39.4%	1.47 [0.74, 2.91]
Zhai 2008	36	42	52	55	16.1%	0.35 [0.08, 1.48]
Total (95% CI)		179		305	100.0%	1.25 [0.64, 2.43]
Total events	107		167			

Heterogeneity: Tau² = 0.17; Chi² = 4.07, df = 2 (P = 0.13); I² = 51%
Test for overall effect: Z = 0.65 (P = 0.52)

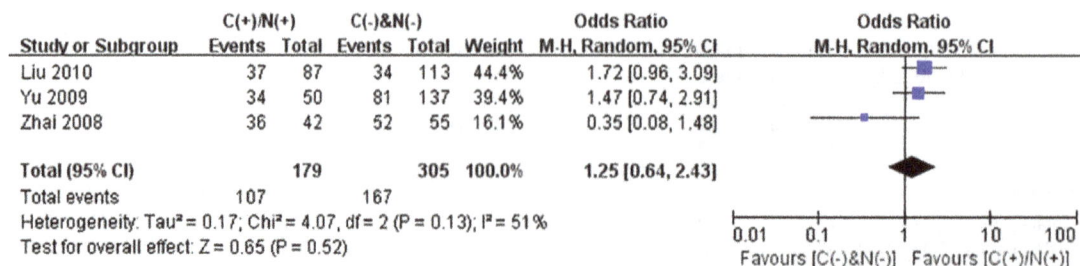

Figure 10. Forest plot of odds ratio for the association of β-catenin expression in cytoplasm and/or nucleus with Tumor encapsulation.

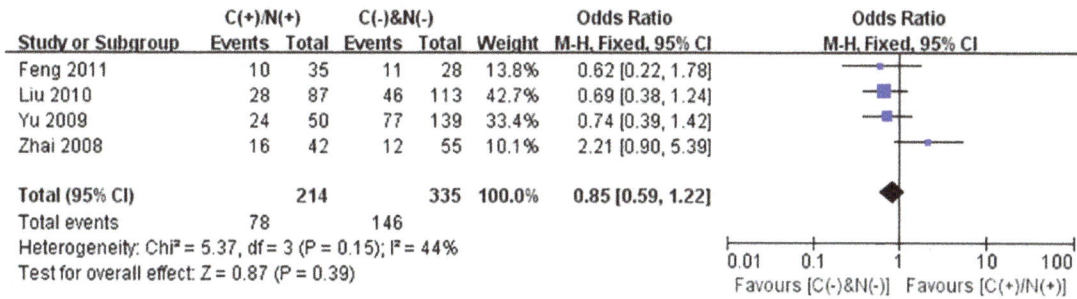

Study or Subgroup	C(+)/N(+) Events	Total	C(-)&N(-) Events	Total	Weight	Odds Ratio M-H, Fixed, 95% CI
Feng 2011	10	35	11	28	13.8%	0.62 [0.22, 1.78]
Liu 2010	28	87	46	113	42.7%	0.69 [0.38, 1.24]
Yu 2009	24	50	77	139	33.4%	0.74 [0.39, 1.42]
Zhai 2008	16	42	12	55	10.1%	2.21 [0.90, 5.39]
Total (95% CI)		214		335	100.0%	0.85 [0.59, 1.22]
Total events	78		146			

Heterogeneity: Chi² = 5.37, df = 3 (P = 0.15); I² = 44%
Test for overall effect: Z = 0.87 (P = 0.39)

Figure 11. Forest plot of odds ratio for the association of β-catenin expression in cytoplasm and/or nucleus with AFP level.

plasmic and/or nuclear β-catenin expression and CTNNB1 mutation. Thus, we couldn't investigate their further relationship by grouping depending on CTNNB1 mutation or not. What's more, during the process of our study selection, we learned that tremendous studies have been done about CTNNB1 mutation and WNT pathway but only a very limited number of clinical studies reported the qualitative relationship between CTNNB1 mutation and its prognostic value. Of the total 22 studies, only 2 ones [36,37] provided the qualitative clinical data. Therefore, we have to screen studies according to cytoplasmic and/or nuclear β-catenin expression though screening basing on CTNNB1 mutation seems more reliable. Moreover, the studies included in this meta-analysis failed to provide symmetric information about location and accumulated percentage of β-catenin expression and prognosis value. Just as depicted in the fifth column of Table 1, some studies provided the number of tissue samples with β-catenin overexpression located in cytoplasm and nucleus respectively but failed to provide the information of prognostic value corresponding to different locations. Some studies only provided the total number of tissue samples with β-catenin overexpression in cytoplasm and/or nucleus but failed to provide

the information about locations in detail. Therefore, it was difficult to evaluate the prognostic value of cytoplasmic or nuclear expression alone by pooling data extracted from each enrolled study in this meta-analysis. We know that nuclear β-catenin expression is clearly linked with activation of the WNT pathway and has significant effect on prognosis but cytoplasmic β-catenin expression alone is not strictly correlated with WNT activation and its prognostic value is inconclusive among researchers. Feng et al [26] and Suzuki et al [40] had reported that cytoplasmic β-catenin expression alone led to metastasis and deeper invasion while Jin et al [21] reported that no changes were observed when β-catenin was ectopically expressed in cytoplasm alone. Therefore, for those included studies combining cytoplasmic with nuclear expression of β-catenin, their conclusion about prognostic values could be bias. Inevitably, the conclusion of this meta-analysis based on these studies could be bias, too. In addition, most of the studies included in this meta-analysis were performed in Asian population, so it was not clear if the results of this meta-analysis will be validated in a western population with HCC. Besides, in this meta-analysis, we mainly analyzed tumors surgically resected rather than palliative HCCs or HCC treated by liver transplan-

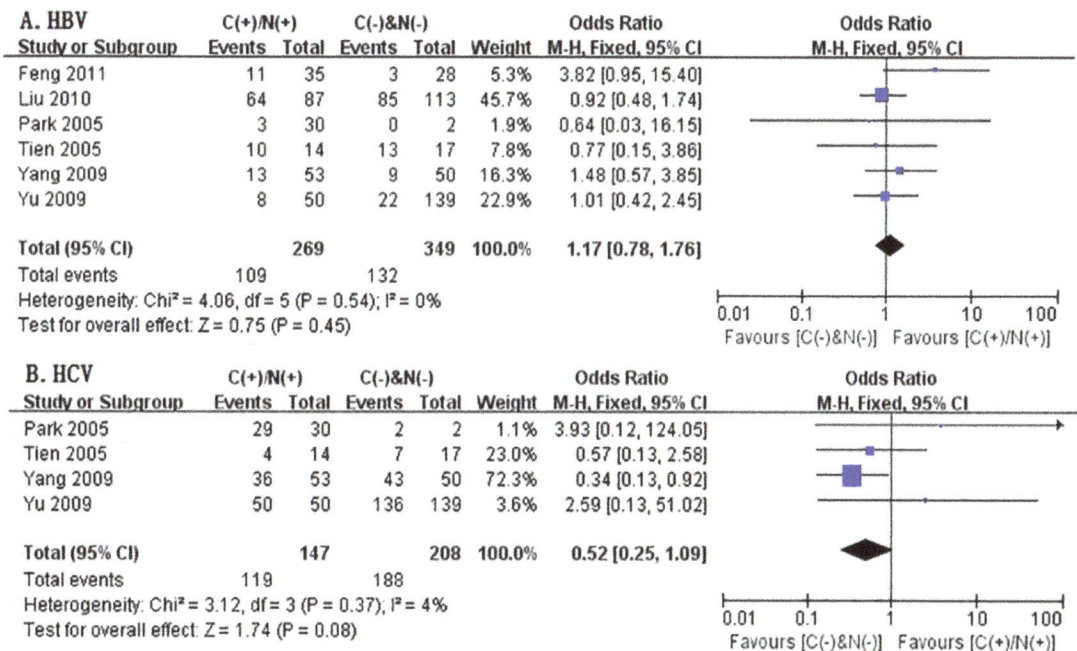

A. HBV

Study or Subgroup	C(+)/N(+) Events	Total	C(-)&N(-) Events	Total	Weight	Odds Ratio M-H, Fixed, 95% CI
Feng 2011	11	35	3	28	5.3%	3.82 [0.95, 15.40]
Liu 2010	64	87	85	113	45.7%	0.92 [0.48, 1.74]
Park 2005	3	30	0	2	1.9%	0.64 [0.03, 16.15]
Tien 2005	10	14	13	17	7.8%	0.77 [0.15, 3.86]
Yang 2009	13	53	9	50	16.3%	1.48 [0.57, 3.85]
Yu 2009	8	50	22	139	22.9%	1.01 [0.42, 2.45]
Total (95% CI)		269		349	100.0%	1.17 [0.78, 1.76]
Total events	109		132			

Heterogeneity: Chi² = 4.06, df = 5 (P = 0.54); I² = 0%
Test for overall effect: Z = 0.75 (P = 0.45)

B. HCV

Study or Subgroup	C(+)/N(+) Events	Total	C(-)&N(-) Events	Total	Weight	Odds Ratio M-H, Fixed, 95% CI
Park 2005	29	30	2	2	1.1%	3.93 [0.12, 124.05]
Tien 2005	4	14	7	17	23.0%	0.57 [0.13, 2.58]
Yang 2009	36	53	43	50	72.3%	0.34 [0.13, 0.92]
Yu 2009	50	50	136	139	3.6%	2.59 [0.13, 51.02]
Total (95% CI)		147		208	100.0%	0.52 [0.25, 1.09]
Total events	119		188			

Heterogeneity: Chi² = 3.12, df = 3 (P = 0.37); I² = 4%
Test for overall effect: Z = 1.74 (P = 0.08)

Figure 12. Forest plot of odds ratio for the association of β-catenin expression in cytoplasm and/or nucleus with etiology. A: HBV; B: HCV.

Table 5. Multivariate analyses of factors associated with survival and recurrence.

Factors	Overall survival			Recurrence free survival		
	HR	95%CI	P value	HR	95%CI	P value
HBeAg (positive vs negative)	0.89	0.54–1.45	0.63	1.36	0.88–2.12	0.17
Liver cirrhosis (no vs yes)	2.02	1.00–4.09	0.17	1.55	0.86–2.80	0.15
AFP level (<20 ng/mL vs ≥21 ng/mL)	1.54	1.10–2.16	0.01	1.29	0.61–2.72	0.51
Tumor differentiation (I–II vs III–IV)	1.34	0.90–1.99	0.15	1.08	0.87–1.34	0.48
Tumor size, (≤5 cm vs >5 cm)	1.08	1.03–1.12	0.001	1.06	1.01–1.10	0.008
Metastasis (no vs yes)	1.36	1.16–1.61	0.0002	1.32	1.15–1.51	<0.0001
Tumor encapsulation (complete vs none)	0.99	0.59–1.69	0.99	0.86	0.56–1.33	0.50
Vascular invasion (no vs yes)	1.53	0.94–2.48	0.09	1.23	0.71–2.12	0.45
TNM stage(I/II vs III/IV)	1.68	1.27–2.22	0.0003	1.67	1.29–2.15	<0.0001
β-catenin (C(+)/N(+) vs C(-)&N(-))	2.73	2.03–3.66	<0.00001	2.56	1.53–4.28	0.0003

tation or radiofrequency ablation, considering the limited retrospective studies, poor representation and thereby inaccuracy of the latter.

In addition, in this meta-analysis, there also remained some limitations worthy of further concern. First, heterogeneity was inevitable among the groups due to differences of patient characteristics such as age, gender and chemotherapies in each study. On the one hand, we used a random-effects model in order to eliminate variations across studies. On the other hand, sensitivity analysis was also used to observe whether omission of any single study would have significant impact on the combined OR estimates. Although the effort could not necessarily rule out the effect of heterogeneity among studies, the adverse influence will be weakened to some degree. Second, bias was unavoidable for clinical evidence because some relevant data were retrieved indirectly from several studies or by reading the survival curve. The inaccurate reading might produce errors and bring about bias. Third, studies performed with positive results or significant outcomes will be apt to be published, suggesting a potential publication bias. Fourth, reports in other languages than English were excluded, so potential language bias may be present in our meta-analysis. Fifth, a significant heterogeneity might also be brought about in this meta-analysis by the difference of the antibodies used for test of ectopic cytoplasmic/nuclear β-catenin expression. Besides, the difference of sample size in each study may induce potential risks of weakening the results of large sample with better quality and strengthening the effect of the small sample with worse quality. All these bias or risks should not be neglected and further investigation should be given to determine whether these factors influence the results of the meta-analysis.

The prognostic and clinicopathological significance of β-catenin expression in cytoplasm or nucleus for patients with HCC was investigated in this meta-analysis. The result suggested that patients with HCC showing cytoplasmic and/or nuclear expression of β-catenin appeared to have a poorer OS and RFS, in comparison with those patients with HCC showing normal membranous expression of β-catenin. Additionally, it showed that nuclear combined with cytoplasmic accumulation of β-catenin significantly correlated with metastasis and vascular invasion, while no significant relationship was observed between β-catenin overexpression in cytoplasm and/or nucleus and advanced differentiation grade, TNM stage, liver cirrhosis, tumor size, tumor encapsulation and AFP level. Besides, no significant

correlation was observed between cytoplasmic and/or nuclear β-catenin expression and etiology (HBV and HCV). Moreover, cytoplasmic and/or nuclear β-catenin expression was an independent prognostic factor. In summary, β-catenin accumulation in cytoplasm and/or nucleus, as an independent prognostic factor, closely associated with poor prognosis and deep invasion for patients with HCC. Thus, cytoplasmic and/or nuclear expression of β-catenin could serve as a potential predictor for progression and prognosis of patients with HCC and act as a novel target of the developed therapies.

Supporting Information

Checklist S1   PRISMA checklist

File S1   Supporting figures. Figure S1, Forest plot of odds ratio for the association of β-catenin expression in cytoplasm and/or nucleus with 1-year overall survival by subgroup analysis. Sub1: ≥50% expression rate; Sub 2: <50% expression rate. Figure S2, Forest plot of odds ratio for the association of β-catenin expression in cytoplasm and/or nucleus with 3-year overall survival by subgroup analysis. Sub1: ≥50% expression rate; Sub 2: <50% expression rate. Figure S3, Forest plot of odds ratio for the association of β-catenin expression in cytoplasm and/or nucleus with 5-year overall survival by subgroup analysis. Sub1: ≥50% expression rate; Sub 2: <50% expression rate. Figure S4, Forest plot of odds ratio for the association of β-catenin expression in cytoplasm and/or nucleus with 1-year recurrence-free survival by subgroup analysis. Sub1: ≥50% expression rate; Sub 2: <50% expression rate. Figure S5, Forest plot of odds ratio for the association of β-catenin expression in cytoplasm and/or nucleus with 3-year recurrence-free survival by subgroup analysis. Sub1: ≥ 50% expression rate; Sub 2: <50% expression rate. Figure S6, Forest plot of odds ratio for the association of β-catenin expression in cytoplasm and/or nucleus with 5-year recurrence-free survival by subgroup analysis. Sub1: ≥50% expression rate; Sub 2: <50% expression rate. Figure S7, Forest plot of odds ratio for the association of β-catenin expression in cytoplasm and/or nucleus with metastasis by subgroup analysis. Sub1: ≥50% expression rate; Sub 2: <50% expression rate. Figure S8, Forest plot of odds ratio for the association of β-catenin expression in cytoplasm and/or nucleus with vascular invasion by subgroup analysis. Sub1: ≥ 50% expression rate; Sub 2: <50% expression rate. Figure S9,

Funnel plot to assess publication bias. A, Begg's publication bias plot showed no publication bias for studies regarding cytoplasmic and/or nuclear expression of β-catenin and 1-year overall survival (OS) in the meta-analysis. B, Begg's publication bias plot showed the presence of publication bias for studies regarding cytoplasmic and/or nuclear expression of β-catenin and 3-year OS in the meta-analysis. C, Begg's publication bias plot showed the presence of publication bias for studies regarding cytoplasmic and/or nuclear expression of β-catenin and 5-year OS in the meta-analysis. Figure S10, Funnel plot to assess publication bias. A, Begg's publication bias plot showed no publication bias for studies regarding cytoplasmic and/or nuclear expression of β-catenin and 1-year reccurrence-free survival (RFS) in the meta-analysis. B, Begg's publication bias plot showed no publication bias for studies regarding cytoplasmic and/or nuclear expression of β-catenin and 3-year RFS in the meta-analysis. C, Begg's publication bias plot showed no publication bias for studies regarding cytoplasmic and/or nuclear expression of β-catenin and 5-year RFS in the meta-analysis. Figure S11, Funnel plot to assess publication bias. Begg's publication bias plot showed no publication bias for studies regarding cytoplasmic and/or nuclear expression of β-catenin and metastasis in the meta-analysis. Figure S12, Funnel plot to assess publication bias. Begg's publication bias plot showed no publication bias for studies regarding cytoplasmic and/or nuclear expression of β-catenin and vascular invasion in the meta-analysis. Figure S13, Funnel plot to assess publication bias. Begg's publication bias plot showed the presence of publication bias for studies regarding cytoplasmic and/or nuclear expression of β-catenin and differentiation grade in the meta-analysis. Figure S14, Funnel plot to assess publication bias. Begg's publication bias plot showed no publication bias for studies regarding cytoplasmic and/

or nuclear expression of β-catenin and TNM stage ((III/IV versus I/II)) in the meta-analysis. Figure S15, Funnel plot to assess publication bias. Begg's publication bias plot showed no publication bias for studies regarding cytoplasmic and/or nuclear expression of β-catenin and liver cirrhosis in the meta-analysis. Figure S16, Funnel plot to assess publication bias. Begg's publication bias plot showed the presence of publication bias for studies regarding cytoplasmic and/or nuclear expression of β-catenin and tumor size in the meta-analysis. Figure S17, Funnel plot to assess publication bias. Begg's publication bias plot showed the presence of publication bias for studies regarding cytoplasmic and/or nuclear expression of β-catenin and tumor encapsulation in the meta-analysis. Figure S18, Funnel plot to assess publication bias. Begg's publication bias plot showed no publication bias for studies regarding cytoplasmic and/or nuclear expression of β-catenin and AFP in the meta-analysis. Figure S19, Funnel plot to assess publication bias. A, publication bias plot showed no publication bias for studies regarding cytoplasmic and/or nuclear expression of β-catenin and HBV in the meta-analysis. B, Begg's publication bias plot showed no publication bias for studies regarding cytoplasmic and/or nuclear expression of β-catenin and HCV in the meta-analysis.
(RAR)

Author Contributions

Conceived and designed the experiments: JC XJC. Performed the experiments: JC JHL RAJ JLS YLL RM HL XL HY. Analyzed the data: JC JHL RAJ JLS. Contributed reagents/materials/analysis tools: JC JHL RAJ JLS YLL HL XL HY. Wrote the paper: JC.

References

1. Dahmani R, Just PA, Perret C (2011) The Wnt/beta-catenin pathway as a therapeutic target in human hepatocellular carcinoma. Clin Res Hepatol Gastroenterol 35: 709–713.
2. El-Serag HB (2012) Epidemiology of viral hepatitis and hepatocellular carcinoma. Gastroenterology 142 : 1264–1273e1261.
3. Ferlay J, Shin HR, Bray F, Forman D, Mathers C, et al. (2010) Estimates of worldwide burden of cancer in 2008: GLOBOCAN 2008. International journal of cancer 127: 2893–2917.
4. Altekruse SF, McGlynn KA, Dickie LA, Kleiner DE (2012) Hepatocellular Carcinoma Confirmation, Treatment, and Survival in Surveillance, Epidemiology, and End Results Registries, 1992-2008. Hepatology 55: 476–482.
5. Inuzuka T, Nishikawa H, Sekikawa A, Takeda H, Henmi S, et al. (2011) Complete response of advanced hepatocellular carcinoma with multiple lung metastases treated with sorafenib: a case report. Oncology 81: 152–157.
6. Sposito C, Mariani L, Germini A, Flores Reyes M, Bongini M, et al. (2013) Comparative efficacy of sorafenib versus best supportive care in recurrent hepatocellular carcinoma after liver transplantation: A case-control study. Journal of hepatology 59: 59–66.
7. Villanueva A, Newell P, Chiang DY, Friedman SL, Llovet JM. (2007) Genomics and signaling pathways in hepatocellular carcinoma. Copyright© 2007 by Thieme Medical Publishers, Inc., 333 Seventh Avenue, New York, NY 10001, USA.pp.055–076.
8. Clevers H (2006) Wnt/β-catenin signaling in development and disease. Cell 127: 469–480.
9. Ding X, Yang Y, Han B, Du C, Xu N, et al. (2014) Transcriptomic Characterization of Hepatocellular Carcinoma with CTNNB1 Mutation. PLoS One 9: e95307.
10. Weis WI, Nelson WJ (2006) Re-solving the cadherin-catenin-actin conundrum. Journal of biological chemistry 281: 35593–35597.
11. Gumbiner BM (1996) Cell adhesion: the molecular basis of tissue architecture and morphogenesis. Cell 84: 345–357.
12. Chen Z, He X, Jia M, Liu Y, Qu D, et al. (2013) beta-catenin overexpression in the nucleus predicts progress disease and unfavourable survival in colorectal cancer: a meta-analysis. PLoS One 8: e63854.
13. Wands JR, Kim M (2014) WNT/beta-catenin signaling and hepatocellular carcinoma. Hepatology.
14. Austinat M, Dunsch R, Wittekind C, Tannapfel A, Gebhardt R, et al. (2008) Correlation between beta-catenin mutations and expression of Wnt-signaling target genes in hepatocellular carcinoma. Molecular Cancer 7.
15. Lee JM, Yang J, Newell P, Singh S, Parwani A, et al. (2014) beta-Catenin signaling in hepatocellular cancer: Implications in inflammation, fibrosis, and proliferation. Cancer Lett 343: 90–97.
16. Chua M-S, Ma L, Wei W, So S (2014) WNT/β-catenin pathway activation in hepatocellular carcinoma: a clinical perspective. Gastrointestinal Cancer: Targets and Therapy: 49.
17. Breuhahn K, Schirmacher P (2009) Signaling networks in human hepatocarcinogenesis—novel aspects and therapeutic options. Progress in molecular biology and translational science 97: 251–277.
18. Zhan P, Ji YN (2014) Prognostic significance of TP53 expression for patients with hepatocellular carcinoma: a meta-analysis. Hepatobiliary Surg Nutr 3: 11–17.
19. Mei XD, Su H, Song J, Dong L (2013) Prognostic significance of beta-catenin expression in patients with non-small cell lung cancer: a meta-analysis. Biosci Trends 7: 42–49.
20. Chen J, Sun MX, Hua YQ, Cai ZD (2014) Prognostic significance of serum lactate dehydrogenase level in osteosarcoma: a meta-analysis. J Cancer Res Clin Oncol.
21. Jin J, Jung H, Wang Y, Xie J, Yeom YI, et al. (2014) Nuclear Expression of Phosphorylated TRAF2- and NCK-interacting Kinase in Hepatocellular Carcinoma is Associated with Poor Prognosis. Pathology - Research and Practice.
22. Zhao N, Sun BC, Zhao XL, Liu ZY, Sun T, et al. (2012) Coexpression of Bcl-2 with epithelial-mesenchymal transition regulators is a prognostic indicator in hepatocellular carcinoma. Med Oncol 29: 2780–2792.
23. Yu B, Yang X, Xu Y, Yao G, Shu H, et al. (2009) Elevated expression of DKK1 is associated with cytoplasmic/nuclear beta-catenin accumulation and poor prognosis in hepatocellular carcinomas. J Hepatol 50: 948–957.
24. Yang MH, Chen CL, Chau GY, Chiou SH, Su CW, et al. (2009) Comprehensive analysis of the independent effect of twist and snail in promoting metastasis of hepatocellular carcinoma. Hepatology 50: 1464–1474.
25. Witjes CD, ten Kate FJ, Verhoef C, de Man RA, JN IJ (2013) Immunohistochemical characteristics of hepatocellular carcinoma in non-cirrhotic livers. J Clin Pathol 66: 687–691.
26. Feng Z, Fan X, Jiao Y, Ban K (2011) Mammalian target of rapamycin regulates expression of beta-catenin in hepatocellular carcinoma. Hum Pathol 42: 659–668.
27. Zulehner G, Mikula M, Schneller D, van Zijl F, Huber H, et al. (2010) Nuclear beta-catenin induces an early liver progenitor phenotype in hepatocellular carcinoma and promotes tumor recurrence. Am J Pathol 176: 472–481.

28. Liu L, Zhu XD, Wang WQ, Shen Y, Qin Y, et al. (2010) Activation of beta-catenin by hypoxia in hepatocellular carcinoma contributes to enhanced metastatic potential and poor prognosis. Clin Cancer Res 16: 2740–2750.

29. Inagawa S, Itabashi M, Adachi S, Kawamoto T, Hori M, et al. (2002) Expression and prognostic roles of beta-catenin in hepatocellular carcinoma: correlation with tumor progression and postoperative survival. Clin Cancer Res 8: 450–456.

30. Endo K, Ueda T, Ueyama J, Ohta T, Terada T (2000) Immunoreactive e-cadherin, alpha-catenin, beta-catenin, and gamma-catenin proteins in hepatocellular carcinoma: Relationships with tumor grade, clinicopathologic parameters, and patients. Human Pathology 31: 558–565.

31. Geng M, Cao YC, Chen YJ, Jiang H, Bi LQ, et al. (2012) Loss of Wnt5a and Ror2 protein in hepatocellular carcinoma associated with poor prognosis. World J Gastroenterol 18: 1328–1338.

32. Cheng AS, Lau SS, Chen Y, Kondo Y, Li MS, et al. (2011) EZH2-mediated concordant repression of Wnt antagonists promotes beta-catenin-dependent hepatocarcinogenesis. Cancer Res 71: 4028–4039.

33. Du GS, Wang JM, Lu JX, Li Q, Ma CQ, et al. (2009) Expression of P-aPKC-iota, E-cadherin, and beta-catenin related to invasion and metastasis in hepatocellular carcinoma. Ann Surg Oncol 16: 1578–1586.

34. Korita PV, Wakai T, Shirai Y, Matsuda Y, Sakata J, et al. (2008) Overexpression of osteopontin independently correlates with vascular invasion and poor prognosis in patients with hepatocellular carcinoma. Hum Pathol 39: 1777–1783.

35. Tien LT, Ito M, Nakao M, Niino D, Serik M, et al. (2005) Expression of beta-catenin in hepatocellular carcinoma. World J Gastroenterol 11: 2398–2401.

36. Park JY, Park WS, Nam SW, Kim SY, Lee SH, et al. (2005) Mutations of beta-catenin and AXIN I genes are a late event in human hepatocellular carcinogenesis. Liver Int 25: 70–76.

37. Huang H, Fujii H, Sankila A, Mahler-Araujo BM, Matsuda M, et al. (1999) Beta-catenin mutations are frequent in human hepatocellular carcinomas associated with hepatitis C virus infection. Am J Pathol 155: 1795–1801.

38. Ihara A, Koizumi H, Hashizume R, Uchikoshi T (1996) Expression of epithelial cadherin and alpha- and beta-catenins in nontumoral livers and hepatocellular carcinomas. Hepatology 23: 1441–1447.

39. Zhai B, Yan HX, Liu SQ, Chen L, Wu MC, et al. (2008) Reduced expression of E-cadherin/catenin complex in hepatocellular carcinomas. World J Gastroenterol 14: 5665–5673.

40. Suzuki T, Yano H, Nakashima Y, Nakashima O, Kojiro M (2002) Beta-catenin expression in hepatocellular carcinoma: a possible participation of beta-catenin in the dedifferentiation process. J Gastroenterol Hepatol 17: 994–1000.

41. Schmitt-Graff A, Ertelt V, Allgaier HP, Koelble K, Olschewski M, et al. (2003) Cellular retinol-binding protein-1 in hepatocellular carcinoma correlates with beta-catenin, Ki-67 index, and patient survival. Hepatology 38: 470–480.

42. Guan CN, Chen XM, Lou HQ, Liao XH, Chen BY, et al. (2012) Clinical significance of axin and beta-catenin protein expression in primary hepatocellular carcinomas. Asian Pac J Cancer Prev 13: 677–681.

43. Gough NR (2012) Focus issue: Wnt and beta-catenin signaling in development and disease. Sci Signal 5: eg2.

22

CXCL17 Expression Predicts Poor Prognosis and Correlates with Adverse Immune Infiltration in Hepatocellular Carcinoma

Li Li[1,2⑨], Jing Yan[2⑨], Jing Xu[2], Chao-Qun Liu[2], Zuo-Jun Zhen[1]*, Huan-Wei Chen[1], Yong Ji[1], Zhi-Peng Wu[1], Jian-Yuan Hu[1], Limin Zheng[2], Wan Yee Lau[1,3]*

1 Department of Hepatic and Pancreatic Surgery, The First People's Hospital of Foshan, Foshan, Guangdong, P. R. China, **2** State Key Laboratory of Oncology in South China, Sun Yat-sen University Cancer Center, Guangzhou, P. R. China, **3** Faculty of Medicine, The Chinese University of Hong Kong, Shatin, New Territories, Hong Kong SAR, P. R. China

Abstract

CXC ligand 17 (CXCL17) is a novel CXC chemokine whose clinical significance remains largely unknown. In the present study, we characterized the prognostic value of CXCL17 in patients with hepatocellular carcinoma (HCC) and evaluated the association of CXCL17 with immune infiltration. We examined CXCL17 expression in 227 HCC tissue specimens by immunohistochemical staining, and correlated CXCL17 expression patterns with clinicopathological features, prognosis, and immune infiltrate density (CD4 T cells, CD8 T cells, B cells, natural killer cells, neutrophils, macrophages). Kaplan-Meier survival analysis showed that both increased intratumoral CXCL17 ($P = 0.015$ for overall survival [OS], $P = 0.003$ for recurrence-free survival [RFS]) and peritumoral CXCL17 ($P = 0.002$ for OS, $P < 0.001$ for RFS) were associated with shorter OS and RFS. Patients in the CXCL17[low] group had significantly lower 5-year recurrence rate compared with patients in the CXCL17[high] group (peritumoral: 53.1% vs. 77.7%, $P < 0.001$, intratumoral: 58.6% vs. 73.0%, $P = 0.001$, respectively). Multivariate Cox proportional hazards analysis identified peritumoral CXCL17 as an independent prognostic factor for both OS (hazard ratio [HR] = 2.066, 95% confidence interval [CI] = 1.296–3.292, $P = 0.002$) and RFS (HR = 1.844, 95% CI = 1.218–2.793, $P = 0.004$). Moreover, CXCL17 expression was associated with more CD68 and less CD4 cell infiltration (both $P < 0.05$). The combination of CXCL17 density and immune infiltration could be used to further classify patients into subsets with different prognosis for RFS. Our results provide the first evidence that tumor-infiltrating CXCL17[+] cell density is an independent prognostic factor that predicts both OS and RFS in HCC. CXCL17 production correlated with adverse immune infiltration and might be an important target for anti-HCC therapies.

Editor: Cordula M. Stover, University of Leicester, United Kingdom

Funding: This work was supported by project grants from the Ministry of Health of China (LZ; 2012ZX10002-011; http://www.moh.gov.cn/publicfiles//business/htmlfiles/wsb/index.htm); China Postdoctoral Science Foundation (JY; 2013M540676; http://res.chinapostdoctor.org.cn/BshWeb/InnerPages_c5a0971c-60a5-4c35-917c-4b5526056791.shtml); and FoShan Postdoctoral Scientific Research project; (LL; 2013; http://www.fshrss.gov.cn/zwgk/tzgg/201312/t20131223_4501821.html). The funders had no role in study design, data collection and analysis, decision to publish, or preparation of the manuscript.

Competing Interests: The authors have declared that no competing interests exist.

* Email: zzjun@fsyyy.com (ZJZ); josephlau@cuhk.edu.hk (WYL)

⑨ These authors contributed equally to this work.

Introduction

Hepatocellular carcinoma (HCC) is among the most common causes of cancer mortality worldwide and its incidence is increasing [1–3]. Although surgical resection is one of the first priorities for HCC treatment, the frequent postsurgical recurrence is a major obstacle to cure. Besides, the general response of HCC to chemotherapy remains far from satisfactory [4]. Thus, discovering biomarkers that identify patients at high risk for recurrence and combining other postsurgical adjuvant therapies to obtain better outcomes is of great importance [5].

Tumor progression is now recognized as the product of evolving crosstalk among different cell types within the tumor microenvironment. Extensive immune cell infiltration is usually present in HCC due to chronic viral infection [6–8]. Chemokines are key mediators for recruiting various immune cells to the tumor microenvironment. The infiltrating cells provide a secondary source of chemokines that further regulate the immune status of the tumor [9–12]. In addition to promoting leukocyte trafficking to tumors, recent studies indicate that chemokines also play important roles in many aspects, including influencing the tumor immune response, regulating angiogenesis, promoting tumor growth, and mediating tumor metastasis [13,14]. The CXC ligand 5 (CXCL5) and CXC receptor 6 (CXCR6) expression has been shown to significantly influences HCC progression, in part by regulating tumor growth and invasion, and via immune cell infiltration [15,16].

CXCL17 is a novel, 119-amino acid CXC chemokine; its receptor is currently unknown [17,18]. As the last chemokine ligand to be discovered, the clinical significance and regulatory activity of CXCL17 remain largely unknown. CXCL17 is expressed constitutively in the lung, trachea, stomach and colon [17,18]. It is a chemoattractant of monocytes, macrophages, dendritic cells (DC), and immature myeloid-derived cells [18]. Several studies have proposed that CXCL17 might act as a chemokine that accelerates tumor progression. CXCL17 is significantly upregulated in breast carcinoma and colon tumors and is associated with carcinogenesis, tumor proliferation, and angiogenesis [17,19]. Interestingly, another study suggested that CXCL17 might be involved in anti-tumor immune response during pancreatic carcinogenesis. In premalignant intraductal papillary mucinous neoplasm, CXCL17 induces DC accumulation at the tumor site, which promotes tumor cell susceptibility to cytotoxic T cell-mediated cytolysis [20]. Although ectopic CXCL17 expression promotes hepatoma HepG2 cell proliferation, the nature and role of CXCL17 in human HCC has not been elucidated [21].

In the present study, we investigated the prognostic significance of CXCL17 in HCC. We then explored the possible regulatory activity of CXCL17 by correlating CXCL17 expression with immune cell infiltration. We also tried to find out whether tumor-infiltrating CXCL17$^+$ cells were an independent prognostic factor of survival and whether they were correlated with immune infiltration in HCC.

Materials and Methods

Patients and Specimens

We used archived formalin-fixed, paraffin-embedded tissues from 8 patients with chronic hepatitis and 227 patients who had undergone curative resection for HCC between 2007 and 2010 at the Sun Yat-sen University Cancer Center. The diagnosis of HCC was confirmed histopathologically in each patient. No patient received anti-cancer therapies or had distant metastasis prior to surgery. Curative resection for HCC was defined as complete resection of all tumor nodules, with a resection margin of at least 1 cm, and leaving the cut surface being free of tumor based on histological examination. Intraoperative ultrasound and postsurgical contrast-enhanced computed tomography (CT) were routinely used to ensure complete removal of HCC [7,22]. Tumor stages were determined according to the tumor-nodes-metastasis (TNM) classification of the International Union Against Cancer (Edition 6) and the Barcelona Clinic Liver Cancer (BCLC) staging classification [23]. Tumor differentiation was graded according to the Edmondson grading system. The clinicopathological characteristics of the patients were summarized in Table 1.

Follow-up and Postoperative Treatment

All patients were followed-up after surgery, undergoing regular surveillance for recurrence with chest radiography, serum alpha-fetoprotein (AFP) level, and abdominal ultrasonography at 2–4-month intervals [7,22,24,25]. If tumor recurrence or metastasis was suspected, further examinations, including CT, magnetic resources imaging (MRI) and hepatic angiography, were performed. Biopsies were obtained when necessary. Patients with confirmed recurrence received further treatment, such as a second surgical resection, radiofrequency ablation, transcatheter arterial chemoembolization, or percutaneous ethanol injection. The median follow-up was 36 months (range, 2–83 months). Of the 227 patients, 97 patients (42.7%) died, 143 patients (63.0%) were diagnosed with tumor recurrence, and 84 patients (37.0%) remained alive without recurrence on follow-up. Data were censored at the last follow-up for patients without recurrence or death. Overall survival (OS) was defined as the interval between the dates of surgery and the date of death or the last follow-up. Recurrence-free survival (RFS) was defined as the interval between the dates of surgery and recurrence or the last follow-up if no recurrence was observed.

Ethics Statement

Written informed consents were obtained from all patients. All samples were coded anonymously, in strict accordance with local ethical guidelines and as stipulated by the Declaration of Helsinki. Before the study, the protocol was approved by the Research Ethics Committee of Sun Yat-sen University Cancer Center.

Tissue Microarray, Immunohistochemistry and Immunocytochemistry

Tissue microarray (TMA) was constructed as described previously [22,24]. Briefly, representative areas away from necrotic and hemorrhagic materials were premarked in the paraffin-embedded blocks by hematoxylin-eosin staining. Duplicates of 1-mm diameter cylinders from the center of the tumor and nontumor liver tissues were obtained from each case to ensure reproducibility and homogeneity. Immunohistochemistry (IHC) for CXCL17 was carried out on paraffin-embedded sections from the 227 patients to better define the anatomical localization of CXCL17 signals. IHC for CD4 (CD4 T cells), CD8 (CD8 T cells), CD20 (B cells), CD57 (natural killer cells), CD15 (neutrophils), and CD68 (macrophages) was performed on TMA sections from 101 specimens randomly selected from the 227 specimens.

IHC and immunocytochemistry (ICC) was carried out using a 2-step protocol (DakoCytomation, Glostrup, Denmark). For IHC, after dewaxing, hydration and endogenous peroxidase blocking was carried out (0.3% H_2O_2 for 10 min). Antigen retrieval was performed by steaming the sections in 10 mM citrate buffer (pH 6.0) for 10 min. Sections were incubated overnight at 4°C with mouse anti-CXCL17 (Monoclonal Mouse IgG2B; clone 422208; R&D Systems, Minneapolis, MN) anti-CD4, anti-CD8, anti-CD57 (Neomarkers, Fremont, CA), anti-CD20, anti-CD15 (Beijing Zhongshan Golden Bridge Biotechnology, Beijing, China), and anti-CD68 (DakoCytomation) antibodies. Horseradish peroxidase-conjugated anti-mouse and anti-rabbit Dako EnVision systems (DakoCytomation) were used as secondary detection reagents and developed with 3,3'-diaminobenzidine (DAB). All sections were counterstained with Mayer's hematoxylin and mounted in non-aqueous mounting medium. Appropriate negative controls were used, in which the primary antibodies were replaced by the same concentration of irrelevant, isotype-matched antibodies. For ICC, leukocytes were isolated from peripheral blood of healthy donors. Density-gradient separation on polymorphprep was performed. The pale-red granulocyte layer was washed and the contaminated erythrocytes were lysed by a brief hypotonic lysis. The cells were then cytospun and cultured in medium alone or with 20% culture supernatants from hepatoma cell-line cells (HepG2 and Huh7) or LPS (50 ng/mL) respectively for 12 h. CXCL17 was stained as IHC staining as described above.

Immunofluorescent Staining and Quantification

Paraffin-embedded HCC sections were incubated overnight at 4°C with primary mouse anti-CXCL17 and rabbit anti-myeloperoxidase (MPO; DakoCytomation), followed by Alexa Fluor 488 donkey anti-mouse and Alexa Fluor 555 donkey anti-rabbit antibodies, respectively (Invitrogen, Carlsbad, CA). Nuclei were stained with 4',6-diamidino-2-phenylindole (DAPI). Slides were mounted with anti-fade mounting medium, dried for 24 h at room

Table 1. Clinical characteristics of 227 patients with HCC.

Variables	Group 1 (CXCL17)	Group 2 (TMA)
Cases (n)	227	101
Age, years (median, range)	51, 13–79	52, 23–73
Gender (male/female)	197/30	90/11
HBsAg (negative/positive)	18/209	1/100
Cirrhosis (absent/present)	85/142	38/63
ALT (U/liter, ≤42/>42)	138/89	60/41
AST (U/liter, ≤42/>42)	131/96	60/41
AFP (ng/ml, ≤25/>25)	78/149	29/72
Tumor size (cm, ≤5/>5)	96/131	37/64
Tumor differentiation (I–II/III–IV)	129/98	44/57
Vascular invasion (absent/present)	186/41	83/18
Tumor multiplicity (solitary/multiple)	170/57	71/30
Capsulation (absent/present)	52/175	23/78
TNM stage (I–II/III–IV)	122/105	51/50
BCLC stage (0–A vs. B–C)	136/91	57/44

Abbreviations: AFP: alpha-fetoprotein; ALT: alanine aminotransferase; AST: aspartate aminotransferase; BCLC: Barcelona Clinic Liver Cancer; HBsAg: hepatitis B surface antigen; TMA: Tissue microarray; TNM: tumor-nodes-metastasis.

temperature, and then stored at $-20°C$ for future use. Images were captured and analyzed using an Olympus FV1000 confocal laser scanning microscope (Center Valley, PA). To quantify the proportion of $CXCL17^+$ cells, numbers of single-positive or double-positive cells in each of five representative fields at ×400 magnification were counted manually by two independent, blinded observers.

Automated Image Acquisition and Quantification of IHC Staining

To detect and evaluate the CXCL17 signal in HCC tumors without bias, we established an automated and standardized quantification method using the Vectra-Inform image analysis system (Perkin-Elmer Applied Biosystems, Foster City, CA) [26–28]. Stained sections were captured with the Nuance VIS-FL Multispectral Imaging System and analyzed with InForm 2.0.1 image analysis software (Perkin-Elmer Applied Biosystems). Images were acquired at 440–700 nm at 20-nm intervals. The spectrum for each chromogen was determined on single-stained control slides and was analyzed by multispectral imaging analysis. A spectral unmixing algorithm separated the grayscale images representing each spectral component quantitatively (Fig. S1A–D). The InForm software enabled tissue compartment (tumor tissue, peritumoral stroma tissue, blank) and cell compartment (cytoplasm, nucleus) segmentation (Fig. S1E–H). The DAB object density counts per megapixel for each tissue category were used for further analysis. Examination of immune infiltrate densities (CD4, CD8, CD20, CD57, CD15, CD68) on TMA were also performed using a method similar to that established for quantifying CXCL17. The total number of CD4, CD8, CD20, CD57, CD15, and CD68 positive cells was deemed identified as the total immune cell infiltrations in the tissue. The percentage of each immune cell subset was calculated by dividing the absolute number of each subset by the total numbers of all these cells.

Statistical Analysis

Subgroups of each immunostaining parameter were divided by their median values. Correlations between immunostaining parameters and clinicopathological features were analyzed by χ^2 tests or Fisher's exact test where appropriate. The association between the numbers of tumor-infiltrating immune cells and CXCL17 was calculated with the Pearson test. Survival analysis was carried out with the Kaplan-Meier method and was compared using the log-rank test. A multivariate Cox proportional hazards regression model was applied to estimate the adjusted hazard ratio (HR) and 95% confidence interval (CI) and to identify independent prognostic factors. For each analysis, 2-sided $P<0.05$ was considered statistically significant. All statistical analyses were performed with SPSS 17.0.

Results

CXCL17 Expression in HCC Tissue

We performed IHC staining of CXCL17 in paraffin-embedded sections to detect CXCL17 in HCC tumors. CXCL17 signals were mainly located in the cytoplasm of stromal cells, but were also observed occasionally in the cytoplasm or nuclei of tumor cells (Fig. 1A). There were CXCL17-producing cells in the nontumor, peritumoral stroma, and intratumoral regions with mean (± SEM) density of 100.0 ± 12.06, 100.5 ± 8.65, 99.3 ± 12.07, respectively (Fig. 1A). The CXCL17 expression was also been examined on human hepatitis tissues (n = 8) with mean (± SEM) density of 29.05 ± 11.13 (Fig. 1A). To determine the source of CXCL17 in HCC tissue, we performed double staining for CXCL17 and various immune cell markers. Confocal microscopic analysis showed that CXCL17 was mainly produced by MPO-positive neutrophils ($68.8\%\pm2.7\%$), and most of MPO-positive neutrophils produced CXCL17 ($78.3\%\pm1.8\%$) (Fig. 1C). Stromal cells with mononuclear morphology and tumor cells also produced CXCL17 (Fig. 1B).

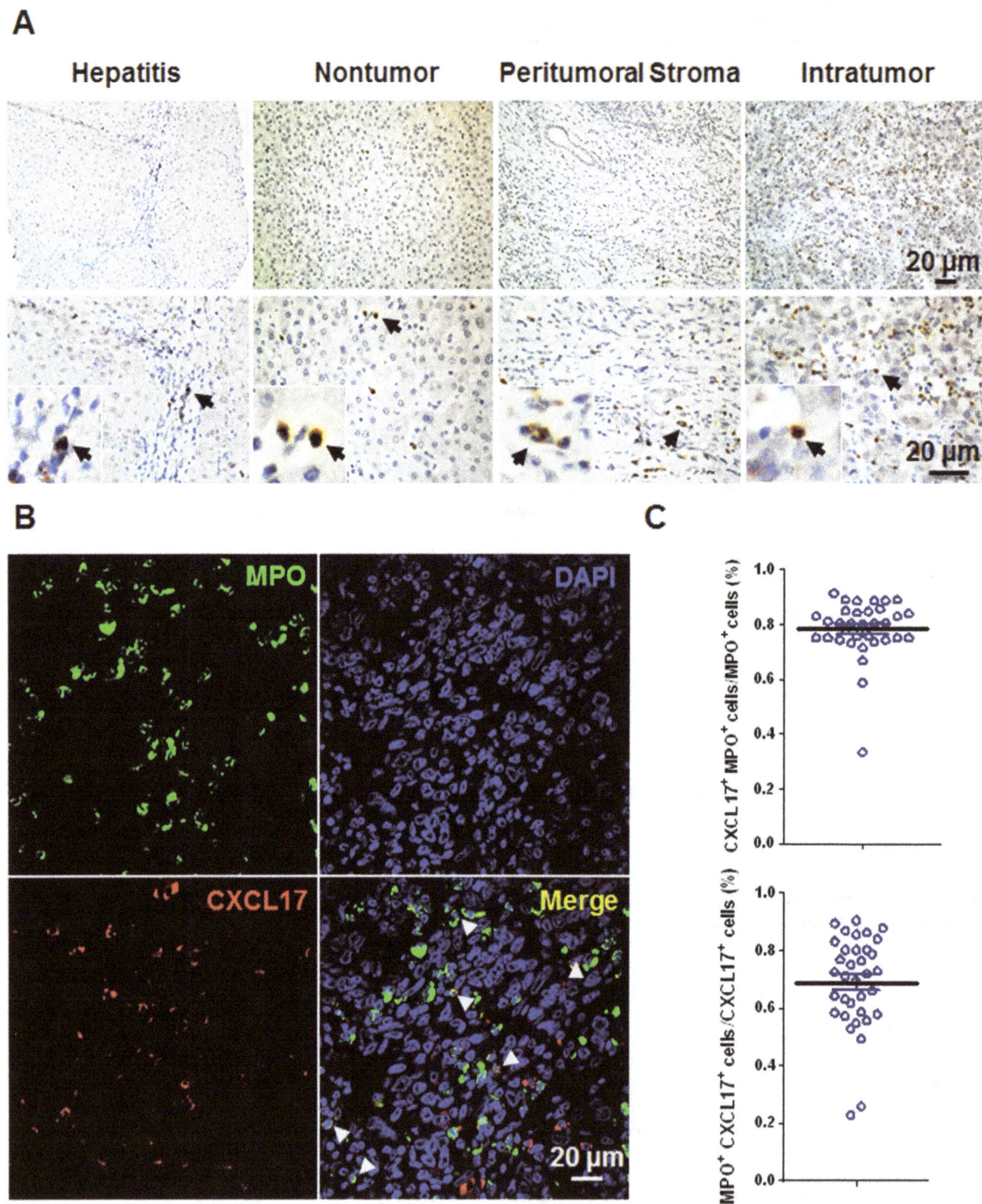

Figure 1. CXCL17 expression *in situ* in HCC tumors. (A) Representative sites depicting CXCL17-producing cells stained brown in human chronic hepatitis liver, nontumor, peritumoral stroma, and intratumoral regions in HCC. Representative sites with low (upper panels) and high (lower panels) magnification were shown. Black arrows indicated CXCL17$^+$ cells. (B) Multiple staining of MPO (green), CXCL17 (red), and DAPI (blue, nuclei) in paraffin-embedded sections analyzed by confocal microscopy. The coexistence of MPO and CXCL17 confirmed that a proportion of MPO$^+$ neutrophils expressed CXCL17. White arrows indicated representative neutrophils expressed CXCL17. (C) Proportions of CXCL17$^+$MPO$^+$ cells in CXCL17$^+$ cells or MPO$^+$ cells of HCC tissue. Results are expressed as mean $\pm$ SEM (bars).

Increased CXCL17 Predicted Poor Survival

To determine whether CXCL17 can be a prognostic marker for HCC, we plotted Kaplan-Meier survival curves to investigate the correlation between CXCL17 expression and survival. Follow-up was completed on January 8, 2014, with a median follow-up duration of 36 months (range, 2–83 months). The 1-, 3-, 5-year OS and RFS rates were 82.7%, 61.8%, 51.2% and 59.9%, 39.2%, 34.4%, respectively. The CXCL17[high] and CXCL17[low] subgroups were divided by the median CXCL17 object density per megapixel (median intratumoral, peritumoral, nontumoral CXCL17 = 20.7, 46.4, 30.1, respectively).

Univariate analysis revealed that both increased intratumoral CXCL17 ($P = 0.017$ for OS, $P = 0.005$ for RFS, Table 2) and higher peritumoral CXCL17 ($P = 0.002$ for OS, $P < 0.001$ for RFS, Table 2) were associated with shorter OS (intratumoral: 50 months vs. >72 months; peritumoral: 35 months vs. >72 months, respectively) and RFS (intratumoral: 13 months vs. 33 months; peritumoral: 13 months vs. 45 months, respectively). Patients in the CXCL17[low] group had a significantly lower 5-year recurrence rate compared with patients in the CXCL17[high] group (peritumoral: 53.1% vs. 77.7%, $P < 0.001$, intratumoral: 58.6% vs. 73.0%, $P = 0.003$, log-rank test, Fig. 2). When stratified by tumor multiplicity, the peritumoral CXCL17 density remained a good predictor of OS (all $P < 0.05$, Fig. S5). Moreover, regardless of tumor differentiation grade, tumor size, TNM stage, and aspartate transaminase (AST) and AFP levels, peritumoral CXCL17 was a good predictor of recurrence (all $P < 0.05$, Fig. S5).

We next assessed whether CXCL17 could serve as an independent predictor of survival by performing multivariate Cox proportional hazards analysis. Clinicopathological variables demonstrated to be significant in the univariate analysis were used as covariates, and peritumoral CXCL17 was found to be an independent prognostic factor for both OS and RFS (Table 2). Peritumoral CXCL17 was associated with elevated risk of death (HR = 2.066, 95% CI = 1.296–3.292, $P = 0.002$) and recurrence (HR = 1.844, 95% CI = 1.218–2.793, $P = 0.004$). Other than CXCL17, the multivariate Cox proportional hazards analysis demonstrated that serum AFP level was an independent predictor of both OS and RFS ($P = 0.002$, $P = 0.002$, respectively).

To evaluate the correlation between CXCL17 expression and tumor development, we also analyzed the association between CXCL17 expression and the clinicopathological parameters. Table 3 shows that increased peritumoral CXCL17 significantly correlated with presence of liver cirrhosis ($P = 0.045$) and less advanced tumor differentiation ($P = 0.004$).

Association between CXCL17 Expression and Local Immune Cell Infiltration

Chemokines are best known for their ability to recruit cells by forming chemokine gradients. To determine the potential role of CXCL17 in immune cell regulation in HCC, we performed comprehensive analyses of immune cell infiltration and examined the correlation between CXCL17 expression and CD4[+], CD8[+], CD20[+], CD57[+], CD15[+], and CD68[+] cell density in HCC tissues using the Pearson correlation test. There was a negative correlation between the intracellular number of CD4 cells and CXCL17 expression (correlation coefficient, R = −0.254, $P < 0.05$, Fig. 3B). Using the percentage of each immune cell subset in the total immune cell infiltrate as an index, we found a negative association between the intracellular percentages of CD4 versus CXCL17 (R = −0.271, $P < 0.05$, Fig. 3C) and a positive correlation between the intracellular percentages of CD68 and CXCL17 (R = 0.213, $P < 0.01$, Fig. 3C). These results indicated that CXCL17 may negatively regulated CD4[+] T cell infiltration while

positively regulated CD68[+] macrophage accumulation in HCC tumors.

Prognostic Value of Combined CXCL17 Expression and Immune Cell Infiltration

Recent studies by other groups and by us have shown that immune infiltrates influence HCC progression significantly [7,24,29–31]. Immunoscore that delineate multiple immune cell infiltrate is a powerful prognostic index [32]. Therefore, we also assessed the combined influence of CXCL17 expression and immune cell densities on prognosis. Patients with more intratumoral CD4[+], CD8[+], CD20[+], and CD57[+] cells tended to have better OS and RFS, while patients with more CD15[+] and CD68[+] cell infiltration had less favorable prognosis (Fig. S7 and S8). In the CXCL17[high] group, patients with more intratumoral CD4[+], CD8[+], CD20[+], and CD57[+] cells had longer survival, while those with more CD15[+] and CD68[+] cell infiltration had shorter survival ($P < 0.05$, Fig. S7). In patients with similar immune infiltrates, for example more CD8[+], CD20[+], or CD57[+] cell infiltration, CXCL17 could be used to further classify patients into subsets with different prognoses for RFS ($P = 0.022$, $P = 0.015$, $P = 0.010$, respectively, Fig. S8). For patients with higher CD20[+] and CD68[+] cell infiltration, CXCL17 could be used to further classify patients into subsets with different prognoses for OS, although the differences were not statistically significant ($P = 0.064$, $P = 0.079$, respectively, Fig. S7).

Discussion

In our study, we identified CXCL17 as an independent prognostic factor for HCC after resection. Patients with less CXCL17[+] cells within the tumor had significantly prolonged OS and RFS compared with the CXCL17[high] subgroup. Multivariate analysis showed that tumor-infiltrating CXCL17 could also serve as a new biomarker for predicting HCC prognosis. Furthermore, analyzing the association between CXCL17 expression and immune cell infiltration revealed a significant correlation between CXCL17 expression and CD4 and CD68 infiltration. The combined CXCL17 expression and immune cell infiltration could be used to further classify patients into subsets with different prognoses for survival. These results support the idea that CXCL17 is a substantial contributor to tumor progression.

Chemokines play critical roles in recruiting a number of different cell types to the tumor microenvironment and are involved in many aspects of tumor progression [9,33]. In the liver, the CXCL12-CXCR4, CX3CL1-CX3CR1, and CCL20-CCR6 axes have received much attention due to their regulation of tumor metastasis, tumor proliferation, and immune cell infiltration [34]. CXCL17 is a newly identified orphan chemokine whose function and clinical significance in human tumors remain unclear [17,18]. In breast cancer and colon tumor, CXCL17 is coregulated with vascular endothelial growth factor (VEGF) and it increases vasculature in vivo, suggesting that it might promote tumor progression by enhancing angiogenesis [17–19]. CXCL17 overexpression increased the number of CD11b[+]/Gr-1[+] myeloid-derived cells in colon tumor and was accompanied by enhanced tumorigenicity, implying that CXCL17 plays a tumor-promoting role by regulating immune cell recruitment [35]. Moreover, CXCL17 overexpression in HepG2 cells inhibits cisplatin-induced apoptosis, thus providing evidence that CXCL17 might be a potential cellular target for enhancing chemotherapy efficiency [21]. Interestingly, CXCL17 may also be involved in anti-tumor immune response. CXCL17 is upregulated in premalignant intraductal papillary mucinous neoplasm, suggesting that it acts

Table 2. Univariate and multivariate analyses of factors associated with survival and recurrence.

Variables	OS Univariate P	OS Multivariate HR	OS Multivariate 95% CI	OS Multivariate P	RFS Univariate P	RFS Multivariate HR	RFS Multivariate 95% CI	RFS Multivariate P
Age (>51 vs. ≤51 years)	0.413			NA	0.145			NA
Gender (male vs. female)	0.755			NA	0.261			NA
HBsAg (positive vs. negative)	0.533			NA	0.079			NA
Cirrhosis (present vs. absent)	0.321			NA	0.310			NA
ALT (>42 vs. ≤42 U/L)	0.250			NA	0.620			NA
AST (>42 vs. ≤42 U/L)	0.003	1.468	0.960–2.246	0.077	0.010	1.348	0.948–1.917	0.097
AFP (>25 vs. ≤25 ng/ml)	0.001	2.181	1.331–3.574	0.002	0.004	1.738	1.190–2.540	0.004
Tumor size (>5 vs. ≤5 cm)	0.005	1.367	0.841–2.224	0.208	0.008	1.215	0.818–1.803	0.334
Tumor differentiation (III–IV vs. I–II)	0.154			NA	0.354			NA
Vascular invasion (present vs. absent)	0.001	1.367	0.706–2.645	0.354	0.025	1.110	0.626–1.966	0.721
Tumor multiplicity (multiple vs. solitary)	≤0.001	1.269	0.647–2.490	0.488	≤0.001	1.515	0.859–2.670	0.151
Capsulation (present vs. absent)	0.107			NA	0.073			NA
TNM stage (III–IV vs. I–II)	≤0.001	1.031	0.593–1.794	0.914	0.001	1.025	0.646–1.627	0.915
BCLC stage (B–C vs. 0–A)	≤0.001	1.656	0.737–3.718	0.222	≤0.001	1.352	0.699–2.614	0.370
Nontumoral CXCL17 (high vs. low)	0.118			NA	0.003	1.289	0.868–1.916	0.208
Peritumoral CXCL17 (high vs. low)	0.002	2.066	1.296–3.292	0.002	≤0.001	1.844	1.218–2.793	0.004
Intratumoral CXCL17 (high vs. low)	0.017	1.344	0.845–2.137	0.212	0.005	1.223	0.836–1.788	0.299

Note: Cox proportional hazards regression model was used. Variables used in multivariate analysis were adopted by univariate analysis. Underlined terms indicate statistical significance. Abbreviations: AFP: alpha-fetoprotein; ALT: alanine aminotransferase; AST: aspartate aminotransferase; BCLC: Barcelona Clinic Liver Cancer; CI: confidence interval; HBsAg: hepatitis B surface antigen; HR: hazard ratio; NA: not adopted; TNM: tumor-nodes-metastasis.

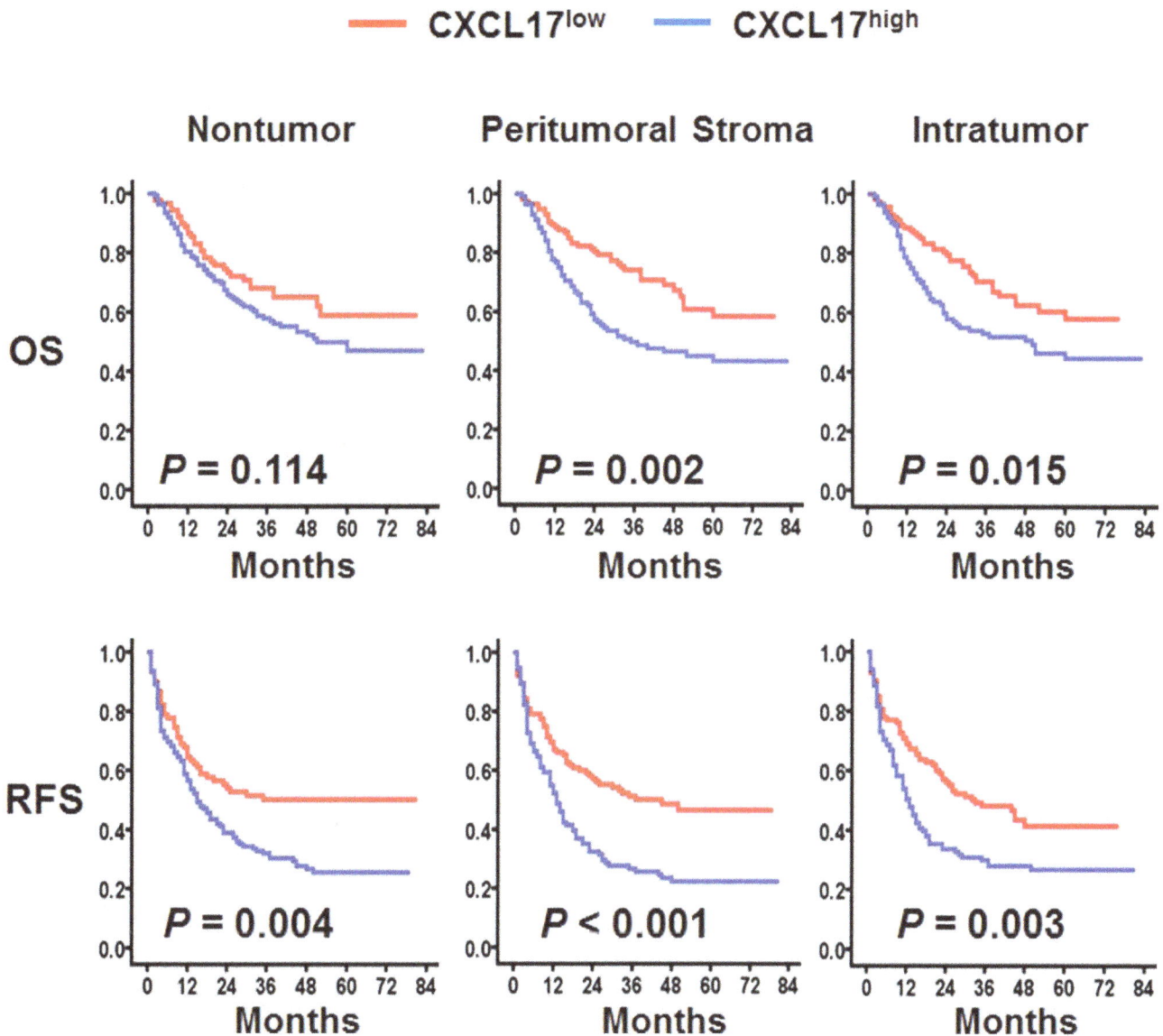

Figure 2. Accumulation of CXCL17-producing cells predicted poor survival in HCC. OS (top) and RFS (bottom) were estimated by the Kaplan-Meier method and compared using the log-rank test (n = 227).

as a danger signal during the early stages of pancreatic carcinogenesis. In malignant intraductal papillary mucinous carcinoma, CXCL17 is downregulated and is associated with decreased DC infiltration, implying that it might be one strategy for tumor escape from immune surveillance [20]. In the present study, we found abundant CXCL17+ cell infiltrated in HCC tumor but were relatively rare in hepatitis liver. The CXCL17 expression was a significant predictor of unfavorable RFS and OS in HCC patients, implying that CXCL17 functions as a pro-tumor factor in HCC. However, we found no correlation between CXCL17 expression and Ki-67 (Fig. S9A), a marker indicating tumor cell proliferation activity or between CD34+ vessel area (Fig. S9B), which indicated the angiogenesis of tumor. These data suggested that CXCL17 may not promote tumor growth or angiogenesis directly, but rather may exhibit pro-tumor abilities by regulating immunological responses in HCC.

To answer the question of whether CXCL17 regulates other immune cell subsets in HCC tumors, we evaluated the association between CXCL17 expression and local immune cell infiltration. We found a positive correlation between the intratumoral percentages of CD68 and CXCL17. CXCL17 was a chemoattractant of monocytes and macrophages. Other groups and ours have demonstrated that tumor-associated macrophage (TAM) number is a poor prognostic marker in HCC [30,31,36–38]. TAM accumulating at tumor sites exhibit immunosuppressive activity by expressing high levels of interleukin 10 and programmed death ligand 1, and promote angiogenesis by producing metalloelastase and VEGF [6,39]. A previous study showed that CXCL17 significantly suppressed the production of proinflammatory cytokines and factors by murine J774 macrophage or primary macrophage [40]. In addition, CXCL17 induced the production of proangiogenic factors such as VEGF by treated monocytes, suggesting an indirect proangiogenic effect of CXCL17 [17]. Thus, the positive correlation between CXCL17 and macrophages in HCC indicates that CXCL17 may promote HCC progression

Table 3. Association of CXCL17 with clinicopathological characteristics.

Variable		Nontumoral CXCL17			Peritumoral CXCL17			Intratumoral CXCL17		
		Low	High	P	Low	High	P	Low	High	P
Age (year)	≤51	58	58	0.946	62	54	0.320	60	56	0.549
	>51	56	55		52	59		53	58	
Gender	Male	99	98	0.979	100	97	0.676	98	99	0.979
	Female	15	15		14	16		15	15	
HBsAg	Negtive	8	10	0.610	9	9	0.984	9	9	0.984
	Positive	106	103		105	104		104	105	
Cirrhosis	Absent	47	38	0.237	50	35	0.045	49	36	0.067
	Present	67	75		64	78		64	78	
ALT (U/liter)	≤42	67	71	0.531	68	70	0.723	70	68	0.723
	>42	47	42		46	43		43	46	
AST (U/liter)	≤42	62	69	0.309	60	71	0.120	64	67	0.745
	>42	52	44		54	42		49	47	
AFP (ng/ml)	≤25	38	40	0.743	35	43	0.244	33	45	0.103
	>25	76	73		79	70		80	69	
Tumor size (cm)	≤5	51	45	0.454	48	48	0.955	49	47	0.745
	>5	63	68		66	65		64	67	
Tumor differentiation	I + II	58	71	0.069	54	75	0.004	63	66	0.745
	III + IV	56	42		60	38		50	48	
Vascular invasion	Absent	93	93	0.888	95	91	0.583	95	91	0.406
	Present	21	20		19	22		18	23	
Tumor multiplicity	Solitary	83	87	0.467	83	87	0.467	84	86	0.848
	Multiple	31	26		31	26		29	28	
Capsulation	Absent	23	29	0.325	21	31	0.106	23	29	0.362
	Present	91	84		93	82		90	85	
TNM stage	I + II	67	55	0.127	68	54	0.073	66	56	0.161
	III + IV	47	58		46	59		47	58	
BCLC stage	0–A	68	68	0.935	69	67	0.850	69	67	0.725
	B–C	46	45		45	46		44	47	

Note: Underlined terms indicate statistical significance. Abbreviations: AFP: alpha-fetoprotein; ALT: alanine aminotransferase; AST: aspartate aminotransferase; BCLC: Barcelona Clinic Liver Cancer; CI: confidence interval; HBsAg: hepatitis B surface antigen; TNM: tumor-nodes-metastasis.

A

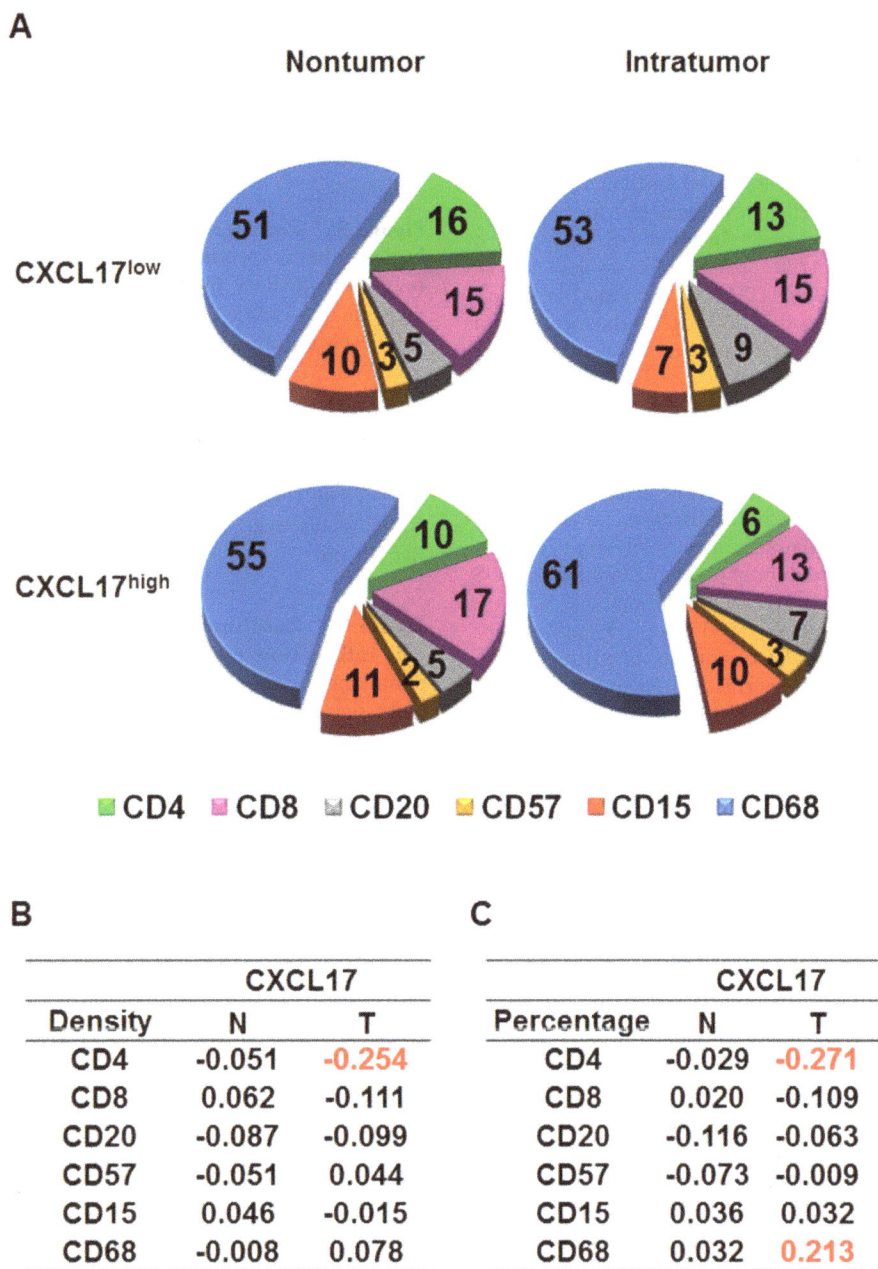

Figure 3. Composition of immune infiltrates according to CXCL17 expression. (A) Pie charts summarized the percentages of nontumor-infiltrating (N, left) and tumor-infiltrating (T, right) CD4, CD8, CD20, CD57, CD15, and CD68 cells in CXCL17[low] and CXCL17[high] groups. (B, C) Correlation coefficients between the density or percentage of CXCL17 and the density of each immune cell subset were shown.

B

	CXCL17	
Density	N	T
CD4	-0.051	-0.254
CD8	0.062	-0.111
CD20	-0.087	-0.099
CD57	-0.051	0.044
CD15	0.046	-0.015
CD68	-0.008	0.078

C

	CXCL17	
Percentage	N	T
CD4	-0.029	-0.271
CD8	0.020	-0.109
CD20	-0.116	-0.063
CD57	-0.073	-0.009
CD15	0.036	0.032
CD68	0.032	0.213

by regulating TAM homing, cytokine production, and proangiogenic activity.

We found a negative association between the intracellular percentages of CD4 and CXCL17. However, we did not examine specific CD4 T cell subpopulations, such as T helper 1 cells, T helper 17 cells, and regulatory T cells. CD4 T cells in the tumor comprised of cell populations with both positive and negative effects on tumor immunity [29,41,42]. Overall, CD4 cells tended to predict favorable prognosis in HCC. Therefore, the negative association between CXCL17 and CD4 cells also indicated the pro-tumor effect of CXCL17 in HCC.

The lineage of CXCL17-producing cells in HCC has not been explored before. CXCL17 is expressed by CD68[+] macrophages and CD138[+] plasma cells in mucosal tissue of the intestine or bronchus [18]. By using multiple immunofluorescence staining we revealed that CXCL17 was mainly expressed by stromal cells in the peritumoral region, while tumor cells expressed CXCL17 with lower intensity. In the peritumoral stroma, neutrophils were the major source of CXCL17 production, which has not been described previously. Cells with macrophage morphology also produced CXCL17, as previously reported. To determine whether CXCL17 was induced in HCC, we also examined whether neutrophils from human peripheral blood could express CXCL17. Considering <1% of peripheral neutrophils produce CXCL17 (data not shown), CXCL17 might be induced in HCC *in situ*. To determine whether CXCL17 could be induced in HCC, we examined leukocytes from human peripheral blood exposed to 20% TSNs from two human hepatoma cells (HepG2 and Huh7). The expression of CXCL17 on neutrophils was up-regulated by TSN treatment and to a less extend by LPS stimulation (Fig. S10). Alternatively, CXCL17$^+$ cells other than CXCL17$^-$ neutrophils may be specifically recruited to the tumor microenvironment. CXCL17 is predicted to be structurally and functionally related to CXCL8, which is a strong, well-known chemokine for neutrophil recruitment [18]. CXCL17 expression by tumor cells was reported to recruit CD11b$^+$Gr1^{high}F4/80$^-$ neutrophilic myeloid-derived suppressor cells [35]. Therefore, CXCL17 expression in tumor-infiltrating neutrophils implies that CXCL17$^+$ neutrophils might regulate neutrophil infiltration in an autocrine manner. In addition, other groups and ours have revealed that tumor-infiltrating neutrophils are a poor prognostic factor for HCC following resection [7,31]. Thus, CXCL17 might be responsible for neutrophil accumulation in tumor and contribute to the immunosuppressive microenvironment in the tumor.

In conclusion, we demonstrate for the first time that CXCL17 is mainly produced by tumor-infiltrating neutrophils and that it can be used as an independent indicator of poor prognosis for both OS and RFS in HCC. CXCL17 expression correlates with unfavorable immune infiltration, and combined CXCL17 and immune cell density further classifies HCC patients into subsets with different prognosis. Therefore, patients with increased CXCL17 may require closer follow-up after surgery. Further studies that define the potential regulatory role of CXCL17 in tumor-infiltrating neutrophils/macrophages in HCC may provide new insights into therapeutic strategies aimed at forming an effective immune response in HCC.

Supporting Information

Figure S1 Details of automated quantification method for IHC staining. (A) Raw image acquired using the 20× objective lens on the Vectra scanner. (B) DAB and (C) hematoxylin staining unmixed according to their respective spectra. (D) Composite of unmixed stains reassigned with different colors for easier interpretation. (E) Representative image trained to establish the tissue segmentation algorithm. User-drawn training regions indicate tumor tissue (yellow), peritumoral stroma (blue), and blank (red) categories. (F) Representative compartment map following automated segmentation. (G) Object segmentation map for DAB staining (brown). The background color was removed for better visualization of the illustrated compartment. (H) Final composite map of the automated tissue and object segmentation.

Figure S2 Representative images for isotype control and CXCL17 staining. A mouse IgG2B isotype control was used for CXCL17 antibody. Bar: 20 μm.

Figure S3 Representative images for double-color immunofluorescence. Multiple staining of (A) macrophage marker CD163 (green), or (B) the T cell marker CD3 (green) CXCL17 (red), and DAPI (blue, nuclei) in paraffin-embedded sections analyzed by confocal microscopy.

Figure S4 The dynamic change of CXCL17 expression in different regions of HCC tissue. Paraffin-embedded HCC sections were stained with CXCL17 antibody. The density of CXCL17$^+$ cells in nontumor (N), peritumor (P) and intratumor (T) regions of the same block were calculated (n = 227). Results are expressed as mean ± SEM (bars) of groups.

Figure S5 Patients were stratified according to pathological characteristics and peritumoral CXCL17 density. OS and RFS in relation to tumor multiplicity, tumor differentiation grade, tumor size, TNM stage, and AST and AFP levels in each subgroup were analyzed.

Figure S6 Immunohistochemisty staining for the various immune cell subsets in CXCL17 low versus CXCL17 high tumors. Immunohistochemisty for CD4 (CD4 T cells), CD8 (CD8 T cells), CD20 (B cells), CD57 (natural killer cells), CD15 (neutrophils), and CD68 (macrophages) was performed. Bar: 20 μm.

Figure S7 Combined CXCL17 expression and immune cell infiltration correlated with OS. Kaplan-Meier curves illustrating the duration of OS and RFS according to CXCL17 expression and density of CD4, CD8, CD20, CD57, CD15, and CD68 cells in the tumor region. Statistically significant differences are indicated in red.

Figure S8 Combined CXCL17 expression and immune cell infiltration correlated with RFS. Kaplan-Meier curves illustrating the duration of OS and RFS according to CXCL17 expression and density of CD4, CD8, CD20, CD57, CD15, and CD68 cells in the tumor region. Statistically significant differences are indicated in red.

Figure S9 CXCL17 expression and tumor cell proliferation and angiogenesis. Correlation between intratumoral CXCL17 expression and tumor cell proliferation rate determined by Ki-67 immunostaining (A) and tumor angiogenesis determined by CD34-vessel area (object density) (B).

Figure S10 Hepatoma TSN induced CXCL17 expression in neutrophil in vitro. Leukocytes were isolated from healthy donor peripheral blood. Cells were cultured in complete medium with 20% of tumor supernatant from HepG2 and Huh7 cells, or 50 ng/mL LPS for 12 h respectively. Control group was left untreated for 12 h. Cells were then cytospin and immunocytochemistry for CXCL17 was performed. Bar: 20 μm.

Author Contributions

Conceived and designed the experiments: LL JY LZ ZJZ WYL. Performed the experiments: LL JY JX CQL. Analyzed the data: LL JY HWC YJ ZPW JYH. Contributed reagents/materials/analysis tools: LL JY JX. Contributed to the writing of the manuscript: LL JY JX WYL LZ.

References

1. Jemal A, Bray F, Center MM, Ferlay J, Ward E, et al. (2011) Global cancer statistics. CA: a cancer journal for clinicians 61: 69–90.
2. Yang JD, Roberts LR (2010) Hepatocellular carcinoma: a global view. Nature Reviews Gastroenterology and Hepatology 7: 448–458.
3. Poon D, Anderson BO, Chen L-T, Tanaka K, Lau WY, et al. (2009) Management of hepatocellular carcinoma in Asia: consensus statement from the Asian Oncology Summit 2009. The lancet oncology 10: 1111–1118.

4. Llovet JM, Bruix J (2008) Molecular targeted therapies in hepatocellular carcinoma. Hepatology 48: 1312–1327.

5. Villanueva A, Hoshida Y, Toffanin S, Lachenmayer A, Alsinet C, et al. (2010) New strategies in hepatocellular carcinoma: genomic prognostic markers. Clinical Cancer Research 16: 4688–4694.

6. Kuang D-M, Zhao Q, Peng C, Xu J, Zhang J-P, et al. (2009) Activated monocytes in peritumoral stroma of hepatocellular carcinoma foster immune privilege and disease progression through PD-L1. The Journal of experimental medicine 206: 1327–1337.

7. Kuang D-M, Zhao Q, Wu Y, Peng C, Wang J, et al. (2011) Peritumoral neutrophils link inflammatory response to disease progression by fostering angiogenesis in hepatocellular carcinoma. Journal of hepatology 54: 948–955.

8. Bjorkstrom NK, Ljunggren HG, Sandberg JK (2010) CD56 negative NK cells: origin, function, and role in chronic viral disease. Trends Immunol 31: 401–406.

9. Balkwill F (2004) Cancer and the chemokine network. Nature Reviews Cancer 4: 540–550.

10. Mishra P, Banerjee D, Ben-Baruch A (2011) Chemokines at the crossroads of tumor-fibroblast interactions that promote malignancy. Journal of leukocyte biology 89: 31–39.

11. Mantovani A (2009) The yin-yang of tumor-associated neutrophils. Cancer cell 16: 173–174.

12. Lazennec G, Richmond A (2010) Chemokines and chemokine receptors: new insights into cancer-related inflammation. Trends in molecular medicine 16: 133–144.

13. Rotondi M, Chiovato L, Romagnani S, Serio M, Romagnani P (2007) Role of chemokines in endocrine autoimmune diseases. Endocrine reviews 28: 492–520.

14. Abastado JP (2012) The next challenge in cancer immunotherapy: controlling T-cell traffic to the tumor. Cancer Res 72: 2159–2161.

15. Zhou SL, Dai Z, Zhou ZJ, Wang XY, Yang GH, et al. (2012) Overexpression of CXCL5 mediates neutrophil infiltration and indicates poor prognosis for hepatocellular carcinoma. Hepatology 56: 2242–2254.

16. Gao Q, Zhao Y-J, Wang X-Y, Qiu S-J, Shi Y-H, et al. (2012) CXCR6 upregulation contributes to a proinflammatory tumor microenvironment that drives metastasis and poor patient outcomes in hepatocellular carcinoma. Cancer research 72: 3546–3556.

17. Weinstein EJ, Head R, Griggs DW, Sun D, Evans RJ, et al. (2006) VCC-1, a novel chemokine, promotes tumor growth. Biochemical and biophysical research communications 350: 74–81.

18. Pisabarro MT, Leung B, Kwong M, Corpuz R, Frantz GD, et al. (2006) Cutting edge: novel human dendritic cell-and monocyte-attracting chemokine-like protein identified by fold recognition methods. The Journal of Immunology 176: 2069–2073.

19. Mu X, Chen Y, Wang S, Huang X, Pan H, et al. (2009) Overexpression of VCC-1 gene in human hepatocellular carcinoma cells promotes cell proliferation and invasion. Acta biochimica et biophysica Sinica 41: 631–637.

20. Hiraoka N, Yamazaki-Itoh R, Ino Y, Mizuguchi Y, Yamada T, et al. (2011) CXCL17 and ICAM2 are associated with a potential anti-tumor immune response in early intraepithelial stages of human pancreatic carcinogenesis. Gastroenterology 140: 310–321. e314.

21. Zhou Z, Lu X, Zhu P, Zhu W, Mu X, et al. (2012) VCC-1 over-expression inhibits cisplatin-induced apoptosis in HepG2 cells. Biochemical and biophysical research communications 420: 336–342.

22. Xu J, Ding T, He Q, Yu X-J, Wu W-C, et al. (2012) An in situ molecular signature to predict early recurrence in hepatitis B virus-related hepatocellular carcinoma. Journal of hepatology 57: 313–321.

23. Bruix J, Llovet JM (2002) Prognostic prediction and treatment strategy in hepatocellular carcinoma. Hepatology 35: 519–524.

24. Gao Q, Qiu S-J, Fan J, Zhou J, Wang X-Y, et al. (2007) Intratumoral balance of regulatory and cytotoxic T cells is associated with prognosis of hepatocellular carcinoma after resection. Journal of Clinical Oncology 25: 2586–2593.

25. Ding T, Xu J, Zhang Y, Guo RP, Wu WC, et al. (2011) Endothelium-coated tumor clusters are associated with poor prognosis and micrometastasis of hepatocellular carcinoma after resection. Cancer 117: 4878–4889.

26. Huang W, Hennrick K, Drew S (2013) A colorful future of quantitative pathology: validation of Vectra technology using chromogenic multiplexed immunohistochemistry and prostate tissue microarrays. Human pathology 44: 29–38.

27. Nicholson TM, Sehgal PD, Drew SA, Huang W, Ricke WA (2013) Sex steroid receptor expression and localization in benign prostatic hyperplasia varies with tissue compartment. Differentiation 85: 140–149.

28. Abel EJ, Bauman TM, Weiker M, Shi F, Downs TM, et al. (2014) Analysis and validation of tissue biomarkers for renal cell carcinoma using automated high throughput evaluation of protein expression. Human pathology. 45: 1092–1099.

29. Zhang J-P, Yan J, Xu J, Pang X-H, Chen M-S, et al. (2009) Increased intratumoral IL-17-producing cells correlate with poor survival in hepatocellular carcinoma patients. Journal of hepatology 50: 980–989.

30. Ding T, Xu J, Wang F, Shi M, Zhang Y, et al. (2009) High tumor-infiltrating macrophage density predicts poor prognosis in patients with primary hepatocellular carcinoma after resection. Human pathology 40: 381–389.

31. Li Y-W, Qiu S-J, Fan J, Zhou J, Gao Q, et al. (2011) Intratumoral neutrophils: a poor prognostic factor for hepatocellular carcinoma following resection. Journal of hepatology 54: 497–505.

32. Galon J, Angell HK, Bedognetti D, Marincola FM (2013) The continuum of cancer immunosurveillance: prognostic, predictive, and mechanistic signatures. Immunity 39: 11–26.

33. Mantovani A, Allavena P, Sica A, Balkwill F (2008) Cancer-related inflammation. Nature 454: 436–444.

34. Huang F, Geng X-P (2010) Chemokines and hepatocellular carcinoma. World journal of gastroenterology: WJG 16: 1832.

35. Matsui A, Yokoo H, Negishi Y, Endo-Takahashi Y, Chun NA, et al. (2012) CXCL17 Expression by Tumor Cells Recruits CD11b+ Gr1highF4/80− Cells and Promotes Tumor Progression. PLoS One 7: e44080.

36. Zhu X-D, Zhang J-B, Zhuang P-Y, Zhu H-G, Zhang W, et al. (2008) High expression of macrophage colony-stimulating factor in peritumoral liver tissue is associated with poor survival after curative resection of hepatocellular carcinoma. Journal of Clinical Oncology 26: 2707–2716.

37. Shirabe K, Mano Y, Muto J, Matono R, Motomura T, et al. (2012) Role of tumor-associated macrophages in the progression of hepatocellular carcinoma. Surgery today 42: 1–7.

38. Sica A, Larghi P, Mancino A, Rubino L, Porta C, et al. (2008) Macrophage polarization in tumour progression. Semin Cancer Biol 18: 349–355.

39. Kuang D-M, Wu Y, Chen N, Cheng J, Zhuang S-M, et al. (2007) Tumor-derived hyaluronan induces formation of immunosuppressive macrophages through transient early activation of monocytes. Blood 110: 587–595.

40. Lee W-Y, Wang C-J, Lin T-Y, Hsiao C-L, Luo C-W (2013) CXCL17, an orphan chemokine, acts as a novel angiogenic and anti-inflammatory factor. American journal of physiology Endocrinology and metabolism 304: E32–40.

41. Fridman WH, Pagès F, Sautès-Fridman C, Galon J (2012) The immune contexture in human tumours: impact on clinical outcome. Nature Reviews Cancer 12: 298–306.

42. Yan J, Zhang Y, Zhang J-P, Liang J, Li L, et al. (2013) Tim-3 expression defines regulatory T cells in human tumors. PLoS One 8: e58006.

Permissions

All chapters in this book were first published in PLOS ONE, by The Public Library of Science; hereby published with permission under the Creative Commons Attribution License or equivalent. Every chapter published in this book has been scrutinized by our experts. Their significance has been extensively debated. The topics covered herein carry significant findings which will fuel the growth of the discipline. They may even be implemented as practical applications or may be referred to as a beginning point for another development.

The contributors of this book come from diverse backgrounds, making this book a truly international effort. This book will bring forth new frontiers with its revolutionizing research information and detailed analysis of the nascent developments around the world.

We would like to thank all the contributing authors for lending their expertise to make the book truly unique. They have played a crucial role in the development of this book. Without their invaluable contributions this book wouldn't have been possible. They have made vital efforts to compile up to date information on the varied aspects of this subject to make this book a valuable addition to the collection of many professionals and students.

This book was conceptualized with the vision of imparting up-to-date information and advanced data in this field. To ensure the same, a matchless editorial board was set up. Every individual on the board went through rigorous rounds of assessment to prove their worth. After which they invested a large part of their time researching and compiling the most relevant data for our readers.

The editorial board has been involved in producing this book since its inception. They have spent rigorous hours researching and exploring the diverse topics which have resulted in the successful publishing of this book. They have passed on their knowledge of decades through this book. To expedite this challenging task, the publisher supported the team at every step. A small team of assistant editors was also appointed to further simplify the editing procedure and attain best results for the readers.

Apart from the editorial board, the designing team has also invested a significant amount of their time in understanding the subject and creating the most relevant covers. They scrutinized every image to scout for the most suitable representation of the subject and create an appropriate cover for the book.

The publishing team has been an ardent support to the editorial, designing and production team. Their endless efforts to recruit the best for this project, has resulted in the accomplishment of this book. They are a veteran in the field of academics and their pool of knowledge is as vast as their experience in printing. Their expertise and guidance has proved useful at every step. Their uncompromising quality standards have made this book an exceptional effort. Their encouragement from time to time has been an inspiration for everyone.

The publisher and the editorial board hope that this book will prove to be a valuable piece of knowledge for researchers, students, practitioners and scholars across the globe.

List of Contributors

Qi-wen Chen, Hao Chen, Zhou-yu Ning, Xiao-yan Zhu, Ye-hua Shen, Yong-qiang Hua, Jing Xie, Wei-dong Shi, Huifeng Gao, Li-tao Xu, Lan-yun Feng, Jun-hua Lin, Zhen Chen, Lu-ming Liu and Zhiqiang Meng
Department of Integrative Oncology, Fudan University Shanghai Cancer Center, Shanghai, China, Department of Oncology, Shanghai Medical College, Fudan University, Shanghai, China

Chien-shan Cheng
School of Chinese Medicine, the University of Hong Kong, Pokfulam, Hong Kong, China

Shi-feng Tang
First Department, Cancer Treatment Center, Weifang Hospital of Traditional Chinese Medicine, Weifang, Shandong Province, China

Xun Zhang
Department of Ultrasound, Fudan University Shanghai Cancer Center, Shanghai, China
Department of Oncology, Shanghai Medical College, Fudan University, Shanghai, China

Sonya Vargulick
Albany College of Pharmacy and Health Sciences, Albany, New York, United States of America

Bo Ping
Department of Pathology, Fudan University Shanghai Cancer Center, Shanghai, China Department of Oncology, Shanghai Medical College, Fudan University, Shanghai, China

Tomoko Yamazaki, Mayumi Mori, Satoko Arai, Akemi Nishijima, Toshihiro Kai, Kayo Aoyama and Toru Miyazaki
Laboratory of Molecular Biomedicine for Pathogenesis, Center for Disease Biology and Integrative Medicine, Faculty of Medicine, The University of Tokyo, Tokyo, Japan

Ryosuke Tateishi and Kazuhiko Koike
Department of Gastroenterology, Graduate School of Medicine, The University of Tokyo, Tokyo, Japan

Masanori Abe and Yoichi Hiasa
Department of Gastroenterology and Metabology, Ehime University Graduate School of Medicine, Ehime, Japan

Mihoko Ban, Maki Maeda, Kiyohiro Izumino, Jun Takahashi, Shinji Seto and Ken-ichiro Inoue
Shunkaikai, Inoue Hospital, Nagasaki, Japan

Takeharu Asano and Yukio Yoshida
Department of Gastroenterology, Jichi Medical University, Saitama Medical Center, Omiya, Japan

Sei Harada and Toru Takebayashi
Department of Preventive Medicine and Public Health, School of Medicine, Keio University, Tokyo, Japan

Toshiaki Gunji
Center for Preventive Medicine, NTT Medical Center Tokyo, Tokyo, Japan

Shin Ohnishi
National Center for Global Health and Medicine, Tokyo, Japan

Ken-ichi Yamamura
Center for Animal Resources and Development, Kumamoto University, Kumamoto, Japan

Toru Miyazaki
Max Planck-The University of Tokyo Center for Integrative Inflammology, Tokyo, Japan CREST, Japan Science and Technology Agency, Tokyo, Japan

Xiankun Zhao, Shuxiang Hu, Lu Wang, Qing Zhang, Xiaodan Zhu, Chaoqun Wang, Ruiyang Tao, Siping Guo, Jing Wang and Yuzhen Gao
Department of Forensic Medicine, Medical College of Soochow University, Suzhou, Jiangsu, P. R. China

Hua Zhao
Department of General Surgery, the First Affiliated Hospital of Soochow University, Suzhou, Jiangsu, P. R. China

Jiejie Xu
Key Laboratory of Medical Molecular Virology, MOE & MOH, School of Basic Medical Sciences, Shanghai Medical College, Fudan University, Shanghai, China

Yan He
Department of Epidemiology, Medical College of Soochow University, Suzhou, Jiangsu, P. R. China

Yi Zhang and Guoqing Liao
Department of Gastrointestinal Surgery, Xiangya Hospital, Central South University, Changsha, P. R. China

Changwei Lin
Department of Gastrointestinal Surgery, Third Xiangya Hospital, Central South University, Changsha, P. R. China

Jie Ding
Department of Gastrointestinal Surgery, Guizhou Provincial People's Hospital, Guiyang, P.R. China

Yang Li and Bo Tang
Department of Hepatobiliary Surgery, Affiliated Hospital of Guilin Medical University, Guilin, P. R. China

Hongming Liu and Bin Xie
Department of Hepatobiliary Surgery, Daping Hospital & Institute of Surgery Research, The Third Military Medical University, Chongqing, China

Guiyu Lou, Chongyi Li and Lixia Gan
Department of Biochemistry and Molecular Biology, The Third Military Medical University, Chongqing, China

Xiaodong Wang and Arthur I. Cederbaum
Department of Pharmacology and Systems Therapeutics, Icahn School of Medicine at Mount Sinai, New York, New York, United States of America

Xiaodong Wang
Chongqing Biomean Technology Co., Ltd, Chongqing, China

Xuefeng Gu, Maoying Fu, Yuqin Ding, Huihui Ni, Wei Zhang and Yanfang Zhu
Department of Infectious Diseases, The First People's Hospital of Kunshan Affiliated with Jiangsu University, Suzhou, China

Xiaojun Tang and Jin Zhu
The Key Laboratory of Cancer Biomarkers, Prevention & Treatment Cancer Center and The Key Laboratory of Antibody Technique of Ministry of Health, Nanjing Medical University, Nanjing, China

Lin Xiong
Department of Pathology, The Second Affiliated Hospital of Nanjing Medical University, Nanjing, China

Jiang Li and Liang Qiu
Department of Pathology, Jiangsu Province Geriatric Institute, Nanjing, China

Jiaren Xu
Department of Hematology and Oncology, Jiangsu Provincial Hospital, Nanjing, China

Jin Zhu
Huadong Medical Institute of Biotechniques, Nanjing, China

Mei Liu, Hongxia Zhu and Ningzhi Xu
Laboratory of Cell and Molecular Biology & State Key Laboratory of Molecular Oncology, Cancer Institute & Cancer Hospital, Chinese Academy of Medical Sciences & Peking Union Medical College, Beijing, P. R. China

Jibing Liu, Huiyong Wu and Yinfa Xie
Department of Interventional Surgical Oncology, Cancer Hospital of Shandong Province, Shandong Academy of Medical Sciences, Jinan, Shandong, China

Liming Wang
Department of Abdominal Surgery, Cancer Institute & Cancer Hospital, Chinese Academy of Medical Sciences & Peking Union Medical College, Beijing, P. R. China

Changchun Zhou
Clinical Laboratory, Cancer Hospital of Shandong Province, Shandong Academy of Medical Sciences, Jinan, Shandong, China

Tao Zhou, Lili Ye, Yu Bai, Dahai Liu, Yong Li and Bei Huang
School of life Sciences, Anhui University, Hefei, China

Aiming Sun, Bryan Cox, Dennis Liotta and James P. Snyder
Department of Chemistry, Emory University, Atlanta, Georgia, United States of America

Aiming Sun, Dennis Liotta and James P. Snyder
Emory Institute for Drug Development (EIDD), Emory University, Atlanta, Georgia, United States of America

Haian Fu
Department of Pharmacology and Emory Chemical Biology Discovery Center, Emory University, Atlanta, Georgia, United States of America

Dahai Liu and Bei Huang
Center for Stem Cell and Translational Medicine, Anhui University, Hefei, China

Tong-Chun Xue, Ning-Ling Ge, Lan Zhang, Jie-Feng Cui, Rong-Xin Chen, Yang You, Sheng-Long Ye and Zheng-Gang Ren
Liver Cancer Institute, Zhongshan Hospital, Fudan University, Shanghai, P. R. China
Key Laboratory of Carcinogenesis and Cancer Invasion (Fudan University), Ministry of Education, Shanghai, P. R. China

Hui Wang, Meng Fang, Xing Gu, Qiang Ji and Chun-Fang Gao
Department of Laboratory Medicine, Eastern Hepatobiliary Surgery Hospital, Second Military Medical University, Shanghai, P. R. China

Dongdi Li
Research School of Chemistry, The Australian National University, Canberra ACT, Australia

Shu-Qun Cheng
Department of Hepatic Surgery (VI), Eastern Hepatobiliary Surgery Hospital, Second Military Medical University, Shanghai, P. R. China

Feng Shen
Department of Hepatic Surgery (IV), Eastern Hepatobiliary Surgery Hospital, Second Military Medical University, Shanghai, P. R. China

Daniele Santini and Francesco Pantano
Medical Oncology Unit - University Campus Bio-Medico, Rome, Italy

Ferdinando Riccardi
Medical Oncology Unit, Cardarelli Hospital, Naples, Italy

Giovan Giuseppe Di Costanzo
Liver Unit, Cardarelli Hospital, Naples, Italy

Antonio Gnoni
Medical Oncology Unit – Hospital of Lecce, Lecce, Italy

Alessandro Comandone
Department of Oncology, Gradenigo Hospital and Gruppo Piemontese Sarcomi, Turin, Italy

Nicola Fazio
Unit of Gastrointestinal and Neuroendocrine Tumor, European Institute of Oncology, Milan, Italy

Alessandro Conti
Department of Clinical and Specialist Sciences, Urology, Polytechnic University of the Marche Region, AOU Ospedali Riuniti Umberto I-GM Lancisi and G Salesi, Ancona, Italy

Cosmo Damiano Gadaleta
Interventional Radiology Unit with Integrated Section of Translational Medical Oncology – National Cancer Institute "Giovanni Paolo II", Bari, Italy

Anna Elisabetta Brunetti, Vito Lorusso and Nicola Silvestris
Medical Oncology Unit – National Cancer Institute "Giovanni Paolo II", Bari, Italy

Yanqiong Liu, Yu He, Taijie Li, Li Xie, Jian Wang, Xue Qin and Shan Li
Department of Clinical Laboratory, First Affiliated Hospital of Guangxi Medical University, Nanning, Guangxi Zhuang Autonomous Region, China

Maja Thiele, Annette Dam Fialla, Emilie Kirstine Dahl and Aleksander Krag
Department of Gastroenterology and Hepatology, Odense University Hospital, Odense, Denmark

Lise Lotte Gluud
Gastrounit, Medical Division, Copenhagen University Hospital, Hvidovre, Denmark

Thomas W. Powers, Benjamin A. Neely and Richard R. Drake
Department of Cell and Molecular Pharmacology and Experimental Therapeutics and MUSC Proteomics Center, Medical University of South Carolina, Charleston, South Carolina, United States of America

Yuan Shao and Richard R. Drake
Hollings Cancer Center Biorepository and Tissue Analysis Resource, Medical University of South Carolina, Charleston, South Carolina, United States of America

Dean A. Troyer
Departments of Pathology and Microbiology and Molecular Cell Biology, Eastern Virginia Medical School, Norfolk, Virginia, United States of America

Anand S. Mehta
Drexel University College of Medicine, Department of Microbiology and Immunology and Drexel Institute for Biotechnology and Virology, Doylestown, Pennsylvania, United States of America

Huiyuan Tang and Brian B. Haab
Laboratory of Cancer Immunodiagnostics, Van Andel Research Institute, Grand Rapids, Michigan, United States of America

Tianhua Liu, Shu Zhang, Jie Chen, Kai Jiang, Qinle Zhang, Kun Guo and Yinkun Liu
Liver Cancer Institute, Zhongshan Hospital, Fudan University, Shanghai, People's Republic of China

Tianhua Liu, Kai Jiang, Qinle Zhang and Yinkun Liu
Cancer Research Center, Institute of Biomedical Science, Fudan University, Shanghai, People's Republic of China

Hongxiu Yu, Huali Shen, Yang Zhang, Fan Zhong, Yinkun Liu, Lunxiu Qin and Pengyuan Yang
Institutes of Biomedical Sciences of Shanghai Medical School, Fudan University, Shanghai, P. R. China

Yinkun Liu and Lunxiu Qin
Zhongshan Hospital, Fudan University, Shanghai, P. R. China

Pengyuan Yang
Department of Chemistry, Fudan University, Shanghai, P. R. China

Yu Lu, Qiliu Peng, Liping Ma, Xiaolian Zhang, Jiangyang Zhao, Xue Qin and Shan Li
Department of Clinical Laboratory, First Affiliated Hospital of Guangxi Medical University, Nanning, Guangxi, China

Zhitong Wu
Department of Clinical Laboratory, Guigang People's Hospital, Guigang, Guangxi, China

Bettina Maiwald, Donald Lobsien, Thomas Kahn and Patrick Stumpp
Department of Diagnostic and Interventional Radiology, University of Leipzig, Leipzig, Germany

Jiugang Song
Department of Gastroenterology, the 309th Hospital of Chinese People's Liberation Army, Beijing, P. R. China

Jiugang Song, Liucun Gao, Shanhong Tang, Huahong Xie, Jingbo Wang, Jiang Jin, Yawen Gou, Zhiping Yang, Zheng Chen, Kaichun Wu and Daiming Fan
State Key Laboratory of Cancer Biology, Xijing Hospital of Digestive Diseases, Fourth Military Medical University, Xi'an, P. R. China

Liucun Gao
Department of Pharmacology and Toxicology, Beijing Institute of Radiation Medicine, Beijing, P. R. China

Guang Yang
Department of XiShan Outpatient Clinic, the 309th Hospital of Chinese People's Liberation Army, Beijing, P. R. China

Shanhong Tang
Department of Digestion, General Hospital of Chengdu Military Command, Chengdu, Sichuan Province, P. R. China

Yongji Wang
Department of Medical, the 309th Hospital of Chinese People's Liberation Army, Beijing, P. R. China,

Yanping Zhang
Asian Games Village Clinic of Logistics Department, the General Armament Department of PLA, Beijing, P. R. China

Jie Liu
Department of Digestive Diseases, Huashan Hospital, Fudan University, Shanghai, P. R. China

Miyuki Takasu, Takuji Yamagami, Yuko Nakamura, Daisuke Komoto, Yoko Kaichi, Chihiro Tani, Shuji Date, Masao Kiguchi and Kazuo Awai
Department of Diagnostic Radiology, Graduate School of Biomedical Sciences, Hiroshima University, Hiroshima, Japan

Jiang Chen, Jinghua Liu, Renan Jin, Jiliang Shen, Yuelong Liang, Hui Lin, Xiao Liang, Hong Yu and Xiujun Cai
Department of General Surgery, Sir Run Run Shaw Hospital of Zhejiang University, Hangzhou, Zhejiang, China

Rui Ma
Department of Surgery, Zhejiang University Hospital, Hangzhou, Zhejiang, China

Li Li, Zuo-Jun Zhen, Huan-Wei Chen, Yong Ji, Zhi-Peng Wu, Jian-Yuan Hu and Wan Yee Lau
Department of Hepatic and Pancreatic Surgery, The First People's Hospital of Foshan, Foshan, Guangdong, P. R. China

Li Li, Jing Yan, Jing Xu, Chao-Qun Liu and Limin Zheng
State Key Laboratory of Oncology in South China, Sun Yat-sen University Cancer Center, Guangzhou, P. R. China

Wan Yee Lau
Faculty of Medicine, The Chinese University of Hong Kong, Shatin, New Territories, Hong Kong SAR, P. R. China

Index